Advances in Experimental Medicine and Biology

Volume 1500

Advances in Experimental Medicine and Biology provides a platform for scientific contributions in the main disciplines of the biomedicine and the life sciences. This series publishes thematic volumes on contemporary research in the areas of microbiology, immunology, neurosciences, biochemistry, biomedical engineering, genetics, physiology, and cancer research. Covering emerging topics and techniques in basic and clinical science, it brings together clinicians and researchers from various fields.

Advances in Experimental Medicine and Biology has been publishing exceptional works in the field for over 40 years, and is indexed in SCOPUS, Medline (PubMed), EMBASE, Reaxys, EMBiology, the Chemical Abstracts Service (CAS), and Pathway Studio.

2023 CiteScore: 5.9

Anna N. Bukiya • Declan W. Ali
Editors

Molecular Mechanisms and Lifelong Consequences of Prenatal Exposure to Psychoactive Substances

Springer

Editors
Anna N. Bukiya
Department of Pharmacology
Addiction Science and Toxicology
University of Tennessee Health
Science Center
Memphis, TN, USA

Declan W. Ali
University of Alberta Edmonton
Edmonton, AB, Canada

ISSN 0065-2598 ISSN 2214-8019 (electronic)
Advances in Experimental Medicine and Biology
ISBN 978-3-032-12740-2 ISBN 978-3-032-12741-9 (eBook)
https://doi.org/10.1007/978-3-032-12741-9

This Springer imprint is published by the registered company Springer Nature Switzerland AG
The registered company address is: Gewerbestrasse 11, 6330 Cham, Switzerland

Contents

About the Editors

Anna N. Bukiya, PhD, is a Professor at the Department of Physiology, Addiction Science and Toxicology, University of Tennessee Health Science Center. Her laboratory is focusing on lipid modulation of ion channel function in excitable tissues and sensitivity to drugs of abuse. Her work has been consistently funded by National Institutes of Health and private foundations. She has published 53 original research articles, authored or co-authored 10 reviews and 14 book chapters. She also co-edited three books and served as a sole editor on one book, all focused on the role of lipids in modulation of protein function during normal physiology and pathological conditions. Her lab utilizes mouse and nonhuman primate models of prenatal alcohol exposure, computational modeling of lipid-protein interactions, biochemical and fluorescence microscopy-based quantification of cellular processes, as well as cerebral artery diameter monitoring approaches ex vivo and in vivo. She is a current member of several societies, including Research Society on Alcohol, International Drug Abuse Research Society, American Society for Pharmacology and Experimental Therapeutics, and Biophysical Society.

Declan W. Ali, PhD, is a Full Professor and Dean at the University of Alberta, Faculty of Science. His research is multi-fold but largely focuses on developmental neurobiology, neurophysiology, and cell biology. His investigations are primarily in zebrafish, where he provides expertise in patch-clamp electrophysiology. His current research focuses on the mechanisms that underlie synaptic development in the central and peripheral nervous systems. Early research focused on synaptic plasticity in the rodent hippocampus and specifically, the effects of tyrosine kinases in CA1 LTP, but over the last 25 years, he has made contributions identifying the mechanisms that underlie synapse formation and maturation, determining how the excitability properties of neurons and muscle fibers change during early development, and how this relates to animal behavior. Recent work has focused on the effects of alcohol and cannabinoids (THC, CBD, and CBN) on neurodevelopment and pain/analgesia, showing that these compounds alter synaptic activity in the CNS and the peripheral nervous system when administered early in development, with effects (in some cases) that last into adulthood and the next generation of animals. Key collaborations have resulted in significant contributions in the field of cell biology and cancer research, particularly on the effects of tyrosine kinases and transient receptor potential channels.

He has published 77 peer-reviewed publications, 4 book chapters and has peer reviewed more than 200 grant applications (NSERC, NIH, NSF, NRC) and more than 150 manuscripts. He has been invited to give more than 30 seminars and has sat on the Editorial Boards of four journals. His research is funded by Canadian federal and provincial funding agencies, and he is a member of several societies, including the Society for Neuroscience, the Canadian Society for Neuroscience, and the International Drug Abuse Research Society.

Animal Models of Prenatal Alcohol Exposure

1

Hannah M. O. Reid, Hanna Elford, Mia A. C. Till, and Brian R. Christie

Abstract

This chapter provides an introduction and overview of animal models that have been used to investigate the teratogenic effects of alcohol. Since the first model was developed in 1899, prenatal alcohol exposure (PAE) has been studied in species ranging from invertebrates to primates. Here, we contextualize and outline critical experimental considerations, including blood alcohol concentration, timing of exposure, and routes of ethanol administration. Detailed comparisons of vertebrate and invertebrate models, particularly rodents, guinea pigs, and non-human primates, highlight their translational relevance and limitations in replicating human gestational processes, and the pathophysiology of fetal alcohol spectrum disorder (FASD). This chapter also examines behavioral outcomes across motor, executive, cognitive, and social domains, illustrating how PAE disrupts neural development and function throughout the lifespan. Collectively, we emphasize the importance of recognizing the pros and cons when selecting an animal model and experimental paradigm.

Keywords

Fetal alcohol spectrum disorder (FASD) · Prenatal alcohol exposure (PAE) · Neurodevelopment · Animal models

1.1 Introduction

Ethanol, referred to colloquially as alcohol, has been consumed liberally throughout human history and consequently is one of the most heavily studied teratogens. Many animal models have been used to study the effects of ethanol on development (Fig. 1.1), and this chapter will give an overview of each. Ethanol is a teratogen that interferes with normal development, though its precise effects on brain and body development remain an active area of research. Exposure to ethanol in utero, known as prenatal alcohol exposure (PAE) or prenatal ethanol exposure (PNEE) can lead to a gradient of disorders. These are four

H. M. O. Reid · M. A. C. Till
Department of Medical Neuroscience, Dalhousie University, Halifax, NS, Canada

School of Medical Sciences, University of Victoria, Victoria, BC, Canada

H. Elford · B. R. Christie (✉)
School of Medical Sciences, University of Victoria, Victoria, BC, Canada

Cellular and Physiological Sciences, University of British Columbia, Vancouver, BC, Canada
e-mail: brain64@uvic.ca

A. N. Bukiya, D. W. Ali (eds.), *Molecular Mechanisms and Lifelong Consequences of Prenatal Exposure to Psychoactive Substances*, Advances in Experimental Medicine and Biology 1500,
https://doi.org/10.1007/978-3-032-12741-9_1

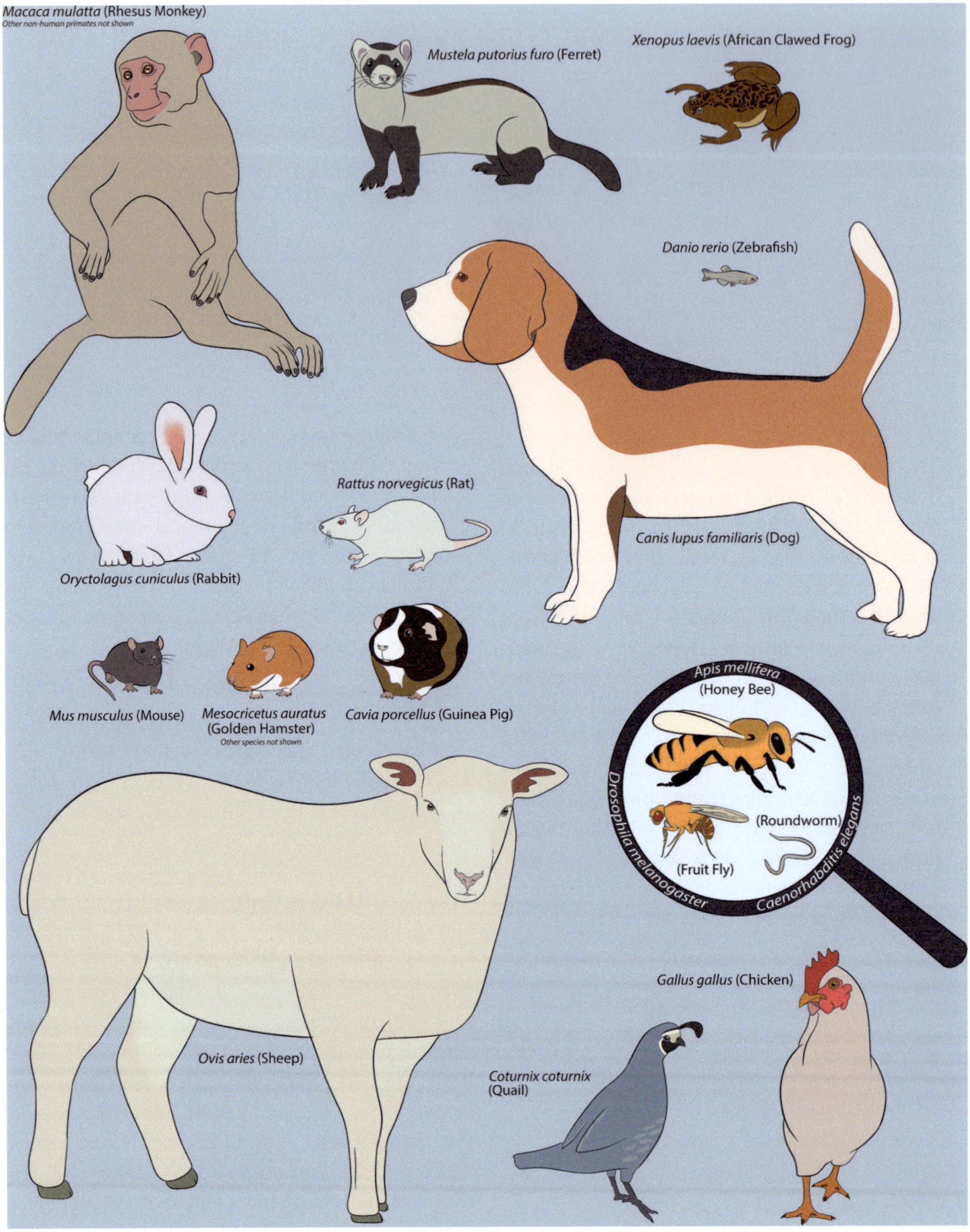

Fig. 1.1 Common animal models used to study prenatal alcohol exposure (PAE). Illustrations of representative species across vertebrate and invertebrate taxa commonly used to investigate the effects of prenatal alcohol exposure and fetal alcohol spectrum disorder

subtypes currently recognized: FASD (fetal alcohol spectrum disorder), FAS (fetal alcohol syndrome), pFAS (partial fetal alcohol syndrome), and ARND/other (alcohol-related neurodevelopmental disorder) (Akison et al. 2024). Fetal alcohol syndrome (FAS) is the most severe disorder resulting from PNEE, characterized by facial dysmorphologies (such as midfacial hypoplasia, wide spaced eyes, and a smooth philtrum), growth retardation, and central nervous system (CNS) dysfunction (Sokol 2003). These developmental abnormalities often lead to cognitive, motor, and behavioral impairments, and have an associated diagnosis in the DSM-5 as Neurobehavioral Disorder Associated with Prenatal Alcohol Exposure (ND-PAE) (Diagnostic and Statistical Manual of Mental Disorders : DSM-5-TR 2022). However, not all incidences of PNEE result in the facial dysmorphology required for diagnosis, but are nonetheless the result of exposure to this teratogen during development (Sokol 2003; Burd and Martsolf 1989). Since FAS was first defined in the 1970's, researchers have realized that the effects of PNEE can vary due to the timing, frequency, and amount of ethanol consumed (Jones 1975; Jones and Smith 1973). Additionally, genetic factors and maternal metabolism can also influence the severity and presentation of PNEE, leading to considerable variability in symptoms (Kleiber et al. 2014).

1.2 A Historical Perspective

Humans have been consuming alcohol for approximately 7000 years, and written references to its connection with birth defects can be found in the works of Plato, Aristotle, and the Old Testament (Jones and Smith 1973; Brown et al. 2019; Warner and Rosett 1975; Calhoun and Warren 2007). While some of this attribution remains tenuous, it is unequivocally recorded that in 1899, Dr. William Sullivan established a link between alcohol consumption and infant mortality in a population of incarcerated women (Sanders 2011; Abel 1999). This publication spurred the temperance movement, and much of the literature from the next several decades became intrinsically linked with morality (Warner and Rosett 1975). During this period, the first known animal model of fetal alcohol exposure was created; in 1903, C. F. Hodge gave cocker spaniels alcohol but observed no effects (Warner and Rosett 1975). It was not until 9 years later that L. B. Nice introduced another animal model using white mice (Warner and Rosett 1975). In the following years, additional animal models were established, including guinea pigs, rats, rabbits, and chickens (Warner and Rosett 1975).

Prohibition and its subsequent repeal effectively halted research in the field, and teratology did not regain momentum until the mid-twentieth century (Brown et al. 2019). Jacqueline Rouquette first described the phenotype now known as fetal alcohol spectrum disorder in 100 hospitalized French children; and while her thesis was documented, it was never submitted for peer review (Rouquette 1957). In 1964 her thesis supervisor, Paul Lemoine, was credited with the discovery when he published on the subject (Brown et al. 2019). Though he acknowledged her contributions in a letter to the editor in 1994, his work, published in French, did not gain widespread recognition (Lemoine 1994). Fetal alcohol exposure only became widely acknowledged after the work of Jones and Smith, who introduced the term fetal alcohol syndrome (Brown et al. 2019). This marked the beginning of the modern era of fetal alcohol exposure research, and with advancements in laboratory techniques, a wide range of animal models have been developed.

1.3 Factors to Consider When Modeling FASD

1.3.1 Blood Alcohol Concentration (BAC)

In Canada and the USA, a BAC of 80 mg/dl is often considered to be the lower limit of legal limit of intoxication. In human studies, maternal BAC data is typically unavailable; however, estimates suggest that BACs exceeding 200 mg/dl—which could be achieved by a 150 lb. woman consuming six alcoholic beverages in 2 h—may contribute to the severe FAS phenotype, while lower BACs may result in milder forms of FASD (Maier and West 2001). Despite the lack of direct BAC data in humans, this measure is commonly used to compare ethanol exposure across species. Since the absolute dose of ethanol administered (in grams of ethanol per kilogram [g/kg]) can vary greatly between species, using BAC is a more standardized and reliable measure of intoxication (Driscoll et al. 1990).

Most animal studies administer alcohol doses that result in BACs ranging from 100 to 400 mg/dl, representing moderate to binge-like levels of exposure and also reflect different rates of ethanol metabolism across species (Livy et al. 2003a). These BACs are typically reported as the highest, or peak BAC that is achieved by the paradigm. The peak BAC achieved depends on both the dose and pattern of administration (Pierce and West 1986; Bonthius et al. 1988). To achieve a low to moderate BAC (80 to 150 mg/dl), researchers typically use liquid diets, voluntary drinking paradigms, or vapor inhalation (Reid et al. 2020). In contrast, higher binge-like BACs (over 200 mg/dl) are normally achieved through oral intubation (gavage) or direct injections.

High BACs are generally linked to greater neurotoxicity, and even one high ethanol dose during critical periods of brain development can lead to significant structural impairments if BAC levels are sufficiently elevated (Boschen et al. 2024; Ieraci and Herrera 2007; Parnell et al. 2009). Low to moderate BACs can also cause significant neuronal damage. While longer exposure periods throughout gestation are commonly used in these models, shorter periods of exposure can still cause significant deficits (Choi et al. 2005; Redila et al. 2006; Wigal and Amsel 1990; Miller 1996). Thus, continuous low-level exposure to ethanol may be as damaging as a single high-level exposure, though the types of deficits incurred may differ. The deficits observed with either mode of administration can be affected by the timing of ethanol exposure.

1.3.2 Developmental Timing of Ethanol Exposure

The timing of ethanol exposure can crucially influence the outcome of the fetus. Mammalian brain development occurs in seven major phases: formation of the neural tube, neurogenesis, neuronal migration, glial cell proliferation, axon and dendrite growth, synaptogenesis followed by extensive pruning and cell death, and axonal myelination (Erecinska et al. 2004). These steps occur throughout the brain, but different regions develop at different times depending on their location along the rostrocaudal axis. Given the dynamic nature of brain development, it is important to consider the developmental timing of alcohol exposure when selecting a model, based on regional and temporal windows of vulnerability.

Gestation and development differ significantly between species, including simple organisms (e.g., *Xenopus, C. elegans,* or zebrafish) and mammals such as rodents (e.g., mice, rats, or guinea pigs) relative to humans. In humans, gestation is divided into three trimesters, all occurring prenatally. The first trimester involves neural tube formation and gastrulation, the second trimester is characterized by extensive cell proliferation and migration, and the third trimester features a rapid "brain growth spurt" marked by substantial growth and differentiation (Dobbing and Sands 1979).

Rodents are the most commonly used animal model in FASD research; despite the fact their gestational period is much shorter than that of humans—18 to 23 days for mice and rats, and approximately 68 days for guinea pigs., As a result, a significant portion of brain development occurs postnatally in these species (Cronise et al. 2001; Tran et al. 2000). The development of the rodent brain is also divided into trimester equivalents. In the guinea pig, the trimester equivalents largely occur prenatally, therefore making their brain development more comparable to humans. In rats and mice, the first trimester equivalent spans gestational days (GD) 1 to 10, the second trimester equivalent corresponds to GD 10 to 20 (just prior to birth) and the third trimester equivalent and the "brain growth spurt" occurs following birth, from postnatal day (PND) 1 to 10 (West 1987). To achieve ethanol exposure across all three trimester equivalents, alcohol must be administered to neonate pups, typically via oral intubation. However, the mechanisms of exposure, absorption, and elimination differ during the prenatal and postnatal periods. For example, ethanol-metabolizing enzymes such as alcohol dehydrogenase are only at 25% of adult levels at birth (Räihä et al. 1967). In utero, the fetus is partially protected by maternal ethanol metabolism, but in neonates, the absence of maternal metabolism leads to higher BAC levels from lower ethanol doses than those used in pregnant dams (Livy et al. 2003b; Brocardo et al. 2012; Gil-Mohapel et al. 2011; Boehme et al. 2011). Further, peri-gestational alcohol exposure has been linked to placental abnormalities which subsequently also effects development (Gualdoni et al. 2022).

1.3.3 Route of Administration

There are several different methods for alcohol administration during pregnancy. In invertebrates and simple vertebrates (e.g., *C. elegans, Xenopus,* and zebrafish), ethanol exposure is usually achieved by bath application. In more complex models, such as rodents and primates, three major methods are employed: ingestion (i.e., through diet, water, or intubation), injection, or inhalation (Reid et al. 2020; Gil-Mohapel et al. 2010; Kelly and Lawrence 2008; Riley and Meyer 1984).

1.3.3.1 Ingestion

The liquid diet model is one of the most used routes of ethanol administration in mouse and rat models and was among the first to be developed (Lieber and DeCarli 1982; Sherwin et al. 1979; Weinberg 1984). In this approach, pregnant dams are provided with a liquid diet throughout gestation, with approximately 35% of the caloric intake (equates to 6.61% v/v ethanol) derived from ethanol. This diet serves as the sole source of nutrition throughout the pregnancy. Using this method, rats can consume an average of 12 g of ethanol/kg/day, with intake reaching up to 18 g/kg/day (Gil-Mohapel et al. 2010). The diet usually begins on gestational day (GD) 1 and is introduced gradually over 3 days: one-third of the final ethanol concentration on GD 1, two-thirds on GD 2, the full concentration from GD 3 and onwards. To control for caloric differences, pair-fed control groups are often included. Pair-fed animals receive an isovolumetric, isocaloric replacement (e.g., maltose dextrin) while having their food intake restricted to match that of the ethanol-consuming group (Berman and Hannigan 2000). The liquid diet model reliably produces BACs between 80 and 180 mg/dl in rats, corresponding to low to moderate levels of exposure (Streissguth et al. 1990, 1994; Christie et al. 2005; Lan et al. 2006; Sickmann et al. 2014; Patten et al. 2013a, b). This results in neurological deficits like those observed in children with FASD.

Ethanol can also be administered through the drinking water, which is usually achieved by training female mice or rats to voluntarily consume a saccharin-sweetened 10% ethanol solution prior to pregnancy (Choi et al. 2005; Allan et al. 2003). Control groups are provided with saccharin-sweetened water only. During pregnancy the rodents have unlimited access to regular rat chow. Following birth, ethanol is gradually removed from the water to minimize withdrawal effects. Using this paradigm, rodents tend to consume approximately 14 g ethanol/kg/day, resulting in a BAC of approximately 120 mg/dl (Choi et al. 2005; Allan et al. 2003).

The liquid diet and voluntary drinking models are advantageous in that they are simple techniques, have reduced time and labor requirements, and decrease animal handling, which minimizes stress and risk of fatality. A disadvantage is that these methods do not allow for the precise control over the dosage or timing of ethanol exposure, leading to increased variability in achieved BACs, as ethanol consumption depends on the animal's voluntary food intake throughout the day. For example, a study found that ethanol consumption among a group of 221 rats on a liquid diet varied significantly, ranging from 4 to 18 g/kg/day (Mankes et al. 1992). Additionally, it is important to note that these models do not include alcohol exposure during the third trimester equivalent, as this occurs after birth. While pregnant dams could continue a liquid diet during the suckling period, the extent to which ethanol crosses into breast milk is uncertain, and the actual dose consumed by the pups cannot be controlled for. Furthermore, dams consuming ethanol during this period may exhibit less attentiveness to their pups and may not engage in appropriate maternal behavior, potentially leading to social and nutritional stress (Gil-Mohapel et al. 2010). Therefore, the liquid diet and voluntary drinking models are typically only used to examine exposure during the first and second trimester equivalents. Despite their limitations, these models retain significant relevance to the human condition, as human mothers may unknowingly consume alcohol during the early stages of pregnancy.

Ethanol can also be delivered directly to the stomach using an intubation method (Cronise et al. 2001; Tran et al. 2000; Brocardo et al. 2012; Gil-Mohapel et al. 2011; Boehme et al. 2011; Kelly and Tran 1997; Serbus et al. 1986). Typically, a syringe is attached to a curved steel gavage needle or plastic tubing, which is inserted down the esophagus to the entrance to the stomach. This method allows ethanol to be administered to pregnant females (usually diluted in water or saline) and to neonatal pups (usually diluted in a nutritional formula). An isocaloric control liquid (e.g., maltose dextrin or sucrose) can also be administered by gavage to control for the stress and nutritional effects of this procedure. This method is commonly used in rodents, including rats (Tran et al. 2000; Brocardo et al. 2012; Gil-Mohapel et al. 2011; Boehme et al. 2011; Kelly and Lawrence 2008; Hamilton et al. 2011; Thomas et al. 2008; Helfer et al. 2009; Klintsova et al. 2007) and guinea pigs (Catlin et al. 1993; Byrnes et al. 2004; Green et al. 2005; Iqbal et al. 2004; Richardson et al. 2002), as well as primates (Clarren and Bowden 1982; Clarren et al. 1987, 1992; Clarren and Astley 1992). The typical dose of ethanol ranges from 2 to 6 g ethanol/kg/day, resulting in BACs generally exceeding 200 mg/dl. Often, the daily dose of ethanol is divided into two administrations, given 4–8 h apart, creating two lower peak BACs within a 24 h period (Driscoll et al. 1990). Advantages are the precise control over dosage and peak BAC achieved, and neonatal exposure to ethanol permits the study of its effects during the third trimester "brain growth spurt." However, care must be taken to ensure that neonates adequately gain weight during ethanol exposure, and often a milk supplement is necessary to maintain healthy body weight (Gil-Mohapel et al. 2010). Significant disadvantages are that this is an invasive, time-consuming procedure associated with increased stress and mortality rates, and that those performing this procedure require specific training to gain competency.

To provide neonate pups with ethanol during the third trimester equivalent, an artificial rearing method known as "pup-in-the-cup" can be employed (Gil-Mohapel et al. 2010). In this procedure, the pup receives intragastric ethanol or a control solution while being kept in a warm cup filled with nesting material, simulating the cage environment and maternal interaction early in life (Samson and Diaz 1981; Bonthius and West 1990). While this method allows for reliable administration of known amounts of food and ethanol, it is invasive, expensive, and isolating, removing many social factors that are crucial for normal neonatal development, such as the presence of littermates and maternal grooming.

1.3.3.2 Injection

Ethanol is frequently administered to rodents through subcutaneous (s.c.) (Ikonomidou et al. 2000; Wozniak et al. 2004; Izumi et al. 2005) or intraperitoneal (i.p.) injections (Boschen et al. 2024; de Licona et al. 2009; Dunty et al. 2001; Webster et al. 1983) either acutely or over multiple days during gestation. This method is particularly useful for examining the acute effects of ethanol on specific developmental stages and allows for a rapid increase in BAC with minimal handling-induced stress. However, this administration method does not resemble human ethanol consumption and may fail to replicate several important aspects of human PNEE. For example, i.p. injections of ethanol during the first trimester equivalent in mice have been associated with a higher incidence of malformations compared to the same ethanol dose delivered via intubation (Webster et al. 1983). Additionally, ethanol administered i.p. to pregnant guinea pigs can quickly cross from the intraperitoneal space into the uterus, chorioamniotic membranes and amniotic fluid, as well as being absorbed into the mother's circulation (Clarke et al. 1985). This suggests the fetus is exposed to high levels of ethanol shortly after injection, which does not accurately mimic what is observed during oral ingestion.

1.3.3.3 Inhalation

The inhalation mode of administration is less common compared to other approaches, but it warrants a brief overview due to its unique advantages and limitations. In this method, pregnant dams, neonatal pups, or both the dam and her litter are placed in a sealed inhalation chamber filled with ethanol vapor for several hours (Reid et al. 2021; Karanian et al. 1986; Miki et al. 2008; Pal and Alkana 1997; Rogers et al. 1979). This method results in a rapid, reliable increase in BAC without the stress of intubation. It is also less labor-intensive than other methods, and multiple animals can be exposed simultaneously. However, this method does not mimic the typical route of ethanol intake in humans, reducing its translational relevance. Another concern is the potential for irritation to the upper respiratory tract by vaporized ethanol, which could introduce additional variables affecting outcomes. Furthermore, if used to expose pups to ethanol during the third trimester equivalent, it often requires prolonged maternal separation, which can result in reduced food intake and stress, and in turn lifelong impacts (Miki et al. 2008; Marais et al. 2008; Kalinichev et al. 2002). New alcohol vapor chambers have constant airflow, to avoid stress associated with carbon-dioxide accumulation (Reid et al. 2021).

1.4 Animal Models of FASD

1.4.1 Rodents

Rodents are the most used models in FASD research, providing valuable insights into molecular biology, synaptic plasticity and cognition. Their widespread use is supported by an extensive body of literature on rodent physiology, behavior, anatomy, development, reproduction, and teratology (Gil-Mohapel et al. 2010; Cudd 2005; Olivares-Costa et al. 2024). The following section discusses the advantages and disadvantages of each model, and the main routes of exposure.

1.4.1.1 *Mus musculus* (Mouse)

Mice are the most commonly used mammals in scientific research due to their ease of care, availability of transgenic and disease models, short life span, and genetic and physiological similarities to humans (Hickman et al. 2017). Although mice were used in early twentieth century research, FASD models only emerged in the early 1980s with the groundbreaking work of Dr. Kathleen Sulik (Sulik et al. 1981). While C57BL/6 is the most common mouse strain used, other strains are also utilized. The ability to genetically manipulate mice can be a huge advantage, and many studies investigating the genetic components of FASD have leveraged mouse models (Kleiber et al. 2011; Gilliam et al. 1987; Hard et al. 2005; Laufer et al. 2013).

Routes of ethanol administration vary across studies, with common methods including i.p. injection (Dunty et al. 2001; Sulik et al. 1981; O'Leary-Moore et al. 2010; Vink et al. 2005), s.c. injection (Wozniak et al. 2004; Olney et al. 2002; Wagner et al. 2014), voluntary drinking paradigms (Allan et al. 2003; Kleiber et al. 2011; Brady et al. 2012), liquid diets (Middaugh and Boggan 1991; Wainwright et al. 1990; Weathersby et al. 1994), and oral intubation (Gilliam et al. 1987). Most studies use chronic exposure paradigms, either throughout pregnancy or the third trimester equivalent. Intermittent exposure is also common, particularly in studies using i.p. ethanol administration to examine critical periods of vulnerability (Dunty et al. 2001; Sulik et al. 1981; Hard et al. 2005; Olney et al. 2002; Wagner et al. 2014; Middaugh and Boggan 1991, 1995). There have also been studies performed where neonates have been administered ethanol before being returned to their mothers for rearing (Kane et al. 2011). The BACs achieved typically range from 80 to 180 mg/dl for voluntary drinking or liquid diet paradigms and exceed 200 mg/dl for i.p. injections or oral intubation. When assessing the variability in doses across these models it is also important to note that different strains of mice can have different susceptibilities to alcohol. For example one study showed that C57BL/6 J mice are more susceptible to morphological malformations and gene-expression disruptions, compared with DBA/2 J mice who show relative resistance (Downing et al. 2012).

A limitation of this animal model is that the third trimester equivalent of brain development occurs postnatally rather than in utero. To overcome this, ethanol can be administered during the early postnatal period (PND 1 to 10) to mimic third-trimester exposure. However, the absence of the placental barrier alters ethanol kinetics and metabolism in pups compared to in utero exposure, requiring an increased maternal dosage to achieve comparable postnatal effects. Further, the placental phenotype differs between species—mice have a hemotrichorial placenta, whereas humans have a hemomonochorial placenta—which may further limit the translatability of mouse models to human FASD (Andersen et al. 2018). This is due to the fact that the placental barrier in mice has three cell layers as opposed to one in humans, which means that the barrier to diffusion is not congruous between us and mice.

Despite these limitations, mice remain a widely used model for FASD research, and many common features observed in human subjects are also observed in mice. This includes cranio-facial abnormalities (Dunty et al. 2001; Sulik et al. 1981; O'Leary-Moore et al. 2010), eye malformation (Sulik et al. 1981), growth retardation (Middaugh and Boggan 1991, 1995 Wainwright et al. 1990), and cognitive deficits (Wozniak et al. 2004; Kleiber et al. 2011; Gilliam et al. 1987; Vink et al. 2005; Wagner et al. 2014; Brady et al. 2012; Wainwright et al. 1990). These deficits are documented across the lifespan—from neonatal stages to adulthood—and with all routes of ethanol exposure. However, severe growth malformations and facial deficits are often not apparent in models with lower BACs. Beyond studying the pathology of PNEE, mouse models are also useful for examining potential therapeutics (Vink et al. 2005).

1.4.1.2 *Rattus norvegicus* (Rat)

Rats are another common model used to study FASD, sharing many similarities with mice. They have relatively short lifespans, a gestational period like the first two human trimesters, and a hemotrichorial placenta that does not fully replicate the role of the human placenta in PNEE. They offer several advantages in terms of their larger size, which facilitates easier handling and sampling, and their more complex behavioral repertoire. This makes them particularly useful for studying higher order behaviors such as social interactions, learning and memory, fear and anxiety, and depression, areas where mice are lacking behaviorally.

Various ethanol administration methods have been used in rat models. Like mice, chronic exposure throughout gestation is achieved with liquid diet and voluntary drinking paradigms, producing moderate stable BACs. High BACs are achieved with oral intubation, either during the gestation period (Qiang et al. 2002), the third trimester equivalent only (Hamilton et al. 2011; Helfer et al. 2009; Thomas et al. 1996, 2008, 2010; Pierce et al. 1993; Goodlett and Peterson 1995; Johnson and Goodlett 2002; Kelly et al. 1988; Stanton and Goodlett 1998), or through all three trimester equivalents (Brocardo et al. 2012; Gil-Mohapel et al. 2011; Boehme et al. 2011). Vapor inhalation is seldom used (Ryabinin et al. 1995; Puglia and Valenzuela 2010), and injection of ethanol tends to be reserved for mouse models (Parnell et al. 2009; Sulik et al. 1981; O'Leary-Moore et al. 2010).

Rat models of FASD rarely exhibit craniofacial abnormalities, but do present hallmark features such as growth retardation (Ryabinin et al. 1995; Abel 1989), structural abnormalities (Miller 1996; Gil-Mohapel et al. 2011; Boehme et al. 2011; Qiang et al. 2002; Pierce et al. 1993; West et al. 1984, 1986; West and Hamre 1985), CNS dysfunction (Sickmann et al. 2014; Patten et al. 2013a; Puglia and Valenzuela 2010; Titterness and Christie 2012; Sutherland et al. 1997; Varaschin et al. 2010; Swartzwelder et al. 1988), and cognitive deficits (Brocardo et al. 2012; Christie et al. 2005; Thomas et al. 2008, 2010; Goodlett and Peterson 1995; Johnson and Goodlett 2002; Kelly et al. 1988; Stanton and

Goodlett 1998; Abel 1989; Blanchard et al. 1987; Nagahara and Handa 1997; Popović et al. 2006; Stone et al. 1996). While many of these impairments are dose- and timing-dependent, they are observed across the lifespan and with all routes of administration. Strain-dependent vulnerabilities have also been observed, although some early studies found no strain differences (Sellin and Laakso 1987; Popoola et al. 2017; Khanna et al. 1990). Long-Evans rats appear more susceptible to ethanol-induced motor impairments than in Wistar rats, as shown in tilting plane tests (Sellin and Laakso 1987). Additionally, hippocampal slices from Long-Evans rats demonstrate a greater ethanol-induced reduction in population spikes (in vitro) compared to Wistar rats (Sellin and Laakso 1987). Differences in ethanol consumption patterns have also been found between different strains (Abel 1999).

1.4.1.3 *Cavia porcellus* (Guinea Pig)

Guinea pigs are a true in utero exposure model, as all three trimester equivalents of brain development occur during gestation. Additionally, their hemomonochorial placenta, like humans, enhances their relevance for translational research (Andersen et al. 2018). The oral intubation route of ethanol administration is most used with guinea pigs, with doses ranging from 3 to 6 g/kg/day (Byrnes et al. 2004; Iqbal et al. 2004; Richardson et al. 2002; McAdam et al. 2008; Burdge and Postle 1995). While some studies begin ethanol administration prior to gestation, most studies begin on GD 1 to 2 (Catlin et al. 1993; Iqbal et al. 2004; Richardson et al. 2002; Burdge and Postle 1995; Abdollah et al. 1993; Kimura et al. 1996). Many of these studies incorporate a nutrition/stress control group that receives sucrose by oral intubation.

Findings from guinea pig models suggest PNEE leads to structural (Green et al. 2005; Burdge and Postle 1995; Abdollah et al. 1993; Kimura et al. 1996), functional (Richardson et al. 2002), and cognitive deficits (Iqbal et al. 2004; Richardson et al. 2002; McAdam et al. 2008) which resemble those seen with the human condition. These deficits have been documented across different developmental stages, including neonates (Green et al. 2005; Iqbal et al. 2004; Burdge and Postle 1995; Kimura et al. 1996), adolescents (Abdollah et al. 1993; Kimura et al. 1996), and adults (Iqbal et al. 2004; Richardson et al. 2002; Abdollah et al. 1993; Kimura et al. 1996). A study restricted ethanol administration to the third trimester equivalent (GD 43 to 62) and found no significant effects on hippocampal synaptic plasticity or spatial learning in adulthood, even with BACs of 245 mg/dl (Byrnes et al. 2004).

Recent studies have investigated FASD biomarkers in guinea pigs, specifically the accumulation of fatty acid ethyl esters accumulation in neonatal hair as an indicator of PNEE, which forms during non-oxidative metabolism of ethanol (Kulaga et al. 2006). Guinea pigs are the only rodents born with neonatal hair, which may increase their utility in the FASD field. Limitations of guinea pigs as a model of FASD include their small litter size and longer gestational period, which can increase the time and costs relative to rat and mouse models. Additionally, guinea pigs are less exploratory which makes them less useful for behavioral testing in comparison to rats (Dringenberg et al. 2001).

1.4.1.4 *Mesocricetus auratus* (Hamster)

Research using hamster models for FASD is extremely limited, with few studies conducted and almost none published since the early 2000s. Like mice and rats, hamsters undergo third-trimester equivalent development postnatally and possess a hemotrichorial placenta (Buse et al. 2014). One study investigated alcohol-induced neural tube defects in golden hamsters, using a 25% ethanol i.p. injection on GD 8, when neural tube closure occurs (Graham and Ferm 1985). Another study examined short- and long-term ethanol-induced excitotoxicity, also in golden hamsters- administering a 7% ethanol solution via liquid diet either during the last 9 to 12 days of gestation or from at least 3 months prior to mating up until PND 5, when pups were euthanized (Adde-Michel et al. 2005). Due to the scarcity of research, hamsters remain an underutilized model for studying FASD.

1.4.1.5 *Mustela putorius furo* (Ferret)

Like hamsters, ferrets have been subjected to few FASD studies. Domestic ferrets typically give birth to eight kits on average, have a longer gestation period of 42 days, and experience a postnatal third trimester equivalent lasting 30 days (Lindeberg 2008). Researchers found that i.p. injections of 3.5 g/kg ethanol in the third trimester equivalent disrupted multisensory integration (Keum and Medina 2024; Keum et al. 2023). Additionally, PNEE leads to a reduction in whole brain volume, an enlarged frontal lobe, and altered connectivity in the posterior parietal lobe (Tang et al. 2018). The literature on ferrets primarily utilizes a third trimester early postnatal exposure paradigm, and they are longer lived than smaller rodents such as mice and rats. These are both limits of the literature and model, however this is counterbalanced by the fact that they are the simplest model to have developed gyri and lend themselves well to the study of neocortical development (Gilardi and Kalebic 2021).

1.4.1.6 *Oryctolagus cuniculus* (Rabbit)

While rabbits were among the earliest models of PNEE, only a single study has utilized them as a model since (Davis 1914; Fuchs 1966). This study revealed that ethanol exposure decreased oxytocin release during parturition (Davis 1914).

1.4.2 Non-Human Primate

Primate models of FASD are considered the gold standard due to their close evolutionary relationship to humans, as well as their similar gestational development and more complex behaviours (Schneider et al. 2011). However, research on PNEE using primates is limited due to ethical considerations, high costs, and the time-consuming nature of these studies. As a result, existing studies often have small sample sizes and use a variety of ethanol dosages and administration methods.

For example, one study allowed four pig-tailed macaques to voluntarily consume ethanol prior to conception and throughout pregnancy (Elton and Wilson 1977). Three monkeys consumed little alcohol and gave birth to normal infants, while one drank heavily throughout her pregnancy, resulting in a hyperactive and tremulous infant (Elton and Wilson 1977). Most primate studies use oral intubation to administer ethanol (Clarren and Bowden 1982; Clarren et al. 1987, 1992; Clarren and Astley 1992), with many studies only delivering alcohol once weekly rather than daily, which may more closely reflect human drinking patterns during pregnancy (Clarren and Bowden 1982; Clarren et al. 1987; Clarren and Astley 1992). Dosage ranges from 0.3 to 5 g/kg, with reported BACs ranging from 150 to 250 mg/dl (Clarren and Astley 1992; Altshuler and Shippenberg 1981). Voluntary drinking paradigms of 0.6 g ethanol/kg/day have also been used, resulting in much lower BACs of 20 to 50 mg/dl (Schneider et al. 2001a, b, 2008). One notable study in baboons which used three mid-gestation binge exposures achieved a maternal BAC of 80 mg/dL, and an ethanol concentration of 63 mg/dL in the amniotic fluid, elucidating how ethanol crosses the placental barrier in an animal model with a placenta similar to humans (Seleverstov et al. 2017).

The timing of ethanol exposure varies widely among studies. Some studies administer ethanol throughout pregnancy (Elton and Wilson 1977; Schneider et al. 2001a; Scott and Fradkin 1984), others begin in the first month of pregnancy (Andersen et al. 2018), and some use intermittent exposure (Clarren and Bowden 1982; Clarren and Astley 1992; Schneider et al. 2001b). Primate studies show that PNEE during development produces growth retardation (Clarren and Bowden 1982; Clarren and Astley 1992; Clarren et al. 1992) and behavioral deficits in adolescence and adulthood (Clarren and Astley 1992; Clarren et al. 1992; Schneider et al. 2001a, b, 2008), resembling those observed with human FASD. As an example, one study in baboons showed fetal growth delay similar to what is seen in humans (Tobiasz et al. 2018).

1.4.3 Other Mammals

1.4.3.1 *Canis lupus familiaris* (Dogs)

Dogs have seldom been used as an animal model to study FASD. One study involving beagles used a gastric intubation method to administer several doses of ethanol (Ellis and Pick 1980). In the groups that achieved BACs of 255 mg/dl and 350 mg/dl, none of the dogs produced live offspring (Ellis and Pick 1980). The lowest exposure group, with BACs of 100 mg/dl, exhibited some level of spontaneous abortion. Low birth weights and few external abnormalities were observed (Ellis and Pick 1980). Overall, canine FASD models do not seem to yield significant novel effects that would make them more valuable than other animal models.

1.4.3.2 *Ovis aries* (Sheep)

Sheep have been shown to exhibit lung defects with PNEE in several studies (Naik et al. 2025). Additionally, they have been used to explore the potential for choline to ameliorate FASD-related learning and memory deficits (Washburn et al. 2025). Further, sheep have been used to investigate the effects of choline supplementation on cerebellar Purkinje neurons in a first trimester binge exposure model (Carugati et al. 2022).

In addition to lung and neuronal outcomes, sheep models have been used to study the circulatory effects of prenatal ethanol exposure. One paper used high-dose binge ethanol in late gestation showed increased fetal cerebral blood flow under acidemic and hypercapnic conditions (Parnell et al. 2007). Conversely, moderate early gestation exposure attenuated the neonatal cerebral vasodilatory response to hypoxia, indicating impaired cerebrovascular reactivity (Gleason et al. 1997).

1.4.4 Avian

1.4.4.1 *Gallus gallus* (Chicken)

Chickens have long been a valuable model organism in embryology due to their accessibility and ease of physical and surgical manipulation. They were among some of the first animals used to study the relationship between PNEE and birth defects (Fere 1895, 1898, 1899; Stockard 1910, 1914). Research conducted in the mid-twentieth century identified various physical abnormalities, including deficits in septal morphogenesis, heart development, and neural tube formation (Flentke and Smith 2018). While contemporary research primarily focuses on the effects of ethanol on chickens intended for human consumption rather than their role as model organisms, a study utilized chickens for transcriptomics analysis (Berres et al. 2017). However, a Canadian research group has used the chicken model to study the genetic underpinnings of the craniofacial abnormalities characteristic of prenatal alcohol exposure (Su et al. 2001).

1.4.4.2 *Coturnix coturnix* (Quail)

Quail have been used as a model organism in two studies investigating PNEE. In one study. Quail eggs were injected with a 50% ethanol solution during the equivalent of day 3 to 4 of human gestation, resulting in deficits in heart development which were ameliorated with folic acid supplementation (Ford et al. 2021). Another study employed a similar method to assess effects of PNEE on DNA hypomethylation, glutathione, and heart defects (Jawaid et al. 2021).

1.4.5 Invertebrates

1.4.5.1 *Caenorhabditis elegans* (Roundworm)

The microscopic nematode worm *Caenorhabditis elegans* is commonly used as an invertebrate model for FASD research, and is useful for studying basic development at the cellular, molecular, and genetic levels (Davis et al. 2008). The *C. elegans* genome has been sequenced, and it has a simple nervous system of 302 neurons with approximately 5000 synapses. The well-characterized stages and timing of embryonic development can be easily visualized due to the transparency of the egg.

There are notable disadvantages of this model. Development of *C. elegans* differs from humans. The egg develops externally, thus alcohol exposure cannot occur in the same manner as humans. Instead, eggs or larvae are exposed to ethanol by bath application (Davis et al. 2008). Additionally, BACs cannot be directly measured. However, studies have shown that if ethanol is applied at a 0.4 M concentration to adult *C. elegans,* this results in an internal ethanol concentration equivalent to 100 mg/dl (Davies et al. 2004).

Research using this model has demonstrated that ethanol exposure produces significant growth retardation, slowed development, impaired reproduction, and death in a dose dependent manner, indicating similar developmental effects to humans (Davis et al. 2008; Lin et al. 2013). Future research with this model may provide insights into the genetic mechanisms of PNEE, and identify specific genes that may confer sensitivity or resistance to the toxic effects of ethanol during development (Davis et al. 2008; Lin et al. 2013).

1.4.5.2 *Drosophila melanogaster* (Fruit Fly)

In *Drosophila* models of FASD, ethanol exposure is typically achieved by allowing eggs to come into direct contact with an agar dish containing alcohol, like the method used with *C. elegans* (Edri et al. 2023). This model is cost-effective and efficient due to the animal's short lifespan, allowing for rapid experimental turnover. A significant advantage is that the entire *Drosophila* genome has been sequenced, and its neural circuitry has been extensively mapped, making it useful for understanding the genetic and phenotypic effects of PNEE. Studies utilizing this model have focused on the effects of ethanol on the transcriptome, as well as visible phenotypes and effects on the nervous system (Mokashi et al. 2021; Morozova et al. 2022; Belhorma et al. 2021). However, this model has some drawbacks—including its lack of complex brain structures such as the hippocampus.

1.4.5.3 *Apis mellifera* (Honeybee)

A single study published an FASD model using honeybees. In this model, larvae were exposed to three different concentrations of ethanol, ranging from 3 to 10%, with the aim of investigating social behaviour (Camilli et al. 2024). Body weight deficits like rodent models of FASD were observed, as well as delays in motor function (Camilli et al. 2024).

1.4.6 Aquatic

1.4.6.1 *Danio rerio* (Zebrafish)

Zebrafish are cost-effective vertebrate models which are easy to house, have a short developmental period, and can produce large numbers of offspring (Ali et al. 2011). Their developmental stages are well characterized, and both their embryonic and mature forms are transparent, allowing for direct visualization of internal structures (Alsakran and Kudoh 2021). This enables precise ethanol exposure during distinct developmental windows, which can be very important in determining critical periods for ethanol exposure (Bilotta et al. 2002). While their genome has been completely sequenced and shares many homologous genes with mammals, their developmental processes and physiology differ significantly from humans.

Compared to invertebrates such as *C. elegans,* Zebrafish offer the advantage of behavioural testing, allowing for the assessment of functional deficits following PNEE alongside anatomical or physiological deficits (Ali et al. 2011). However, ethanol application occurs through bath application, requiring it to penetrate the chorion of the egg, resulting in variability in actual exposure levels. To ensure adequate amounts cross into the embryo, high concentrations are often used, mimicking binge-like exposure (Yelin et al. 2005, 2007).

1.4.6.2 *Xenopus laevis* (African Clawed Frog)

Clawed frogs, like Zebrafish, are simple vertebrates that are cheap, small, develop quickly, and produce large amounts of offspring. Their transparent embryos and immature tadpoles allow for easy visualization of internal structures during distinct developmental stages. They also have fully sequenced genomes with many homologous genes to mammals and can undergo simple behavioral assessments. However, like *C. elegans,* their developmental process and physiology differ from humans. Ethanol exposure also occurs through bath application, requiring high concentrations for sufficient uptake (Yelin et al. 2005, 2007).

Studies utilizing zebrafish and clawed frog models for PNEE have demonstrated that developmental ethanol exposure can cause growth retardation, including reduced body length, microcephaly, skeletal deficits, and eye malformation (Bilotta et al. 2002; Yelin et al. 2005, 2007; Loucks and Ahlgren 2012; Zhang et al. 2014; Peng et al. 2004; Marrs et al. 2010). Cognitive dysfunction has also been observed in simple behavioral tasks such as visual acuity tests (Bilotta et al. 2002), associative learning (Fernandes et al. 2014), and social behavior (Fernandes and Gerlai 2009), even in the absence of physical abnormalities (Fernandes et al. 2014; Fernandes and Gerlai 2009). These effects were accompanied by changes in gene expression (Yelin et al. 2007; Loucks and Ahlgren 2012; Peng et al. 2004) and are dependent on the ethanol dose, developmental timing, and duration of exposure (i.e., chronic vs. acute), with the blastula, gastrulation and somitogenesis periods being particularly sensitive (Yelin et al. 2005; Marrs et al. 2010).

1.5 Behavioral Manipulations

Many behavioral manipulations have characterized the functional consequences of PNEE in animal models, which often correlate with known human dysfunctions (Mattson et al. 2011). Behavioral experiments are necessary tools for assessing the efficacy of novel therapeutic approaches for PNEE offspring. While there are other types of behaviors that have been studied after PNEE, such as anxiety and hyperactivity, this review will focus on five major classes of behavior, including several key behavioral tasks where performance is affected by prenatal ethanol ingestion, injection, and inhalation.

1.5.1 Motor Skills

The cerebellum is a region of the fetal brain that is particularly vulnerable to damage by ethanol in utero. Motor hyperactivity is often reported in children with FASD, who also perform poorly on fine motor coordination and reaching tasks and have deficits in postural balance (Domellöf et al. 2011; Mitoma et al. 2024; Roebuck et al. 1998). Recently, children diagnosed with FASD were found to have poor saccade accuracy, a task dependent on the cerebellum (Paolozza et al. 2013; Quaia et al. 1999). Motor performance can readily be evaluated in animal models using standardized tasks that include the rotarod, runway, directed reaching, and gait analyses.

In rat pups exposed to ethanol via intubation throughout all stages of pregnancy and during the early postnatal period, the overall volume of the cerebellum and Purkinje cell (PC) numbers were reduced (Maier et al. 1999). Other studies have identified the third trimester equivalent as a period of vulnerability for PCs (Marcussen et al. 1994). PC density is reduced in PND 10 rat offspring exposed to ethanol (gestational intubation) and the ultrastructure of this neural population is modified, indicating a delay in cellular development (Lewandowska et al. 2012). The widely reported damage to the cerebellum has observable, functional consequences on motor-related behaviors.

Behavioral tasks such as the rotarod, runway tasks and gait analysis software may be used to examine damage to the cerebellum and related motor structures. In the rotarod task, a rodent is placed on a rotating rod and is required to run on the rod for as long as possible. The rotational speed of the bar can be increased, and the experimenter can then measure the duration of time that the animal can remain on the bar at various speeds. In rodents, it is thought that the motor deficits caused by PNEE are most apparent early in life, and in most cases unseen at adulthood. A study (gestational liquid diet) showed these age effects with the anticipated motor hyperactivity in PND 28 and 56 rat offspring, while seeing no evidence of motor impairment at PND

112 (Bond and Digiusto 1977). Similarly, adult rat offspring (intubation, GD 7–20) show no evidence of motor dysfunction or hyperactivity on a rotarod or open field task (Dursun et al. 2006). During this early window of observation, rats (gestational liquid diet) have been found to be ataxic, exhibiting asymmetrical gait, shorter stride length and greater step angle than their respective controls (Hannigan and Riley 1988). Young mice (< PND 60, gestational ethanol in drinking water) perform poorly on the runway and rotarod tasks (Cebolla et al. 2009). However, when ethanol administration was restricted to the postnatal period (intubation PND 4–9) as adults (> PND 70), these animals perform poorly on an eyeblink conditioning task, a form of classical conditioning where a light is paired with a puff of air on the eye, causing the animal to blink (Lindquist et al. 2013). The impaired performance on this hippocampal-independent task is thought to be due to ethanol-induced damage to the interpositus nucleus of the cerebellum via cell loss and altered firing (Young et al. 2010; Green 2004). A study examined the specific timing of postnatal exposure to ethanol (via gastronomy) in relation to cerebellar damage and motor performance. The authors identified PND 4/5 as a critical period for ethanol exposure where the greatest deficits could be seen on a parallel bar task at PND 30 and 52, where the width between bars that the animal was required to cross over was gradually widened. This time point also produced the greatest decreases in cerebellar and brainstem weights at PND 55 (Thomas et al. 1996). Others have shown that when ethanol is restricted to the postnatal period (intragastric ethanol, PND 2–10), motor hyperactivity in rats persists into adulthood, at least until PND 91 (Tran et al. 2000).

These studies stress the importance of considering the timing of ethanol administration, and the age of the offspring when conducting motor behavior studies. They also highlight the need for additional studies in this area in aged animals.

1.5.2 Executive Function

Executive functioning is the ability to use appropriate problem solving in goal-directed behaviors, and includes behaviors such as response inhibition, working memory, and set shifting. These functions have long been thought to be dependent on frontal lobe structures, such as the prefrontal cortex (Gursky et al. 2021; Ridderinkhof et al. 2004), though some argue that extra-frontal-lobe structures may also be involved (Alvarez and Emory 2006). In humans, these behaviors can easily be measured through standardized tests, and they appear to be gravely impacted by prenatal alcohol use (Rasmussen 2005). Children with FASD have difficulties inhibiting responses on the Stroop Test a task where an individual must inhibit the natural tendency to read words, being required instead to state the color of the font (Connor et al. 2000). In addition, these individuals have difficulty in suppressing saccade responses in visual tasks while waiting for the proper initiating signal (Paolozza et al. 2013) and exhibit poor working memory when asked to recall digit spans backwards (Aragón et al. 2008). On the Wisconsin Card Sorting Task, where the subject must detect, use and change card sorting strategies, individuals with FASD make more errors related to shifting sort strategies (Vaurio et al. 2008). In rodents, executive function tasks are complex, and a single task often requires the use of response inhibition, working memory, and set shifting among others.

Response inhibition tasks require the subjects to inhibit responses they may be naturally predisposed to perform in specific environments. For example, in rodents, passive avoidance is a task commonly used to show response inhibition. In these tasks, the rodent is placed in a box that contains a "safe" area, adjacent to a grid floor that will provide a shock if the animal steps onto the grid within a trial. The animal must learn to inhibit the natural tendency to explore new environments and remain on the "safe" side of the test chamber for the entire trial. Rats prenatally exposed to ethanol (liquid diet, GD 6–16) show impairments in these passive avoidance tasks, at both PND 18 and PND 41–53 (Riley et al. 1979). In a large rat study, offspring exposed to ethanol (liquid diet, GD 5–20) again exhibited impaired passive avoidance of a shock at both PND 17 and PND 48, but not at PND 114, and took longer to spontaneously alter their exploratory strategy on a T-maze where the animal would be confined after visiting a particular arm when tested at PND 16 and PND 63 but not at PND 112 (Abel 1982). Rats exposed prenatally to ethanol (liquid diet, GD 1–20) have fewer cells in layers II and V of the medial prefrontal cortex, which was correlated with poor performance on a reversal learning task in adulthood (> PND 90) (Mihalick et al. 2001).

Working memory is a short form of memory where information from a recent experience must be used to perform the appropriate response on a following trial or task. Working memory is a form of memory that is known to primarily require the functional activity of the prefrontal cortex, differentiating it from other forms of memory (Goldman-Rakic 1995; Kane and Engle 2002). Behavioral tasks that evaluate working memory include delayed matching to sample tasks where a stimulus is provided, followed by a delay then a choice between multiple different stimuli. In these experiments the organism must remember the initial stimulus then pick the matching stimulus when given a choice after the delay, and is readily adapted for rodent, non-human primates, and humans. For rodents, the task can be modified to a delayed matching-to-place task in a Morris water maze (MWM) where a platform is located in an arm during a search trial, then after a delay the animal must return to the location of the platform during the search session. When ethanol administration occurs in the third trimester equivalent (gastronomy, PND 6–9), these rats perform poorly on the matching-to-place task at PND 35, PND 105, and PND 180, when the delay between the search and test trials is 2 h, though this task requires both intact working and spatial memory (Girard et al. 2000).

Set shifting is a complex task that can readily be performed by human and non-human primates, with variable evidence from rodents. In rats, set shifting tasks are not as well established as human and non-human primate work. In delayed non-matching-to-sample tasks, the subject not only requires functional working memory and inhibitory control but also set shifting where the organism must be able to observe the sample stimulus then shift their attention to choose the non-matching option during the subsequent test trial. In one rat study of delayed non-matching-to-sample, adult PNEE animals (liquid diet, GD 1–22) showed no impairments in set shifting (Kim et al. 1997). Future rodent work in this area may use a unique behavioral task adapted from primate studies to fully understand how set shifting may be altered by PNEE in rodents and shed light on the underlying neural substrates for these behaviors (Birrell and Brown 2000). In a study of rhesus monkeys exposed to ethanol (GD 5—parturition, voluntary drinking), the 32- to 34-month-old offspring had difficulty acquiring a delayed non-matching to sample task (Schneider et al. 2001a).

When using animal models to examine the effect of PNEE on executive functions, it is critical to design appropriate tasks for the model in question. Tasks used for one species may not be easily applied to other without modifications for the species in question.

1.5.3 Learning and Memory

The damaging effects of PNEE on learning and memory have been reliably reported in many species. Here we will focus on hippocampal-specific learning and memory in rodents and in humans. We primarily discuss the behavior research but will also touch on some electrophysiological underpinnings of these behaviors. In spatial object memory tasks where a child must remember the location of multiple objects on a semi-random grid, children with FAS were unable to recall objects after a delay and exhibited distorted spatial array when asked to recall where the objects were (Uecker and Nadel 1996). Additional work with humans with FASD is necessary to understand the manifestations of neural damage caused by PNEE. Future studies of spatial memory may utilize virtual 3D object recognition tasks where the subject can undergo PET or fMRI scans while virtually exploring a space (Maguire et al. 1998; Spadoni et al. 2009).

In rodents, hippocampal-dependent memory can be assessed in a variety of behavioral tasks including tasks such as the MWM and fear conditioning. PNEE-induced hippocampal damage has been widely reported in rodents (Gil-Mohapel et al. 2010; Berman and Hannigan 2000; Swartzwelder et al. 1988; Barnes and Walker 1981; Grafe et al. 2021; Nixon and Crews 2002). The MWM is a standard task where a T, plus or open field maze can be submerged in cloudy water. A platform can then be hidden below the surface, with visual detection of the rodent when swimming in the maze. The animal must swim to explore the maze and find the submerged platform to escape the water in multiple training trials where variables such as latency to the platform, swim speed, and distance travelled to the platform can be measured. The MWM can be adapted for many functions, such as delayed matching-to-place, which are readily learned by healthy rodents (Girard et al. 2000). However, PNEE rodents exhibit significant impairments on this task (rats, liquid diet, GD 1–22 (Christie et al. 2005; Blanchard et al. 1987; Gianoulakis 1990); rats, intubation, PND 4–9 (Thomas et al. 2008, 2010; Goodlett and Peterson 1995; Johnson and Goodlett 2002; Kelly et al. 1988); guinea pigs, intubation, GD 2–67 (Iqbal et al. 2004).

Fear conditioning is a behavioral task that is both easily implemented and readily learned by rodents. Trace fear conditioning occurs when an unconditioned stimulus (US), such as a foot shock, follows a conditioned stimulus (CS), such as a tone or a light. Following multiple training sessions, the animal is tested in a novel context, like the training context and freezing responses are recorded in response to presentation of the CS alone. PNEE rats perform poorly on this task when ethanol is given in the third trimester equivalent (intubation, PND 4–9) (Wagner and Hunt 2006), with the poorest performance observed when ethanol administration occurred from PND 4–6 (intubation) (Hunt et al. 2009).

Other forms of hippocampal memory are impaired by PNEE in rodents. A study subjected PNEE offspring exposed to gestational ethanol in a liquid diet during gestation and/or the early postnatal period to an extensive battery of memory tasks to evaluate performance in spatial learning, orientation, and simple and more complex object recognition. Generally, ethanol exposed offspring performed poorly, though the impairments in these animals became increasingly evident as the task difficulty increased, with animals treated during the early postnatal period performing worse than others (Popović et al. 2006).

It would be remiss to discuss learning and memory without mentioning hippocampal plasticity as investigated by electrophysiology. Specifically, learning and memory function can be investigated using ex vivo electrophysiology. Long-term potentiation (LTP) and long-term depression (LTD) are two central mechanisms implicated in learning and memory; LTP is when a strong neural signal causes future signals to be propagated more easily, and LTD is where low frequency inputs cause future signals to be less likely to be propagated (Bliss and Collingridge 1993; Collingridge 2024; Eyolfson et al. 2024). Synaptic plasticity has been shown repeatedly to be impaired in rodent models of FASD (Grafe et al. 2021; Basavarajappa and Subbanna 2023; Goncalves-Garcia and Hamilton 2024).

1.5.4 Social Behavior

Social behaviors in humans and non-humans alike are caused by complex interactions between genetics, early life experiences, and later social learning that can be altered by PNEE (Kelly et al. 2000, 2009; Lussier et al. 2023). For humans, appropriate behavior in a social context is critical for societal integration, and therefore it is critical to consider that PNEE can shape lifelong behavior, and that FASD is not simply a childhood disorder, as highlighted by a longitudinal study examining childhood, adolescents, and adults (Streissguth 1991).

Social dysfunctions in humans with FASD are apparent early in life with altered sleep patterns, increased irritability and feeding difficulties during infancy (Coles and Platzman 1993). Similarly, neonatal rats exposed to ethanol in the early postnatal period (gastronomy, PND 2–12) take longer to attach to the nipple and spend less time suckling than controls (Barron et al. 1991), emit more vocalizations on PND 5 when separated from the dam after pre- and postnatal ethanol exposure (intubation, GD 1–22, and PND 2–10) (Marino et al. 2002), and are not retrieved by the dam as quickly as unexposed pups (drinking water, GD 0–30) (Ness and Franchina 1990). These negative early life experiences can play a role in shaping social development long-term.

For humans, other social behavioral problems associated with fetal ethanol exposure become apparent at school age. When matched with unexposed children with low verbal IQs, children with FAS have poor coping skills and interpersonal relationship skills according to the Vineland Adaptive Behavior Scale (VABS), performing three standard deviations below the norm for their age (Thomas et al. 1998). Others have also reported increased aggression in children with FAS (Brown et al. 1991). In juvenile PNEE rats (liquid diet, GD 6–20) the sexually dimorphic play behaviors were reversed where males displayed female behaviors and vice versa (Meyer and Riley 1986). Prior to puberty, ethanol-exposed rats (intubation, GD 6–19) exhibit more play behavior though males that are more aggressive following puberty than un-exposed controls (Royalty 1990). However, it is important to note that there are great differences between the complexity of social behavior in humans and rodents at this age and beyond when drawing parallels between the two species.

Unlike other previously discussed behaviors, disruptions in the social behaviors of adult humans and rats have been readily shown. In adolescent and adult humans exposed to ethanol in utero, whose average chronological age was 17, the average adaptive functioning as measured by the VABS was equivalent that of a 7-year-old healthy child (Streissguth 1991). In this same study, all adolescents and adults were classified into the significant and intermediate categories of the maladaptive behavior section of the VABS, including behaviors, such as social withdrawal and teasing or bullying of others (Streissguth 1991). A report on secondary disabilities associated with FASD stated that of adult females exposed to ethanol in utero, 40% had drank alcohol while they were pregnant, and over 50% of the children had been removed from the care of the mother (Streissguth et al. 1996). Difficulties in parenting have also been observed in rats that drank ethanol throughout gestation (Hård et al. 1985). In this study, females exposed to ethanol failed to retrieve pups removed from their nests, a task normally accomplished in a short time by control animals. The researchers also observed disorganized and distracted behavior in the mothers. For instance, dams might start carrying a pup part of the way toward the nest, but then drop it and be distracted by self-grooming, eating or drinking and forget about the retrieval effort (Hård et al. 1985). Adult males also show disrupted social behaviors in adulthood. Male rat offspring exposed to ethanol prenatally spend less time sniffing other rats at PND 90 than those exposed to maternal saccharin water (gestational ethanol in drinking water) (Hamilton et al. 2010) and display more aggressive behaviors, including attacks, tail rattling and chasing in the presence of conspecifics (Krsiak et al. 1977). These findings in both rodents and humans stress that the effects of FASD do not exist in childhood alone, and that they can have effects on the next generation of offspring.

1.6 Summary

PNEE remains unfortunately common, though there are a great deal of laboratories around the world delineating the mechanisms behind the teratogenic effects of ethanol and the underlying biochemical, molecular and genetic events that lead to the cognitive deficits characteristic of PNEE. Animal models have been invaluable for this body of work particularly because they allow us to examine different drugs and supplements for their potential therapeutic properties on both neural structures and observable behavior. Since the turn of the last century, a multitude of animals ranging from flies to mice to dogs to chickens have been used to investigate the behavioral phenotypes and molecular mechanisms associated with PNEE. It is critical for both fields to consider the potential life-long implications of PNEE. Moving forward, translational research linking human and animal work is imperative to paint a vivid picture of damage caused by PNEE and to eventually find a way to overcome some of the devastating effects of this condition.

References

Abdollah S, Catlin MC, Brien JF (1993) Ethanol neurobehavioural teratogenesis in the Guinea pig: behavioural dysfunction and hippocampal morphologic change. Can J Physiol Pharmacol 71:776–782

Abel EL (1982) In utero alcohol exposure and developmental delay of response inhibition. Alcohol Clin Exp Res 6:369–376

Abel EL (1989) Paternal and maternal alcohol consumption: effects on offspring in two strains of rats. Alcohol Clin Exp Res 13:533–541

Abel EL (1999) Was the fetal alcohol syndrome recognized by the Greeks and the Romans? Alcohol Alcohol 34:868–872

Adde-Michel C, Hennebert O, Laudenbach V, Marret S, Leroux P (2005) Effect of perinatal alcohol exposure on ibotenic acid-induced excitotoxic cortical lesions in newborn hamsters. Pediatr Res 57:287–293

Akison LK et al (2024) Prenatal alcohol exposure and associations with physical size, dysmorphology and neurodevelopment: a systematic review and meta-analysis. BMC Med 22:467

Ali S, Champagne DL, Spaink HP, Richardson MK (2011) Zebrafish embryos and larvae: a new generation of disease models and drug screens. Birth Defects Res Part C Embryo Today Rev 93:115–133

Allan AM, Chynoweth J, Tyler LA, Caldwell KK (2003) A mouse model of prenatal ethanol exposure using a voluntary drinking paradigm. Alcohol Clin Exp Res 27:2009–2016

Alsakran A, Kudoh T (2021) Zebrafish as a model for fetal alcohol spectrum disorders. Front Pharmacol 12: 721924

Altshuler HL, Shippenberg TS (1981) A subhuman primate model for fetal alcohol syndrome research. Neurobehav Toxicol Teratol 3:121–126

Alvarez JA, Emory E (2006) Executive function and the frontal lobes: a meta-analytic review. Neuropsychol Rev 16:17–42

Andersen MD et al (2018) Animal models of fetal medicine and obstetrics. In: Bartholomew I (ed) *Experimental animal models of human diseases – an effective therapeutic strategy*. InTech. https://doi.org/10.5772/intechopen.74038

Aragón AS et al (2008) Neuropsychological study of FASD in a sample of American Indian children: processing simple versus complex information. Alcohol Clin Exp Res 32:2136–2148

Barnes DE, Walker DW (1981) Prenatal ethanol exposure permanently reduces the number of pyramidal neurons in rat hippocampus. Brain Res 227:333–340

Barron S, Kelly SJ, Riley EP (1991) Neonatal alcohol exposure alters suckling behavior in neonatal rat pups. Pharmacol Biochem Behav 39:423–427

Basavarajappa BS, Subbanna S (2023) Synaptic plasticity abnormalities in fetal alcohol spectrum disorders. Cells 12:442

Belhorma K et al (2021) Developmental ethanol exposure causes central nervous system dysfunction and may slow the aging process in a drosophila model of fetal alcohol spectrum disorder. Alcohol 94:65–73

Berman RF, Hannigan JH (2000) Effects of prenatal alcohol exposure on the hippocampus: spatial behavior, electrophysiology, and neuroanatomy. Hippocampus 10:94–110

Berres ME, Garic A, Flentke GR, Smith SM (2017) Transcriptome profiling identifies ribosome biogenesis as a target of alcohol teratogenicity and vulnerability during early embryogenesis. PLoS One 12:e0169351

Bilotta J, Saszik S, Givin CM, Hardesty HR, Sutherland SE (2002) Effects of embryonic exposure to ethanol on zebrafish visual function. Neurotoxicol Teratol 24: 759–766

Birrell JM, Brown VJ (2000) Medial frontal cortex mediates perceptual attentional set shifting in the rat. J Neurosci 20:4320–4324

Blanchard BA, Riley EP, Hannigan JH (1987) Deficits on a spatial navigation task following prenatal exposure to ethanol. Neurotoxicol Teratol 9:253–258

Bliss TVP, Collingridge GL (1993) A synaptic model of memory: long-term potentiation in the hippocampus. Nature 361:31–39

Boehme F et al (2011) Voluntary exercise induces adult hippocampal neurogenesis and BDNF expression in a rodent model of fetal alcohol spectrum disorders. Eur J Neurosci 33:1799–1811

Bond NW, Digiusto EL (1977) Effects of prenatal alcohol consumption on shock avoidance learning in rats. Psychol Rep 41:1269–1270

Bonthius DJ, West JR (1990) Alcohol-induced neuronal loss in developing rats: increased brain damage with binge exposure. Alcohol Clin Exp Res 14:107–118

Bonthius DJ, Goodlett CR, West JR (1988) Blood alcohol concentration and severity of microencephaly in neonatal rats depend on the pattern of alcohol administration. Alcohol (Fayettev) 5:209–214

Boschen KE et al (2024) Gastrulation-stage alcohol exposure induces similar rates of craniofacial malformations in male and female C57BL/6J mice. Birth Defects Res. 116:e2292

Brady ML, Allan AM, Caldwell KK (2012) A limited access mouse model of prenatal alcohol exposure that produces long-lasting deficits in hippocampal-dependent learning and memory. Alcohol Clin Exp Res 36:457–466

Brocardo PS et al (2012) Anxiety- and depression-like behaviors are accompanied by an increase in oxidative stress in a rat model of fetal alcohol spectrum disorders: protective effects of voluntary physical exercise. Neuropharmacology 62:1607–1618

Brown RT et al (1991) Effects of prenatal alcohol exposure at school age. II Attention and behavior. *Neurotoxicol Teratol* 13:369–376

Brown JM, Bland R, Jonsson E, Greenshaw AJ (2019) A brief history of awareness of the link between alcohol and fetal alcohol spectrum disorder. Can J Psychiatr 64:164–168

Burd L, Martsolf JT (1989) Fetal alcohol syndrome: diagnosis and syndromal variability. Physiol Behav 46:39–43

Burdge GC, Postle AD (1995) Effect of maternal ethanol consumption during pregnancy on the phospholipid molecular species composition of fetal Guinea-pig brain, liver and plasma. Biochim Biophys Acta 1256: 346–352

Buse E et al (2014) The placenta in toxicology. Part I: animal models in toxicology: placental morphology and tolerance molecules in the cynomolgus monkey (Macaca fascicularis). Toxicol Pathol 42:314–326

Byrnes ML, Richardson DP, Brien JF, Reynolds JN, Dringenberg HC (2004) Spatial acquisition in the Morris water maze and hippocampal long-term potentiation in the adult guinea pig following brain growth spurt--prenatal ethanol exposure. Neurotoxicol Teratol 26: 543–551

Calhoun F, Warren K (2007) Fetal alcohol syndrome: historical perspectives. Neurosci Biobehav Rev 31: 168–171

Camilli MP et al (2024) Fetal alcohol spectrum disorder: the honey bee as a social animal model. Life 14:434

Carugati M, Goodlett CR, Cudd TA, Washburn SE (2022) The effects of gestational choline supplementation on cerebellar Purkinje cell number in the sheep model of binge alcohol exposure during the first trimester-equivalent. Alcohol 100:11–21

Catlin MC, Abdollah S, Brien JF (1993) Dose-dependent effects of prenatal ethanol exposure in the Guinea pig. Alcohol 10:109–115

Cebolla AM et al (2009) Effects of maternal alcohol consumption during breastfeeding on motor and cerebellar Purkinje cells behavior in mice. Neurosci Lett 455:4–7

Choi IY, Allan AM, Cunningham LA (2005) Moderate fetal alcohol exposure impairs the neurogenic response to an enriched environment in adult mice. Alcohol Clin Exp Res 29:2053–2062

Christie BR et al (2005) Voluntary exercise rescues deficits in spatial memory and long-term potentiation in prenatal ethanol-exposed male rats. Eur J Neurosci 21:1719–1726

Clarke DW, Steenaart NA, Breedon TH, Brien JF (1985) Differential pharmacokinetics for oral and intraperitoneal administration of ethanol to the pregnant Guinea pig. Can J Physiol Pharmacol 63:169–172

Clarren SK, Astley SJ (1992) Pregnancy outcomes after weekly oral administration of ethanol during gestation in the pig-tailed macaque: comparing early gestational exposure to full gestational exposure. Teratology 45:1–9

Clarren SK, Bowden DM (1982) Fetal alcohol syndrome: a new primate model for binge drinking and its relevance to human ethanol teratogenesis. J Pediatr 101: 819–824

Clarren SK, Bowden DM, Astley SJ (1987) Pregnancy outcomes after weekly oral administration of ethanol during gestation in the pig-tailed macaque (Macaca nemestrina). Teratology 35:345–354

Clarren SK, Astley SJ, Gunderson VM, Spellman D (1992) Cognitive and behavioral deficits in nonhuman primates associated with very early embryonic binge exposures to ethanol. J Pediatr 121:789–796

Coles CD, Platzman KA (1993) Behavioral development in children prenatally exposed to drugs and alcohol. Int J Addict 28:1393–1433

Collingridge GL (2024) Long-term potentiation in the hippocampus: from magnesium to memory. Neuroscience 578:126–131. https://doi.org/10.1016/j.neuroscience.2024.11.069

Connor PD, Sampson PD, Bookstein FL, Barr HM, Streissguth AP (2000) Direct and indirect effects of prenatal alcohol damage on executive function. Dev Neuropsychol 18:331–354

Cronise K, Marino MD, Tran TD, Kelly SJ (2001) Critical periods for the effects of alcohol exposure on learning in rats. Behav Neurosci 115:138–145

Cudd TA (2005) Animal model systems for the study of alcohol teratology. Exp Biol Med (Maywood) 230: 389–393

Davies AG, Bettinger JC, Thiele TR, Judy ME, McIntire SL (2004) Natural variation in the npr-1 gene modifies ethanol responses of wild strains of C. elegans. Neuron 42:731–743

Davis CL (1914) The effect of alcohol on the male germ cells studied by means of double mating. University of Wisconsin

Davis JR, Li Y, Rankin CH (2008) Effects of developmental exposure to ethanol on Caenorhabditis elegans. Alcohol Clin Exp Res 32:853–867

de Licona HK et al (2009) A single exposure to alcohol during brain development induces microencephaly and neuronal losses in genetically susceptible mice, but not in wild type mice. Neurotoxicology 30:459–470

Diagnostic and Statistical Manual of Mental Disorders : DSM-5-TR (2022) Diagnostic and statistical manual of mental disorders : DSM-5-TR. American Psychiatric Association Publishing, Washington, DC

Dobbing J, Sands J (1979) Comparative aspects of the brain growth spurt. Early Hum Dev 3:79–83

Domellöf E, Fagard J, Jacquet A-Y, Rönnqvist L (2011) Goal-directed arm movements in children with fetal alcohol syndrome: a kinematic approach. Eur J Neurol 18:312–320

Downing C et al (2012) Gene expression changes in C57BL/6J and DBA/2J mice following prenatal alcohol exposure. Alcohol Clin Exp Res 36:1519–1529

Dringenberg HC, Richardson DP, Brien JF, Reynolds JN (2001) Spatial learning in the Guinea pig: cued versus non-cued learning, sex differences, and comparison with rats. Behav Brain Res 124:97–101
Driscoll CD, Streissguth AP, Riley EP (1990) Prenatal alcohol exposure: comparability of effects in humans and animal models. Neurotoxicol Teratol 12:231–237
Dunty WC, Chen SY, Zucker RM, Dehart DB, Sulik KK (2001) Selective vulnerability of embryonic cell populations to ethanol-induced apoptosis: implications for alcohol-related birth defects and neurodevelopmental disorder. Alcohol Clin Exp Res 25:1523–1535
Dursun I, Jakubowska-Doğru E, Uzbay T (2006) Effects of prenatal exposure to alcohol on activity, anxiety, motor coordination, and memory in young adult Wistar rats. Pharmacol Biochem Behav 85:345–355
Edri T, Cohen D, Shabtai Y, Fainsod A (2023) Alcohol induces neural tube defects by reducing retinoic acid signaling and promoting neural plate expansion. Front Cell Dev Biol 11:1282273
Ellis FW, Pick JR (1980) An animal model of the fetal alcohol syndrome in beagles. Alcohol Clin Exp Res 4: 123–134
Elton RH, Wilson ME (1977) Changes in ethanol consumption by pregnant pigtailed macaques. J Stud Alcohol 38:2181–2183
Erecinska M, Cherian S, Silver IA (2004) Energy metabolism in mammalian brain during development. Prog Neurobiol 73:397–445
Eyolfson E et al (2024) The effect of traumatic brain injury on learning and memory: a synaptic focus. Neuroscientist 31(2):195–214. https://doi.org/10.1177/10738584241275583
Fere CH (1895) Etudes experimentales sur l'influence teratogene ou degenerative des alcools et des essences sur l'embryon de poulet. J Anat Physiol 31:161–186
Fere CH (1898) Presentation de poulets vivants provenant d'oeufs ayant subi des injections d'alcool ethylique dans l'albumen. C R Seances Soc Biol Ses Fil 46:646
Fere CH (1899) Influence du repos sur les effects de l'exposition préalable aux vapeurs d'alcool avant l'incubation de l'oeuf de poule. Comptes Rendus Séances Société Biol Ses Fil 51:806
Fernandes Y, Gerlai R (2009) Long-term behavioral changes in response to early developmental exposure to ethanol in zebrafish. Alcohol Clin Exp Res 33:601–609
Fernandes Y, Tran S, Abraham E, Gerlai R (2014) Embryonic alcohol exposure impairs associative learning performance in adult zebrafish. Behav Brain Res 265: 181–187
Flentke GR, Smith SM (2018) The avian embryo as a model for fetal alcohol spectrum disorder. Biochem Cell Biol 96:98–106
Ford SM et al (2021) Folic acid prevents functional and structural heart defects induced by prenatal ethanol exposure. Am J Physiol-Heart Circ Physiol 320: H1313–H1320
Fuchs A-R (1966) The inhibitory effect of ethanol on the release of oxytocin during parturition in the rabbit. J Endocrinol 35:125–134
Gianoulakis C (1990) Rats exposed prenatally to alcohol exhibit impairment in spatial navigation test. Behav Brain Res 36:217–228
Gilardi C, Kalebic N (2021) The ferret as a model system for neocortex development and evolution. Front Cell Dev Biol 9:661759
Gilliam DM, Stilman A, Dudek BC, Riley EP (1987) Fetal alcohol effects in long- and short-sleep mice: activity, passive avoidance, and in utero ethanol levels. Neurotoxicol Teratol 9:349–357
Gil-Mohapel J, Boehme F, Kainer L, Christie BR (2010) Hippocampal cell loss and neurogenesis after fetal alcohol exposure: insights from different rodent models. Brain Res Rev 64:283–303
Gil-Mohapel J et al (2011) Altered adult hippocampal neuronal maturation in a rat model of fetal alcohol syndrome. Brain Res 1384:29–41
Girard TA, Xing HC, Ward GR, Wainwright PE (2000) Early postnatal ethanol exposure has long-term effects on the performance of male rats in a delayed matching-to-place task in the Morris water maze. Alcohol Clin Exp Res 24:300–306
Gleason CA, Iida H, Hotchkiss KJ, Northington FJ, Traystman RJ (1997) Newborn cerebrovascular responses after first trimester moderate maternal ethanol exposure in sheep. Pediatr Res 42:39–45
Goldman-Rakic PS (1995) Cellular basis of working memory. Neuron 14:477–485
Goncalves-Garcia M, Hamilton DA (2024) Unraveling the complex relationship between prenatal alcohol exposure, hippocampal LTP, and learning and memory. Front Mol Neurosci 16:1326089
Goodlett CR, Peterson SD (1995) Sex differences in vulnerability to developmental spatial learning deficits induced by limited binge alcohol exposure in neonatal rats. Neurobiol Learn Mem 64:265–275
Grafe EL, Fontaine CJ, Thomas JD, Christie BR (2021) Effects of prenatal ethanol exposure on choline-induced long-term depression in the hippocampus. J Neurophysiol 126:1622–1634
Graham JM, Ferm VH (1985) Heat- and alcohol-induced neural tube defects: interactions with folate in a golden hamster model. Pediatr Res 19:247–251
Green JT (2004) The effects of ethanol on the developing cerebellum and eyeblink classical conditioning. Cerebellum 3:178–187
Green CR et al (2005) Chronic prenatal ethanol exposure increases apoptosis in the hippocampus of the term fetal Guinea pig. Neurotoxicol Teratol 27:871–881
Gualdoni GS, Pérez-Tito L, Barril C, Sobarzo C, Cebral E (2022) Abnormal growth and morphogenesis of placenta at term is linked to adverse fetal development after perigestational alcohol consumption up to early gestation in mouse. Birth Defects Res 114:611–630
Gursky ZH, Savage LM, Klintsova AY (2021) Executive functioning-specific behavioral impairments in a rat

model of human third trimester binge drinking implicate prefrontal-thalamo-hippocampal circuitry in fetal alcohol Spectrum disorders. Behav Brain Res 405: 113208
Hamilton DA et al (2010) Prenatal exposure to moderate levels of ethanol alters social behavior in adult rats: relationship to structural plasticity and immediate early gene expression in frontal cortex. Behav Brain Res 207:290–304
Hamilton GF et al (2011) Neonatal alcohol exposure disrupts hippocampal neurogenesis and contextual fear conditioning in adult rats. Brain Res 1412:88–101
Hannigan JH, Riley EP (1988) Prenatal ethanol alters gait in rats. Alcohol (Fayettev) 5:451–454
Hård E et al (1985) Impaired maternal behaviour and altered central serotonergic activity in the adult offspring of chronically ethanol treated dams. Acta Pharmacol Toxicol (Copenh) 56:347–353
Hard ML, Abdolell M, Robinson BH, Koren G (2005) Gene-expression analysis after alcohol exposure in the developing mouse. J Lab Clin Med 145:47–54
Helfer JL, Goodlett CR, Greenough WT, Klintsova AY (2009) The effects of exercise on adolescent hippocampal neurogenesis in a rat model of binge alcohol exposure during the brain growth spurt. Brain Res 1294:1–11
Hickman DL, Johnson J, Vemulapalli TH, Crisler JR, Shepherd R (2017) Commonly used animal models. In: *Principles of animal research*. Elsevier, pp 117–175. https://doi.org/10.1016/B978-0-12-802151-4.00007-4
Hunt PS, Jacobson SE, Torok EJ (2009) Deficits in trace fear conditioning in a rat model of fetal alcohol exposure: dose-response and timing effects. Alcohol (Fayettev) 43:465–474
Ieraci A, Herrera DG (2007) Single alcohol exposure in early life damages hippocampal stem/progenitor cells and reduces adult neurogenesis. Neurobiol Dis 26: 597–605
Ikonomidou C et al (2000) Ethanol-induced apoptotic neurodegeneration and fetal alcohol syndrome. Science 287:1056–1060
Iqbal U, Dringenberg HC, Brien JF, Reynolds JN (2004) Chronic prenatal ethanol exposure alters hippocampal GABA(A) receptors and impairs spatial learning in the Guinea pig. Behav Brain Res 150:117–125
Izumi Y et al (2005) A single day of ethanol exposure during development has persistent effects on bi-directional plasticity, N-methyl-D-aspartate receptor function and ethanol sensitivity. Neuroscience 136: 269–279
Jawaid S et al (2021) Glutathione protects the developing heart from defects and global DNA hypomethylation induced by prenatal alcohol exposure. Alcohol Clin Exp Res 45:69–78
Johnson TB, Goodlett CR (2002) Selective and enduring deficits in spatial learning after limited neonatal binge alcohol exposure in male rats. Alcohol Clin Exp Res 26:83–93
Jones KL (1975) The fetal alcohol syndrome. Addict Dis 2:79–88
Jones KL, Smith DW (1973) Recognition of fetal alcohol sydrome in early infancy. Lancet 302:999–1001
Kalinichev M, Easterling KW, Plotsky PM, Holtzman SG (2002) Long-lasting changes in stress-induced corticosterone response and anxiety-like behaviors as a consequence of neonatal maternal separation in Long–Evans rats. Pharmacol Biochem Behav 73:131–140
Kane MJ, Engle RW (2002) The role of prefrontal cortex in working-memory capacity, executive attention, and general fluid intelligence: an individual-differences perspective. Psychon Bull Rev 9:637–671
Kane CJM et al (2011) Protection of neurons and microglia against ethanol in a mouse model of fetal alcohol spectrum disorders by peroxisome proliferator-activated receptor-γ agonists. Brain Behav Immun 25 (Suppl 1):S137–S145
Karanian J et al (1986) Characterization of an automated apparatus for precise control of inhalation chamber ethanol vapor and blood ethanol concentrations. Alcohol Clin Exp Res 10:443–447
Kelly SJ, Lawrence CR (2008) Intragastric intubation of alcohol during the perinatal period. Methods Mol Biol Clifton NJ 447:101–110
Kelly SJ, Tran TD (1997) Alcohol exposure during development alters social recognition and social communication in rats. Neurotoxicol Teratol 19:383–389
Kelly SJ, Goodlett CR, Hulsether SA, West JR (1988) Impaired spatial navigation in adult female but not adult male rats exposed to alcohol during the brain growth spurt. Behav Brain Res 27:247–257
Kelly SJ, Day N, Streissguth AP (2000) Effects of prenatal alcohol exposure on social behavior in humans and other species. Neurotoxicol Teratol 22:143–149
Kelly SJ, Goodlett CR, Hannigan JH (2009) Animal models of fetal alcohol spectrum disorders: impact of the social environment. Dev Disabil Res Rev 15:200–208
Keum D, Medina AE (2024) The effect of developmental alcohol exposure on multisensory integration is larger in deeper cortical layers. Alcohol 121:193–198
Keum D, Pultorak K, Meredith MA, Medina AE (2023) Effects of developmental alcohol exposure on cortical multisensory integration. Eur J Neurosci 57:784–795
Khanna JM, Kalant H, Shah G, Sharma H (1990) Comparison of sensitivity and alcohol consumption in four outbred strains of rats. Alcohol 7:429–434
Kim CK et al (1997) Object-recognition and spatial learning and memory in rats prenatally exposed to ethanol. Behav Neurosci 111:985–995
Kimura KA, Parr AM, Brien JF (1996) Effect of chronic maternal ethanol administration on nitric oxide synthase activity in the hippocampus of the mature fetal Guinea pig. Alcohol Clin Exp Res 20:948–953
Kleiber ML, Wright E, Singh SM (2011) Maternal voluntary drinking in C57BL/6J mice: advancing a model for fetal alcohol spectrum disorders. Behav Brain Res 223:376–387

Kleiber ML et al (2014) Long-term genomic and epigenomic dysregulation as a consequence of prenatal alcohol exposure: a model for fetal alcohol spectrum disorders. Front Genet 5:161

Klintsova AY et al (2007) Persistent impairment of hippocampal neurogenesis in young adult rats following early postnatal alcohol exposure. Alcohol Clin Exp Res 31:2073–2082

Krsiak M, Elis J, Pöschlová N, Masek K (1977) Increased aggressiveness and lower brain serotonin levels in offspring of mice given alcohol during gestation. J Stud Alcohol 38:1696–1704

Kulaga V et al (2006) Fatty acid ethyl esters (FAEE); comparative accumulation in human and Guinea pig hair as a biomarker for prenatal alcohol exposure. Alcohol Alcohol 41:534–539

Lan N et al (2006) Prenatal ethanol exposure alters the effects of gonadectomy on hypothalamic-pituitary-adrenal activity in male rats. J Neuroendocrinol 18: 672–684

Laufer BI, Diehl EJ, Singh SM (2013) Neurodevelopmental epigenetic etiologies: insights from studies on mouse models of fetal alcohol spectrum disorders. Epigenomics 5:465–468

Lemoine P (1994) The letter from professor Lemoine. Addiction 89:1021–1023

Lewandowska E et al (2012) Alcohol-induced changes in the developing cerebellum. Ultrastructural and quantitative analysis of neurons in the cerebellar cortex. Folia Neuropathol 50:397–406

Lieber CS, DeCarli LM (1982) The feeding of alcohol in liquid diets: two decades of applications and 1982 update. Alcohol Clin Exp Res 6:523–531

Lin CH, Sa S, Chand J, Rankin CH (2013) Dynamic and persistent effects of ethanol exposure on development: an in vivo analysis during and after embryonic ethanol exposure in Caenorhabditis elegans. Alcohol Clin Exp Res 37(Suppl 1):E190–E198

Lindeberg H (2008) Reproduction of the female ferret (Mustela putorius furo). Reprod Domest Anim 43: 150–156

Lindquist DH, Sokoloff G, Milner E, Steinmetz JE (2013) Neonatal ethanol exposure results in dose-dependent impairments in the acquisition and timing of the conditioned eyeblink response and altered cerebellar interpositus nucleus and hippocampal CA1 unit activity in adult rats. Alcohol (Fayettev) 47:447–457

Livy DJ, Parnell SE, West JR (2003a) Blood ethanol concentration profiles: a comparison between rats and mice. Alcohol 29:165–171

Livy DJ, Miller EK, Maier SE, West JR (2003b) Fetal alcohol exposure and temporal vulnerability: effects of binge-like alcohol exposure on the developing rat hippocampus. Neurotoxicol Teratol 25:447–458

Loucks E, Ahlgren S (2012) Assessing teratogenic changes in a zebrafish model of fetal alcohol exposure. J Vis Exp JoVE 61:3704. https://doi.org/10.3791/3704

Lussier AA, Petrelli B, Hicks GG, Weinberg J (2023) Genetic, epigenetic, and environmental influences on fetal alcohol Spectrum disorder: implications for diagnosis, research and clinical practice. In: Eisenstat DD, Goldowitz D, Oberlander TF, Yager JY (eds) Neurodevelopmental pediatrics: genetic and environmental influences. Springer, Cham, pp 441–456. https://doi.org/10.1007/978-3-031-20792-1_28

Maguire EA, Frith CD, Burgess N, Donnett JG, O'Keefe J (1998) Knowing where things are parahippocampal involvement in encoding object locations in virtual large-scale space. J Cogn Neurosci 10:61–76

Maier SE, West JR (2001) Drinking patterns and alcohol-related birth defects. *Alcohol Res Health J Natl Inst Alcohol Abuse Alcohol* 25:168–174

Maier SE, Miller JA, Blackwell JM, West JR (1999) Fetal alcohol exposure and temporal vulnerability: regional differences in cell loss as a function of the timing of binge-like alcohol exposure during brain development. Alcohol Clin Exp Res 23:726–734

Mankes RF, Battles AH, LeFevre R, van der Hoeven T, Glick SD (1992) Preferential alcoholic embryopathy: effects of liquid diets. Lab Anim Sci 42:561–566

Marais L, Van Rensburg SJ, Van Zyl JM, Stein DJ, Daniels WMU (2008) Maternal separation of rat pups increases the risk of developing depressive-like behavior after subsequent chronic stress by altering corticosterone and neurotrophin levels in the hippocampus. Neurosci Res 61:106–112

Marcussen BL, Goodlett CR, Mahoney JC, West JR (1994) Developing rat Purkinje cells are more vulnerable to alcohol-induced depletion during differentiation than during neurogenesis. Alcohol (Fayettev) 11:147–156

Marino MD, Cronise K, Lugo JN, Kelly SJ (2002) Ultrasonic vocalizations and maternal-infant interactions in a rat model of fetal alcohol syndrome. Dev Psychobiol 41:341–351

Marrs JA et al (2010) Zebrafish fetal alcohol syndrome model: effects of ethanol are rescued by retinoic acid supplement. Alcohol (Fayettev) 44:707–715

Mattson SN, Crocker N, Nguyen TT (2011) Fetal alcohol spectrum disorders: neuropsychological and behavioral features. Neuropsychol Rev 21:81–101

McAdam TD, Brien JF, Reynolds JN, Dringenberg HC (2008) Altered water-maze search behavior in adult Guinea pigs following chronic prenatal ethanol exposure: lack of mitigation by postnatal fluoxetine treatment. Behav Brain Res 191:202–209

Meyer LS, Riley EP (1986) Social play in juvenile rats prenatally exposed to alcohol. Teratology 34:1–7

Middaugh LD, Boggan WO (1991) Postnatal growth deficits in prenatal ethanol-exposed mice: characteristics and critical periods. Alcohol Clin Exp Res 15:919–926

Middaugh LD, Boggan WO (1995) Perinatal maternal ethanol effects on pregnant mice and on offspring viability and growth: influences of exposure time and weaning diet. Alcohol Clin Exp Res 19:1351–1358

Mihalick SM, Crandall JE, Langlois JC, Krienke JD, Dube WV (2001) Prenatal ethanol exposure, generalized

learning impairment, and medial prefrontal cortical deficits in rats. Neurotoxicol Teratol 23:453–462
Miki T et al (2008) Ethanol neurotoxicity and dentate gyrus development. Congenit Anom 48:110–117
Miller MW (1996) Limited ethanol exposure selectively alters the proliferation of precursor cells in the cerebral cortex. Alcohol Clin Exp Res 20:139–143
Mitoma H, Manto M, Shaikh AG (2024) Alcohol toxicity in the developing cerebellum. Diagnostics 14:1415
Mokashi SS et al (2021) Developmental alcohol exposure in drosophila: effects on adult phenotypes and gene expression in the brain. Front Psych 12:699033
Morozova TV, Shankar V, MacPherson RA, Mackay TFC, Anholt RRH (2022) Modulation of the drosophila transcriptome by developmental exposure to alcohol. BMC Genomics 23:347
Nagahara AH, Handa RJ (1997) Fetal alcohol exposure produces delay-dependent memory deficits in juvenile and adult rats. Alcohol Clin Exp Res 21:710–715
Naik VD et al (2025) Sexual dimorphism in lung transcriptomic adaptations in fetal alcohol spectrum disorders. Respir Res 26:6
Ness JW, Franchina JJ (1990) Effects of prenatal alcohol exposure on rat pups' ability to elicit retrieval behavior from dams. Dev Psychobiol 23:85–99
Nixon K, Crews FT (2002) Binge ethanol exposure decreases neurogenesis in adult rat hippocampus. J Neurochem 83:1087–1093
O'Leary-Moore SK et al (2010) Magnetic resonance microscopy-based analyses of the brains of normal and ethanol-exposed fetal mice. Birth Defects Res A Clin Mol Teratol 88:953–964
Olivares-Costa M, Fabio MC, De la Fuente-Ortega E, Haeger PA, Pautassi R (2024) New therapeutics for the prevention or amelioration of fetal alcohol spectrum disorders: a narrative review of the preclinical literature. Am J Drug Alcohol Abuse 50:749–770
Olney JW et al (2002) Ethanol-induced apoptotic neurodegeneration in the developing C57BL/6 mouse brain. Brain Res Dev Brain Res 133:115–126
Pal N, Alkana RL (1997) Use of inhalation to study the effect of ethanol and ethanol dependence on neonatal mouse development without maternal separation: a preliminary study. Life Sci 61:1269–1281
Paolozza A, Titman R, Brien D, Munoz DP, Reynolds JN (2013) Altered accuracy of saccadic eye movements in children with fetal alcohol spectrum disorder. Alcohol Clin Exp Res 37:1491–1498
Parnell SE et al (2007) Chronic ethanol increases fetal cerebral blood flow specific to the ethanol-sensitive cerebellum under normoxaemic, hypercapnic and acidaemic conditions: ovine model. Exp Physiol 92: 933–943
Parnell SE et al (2009) Magnetic resonance microscopy defines ethanol-induced brain abnormalities in prenatal mice: effects of acute insult on gestational day 8. Alcohol Clin Exp Res 33:1001–1011
Patten AR et al (2013a) Impairments in hippocampal synaptic plasticity following prenatal ethanol exposure are dependent on glutathione levels. Hippocampus 23: 1463–1475
Patten AR, Sickmann HM, Dyer RA, Innis SM, Christie BR (2013b) Omega-3 fatty acids can reverse the long-term deficits in hippocampal synaptic plasticity caused by prenatal ethanol exposure. Neurosci Lett 551:7–11
Peng Y et al (2004) A critical role of Pax6 in alcohol-induced fetal microcephaly. Neurobiol Dis 16:370–376
Pierce DR, West JR (1986) Blood alcohol concentration: a critical factor for producing fetal alcohol effects. Alcohol (Fayettev) 3:269–272
Pierce DR, Serbus DC, Light KE (1993) Intragastric intubation of alcohol during postnatal development of rats results in selective cell loss in the cerebellum. Alcohol Clin Exp Res 17:1275–1280
Popoola DO, Nizhnikov ME, Cameron NM (2017) Strain-specific programming of prenatal ethanol exposure across generations. Alcohol 60:191–199
Popović M, Caballero-Bleda M, Guerri C (2006) Adult rat's offspring of alcoholic mothers are impaired on spatial learning and object recognition in the can test. Behav Brain Res 174:101–111
Puglia MP, Valenzuela CF (2010) Repeated third trimester-equivalent ethanol exposure inhibits long-term potentiation in the hippocampal CA1 region of neonatal rats. Alcohol (Fayettev) 44:283–290
Qiang M, Wang MW, Elberger AJ (2002) Second trimester prenatal alcohol exposure alters development of rat corpus callosum. Neurotoxicol Teratol 24:719–732
Quaia C, Lefèvre P, Optican LM (1999) Model of the control of saccades by superior colliculus and cerebellum. J Neurophysiol 82:999–1018
Räihä NC, Koskinen M, Pikkarainen P (1967) Developmental changes in alcohol-dehydrogenase activity in rat and Guinea-pig liver. Biochem J 103:623–626
Rasmussen C (2005) Executive functioning and working memory in fetal alcohol spectrum disorder. Alcohol Clin Exp Res 29:1359–1367
Redila VA et al (2006) Hippocampal cell proliferation is reduced following prenatal ethanol exposure but can be rescued with voluntary exercise. Hippocampus 16: 305–311
Reid HMOHMO et al (2020) A systematic review of the effects of perinatal alcohol exposure and perinatal marijuana exposure on adult neurogenesis in the dentate gyrus. Alcohol Clin Exp Res 44:acer.14332
Reid HMO et al (2021) Prenatal alcohol and cannabis exposure can have opposing and region-specific effects on parvalbumin interneuron numbers in the hippocampus. Alcohol Clin Exp Res 45(11):2246–2255. https://doi.org/10.1111/ACER.14708
Richardson DP, Byrnes ML, Brien JF, Reynolds JN, Dringenberg HC (2002) Impaired acquisition in the water maze and hippocampal long-term potentiation after chronic prenatal ethanol exposure in the Guinea-pig. Eur J Neurosci 16:1593–1598

Ridderinkhof KR, Ullsperger M, Crone EA, Nieuwenhuis S (2004) The role of the medial frontal cortex in cognitive control. Science 306:443–447
Riley EP, Meyer LS (1984) Considerations for the design, implementation, and interpretation of animal models of fetal alcohol effects. Neurobehav Toxicol Teratol 6: 97–101
Riley EP, Lochry EA, Shapiro NR (1979) Lack of response inhibition in rats prenatally exposed to alcohol. Psychopharmacology 62:47–52
Roebuck TM, Simmons RW, Mattson SN, Riley EP (1998) Prenatal exposure to alcohol affects the ability to maintain postural balance. Alcohol Clin Exp Res 22: 252–258
Rogers J, Wiener SG, Bloom FE (1979) Long-term ethanol administration methods for rats: advantages of inhalation over intubation or liquid diets. Behav Neural Biol 27:466–486
Rouquette J (1957) Influence de la toxicomanie alcoolique parentale sur le développement physique & psychique des jeunes enfants. Faculty of Medicine of Paris
Royalty J (1990) Effects of prenatal ethanol exposure on juvenile play-fighting and postpubertal aggression in rats. Psychol Rep 66:551–560
Ryabinin AE, Cole M, Bloom FE, Wilson MC (1995) Exposure of neonatal rats to alcohol by vapor inhalation demonstrates specificity of microcephaly and Purkinje cell loss but not astrogliosis. Alcohol Clin Exp Res 19:784–791
Samson HH, Diaz J (1981) Altered development of brain by neonatal ethanol exposure: zinc levels during and after exposure. Alcohol Clin Exp Res 5:563–569
Sanders JL (2011) Commentary: what might have been: Sullivan may have impacted modern prenatal alcohol research under different circumstances. Int J Epidemiol 40:283–285
Schneider ML, Moore CF, Kraemer GW (2001a) Moderate alcohol during pregnancy: learning and behavior in adolescent rhesus monkeys. Alcohol Clin Exp Res 25: 1383–1392
Schneider ML, Moore CF, Becker EF (2001b) Timing of moderate alcohol exposure during pregnancy and neonatal outcome in rhesus monkeys (Macaca mulatta). Alcohol Clin Exp Res 25:1238–1245
Schneider ML et al (2008) Sensory processing disorder in a primate model: evidence from a longitudinal study of prenatal alcohol and prenatal stress effects. Child Dev 79:100–113
Schneider ML, Moore CF, Adkins MM (2011) The effects of prenatal alcohol exposure on behavior: rodent and primate studies. Neuropsychol Rev 21:186–203
Scott WJ, Fradkin R (1984) The effects of prenatal ethanol in cynomolgus monkeys. Teratology 29:49–56
Seleverstov O et al (2017) Maternal alcohol exposure during mid-pregnancy dilates fetal cerebral arteries via endocannabinoid receptors. Alcohol (Fayettev) 61:51–61
Sellin LC, Laakso PS (1987) Effect of ethanol on motor performance and hippocampal population spikes in some standard and selectively outbred rat strains. Alcohol Clin Exp Res 11:502–505
Serbus DC, Young MW, Light KE (1986) Blood ethanol concentrations following intragastric intubation of neonatal rat pups. Neurobehav Toxicol Teratol 8:403–406
Sherwin BT, Jacobson S, Troxell SL, Rogers AE, Pelham RW (1979) A rat model (using a semipurified diet) of the fetal alcohol syndrome. Curr Alcohol 7:15–30
Sickmann HM et al (2014) Prenatal ethanol exposure has sex-specific effects on hippocampal long-term potentiation. Hippocampus 24:54–64
Sokol RJ (2003) Fetal alcohol spectrum disorder. JAMA 290:2996
Spadoni AD et al (2009) BOLD response during spatial working memory in youth with heavy prenatal alcohol exposure. Alcohol Clin Exp Res 33:2067–2076
Stanton ME, Goodlett CR (1998) Neonatal ethanol exposure impairs eyeblink conditioning in weanling rats. Alcohol Clin Exp Res 22:270–275
Stockard CR (1910) The influence of alcohol and other anaesthetics on embryonic development. Am J Anat 10:369
Stockard CR (1914) The artificial production of eye abnormalities in the chick embryo. Anat Rec 8:31–41
Stone WS et al (1996) Prenatal exposure to alcohol in adult rats: relationships between sleep and memory deficits, and effects of glucose administration on memory. Brain Res 742:98–106
Streissguth AP et al (1991) Fetal alcohol syndrome in adolescents and adults. JAMA 265:1961–1967
Streissguth AP, Barr HM, Sampson PD (1990) Moderate prenatal alcohol exposure: effects on child IQ and learning problems at age 7 1/2 years. Alcohol Clin Exp Res 14:662–669
Streissguth AP et al (1994) Drinking during pregnancy decreases word attack and arithmetic scores on standardized tests: adolescent data from a population-based prospective study. Alcohol Clin Exp Res 18: 248–254
Streissguth AP, Barr HM, Kogan J, Bookstein FL (1996) Understanding the occurrence of secondary disabilities in clients with Fetal Alcohol Syndrome (FAS) and Fetal Alcohol Effects (FAE), pp 1–72
Su B, Debelak KA, Tessmer LL, Cartwright MM, Smith SM (2001) Genetic influences on craniofacial outcome in an avian model of prenatal alcohol exposure. Alcohol Clin Exp Res 25:60–69
Sulik KK, Johnston MC, Webb MA (1981) Fetal alcohol syndrome: embryogenesis in a mouse model. Science 214:936–938
Sutherland RJ, McDonald RJ, Savage DD (1997) Prenatal exposure to moderate levels of ethanol can have long-lasting effects on hippocampal synaptic plasticity in adult offspring. Hippocampus 7:232–238
Swartzwelder HS, Farr KL, Wilson WA, Savage DD (1988) Prenatal exposure to ethanol decreases physiological plasticity in the hippocampus of the adult rat. Alcohol (Fayettev) 5:121–124

Tang S, Xu S, Gullapalli RP, Medina AE (2018) Effects of early alcohol exposure on functional organization and microstructure of a visual-tactile integrative circuit. Alcohol Clin Exp Res 42:727–734

Thomas JD, Wasserman EA, West JR, Goodlett CR (1996) Behavioral deficits induced by bingelike exposure to alcohol in neonatal rats: importance of developmental timing and number of episodes. Dev Psychobiol 29:433–452

Thomas SE, Kelly SJ, Mattson SN, Riley EP (1998) Comparison of social abilities of children with fetal alcohol syndrome to those of children with similar IQ scores and normal controls. Alcohol Clin Exp Res 22:528–533

Thomas JD, Sather TM, Whinery LA (2008) Voluntary exercise influences behavioral development in rats exposed to alcohol during the neonatal brain growth spurt. Behav Neurosci 122:1264–1273

Thomas JD, Idrus NM, Monk BR, Dominguez HD (2010) Prenatal choline supplementation mitigates behavioral alterations associated with prenatal alcohol exposure in rats. Birt. Defects Res. A. Clin. Mol. Teratol. 88:827–837

Titterness AK, Christie BR (2012) Prenatal ethanol exposure enhances NMDAR-dependent long-term potentiation in the adolescent female dentate gyrus. Hippocampus 22:69–81

Tobiasz AM et al (2018) The effect of prenatal alcohol exposure on fetal growth and cardiovascular parameters in a baboon model of pregnancy. Reprod Sci 25:1116–1123

Tran TD, Cronise K, Marino MD, Jenkins WJ, Kelly SJ (2000) Critical periods for the effects of alcohol exposure on brain weight, body weight, activity and investigation. Behav Brain Res 116:99–110

Uecker A, Nadel L (1996) Spatial locations gone awry: object and spatial memory deficits in children with fetal alcohol syndrome. Neuropsychologia 34:209–223

Varaschin RK, Akers KG, Rosenberg MJ, Hamilton DA, Savage DD (2010) Effects of the cognition-enhancing agent ABT-239 on fetal ethanol-induced deficits in dentate gyrus synaptic plasticity. J Pharmacol Exp Ther 334:191–198

Vaurio L, Riley EP, Mattson SN (2008) Differences in executive functioning in children with heavy prenatal alcohol exposure or attention-deficit/hyperactivity disorder. J Int Neuropsychol Soc JINS 14:119–129

Vink J, Auth J, Abebe DT, Brenneman DE, Spong CY (2005) Novel peptides prevent alcohol-induced spatial learning deficits and proinflammatory cytokine release in a mouse model of fetal alcohol syndrome. Am J Obstet Gynecol 193:825–829

Wagner AF, Hunt PS (2006) Impaired trace fear conditioning following neonatal ethanol: reversal by choline. Behav Neurosci 120:482–487

Wagner JL, Zhou FC, Goodlett CR (2014) Effects of one- and three-day binge alcohol exposure in neonatal C57BL/6 mice on spatial learning and memory in adolescence and adulthood. Alcohol (Fayettev) 48: 99–111

Wainwright PE et al (1990) Effects of prenatal ethanol and long-chain n-3 fatty acid supplementation on development in mice. 1. Body and brain growth, sensorimotor development, and water T-maze reversal learning. Alcohol Clin Exp Res 14:405–412

Warner RH, Rosett HL (1975) The effects of drinking on offspring: an historical survey of the American and British literature. J Stud Alcohol 36:1395–1420

Washburn S, Nation K, Cudd T, Stanton M, Goodlett C (2025) Gestational choline supplementation ameliorates T-maze reversal learning deficits induced by first trimester binge alcohol exposure in weanling lambs. Alcohol 123:109–120

Weathersby RT, Becker HC, Hale RL (1994) Reduced sensitivity to the effects of clonidine on ethanol-stimulated locomotor activity in adult mouse offspring prenatally exposed to ethanol. Alcohol (Fayettev) 11: 517–522

Webster WS, Walsh DA, McEwen SE, Lipson AH (1983) Some teratogenic properties of ethanol and acetaldehyde in C57BL/6J mice: implications for the study of the fetal alcohol syndrome. Teratology 27:231–243

Weinberg J (1984) Nutritional issues in perinatal alcohol exposure. Neurobehav Toxicol Teratol 6:261–269

West JR (1987) Fetal alcohol-induced brain damage and the problem of determining temporal vulnerability: a review. Alcohol Drug Res 7:423–441

West JR, Hamre KM (1985) Effects of alcohol exposure during different periods of development: changes in hippocampal mossy fibers. Brain Res 349:280–284

West JR, Dewey SL, Pierce DR, Black AC (1984) Prenatal and early postnatal exposure to ethanol permanently alters the rat hippocampus. Ciba Found Symp 105:8–25

West JR, Hamre KM, Cassell MD (1986) Effects of ethanol exposure during the third trimester equivalent on neuron number in rat hippocampus and dentate gyrus. Alcohol Clin Exp Res 10:190–197

Wigal T, Amsel A (1990) Behavioral and neuroanatomical effects of prenatal, postnatal, or combined exposure to ethanol in weanling rats. Behav Neurosci 104:116–126

Wozniak DF et al (2004) Apoptotic neurodegeneration induced by ethanol in neonatal mice is associated with profound learning/memory deficits in juveniles followed by progressive functional recovery in adults. Neurobiol Dis 17:403–414

Yelin R et al (2005) Ethanol exposure affects gene expression in the embryonic organizer and reduces retinoic acid levels. Dev Biol 279:193–204

Yelin R, Kot H, Yelin D, Fainsod A (2007) Early molecular effects of ethanol during vertebrate embryogenesis. Differ Res Biol Divers 75:393–403

Young BW, Sengelaub DR, Steinmetz JE (2010) MK-801 administration during neonatal ethanol withdrawal attenuates interpositus cell loss and juvenile eyeblink conditioning deficits. Alcohol (Fayettev) 44:359–369

Zhang C et al (2014) Molecular and morphological changes in zebrafish following transient ethanol exposure during defined developmental stages. Neurotoxicol Teratol 44:70–80

Impact of Prenatal Alcohol Exposure on the Cerebral Circulation: Potential Implications for Stroke

2

Partha S. Saha, Denise M. Arrick, and William G. Mayhan

Abstract

Prenatal alcohol exposure (PAE) is recognized as a teratogenic factor that affects neural development, resulting in a range of structural, functional, and cognitive/behavioral abnormalities contributing to the pathogenesis of fetal alcohol spectrum disorder (FASD). FASD is a major preventable cause of developmental delay in humans. There are many molecular and cellular mechanisms by which PAE could contribute to abnormalities seen in individuals with FASD. Understanding these mechanisms will be critical for the development of therapeutic approaches that could benefit not only the developing fetus, but the newborn as they mature into adolescence and adulthood. The goal of this review is to discuss the impact of PAE on neural and vascular development/function and define potential cellular/molecular mechanisms that contribute to the effects of PAE. We believe that an understanding regarding the influence of PAE on cerebral vascular function may provide insights into the pathogenesis of symptoms related to FASD.

Keywords

Microcirculation · Reactivity · Nitric oxide · Oxidative stress

2.1 Introduction

General Considerations Ethanol, often used as a psychotropic drug, can cross the placental barrier potentially leading to teratogenic effects especially during organogenesis. The extent of the harmful consequences of prenatal alcohol exposure (PAE) is influenced by many factors including the concentration of alcohol, the timing of alcohol exposure, and the duration of intake of alcohol. These factors can lead to various negative outcomes in fetal and birth health including stillbirth, stunted preterm growth, early childbirth, lower birth weight, and an increase in infant

Source of Support: Original studies from our laboratory were supported by grants from the National Institute on Alcohol Abuse and Alcoholism (AA11288, AA027206) and funds from the Sanford School of Medicine at the University of South Dakota.

P. S. Saha
School of Science, Technology, Engineering, and Math (STEM), Diné College, Shiprock, NM, USA
e-mail: psaha@dinecollege.edu

D. M. Arrick · W. G. Mayhan (✉)
Division of Biomedical and Translational Sciences, Sanford School of Medicine, University of South Dakota, Vermillion, SD, USA
e-mail: Denise.arrick@usd.edu; william.mayhan@usd.edu

A. N. Bukiya, D. W. Ali (eds.), *Molecular Mechanisms and Lifelong Consequences of Prenatal Exposure to Psychoactive Substances*, Advances in Experimental Medicine and Biology 1500,
https://doi.org/10.1007/978-3-032-12741-9_2

mortality (Aliyu et al. 2008; Fertig and Watson 2009; Jaddoe et al. 2007; Cil 2017; Jacks et al. 2021; O'Leary et al. 2013; Wisborg et al. 2001). Notably, PAE significantly affects the fetal brain, causing developmental, morphological, and functional abnormalities (Mattson et al. 2001; Caputo et al. 2016).

Fetal alcohol spectrum disorder (FASD) is a comprehensive term used to describe the negative consequences that result from exposure to alcohol during pregnancy. These consequences can include various abnormalities in physical appearance, and neurological and behavioral development (Thomas et al. 2010), making FASD a major cause of preventable cognitive deficits in children, adolescents, and adults (May et al. 2009; Amendah et al. 2011; Centers for Disease Control and Prevention n.d.). FASD covers many alcohol-related issues of differing severity. The most extreme variant, fetal alcohol syndrome (FAS), is recognized by specific physical features observed in newborns, that is, abnormal facial features, short height, low body weight, small head size, and vision/hearing deficits. When alcohol exposure during pregnancy is confirmed but the symptoms are insufficient for a full FAS diagnosis, partial fetal alcohol syndrome (pFAS) is identified (Riley et al. 2011).

Despite increased awareness of the risks of PAE, its prevalence remains high. Data indicate that about 8% pregnant women who consume alcohol may have a child affected by FASD, resulting in over 630,000 newborns with FASD annually (Lange 2017). Systematic reviews and meta-analysis have shown that in the United States, 45% of pregnancies were unintended, with 10% of women aged 18 to 44 admitting to alcohol use during the past 30 days, and about 33% of women engaging in binge drinking, that is, a pattern of drinking that brings blood alcohol concentration to 0.08% or higher in about 2 h (Dejong et al. 2019; Finer and Zolna 2016). Research from four US school systems found FASD rates in school-aged children to be between 1% and 5%, with a weighted prevalence estimated to be 3% to about 10% (May et al. 2018). FASD's prevalence in the United States is estimated at 2–5% (May et al. 2009, 2018). The costs for diagnosing and continued care for a child with FASD can escalate to $two million in severe cases. It has been estimated that the cost for healthcare and specialized services for individuals with FASD was near $4 billion in the United States (Amendah et al. 2011; Lupton et al. 2004).

The precise mechanisms that contribute to abnormalities associated with FASD are not completely understood but are multifactorial, involving many molecular/cellular pathways, including pathways that may regulate cerebral vascular function and hence blood flow to the brain. For example, studies have shown that PAE significantly affects functional responses of cerebral arterioles, which are an integral component to the neurovascular unit (Muoio et al. 2014; Iadecola 2017). The impact of PAE on cerebral arterioles, and thus the control of cerebral blood flow during changes in metabolic demand, may have important implications to cognitive and behavioral consequences in childhood, adolescence, and adulthood. This review will address findings that have examined the consequence of PAE on the developing fetus and its implications into adolescence and adulthood, including the potential for an increase in the pathogenesis of stroke.

Lifelong Consequences of FASD The Developmental Origins of Health and Disease (DOHaD) suggests that the environment and experiences during early life stages, particularly during prenatal development and infancy, can influence health and disease risk later in life (Barker 1989). Individuals with FASD are often identified during childhood and there is a considerable body of literature documenting the presence of neurobehavioral deficits in children and adolescents diagnosed with FASD (Mattson et al. 2011; West 1987). Children with FASD exhibit compromised hand-eye coordination (Irner et al. 2011) and a reduced size of the cerebellar vermis when compared to control children of the same age (Archibald et al. 2001; Sowell et al. 1996). Alterations in executive function have been noted in children that have been exposed to alcohol prenatally (Pei et al. 2011; Rasmussen et al. 2011). Children who have been exposed to alcohol during prenatal development may experience negative effects on their ability to solve social problems (Stevens et al. 2012). According to a study conducted by Irner et al. (2011), preschool-aged children who were exposed to prenatal alcohol had lower scores on a specific subscale measuring personality and social skills. Investigators utilizing magnetic resonance imaging (MRI) have shown decreases in total brain volume and white matter among children and adolescents who have been exposed to prenatal alcohol (Lebel et al. 2011; Wozniak and Muetzel 2011). Several studies have documented a correlation between alcohol exposure and a compromise in overall health, that is, diminished immunological function, impaired glucose tolerance, hyperinsulinemia, and an increased incidence of some pediatric malignancies when compared to the general population (Oleson et al. 1998; Johnson et al. 1981; Castells et al. 1981; Burd et al. 2014).

Several physical, cognitive, and neurobehavioral characteristics observed in children with FASD persist throughout adulthood. Young adults with FASD often have secondary difficulties, including school dropouts, involvement in legal issues, and struggles with substance and alcohol addiction [as reviewed in (Moore and Riley 2015)]. While the amount of clinical research conducted in humans is limited, there are many studies that have examined the influence of PAE in various animal models of FASD. These studies have shown an increased susceptibility to autoimmune disorders, diabetes, chronic hypertension, and cancer (McGill et al. 2009; Zhang et al. 2012; Chen and Nyomba 2003; Pennington et al. 2002; Nordestgaard and Varbo 2014; Murugan et al. 2013). In addition, it has been suggested that adult mice and rats that were exposed to prenatal alcohol may have a diminished ability to adapt to brain trauma produced by cerebral ischemia/reperfusion and thus may be more susceptible to ischemic stroke (Bake et al. 2017; Cananzi and Mayhan 2019). Studies in mice demonstrate that PAE reduces cranial blood flow both in utero and in adulthood, adversely affecting behavioral recovery following stroke-like events (Bake et al. 2012, 2017). In addition, impaired cerebral vascular function and presumably the control of cerebral blood flow have been shown to be diminished by PAE (Cananzi and Mayhan 2019), suggesting a possible predisposition to cerebral ischemic events that may contribute to behavioral/cognitive dysfunction observed in humans with FASD.

FASD also causes significant developmental issues for other organ systems including the peripheral nervous, cardiovascular, renal, hepatic, gastrointestinal, and endocrine systems. PAE also has a profound impact on the spinal cord, indicating a broader scope of neurological damage than previously understood (Heaton and Bradley 1995). With regard to the cardiovascular system, investigators have shown that alcohol can have a negative impact on blood flow through the umbilical artery (Jones et al. 1981; Mukherjee and Hodgen 1982), potentially leading to overall growth abnormalities (Abel 1984, 1985). It appears that alcohol has the potential to hinder development by affecting protein synthesis, hormone levels, as well as other growth-influencing factors (Kennedy 1984; Pennington et al. 1983). Further, an increase in oxidative stress (Ornoy 2007; Pollard 2007) and the interference with growth factor signaling (Feng et al. 2005; Miller 2003) may influence overall development of the fetus. PAE has been shown to significantly decrease the distribution of blood flow to the brain and has been linked to serious cardiac issues in newborns, including conotruncal defects (congenital cardiovascular anomalies involving the outflow tracts and great vessels), leading to severe heart muscle damage (Henderson et al. 2007; Yang et al. 2015). Renal abnormalities by PAE include hypoplasia, agenesis, and hydronephrosis (Hofer and Burd 2009). A study using rats found that PAE resulted in reduced number of nephrons at 1 month of age and increased arterial blood pressure at 6 months of age (Gray et al. 2010). In the liver, PAE leads to hyperbilirubinemia, causing jaundice in newborns (Hofer and Burd 2009). Additionally, PAE results in enteric neuropathy, manifesting as chronic intestinal pseudoobstruction in infants (Uc et al. 1997). The endocrine system is also significantly affected by PAE. Cortisol, the hormone regulating the body's response to stress, is altered by in utero exposure to alcohol, with higher evening and lower morning values, which may contribute to chronic depression in early adolescence (Goodyer et al. 2001; McLachlan et al. 2016). PAE impacts the limbic-hypothalamic-pituitary-adrenal axis, altering cortisol activity and sensitivity to the inhibitory effect of testosterone (Ouellet-Morin et al. 2011). Furthermore, differences in insulin-like growth factors (IGF-I, IGF-II) and leptin levels between ethanol-exposed and control groups suggest potential markers for PAE and may be associated with pre- and post-natal growth retardation (Aros et al. 2011). Other organ systems are also not immune to the effects of PAE. In animal models, PAE has been shown to affect both the lung and musculoskeletal system (Gauthier 2015). Within the prostate, PAE leads to abnormal cellular structure in adult rats and increases the incidence of prostate tumors following exposure to carcinogens and testosterone (Murugan et al. 2013). This short overview of the effects of PAE across various organ systems underscores the significant and wide-ranging impacts of alcohol consumption during pregnancy. Thus, it appears that PAE predisposes to many cerebral and systemic abnormalities that are not specific to the fetus but continue into adolescence and adulthood. Further investigation will be necessary to determine the mechanisms of these long-term effects of PAE on multiorgan systems.

Cellular/Molecular Mechanisms Accounting for Effects of PAE In adults, the metabolism of ethanol (ETOH) predominantly occurs through the alcohol dehydrogenase (ADH) and cytochrome P450 2E1 (CYP2E1) pathways, with catalase (CAT) playing a less significant role. ADH accounts for about 90% of ETOH metabolism, while CYP2E1 contributes to about 10% of ETOH metabolism (Koop 2006; Gupta et al. 2016). During human fetal development, CYP2E1 becomes active from the 16th week of gestation, whereas ADH activity initiates around the 26th week of gestation. In the developing fetus, both enzymes exhibit lower cellular levels/activity compared to that measured in adults, thus accounting for elevated and sustained ETOH concentrations in the fetal environment and the increased susceptibility of the fetus to the damaging effects of ETOH (Koop 2006; Gupta et al. 2016). There are several cellular mechanisms by which ETOH contributes to the development of FASD, as outlined in Fig. 2.1. An understanding of the precise role of these mechanisms will be essential for comprehending FASD's etiology and the development of effective interventions.

Oxidative Stress FASD is characterized by distinct neurodevelopmental abnormalities that may arise from an ETOH-induced increase in reactive oxygen species. Oxidative stress, a primary outcome of ETOH metabolism, occurs due to the conversion of ETOH to acetaldehyde, which is facilitated by alcohol dehydrogenase and cytochrome P450 2E1. The formation of reactive oxygen species leads to oxidation of lipids, proteins, and DNA, with subsequent disruption of tissue homeostasis, cellular functions, and DNA integrity, to induce autophagy, apoptosis, and necrosis (Yang and Luo 2015; Miller-Pinsler and Wells 2016; Wong et al. 2008; Wells et al. 2009; Chen et al. 2012; Luo 2014). Long-term studies on PAE have shown an increase in oxidative stress, lipid peroxidation, and markers of apoptosis, which were associated with behavioral disorders in rats (Koop 2006; Hummel et al. 2023; Guerri et al. 2009). These investigators found that the increase in oxidative stress targeted serotonergic neurons, leading to apoptosis, reduced brain volume, and cortical abnormalities, all of which may contribute to cognitive and behavioral dysfunction (Koop 2006; Hummel et al. 2023; Guerri et al. 2009).

The fetal brain has heightened susceptibility to damage from oxidative stress. This is most likely related to an increase in metabolic rate of the brain in the fetus when compared to other developing organ systems, the abundance in unsaturated fatty acids in the brain, and/or the presence of neurotransmitters that can be oxidized, thereby

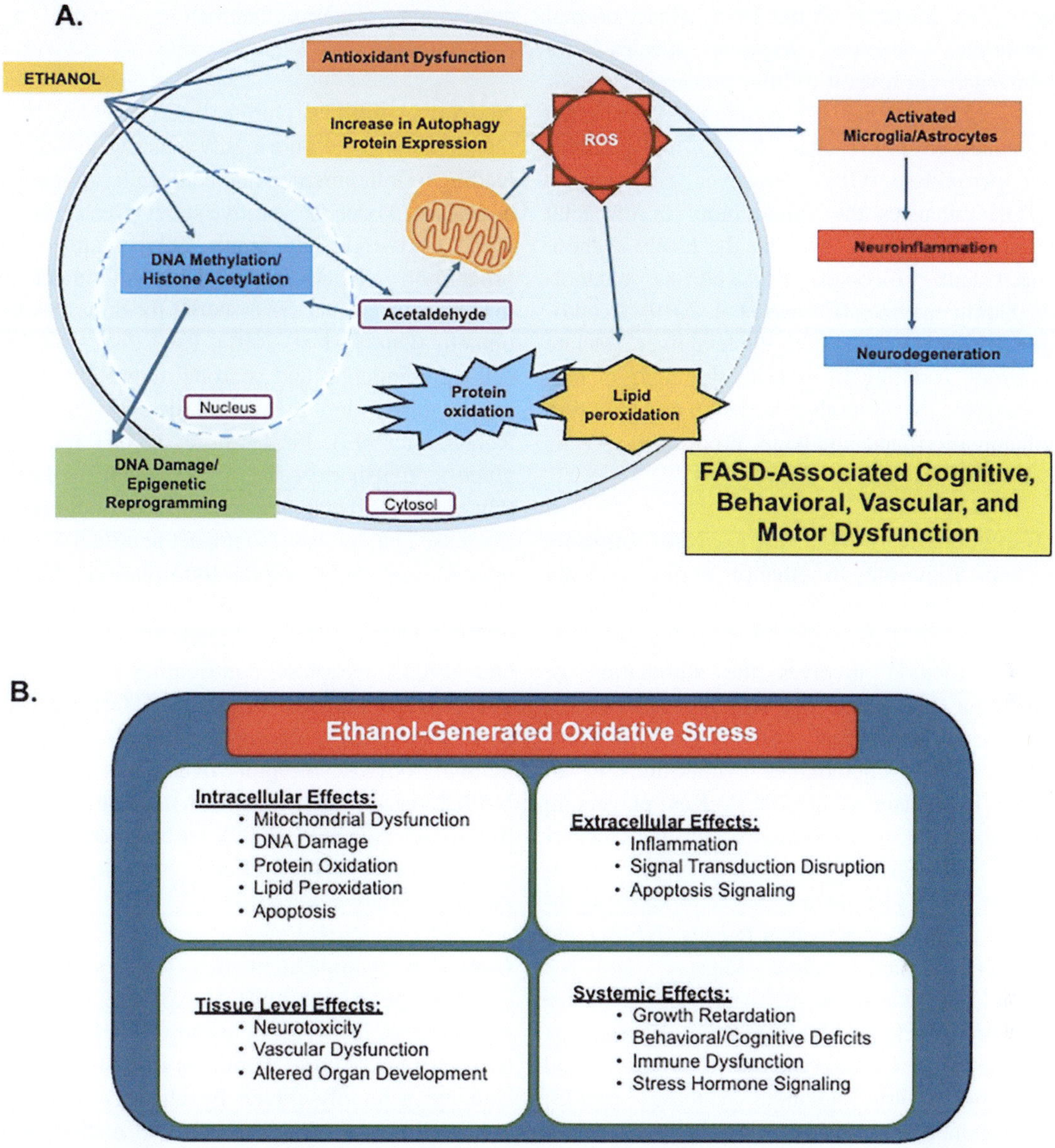

Fig. 2.1 *Panel A: Mechanisms of ethanol-induced cellular damage*. Ethanol exposure triggers multiple intracellular pathways leading to neuroinflammation and associated pathogenesis of FASD. ETOH can directly interact with DNA and histones, potentially causing genetic and epigenetic alterations and promotes the formation of reactive oxygen species (ROS) through the mitochondrial respiratory chain and NADPH oxidase pathways. The imbalance in intracellular redox state results in protein oxidation, lipid peroxidation, and activation of microglia/astrocytes, damaging cellular structures. ETOH-induced antioxidant dysfunction (affecting enzymes such as SOD, CAT, Gpx, and GR) exacerbates oxidative damage. Additionally, ETOH exposure increases autophagy protein expression. These processes collectively contribute to neuroinflammation and neurodegeneration, and FASD-associated consequences. *Panel B: Multilevel impact of ethanol-generated ROS*. Ethanol metabolism generates ROS, leading to a cascade of damaging effects at various levels. These cellular- and tissue-level effects result in systemic manifestations that contribute to the extensive impact of ETOH-induced oxidative stress on the body

serving as substrates (Porter 1984). Under normal conditions, reactive oxygen species are eliminated via several cellular processes, including mitochondrial respiration, superoxide dismutase (SOD), catalase (CAT), and glutathione peroxidase (GPx). However, exposure to ETOH enhances the vulnerability in the fetal brain to damage by lowering the levels of these antioxidant processes, as well as ethanol-degrading enzymes (Ehrhart et al. 2019). In addition, PAE adversely affects the fetal liver's lactate pathway, resulting in glucose shortages in nervous tissue (Streissguth et al. 1980) and initiating inflammation and cytokine production (Wells et al. 2016; Hoyt et al. 2017).

Dysregulation of the Neuroimmune System Exposure to ethanol during prenatal development activates the neuroimmune system, leading to brain damage and neurodegeneration. This activation involves the stimulation of microglia and astrocytes, which results in the increased production of pro-inflammatory cytokines and chemokines (Montesinos et al. 2015; Bjørkhaug et al. 2019). Key players in this inflammatory response are Toll-like receptor 4 and NOD-like receptors, which initiate signaling pathways such as nuclear factor kappa-light-chain-enhancer of activated B cells (NFkB) and mitogen-activated protein kinases (MAPK). These pathways up-regulate inflammatory mediators, including High Mobility Group Box 1 (HMGB1), Cyclooxygenase-2 (COX-2), and Inducible Nitric Oxide Synthase (iNOS) (Montesinos et al. 2015), culminating in considerable damage to synaptic and myelin proteins, as well as neural cells. This damage notably includes apoptotic cell death in the prefrontal cortex as a result of PAE (Alfonso-Loeches et al. 2012). PAE is also detrimental to myelination and the structure of white matter, leading to reductions in myelin-associated proteins and alterations in oligodendrocytes, subsequently impairing neural transmission and cognitive development (Alfonso-Loeches et al. 2012; Cantacorps et al. 2017). The combination of these factors highlights the extensive and multifaceted impact of PAE on the developing brain, particularly concerning neuroinflammation and its consequences.

Neurotransmitters During embryonic development, neuronal cells are highly sensitive to toxins, leading to inflammation and cell death (apoptosis and necrosis) due to oxidative stress (Heaton et al. 2002; Cartwright and Smith 1995). Damage to progenitor cell lines affects the development of mature neurons that are essential for brain development (Dunty et al. 2001). PAE disrupts glial cell differentiation and neuronal migration causing cognitive and motor disorders (Miller and Robertson 1993). Furthermore, ETOH reduces glucose transporters in hippocampal neurons (Hu et al. 1995) and alters neurotransmitter levels (increase and decrease) to impact neuronal development and nerve signal transmission (Maier et al. 1996; Zhou et al. 2005; Ikonomidou et al. 2000). ETOH also inhibits neurosteroid synthesis and NMDA receptors, contributing to synaptic dysfunction (Tokuda et al. 2013). ETOH-induced neurodegeneration during synaptogenesis may involve GABA receptor overexpression and N-Methyl-D-Aspartate (NMDA) receptor inhibition (Sanderson et al. 2009), with age-dependent and lineage-specific effects on developing neurons (Brady et al. 2013).

Gene Expression/Epigenetics The modification of gene expression by ETOH exposure is a complex process, involving both short-term and long-term changes. These alterations in gene expression are primarily driven by changes in DNA methylation, including the cytosine methylation pathway (Ehrhart et al. 2023), which lead to shifts in epigenetic imprinting. These epigenetic changes cause long-term alterations in gene expression leading to modified brain structure and function. Interestingly, initial studies have found that these methylation changes also occur in the germ cells of ETOH-exposed males (Sarkar 2016) suggesting a potential for transgenerational effects. The exploration of these gene expression changes is further advanced through omics data-driven approaches revealing the distinct phenotype of FASD. For instance, gene expression analysis of rat placenta by Rosenberg et al. (2010) identified 22 genes with altered expression in alcohol-consuming dams. Moreover, a comprehensive transcriptomics meta-study highlighted a significant downregulation of many genes (Rogic et al. 2016), indicating widespread alterations in gene expression involving crucial processes like RNA management and chromatin organization. Thus, ETOH-induced epigenetic modifications, primarily via DNA methylation, may have far-reaching implications for brain development and systemic and cerebral vascular function, with potential transgenerational effects.

Epigenetic alterations can influence the behavior of cells by activating or repressing gene expression without directly modifying the genetic code. Research conducted on animal models, cultured neurons, and early human clinical trials suggests that alcohol may have a detrimental effect on epigenetic programming in developing neurobiological systems [reviewed in (Lussier et al. 2017)]. Long-term epigenetic effects of ETOH exposure suggest intricate alterations at the molecular level, particularly in DNA methylation and histone acetylation. Investigators have suggested that alcohol's impact on DNA methylation can be bidirectional, causing either hypomethylation or hypermethylation depending on the specific region, tissue, or loci involved (Ungerer et al. 2013; Nagre et al. 2015; Otero et al. 2012; Perkins et al. 2013; Liu et al. 2009). In one example, PAE induced global DNA hypomethylation in a rodent model, which appeared to be a direct consequence of ETOH's interference in the one-carbon metabolic pathway to inhibit key enzymes (methionine xynthase (MTR), solute carrier family 19 member 1 (SLC19A1), and methionine adenosyltransferase 1A (MAT1A)) (Zeisel 2011). This molecular perturbation in hypomethylation manifested phenotypically by altered coat color in Agouti mice (Kaminen-Ahola et al. 2010). In addition, epigenetic modification correlated with decreased gene expression and heightened incidence of neural tube defects, as elucidated through MEDIP-chip analysis (Liu et al. 2009). These methylation patterns, inherently dynamic during developmental processes, are susceptible to disruption by ETOH, with potential transgenerational inheritance, affecting various phenotypes (Chen et al. 2013; Abbott et al. 2018). Further, PAE may cause hypermethylation to certain physiologically important genes, such as the proopiomelanocortin (POMC) gene, which regulates stress response in mammals. Govorko et al. found that PAE increased methylation of the POMC gene's promoter region in Sprague-Dawley rats leading to reduced expression and a heightened stress response. This effect persisted up to the F3 generation in males but not females (Govorko et al. 2012). In parallel, ETOH's impact extends to histone modifications, characterized by a reduction in methylation and an augmentation in acetylation, altering histone markers such as H3K9ac, H3K27me2,3, and H3K9me2, and modulating the activity of related enzymes, including histone deacetylases (HDACs) and euchromatic histone lysine methyltransferase 2 (EHMT2) (Ehrhart et al. 2017; Chater-Diehl et al. 2017). These modifications, integral to gene regulation, underscore the extensive influence of ETOH on both genetic and epigenetic mechanisms, delineating a complex landscape of molecular changes initiated by PAE.

Impact of PAE on the Developing Brain The impact of PAE on brain development ultimately contributes to structural and functional outcomes observed in individuals with FASD. These insights underline the critical need for understanding the full scope of PAE's impact on brain development, structure, and function to develop effective interventions and support strategies for those with FASD. The following section discusses the various aspects of PAE influence on brain development, structure, and function.

Due to the complex nature by which ETOH can affect multiple cellular processes, its impact on the developing brain is complex. ETOH can potentially lead to the death of brain cells and disrupt intricate cellular and molecular processes. These effects can be attributed to ETOH, both through direct and indirect means. ETOH can potentially impact the development of the embryonic brain by disrupting the proliferation and migration of neurons (Riley and Mcgee 2005; Miller 1986) or by causing cell death (Bonthius and West 1990; Ikonomidou et al. 2001; Marcussen et al. 1994). Furthermore, the consumption of ETOH has been found to increase fetal glutamate levels (Karl et al. 1995; Thomas et al. 1997) and the functioning of glutamate N-methyl-D-aspartate receptors (Hoffman et al. 1989; Hughes et al. 1998). These effects can potentially lead to abnormal migration of neurons and glial cells. PAE can have toxic consequences in the short term and long term. In the short term, ETOH exposure often triggers oxidative stress (Chater-Diehl et al. 2016), significantly affecting genes related to energy metabolism and apoptosis leading to decreased cell proliferation and increased cell death (Li et al. 2001). Additionally, ETOH disrupts mitochondrial bioenergetics in neuronal cells, inhibiting mitochondrial proliferation and differentiation resulting in a reduction of mitochondrial volume and a decrease in the activity of mitochondrial respiratory chain complexes and ATP synthase (Bukiya 2019). In the long-term ETOH exposure may affect growth factors, the cytoskeleton, cell adhesion molecules, and neurotransmitter systems (Gupta et al. 2016). These changes play a pivotal role in the growth, structure, and function of the central nervous system (CNS) and on cerebral blood flow (Jarmasz et al. 2017), and extend their influence on other organs, including the heart, kidney, and immune system (Caputo et al. 2016). Particularly noteworthy is the impact on neuronal crest formation, likely due to the destabilization of β-catenin (Smith et al. 2014).

PAE is associated with a decreased brain volume. For instance, the cerebral cortex shows complex volume alterations that are heterogeneous by region and by age. These changes in brain structure and shape by PAE are rooted in underlying changes to cellular development and migration (Yang et al. 2012). Additionally, regional brain size/structure is influenced by factors like cell proliferation, migration, blood flow, and cell death, and is notably affected by PAE. In developmental areas like the cortical neuroepithelium and ventricular zone, which contain multipotent stem cell populations, PAE results in decreased cell number and prolonged cell cycles. This differential effect on various cell populations leads to significant changes in brain patterning and size (Sun and Hevner 2014). PAE also impacts neurogenesis, with different regions of the brain showing varying levels of vulnerability. ETOH exposure appears to shift the cellular outcome in embryonic stem cells and alters gene expression related to cortical layer or region. This contributes to changes in the generation of neurons across development, potentially resulting in altered molecular identities of neurons within cortical layers and inappropriate cellular function (Ogony et al. 2013).

The cerebral cortex plays an integral role in controlling numerous complex functions. It is primarily responsible for high-level cognitive tasks such as reasoning, language, memory, and consciousness. Beyond these cognitive aspects, the cortex is also essential for sensory perception and motor coordination, effectively acting as the command center for a myriad of actions and decisions. The development of the cerebral cortex is critical for normal brain function. During crucial stages of gestation and early after birth, the cortex experiences significant growth and organization. This period of development is critical for establishing the neural pathways and networks necessary for cortical function, that is, learning, emotional regulation, and complex thinking. Maintaining the functionality of the cortex relies on an adequate vascular development, which provides the blood supply necessary for function. This process involves forming a dense network of blood vessels, ensuring the cortex receives adequate oxygen and nutrients, crucial for supporting its high metabolic demand. In the cerebral cortex, as well as in the entire brain, a balance of blood flow is achieved through the interaction of myogenic, metabolic, and neurogenic mechanisms within the neurovascular unit (NVU), which consists of vascular cells (endothelial cells, pericytes, smooth muscle cells), glia (astrocytes, oligodendroglia, microglia), neurons, and the basal lamina matrix, all working to maintain constant blood flow despite changes in driving pressure. However, any developmental alterations in the cerebral cortex can lead to significant consequences, impacting cognitive abilities, learning processes, and potentially leading to neurological disorders. These developmental abnormalities can arise from genetic factors, environmental influences, or complications during pregnancy and birth, affecting the cortex's structure and function and leading to various developmental disorders. Similarly, PAE may adversely influence vascular hemodynamics. In clinical studies of cases of children who died with a diagnosis of FASD, cerebellar abnormalities were reported, possibly due in part to hydrocephaly (Clarren et al. 1978; Wisniewski et al. 1983). These suggest that PAE can have detrimental effects on cerebral development during fetal growth. These deficits, caused by PAE, are not just temporary but persist into adulthood, indicating long-term consequences. PAE also disrupts cell migration, leading to the presence of cortical heterotopias or clusters of misguided neurons. This disruption affects both radial and tangential migration, impacting the overall structure and connectivity of the brain. Such alterations can lead to long-term effects on brain function and development (Miller 1993).

Impact of PAE on Cerebral Vascular Development During normal development, in the early stages of pregnancy, the neural tube is encircled by a perineural vascular plexus that forms by vasculogenesis. During the mid-gestation period, endothelial cells from the perineural vascular plexus enter neural tissue and utilize fibers from multipotent stem cells to guide their migration toward the ventricular surface. This process marks the beginning of the formation of blood vessels in the brain. Neuronal and vascular development in the embryonic brain during the second trimester is of utmost importance (Bayer et al. 1993; Norman and O'Kusky 1986). During this stage, a network of arteries within the sub-arachnoid region generates microvessels that penetrate the developing fetal brain (Norman and O'Kusky 1986). These microvessels provide the necessary nutrients for growth and development of the fetal brain (Tam and Watts 2010). Previous studies have shown significant alterations in the microstructure of brain capillaries in rats during PAE (Popova 1992; Kelly et al. 1990). During the early- to mid-gestation stage, the growth of blood vessels in the brain is controlled by angiogenesis. Angiogenesis is an intricate process that is carefully regulated by an equilibrium between pro- and anti-angiogenic factors (Bergers and Benjamin 2003). The growth-stimulatory signals include vascular endothelial growth factor (VEGF), integrins, fibronectin, angiopoietins, vascular cell adhesion molecules (VCAM), fibroblast growth factors (FGF), tyrosine kinases (TK), extracellular matrix (ECM) proteins and proteinases, transforming growth factor (TGF), and Wnt signaling factors. In contrast, tumor necrosis factor (TNF) signaling and pro-apoptosis factors serve as inhibitory signals (Carmeliet and Collen 1998; Ulrich et al. 2016; Wang and Kroenke 2015). This process also leads to the formation of the blood–brain barrier through many cellular and molecular events (Walchli et al. 2015; Obermeier et al. 2013; Kim et al. 2006). During the mid-to-late gestation phase, the communication between neural cells and endothelial cells continues and is essential for the growth and development of the nervous system (McConnell et al. 2017). Pericytes enhance vascular stability by the secretion of many stabilizing factors, including angiopoietin-1 (ANG1), platelet-derived growth factor (PDGF-β), and tissue inhibitor of metalloproteinase 3 (TIMP3) (Geudens and Gerhardt 2011). Astrocytes generate chemical substances that can contribute to constriction or relaxation of cerebral arteries/arterioles/capillaries in response to neurological signals and/or chemical mediators. From late-gestation to birth, the blood–brain barrier undergoes maturation that leads to the formation of a basement membrane that is abundant in laminin, collagen IV, and fibronectin, completely enveloping the vasculature of the brain (Siqueira et al. 2021). PAE has profound effects on these processes, ultimately leading to alterations in structure and function of cerebral blood vessels (Solonskii et al. 2008). A recent study using adult nonhuman primates

(Williams et al. 2008) and mice (Radek et al. 2005, 2008) found that ETOH has a negative impact on vasculogenesis and angiogenesis. Microarray analysis has shown that genes involved in angiogenesis, such as the VEGF gene family, are targeted by ETOH toxicity (Wang et al. 2010). PAE not only disrupts the signaling components that govern vascularization and brain development, but it also affects specific molecular targets involved in cerebral vascular development. ETOH can directly impact the molecular and cellular components of the blood–brain barrier from the early stages of development. Additional studies have shown that the developing brain is particularly vulnerable to the effects of ETOH because it contains many proapoptotic proteins and has low levels of proteins involved in stress response mechanisms, such as autophagy or unfolded protein response (Alimov et al. 2013). Furthermore, a proteomics analysis indicated that baboon fetuses exposed to alcohol exhibited alterations in mitochondria and structural proteins within cerebral arteries (Bisen et al. 2019). PAE can also disrupt angiogenesis by impairing endothelial cell function, which is essential for the migration of GABAergic interneurons to the cortex (Won et al. 2013; Luhmann et al. 2015). ETOH, acting as an NMDA receptor antagonist (Zhao et al. 2015), inhibits glutamate-induced matrix metalloproteinase-9 (MMP-9) and tissue-plasminogen activator (t-PA) activities needed for blood vessel development (Legros et al. 2009). This disruption hampers proper angiogenesis and the positioning of interneurons (Léger et al. 2020; Xu et al. 2011), leading to the neurodevelopmental issues observed in those diagnosed with FASD (Jégou et al. 2012; LeLecuyer et al. 2017). Since endothelial cells, along with pericytes, astrocytes, neurons, and microglia, are instrumental in the formation of the blood–brain barrier and are components in the angiogenetic process (Wolburg et al. 2009; Abbott et al. 2010; McCarty 2005), it is plausible that PAE poses a significant risk to blood–brain barrier structure and function. However, while studies have shown that PAE can influence structural components of the blood–brain barrier (tight junctional proteins, endothelium, pericytes, astrocytes, neurons, and microglia) and the expression of pro-inflammatory genes (Siqueira et al. 2022), there is a paucity of information regarding the impact of PAE on functional aspects of the blood–brain barrier. One previous study examined the influence of PAE on the transport of horseradish peroxidase across the blood–brain barrier and found no evidence of alcohol-induced effects (Phillips et al. 1997). Future studies will be necessary to determine the relationship between PAE, the structural components of the blood–brain barrier, and the functional outcomes of these alterations to the blood–brain barrier.

One of the critical effects of PAE is the significant increase in both systemic and brain-specific inflammation (Alfonso-Loeches and Guerri 2011; Brocardo et al. 2011). This is primarily mediated through the activation of microglia, which undergo morphological and functional changes by alcohol. These changes result in an increased release of proinflammatory cytokines and chemokines in vital brain areas. The persistent state of inflammation and microglial activation in response to PAE underscores its impact on the brain's immune environment, with potential long-term consequences for neurodevelopment (Streissguth et al. 1994; Currie et al. 2016; Barker 1995). Astrocytes, which cover about 99% of the cerebral vascular surface (Mathiisen et al. 2010), play a significant role in regulating endothelial cell physiology. This regulation is mediated through the secretion of various cytokines such as Transforming Growth Factor Beta 1 (TGF-β1), Glial Cell Line-Derived Neurotrophic Factor (GDNF), Basic Fibroblast Growth Factor (bFGF), and Angiopoietin 1 (ANG1), all of which are crucial for the specialization of endothelium (Alvarez et al. 2013; Cambier et al. 2005; Diniz et al. 2019). Ethanol exposure also induces cerebral microhemorrhages (Welch et al. 2016) and compromises endothelial cell integrity (Haorah et al. 2005a, b). Moreover, ETOH significantly affects astrocyte biology, impeding their growth and differentiation, deregulating Glial

Fibrillary Acidic Protein (GFAP) expression (Topper et al. 2015; Wilhelm and Guizzetti 2015; Goodlett et al. 1993; Guizzetti et al. 2014), and causing persistent alterations in the profile of proteins secreted by astrocytes. These proteins are critical for cellular function, including cell survival, growth, differentiation, and synaptogenesis (Trindade et al. 2016). These ETOH-induced changes in astrocytes and their interactions with endothelial cells are intrinsically linked to the developmental anomalies observed in FASD (Guerri et al. 2001). Overall, this evidence indicates that consuming alcohol during pregnancy may impact the formation of the cerebral microvascular network at macroscopic and microscopic levels. These defects can be attributed to a disruption in the processes of forming new blood vessels and the growth of existing vessels. Thus, the implications of PAE on the developing neurovascular networks are profound. These effects collectively highlight the critical need to understand and address the extensive impact of PAE on the brain, particularly in the context of cerebral vascular health.

Impact of Prenatal Alcohol Exposure on Functional Responses of Cerebral Blood Vessels Essential for proper brain function is the synchronization of metabolic demand (oxygen and nutrient delivery) to cerebral blood flow. This process involves the ongoing adjustment (dilation versus constriction) of cerebral blood vessels to regulate blood flow to the various regions of the brain. Exposure to ETOH has been shown to alter maternal blood flow to the uterus and fetal cerebral blood flow in mice, sheep, baboons, and human subjects (Bake et al. 2012; Falconer et al. 1990; Mann et al. 1975; Richardson et al. 1985; Gleason and Hotchkiss 1992; Parnell et al. 2007; Kochunov et al. 2010; North et al. 2018; Simakova et al. 2019; Tobiasz et al. 2018; Seleverstov et al. 2017). The response of cerebral blood flow to maternal alcohol consumption appears to be dependent on the concentration of ETOH and the timing of exposure during gestation (May and Gossage 2011; Maier and West 2001; West et al. 1987). For instance, administering 1 g/kg of ETOH through maternal infusion resulted in a decrease in cerebral blood flow in preterm sheep (Richardson et al. 1985) and baboons (Tobiasz et al. 2018). However, no change in fetal cerebral blood flow was seen in sheep throughout the middle stage (gestation day 92, which mimics the human gestation period of 145–150 days) of gestation (Gleason and Hotchkiss 1992). Conversely, a study by Parnell et al. (2007) using a similar ovine model found that administering a higher amount of ETOH (1.75 g/kg) increased cerebral blood flow by greater than 30%. In the cerebellum, the increase in cerebral blood flow 1-h after the administration of ETOH was up to 50 percent higher compared to the control group. These findings emphasize that the impact of ETOH on cerebral blood flow is dependent on concentration and brain region (Parnell et al. 2018). PAE has been shown to alter responses of the cerebral circulation to changes in metabolism. For example, fetal exposure to ETOH during the first and second trimesters decreased cerebral vasodilator responses to hypoxia (Mayock et al. 2007; Gleason et al. 1997) and acidosis (Mayock et al. 2008). Investigators have also examined the influence of PAE on responses to important vasoactive agonists. Vasoactive intestinal peptide (VIP) serves as a neurotransmitter or neuromodulator in both the peripheral and central nervous systems. VIP acts on specific receptors to dilate large and small cerebral arteries (Grant et al. 2006; Gaw et al. 1991; Wei et al. 1980; Dacey et al. 1988) and thus may regulate cerebral blood flow and neurovascular coupling. Investigators have shown that PAE can lead to a permanent decrease in VIP levels in the rat fetal brain (Spong et al. 2002). This decrease could indicate a loss of neuronal connections that carry VIP or a change in the density of VIP receptors in the brain. In addition, in an adult sheep model mimicking binge drinking during pregnancy, alcohol exposure was found to dramatically increase dilator responses of adult intracerebral arterioles to VIP (Ngai et al. 2008). Although the precise mechanism remains unknown, the authors speculated that this effect of PAE on VIP-dependent reactivity was related to a compensatory response to alcohol-induced underdevelopment of neurotransmitter pathways.

In contrast, studies have shown that PAE can lead to long-lasting decreases in reactivity of cerebral and large peripheral arteries. PAE reduced relaxation of the aorta in response to carbamylcholine (an activator of acetylcholine receptors) in rats 25 weeks post-birth, suggesting a role for altered endothelial function, that is, nitric oxide synthesis/production/reactivity (Turcotte et al. 2002). Others have shown a decrease in vasodilation in response to serotonin in alcohol-exposed ovine fetuses (Parkington et al. 2014), which may have been, in part, related to an alteration in the structural components of the vascular wall, that is, elastin and collagen. Similarly, studies from our laboratory have shown that reactivity of cerebral arterioles to an agonist (ADP) that dilates cerebral arterioles via activation of endothelial nitric oxide synthase (eNOS) was diminished in adolescent and adult rats (Cananzi and Mayhan 2019; Cananzi and Mayhan 2017; Saha et al. 2021a) that were exposed to alcohol in utero. However, responses to an eNOS-independent agonist (nitroglycerin) were not altered by PAE. This suggests that there was a specific alteration in endothelial function produced by PAE and not a non-specific effect of PAE on vascular smooth muscle. In addition, we found that responses of cerebral arterioles to an agonist (NMDA) that dilated cerebral arterioles via activation of neuronal nitric oxide synthase (nNOS) were impaired in adolescent and adult rats exposed to alcohol in utero (Cananzi and Mayhan 2017, 2019; Saha et al. 2021a). Further, we have reported that responses of cerebral arterioles to activation of potassium (K+) channels were impaired in rats exposed to alcohol in utero (Saha et al. 2023). Thus, in addition to altering responses to eNOS- and nNOS-dependent agonists, PAE also appears to influence responses to other important cellular pathways that govern the regulation of cerebral blood flow during changes in metabolic demand. We reasoned that impaired dilator responses of cerebral arterioles to eNOS- and nNOS-dependent agonists may have implications to the pathogenesis of ischemic stroke and/or brain damage following an ischemic event. To test this possibility, we examined infarct volume following cerebral ischemia/reperfusion (middle cerebral artery occlusion) in rats exposed to alcohol in utero (Cananzi and Mayhan 2019). We found that infarct volume was greater in rats following PAE. We suggest that there is a coupling between impaired dilator responses of cerebral arterioles to brain damage following an ischemic event and speculate that impaired dilator responses of cerebral arterioles may contribute to functional and structural abnormalities of the brain by PAE. Finally, we examined constrictor response of cerebral arterioles in rats exposed to alcohol in utero (Saha et al. 2021b). We found that constrictor responses of cerebral arterioles to the thromboxane analog (U-46619) and arginine vasopressin, which are physiologically important mediators, were similar in male and female rats regardless of PAE or age. In addition, there was no discernible distinction in the response of adolescent rats, regardless of gender, to angiotensin II following PAE. However, adult females who were exposed to alcohol in utero showed an unexpected increase in dilation of cerebral arterioles in response to a high concentration of angiotensin II, which is presumably related to an increase in angiotensin II-induced increase in oxidative stress (Saha et al. 2021b). Based on these findings, it is conceivable that loss of vasodilation in response to activation of endothelial and neuronal pathways, with preservation of vasoconstriction, may lead to a scenario that favors an alteration in the regulation of cerebral blood flow during changes in metabolic demand. This sequence of events may contribute to an increase in brain damage following an ischemic event and/or may lead to an increase the pathogenesis of stroke in individuals suffering from FASD.

Mechanisms of Impaired Cerebral Vascular Function by PAE Many cellular/molecular mechanisms have been suggested to play a role in impaired cerebral vascular function induced by PAE. A study found that dilation of fetal cerebral arteries during exposure to alcohol in utero is the result of activation of the endocannabinoid system (Seleverstov et al. 2017). In addition, treatment with rimonabant, a CB receptor inverse agonist, could rescue this response and suggests that CB receptors may contribute to the persistent vasodilatory impact of alcohol on fetal cerebral arteries.

Both ETOH and its catabolite acetaldehyde are inherently toxic, with oxidative stress being the primary source of damage. Oxidative stress is defined as the presence of elevated quantities of reactive oxygen species (ROS) within cells, leading to the impairment of lipids, proteins, and DNA. ROS are molecules or ions that result from the incomplete reduction of oxygen by a single electron. The primary ROS consist of superoxide (O2•), hydrogen peroxide (H2O2), and the hydroxyl radical (•OH). Our laboratory examined the generation of superoxide from cerebral tissue of adolescent and adult rats exposed to alcohol in utero (Cananzi and Mayhan 2017, 2019). We found that PAE elevated the basal levels of superoxide in the parietal cortex of rats, even in the presence of NADPH, which was utilized to augment NADPH oxidase activity. NOX-2 and NOX-4 are variants of the NADPH oxidase system that are present in endothelium and vascular smooth muscle, and are responsible for the production of superoxide (Chrissobolis et al. 2012; De Silva and Faraci 2012; Konior et al. 2014; Lynch et al. 2013; Paravicini et al. 2004). We found that PAE enhanced the expression of NOX-2 and NOX-4 in the brain, which presumably contributed to the elevation of superoxide following PAE. Next, we examined the role of oxidative stress in impaired cerebral vascular function in PAE. Apocynin, a potent antioxidant, reduced the levels of superoxide and alleviated impaired eNOS- and nNOS-dependent reactivity in cerebral arterioles in rats exposed to alcohol in utero (Cananzi and Mayhan 2017, 2019; Saha et al. 2021a). In addition, inhibition of oxidative stress with apocynin restored impaired responses of cerebral arterioles to agonists which activate K + channels (Saha et al. 2023). These findings suggest that elevations in the levels of superoxide, presumably from the mitochondria, can account for impaired cerebral vascular function during PAE. Similarly, apocynin was able to lessen brain damage after cerebral ischemia/reperfusion injury during PAE, suggesting that when vascular function is restored this protects the brain from the damaging effects of an ischemic event. Finally, Saha et al. (2021a) utilized rosiglitazone, a gamma subtype agonist for peroxisome proliferator-activated receptors (PPARs), to determine whether activation of PPARγ could prevent impaired cerebral vascular function. These receptors are located on vascular smooth muscle and endothelium (Fukunaga et al. 2001; Marx et al. 1998, 1999). Administration of rosiglitazone to male and female adult rats, whether in acute or chronic therapy, effectively restored cerebral vascular dysfunction in response to eNOS- and nNOS-dependent agonists caused by PAE. Furthermore, rosiglitazone effectively reduced superoxide levels in parietal cortex tissue (Saha et al. 2021a). Although no studies that we are aware of have specifically examined the cellular organelles responsible for an increase in oxidative stress it appears likely that the mitochondria play a significant role. Alcohol can produce anomalies in the mitochondria during prenatal development (Manzo-Avalos and Saavedra-Molina 2010). These abnormalities are due to alcohol directly affecting the mitochondria (Bisen et al. 2019; Manzo-Avalos and Saavedra-Molina 2010) and/or due to alcohol-induced alterations in blood flow to the fetal brain (Parnell et al. 2007; Seleverstov et al. 2017).

Conclusion The impact of PAE on the brain is extensive and multifaceted, affecting structural development, neurogenesis, cell survival, cerebral vascular health, inflammation, cognitive function, and behavior. These changes contribute to a range of disabilities seen in individuals with FASD. Despite heightened consciousness regarding the potential hazards associated with PAE, its incidence continues to increase. This review emphasized the impacts of PAE on the brain and cerebral blood vessels (Fig. 2.2). We believe that impaired cerebral vascular function may provide a key link to behavioral and cognitive dysfunction in individuals suffering from FASD. In addition, PAE appears to activate many cellular pathways

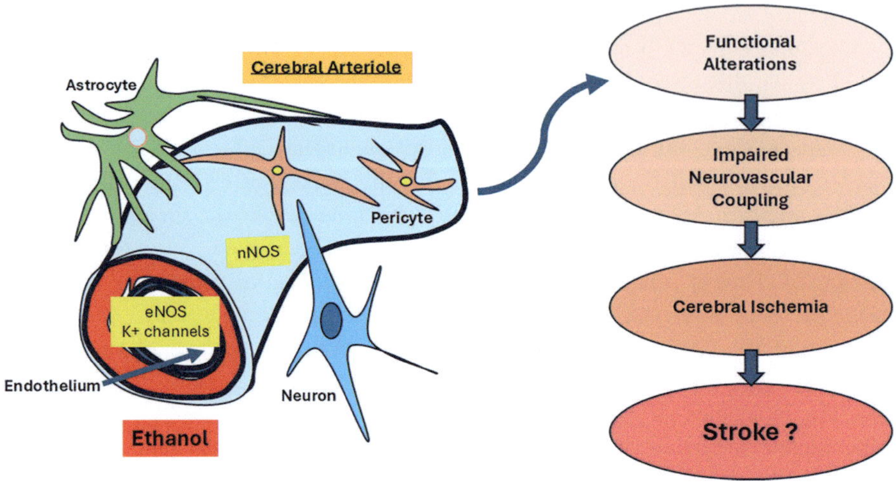

Fig. 2.2 *Impact of prenatal alcohol exposure on neurovascular components and outcomes in FASD*. The left portion of the figure highlights key neurovascular components (astrocytes, pericytes, neurons, and endothelium). ETOH impairs critical cerebral dilator pathways (eNOS, nNOS, and K^+ channels) that could lead to a decrease in blood flow to the brain in response to changes in metabolic demand/chemical mediators/neurotransmitters. Alterations in neurovascular coupling would create a scenario of cerebral ischemia, and thus could contribute to the pathogenesis of stroke in those that suffer from FASD

associated with increasing oxidative stress to negatively impact dilator and constrictor processes. Changes in cerebral vascular function may provide a scenario for the pathogenesis of increased brain damage following cerebral ischemia, and perhaps stroke in newborns, adolescents, and adults suffering from FASD. Future research should focus on targeting processes that regulate cerebral arterial/arteriolar function, and hence the control of cerebral blood flow. We believe that this could greatly influence cognitive and behavioral outcomes for those affected by FASD.

Author Contributions Study conception and design: PS, WM, and DA; Manuscript preparation: PS, WM, and DA. All authors reviewed the contents and approved the final version of the manuscript.

Conflict of Interest The authors declare that the research was conducted in the absence of any commercial or financial relationships that could be construed as a potential conflict of interest.

References

Abbott NJ, Patabendige AA, Dolman DE et al (2010) Structure and function of the blood-brain barrier. Neurobiol Dis 37:13–25. https://doi.org/10.1016/j.nbd.2009.07.030

Abbott CW, Rohac DJ, Bottom RT et al (2018) Prenatal ethanol exposure and neocortical development: a transgenerational model of FASD. Cereb Cortex 28: 2908–2921. https://doi.org/10.1093/cercor/bhx168

Abel EL (1984) Prenatal effects of alcohol. Drug Alcohol Depend 14:1–10. https://doi.org/10.1016/0376-8716(84)90012-7

Abel EL (1985) Prenatal effects of alcohol on growth: a brief overview. Fed Proc 44:2318–2322

Alfonso-Loeches S, Guerri C (2011) Molecular and behavioral aspects of the actions of alcohol on the adult and developing brain. Crit Rev Clin Lab Sci 48: 19–47

Alfonso-Loeches S, Pascual M, Gómez-Pinedo U et al (2012) Toll-like receptor 4 participates in the myelin disruptions associated with chronic alcohol abuse. Glia 60:948–964. https://doi.org/10.1002/glia.22327

Alimov A, Wang H, Liu M et al (2013) Expression of autophagy and UPR genes in the developing brain during ethanol-sensitive and resistant periods. Metab Brain Dis 28:667–676. https://doi.org/10.1007/s11011-013-9430-2

Aliyu MH, Wilson RE, Zoorob R et al (2008) Alcohol consumption during pregnancy and the risk of early stillbirth among singletons. Alcohol 42:369–374. https://doi.org/10.1016/J.ALCOHOL.2008.04.003

Alvarez JI, Katayama T, Prat A (2013) Glial influence on the blood brain barrier. Glia 61:1939–1958. https://doi.org/10.1002/glia.22575

Amendah DD, Grosse SD, Bertrand J (2011) Medical expenditures of children in the United States with

fetal alcohol syndrome. Neurotoxicol Teratol 33:322–324
Archibald S, Fennema-Notestine C, Gamst A et al (2001) Brain dysmorphology in individuals with severe prenatal alcohol exposure. Dev Med Child Neurol 43: 148–154
Aros S, Mills JL, I~niguez G et al (2011) Effects of prenatal ethanol exposure on postnatal growth and the insulin-like growth factor axis. Horm Res Paediatr 75: 166–173
Bake S, Tingling JD, Miranda RC (2012) Ethanol exposure during pregnancy persistently attenuates cranially directed blood flow in the developing fetus: evidence from ultrasound imaging in a murine second trimester equivalent model. Alcohol Clin Exp Res 36:748–758
Bake S, Gardner R, Tingling JD et al (2017) Fetal alcohol exposure alters blood flow and neurological responses to transient cerebral ischemia in adult mice. Alcohol Clin Exp Res 41:117–127. https://doi.org/10.1111/acer.13277
Barker DJP (1989) Weight in infancy and death from Ischaemic heart disease. Lancet 8663:577–580
Barker DJ (1995) Intrauterine programming of adult disease. Mol Med Today 1:418–423
Bayer S, Altman J, Russo R et al (1993) Timetables of neurogenesis in the human brain based on experimentally determined patterns in the rat. Neurotoxicology 14:83–144
Bergers G, Benjamin LE (2003) Tumorigenesis and the angiogenic switch. Nat Rev Cancer 3:401–410. https://doi.org/10.1038/nrc1093
Bisen S, Kakhniashvili D, Johnson DL et al (2019) Proteomic analysis of baboon cerebral artery reveals potential pathways of damage by prenatal alcohol exposure. Mol Cell Proteomics 18:294–307. https://doi.org/10.1074/mcp.RA118.001047
Bjørkhaug ST, Neupane SP, Bramness JG et al (2019) Plasma cytokine levels in patients with chronic alcohol overconsumption: relations to gut microbiota markers and clinical correlates. Alcohol 85:35–40. https://doi.org/10.1016/j.alcohol.2019.10.002
Bonthius DJ, West JR (1990) Alcohol-induced neuronal loss in developing rats: increased brain damage with binge exposure. Alcohol Clin Exp Res 14:107–118. https://doi.org/10.1111/j.1530-0277.1990.tb00455.x
Brady ML, Diaz MR, Iuso A et al (2013) Moderate prenatal alcohol exposure reduces plasticity and alters NMDA receptor subunit composition in the dentate gyrus. J Neurosci 33:1062–1067. https://doi.org/10.1523/JNEUROSCI.1217-12.2013
Brocardo PS, Gil-Mohapel J, Christie BR (2011) The role of oxidative stress in fetal alcohol spectrum disorders. Brain Res Rev 67:209–225
Bukiya AN (2019) Fetal cerebral artery mitochondrion as target of prenatal alcohol exposure. Int J Environ Res Public Health 16:1586. https://doi.org/10.3390/ijerph16091586
Burd L, Peterson L, Kobrinsky N (2014) Fetal alcohol spectrum disorders and childhood cancer: a concise review of case reports and future research considerations. Ped Blood Cancer 61:768–770. [PubMed: 24292988]
Cambier S, Gline S, Mu D et al (2005) Integrin alpha (v)beta8-mediated activation of transforming growth factor-beta by perivascular astrocytes: an angiogenic control switch. Am J Pathol 166:1883–1894
Cananzi SG, Mayhan WG (2017) In utero exposure to alcohol alters reactivity of cerebral arterioles. J Cereb Blood Flow Metab 39:332–341. https://doi.org/10.1177/0271678X17728163
Cananzi SG, Mayhan WG (2019) In utero exposure to alcohol impairs reactivity of cerebral arterioles and increases susceptibility of the brain to damage following ischemia/reperfusion in adulthood. Alcohol Clin Exp Res 43:607–616. https://doi.org/10.1111/acer.13979
Cantacorps L, Alfonso-Loeches S, Moscoso-Castro M et al (2017) Maternal alcohol binge drinking induces persistent neuroinflammation associated with myelin damage and behavioural dysfunctions in offspring mice. Neuropharmacology 123:368–384. https://doi.org/10.1016/j.neuropharm.2017.05.034
Caputo C, Wood E, Jabbour L (2016) Impact of fetal alcohol exposure on body systems: a systematic review. Birth Defects Res C Embryo Today 108:174–180. https://doi.org/10.1002/bdrc.21129
Carmeliet P, Collen D (1998) Vascular development and disorders: molecular analysis and pathogenic insights. Kidney Int 53:1519–1549. https://doi.org/10.1046/j.1523-1755.1998.00936.x
Cartwright MM, Smith SM (1995) Increased cell death and reduced neural crest cell numbers in ethanol-exposed embryos: partial basis for the fetal alcohol syndrome phenotype. Alcohol Clin Exp Res 19:378–386. https://doi.org/10.1111/j.1530-0277.1995.tb01519.x
Castells S, Mark E, Abaci F et al (1981) Growth retardation in fetal alcohol syndrome. Unresponsiveness to growth-promoting hormones. Dev Pharmacol Ther 3: 232–241. [PubMed: 7201377]
Centers for Disease Control and Prevention (n.d.) Alcohol and public health. Available online: http://www.cdc.gov/alcohol/fact-sheets/underage-drinking.htm
Chater-Diehl EJ, Laufer BI, Castellani CA et al (2016) Alteration of gene expression, DNA methylation, and histone methylation in free radical scavenging networks in adult mouse hippocampus following fetal alcohol exposure. PLoS One 11:e0154836
Chater-Diehl EJ, Laufer BI, Singh SM (2017) Changes to histone modifications following prenatal alcohol exposure: an emerging picture. Alcohol 60:41–52
Chen L, Nyomba BL (2003) Effects of prenatal alcohol exposure on glucose tolerance in the rat offspring. Metabolism 52:454–462. [PubMed: 12701058]
Chen G, Ke Z, Xu M et al (2012) Autophagy is a protective response to ethanol neurotoxicity. Autophagy 8: 1577–1589. https://doi.org/10.4161/auto.21376

Chen Y, Ozturk NC, Zhou FC (2013) DNA methylation program in developing hippocampus and its alteration by alcohol. PLoS One 8:e60503

Chrissobolis S, Banfi B, Sobey CG et al (2012) Role of NOX isoforms in angiotensin II induced oxidative stress and endothelial dysfunction in brain. J Appl Physiol 113:184–191. https://doi.org/10.1152/japplphysiol.00455.2012

Cil G (2017) Effects of posted point-of-sale warnings on alcohol consumption during pregnancy and on birth outcomes. J Health Econ 53:131–155. https://doi.org/10.1016/j.jhealeco.2017.03.004

Clarren S, Alvord EJ, Sumi S et al (1978) Brain malformations related to prenatal exposure to ethanol. J Pediatr 92:457–460

Currie BA, Hoy J, Legge L et al (2016) Adults with fetal alcohol spectrum disorder: factors associated with positive outcomes and contact with the criminal justice system. J Popul Ther Clin Pharmacol 23:e37–e52

Dacey RG, Bassett JE, Takayasu M (1988) Vasomotor responses of rat intracerebral arterioles to vasoactive intestinal peptide, substance P, neuropeptide Y, and bradykinin. J Cereb Blood Flow Metab 8:254–261. https://doi.org/10.1038/jcbfm.1988.56

De Silva TM, Faraci FM (2012) Effects of angiotensin II on the cerebral circulation: role of oxidative stress. Front Physiol 3(3):484. https://doi.org/10.3389/fphys.2012.00484

Dejong K, Olyaei A, Lo JO (2019) Alcohol use in pregnancy. Clin Obstet Gynecol 62:142–155. https://doi.org/10.1097/GRF.0000000000000414

Diniz LP, Matias I, Siqueira M et al (2019) Astrocytes and the TGF-beta1 pathway in the healthy and diseased brain: a double-edged sword. Mol Neurobiol 56: 4653–4679. https://doi.org/10.1007/s12035-018-1396-y

Dunty WC, Chen SY, Zucker RM et al (2001) Selective vulnerability of embryonic cell populations to ethanol induced apoptosis: implications for alcohol-related birth defects and neurodevelopmental disorder. Alcohol Clin Exp Res 25:1523–1535. https://doi.org/10.1111/j.1530-0277.2001.tb02156.x

Ehrhart F, Hanspers K, Martens M (2017) Ethanol-effects-on-histone modifications. http://www.wikipathways.org/instance/WP3996

Ehrhart F, Roozen S, Verbeek J et al (2019) Review and gap analysis: molecular pathways leading to fetal alcohol spectrum disorders. Mol Psychiatry 24:10–17. https://doi.org/10.1038/s41380-018-0095-4

Ehrhart F, Kutmon K, Coort S (2023) Cytosine-methylation-pathway. http://www.wikipathways.org/instance/WP3585. Accessed 07 Sept 2023

Falconer J, Leonhardt RA, Agarwal DP et al (1990) Effect of acute ethanol drinking on alcohol metabolism in subjects with different ADH and ALDH genotypes. Alcohol 25:413–418. https://doi.org/10.1016/0741-8329(90)90025-8

Feng MJ, Yan SE, Yan QS (2005) Effects of prenatal alcohol exposure on brain derived neurotrophic factor and its receptor tyrosine kinase B in offspring. Brain Res 1042:125–132. https://doi.org/10.1016/j.brainres.2005.02.017

Fertig AR, Watson T (2009) Minimum drinking age laws and infant health outcomes. J Health Econ 28:737–747. https://doi.org/10.1016/j.jhealeco.2009.02.006

Finer LB, Zolna MR (2016) Declines in unintended pregnancy in the United States, 2008-2011. N Engl J Med 374:843–852. https://doi.org/10.1056/NEJMsa1506575

Fukunaga Y, Itoh H, Doi K et al (2001) Thiazolidinediones, peroxisome proliferator-activated receptor gamma agonists, regulate endothelial cell growth and secretion of vasoactive peptides. Atherosclerosis 158:113–119. https://doi.org/10.1016/s0021-9150(01)00430-0

Gauthier TWMD (2015) Prenatal alcohol exposure and the developing immune system. J Alcohol Res 37:279–285

Gaw AJ, Aberdeen J, Humphrey PP et al (1991) Relaxation of sheep cerebral arteries by vasoactive intestinal polypeptide and neurogenic stimulation: inhibition by L -NG-monomethyl arginine in endothelium-denuded vessels. Br J Pharmacol 102:567–672. https://doi.org/10.1111/j.1476-5381.1991.tb12213.x

Geudens I, Gerhardt H (2011) Coordinating cell behaviour during blood vessel formation. Development 138: 4569–4583. https://doi.org/10.1242/dev.062323

Gleason CA, Hotchkiss KJ (1992) Cerebral responses to acute maternal alcohol intoxication in immature fetal sheep. Pediatr Res 31:645–648. https://doi.org/10.1203/00006450-199206000-00021

Gleason CA, Iida H, Hotchkiss KJ et al (1997) Newborn cerebrovascular responses after first trimester moderate maternal ethanol exposure in sheep. Pediatr Res 42:39–45. https://doi.org/10.1203/00006450-199707000-00007

Goodlett CR, Leo JT, O'Callaghan JP et al (1993) Transient cortical astrogliosis induced by alcohol exposure during the neonatal brain growth spurt in rats. Brain Res Dev Brain Res 72:85–97

Goodyer IM, Park R, Herbert J (2001) Psychosocial and endocrine features of chronic first episode major depression in 8–16 year olds. Biol Psychiatry 50: 351–357

Govorko D, Bekdash RA, Zhang C et al (2012) Germline transmits fetal alcohol adverse effect on hypothalamic proopiomelanocortin gene across generations. Dmitry Biol Psych 72:378–388

Grant S, Lutz EM, McPhaden AR et al (2006) Location and function of VPAC1, VPAC2 and NPR-C receptors in VIP-induced vasodilation of porcine basilar arteries. J Cereb Blood Flow Metab 26:58–67. https://doi.org/10.1038/sj.jcbfm.9600163

Gray SP, Denton KM, Cullen-McEwen L et al (2010) Prenatal exposure to alcohol reduces nephron number and raises blood pressure in progeny. J Am Soc Nephrol 21:1891–1902

Guerri C, Pascual M, Renau-Piqueras J (2001) Glia and fetal alcohol syndrome. Neurotoxicology 22:593–599

Guerri C, Bazinet A, Riley EP (2009) Foetal alcohol spectrum disorders and alterations in brain and behaviour. Alcohol 44:108–114

Guizzetti M, Zhang X, Goeke C et al (2014) Glia and neurodevelopment: focus on fetal alcohol spectrum disorders. Front Pediatr 11(2):123. https://doi.org/10.3389/fped.2014.00123

Gupta KK, Gupta VK, Shirasaka T (2016) An update on fetal alcohol syndrome-pathogenesis, risks, and treatment. Alcohol Clin Exp Res 40:1594–1602

Haorah J, Heilman D, Knipe B et al (2005a) Ethanol-induced activation of myosin light chain kinase leads to dysfunction of tight junctions and blood-brain barrier compromise. Alcohol Clin Exp Res 29:999–1009

Haorah J, Knipe B, Leibhart J et al (2005b) Alcohol-induced oxidative stress in brain endothelial cells causes blood-brain barrier dysfunction. J Leukoc Biol 78:1223–1232. https://doi.org/10.1189/jlb.0605340

Heaton MB, Bradley DM (1995) Ethanol influences on the chick embryo spinal cord motor system: analyses of motoneuron cell death, motility, and target trophic factor activity and in vitro analyses of neurotoxicity and trophic factor neuroprotection. J Neurobiol 26:47–61

Heaton M, Paiva M, Mayer J et al (2002) Ethanol-mediated generation of reactive oxygen species in developing rat cerebellum. Neurosci Lett 334:83–86. https://doi.org/10.1016/S0304-3940(02)01123-0

Henderson J, Gray R, Brocklehurst P (2007) Systematic review of effects of low-moderate prenatal alcohol exposure on pregnancy outcome. BJOG 114:243–252

Hofer R, Burd L (2009) Review of published studies of kidney, liver, and gastrointestinal birth defects in fetal alcohol spectrum disorders. Birth Defects Res A Clin Mol Teratol 85:179–183

Hoffman PL, Rabe CS, Moses F et al (1989) N-methyl-D-aspartate receptors and ethanol: inhibition of calcium flux and cyclic GMP production. J Neurochem 52: 1937–1940. https://doi.org/10.1111/j.1471-4159.1989.tb07280.x

Hoyt LR, Randall MJ, Ather JL et al (2017) Mitochondrial ROS induced by chronic ethanol exposure promote hyper-activation of the NLRP3 inflammasome. Redox Biol 12:883–896. https://doi.org/10.1016/j.redox.2017.04.020

Hu IC, Singh SP, Snyder AK (1995) Effects of ethanol on glucose transporter expression in cultured hippocampal neurons. Alcohol Clin Exp Res 19:1398–1402. https://doi.org/10.1111/j.1530-0277.1995.tb00998.x

Hughes PD, Kim YN, Randall PK et al (1998) Effect of prenatal ethanol exposure on the developmental profile of the NMDA receptor subunits in rat forebrain and hippocampus. Alcohol Clin Exp Res 22:1255–1261. https://doi.org/10.1111/j.1530-0277.1998.tb03906.x

Hummel J, Pico A, Willighagen E et al (2023) DNA-damage-response-pathway. http://www.wikipathways.org/instance/WP707. Accessed 08 Sept 2023

Iadecola C (2017) The neurovascular unit coming of age: a journey through neurovascular coupling in health and disease. Neuron 96:17–42. https://doi.org/10.1016/j.neuron.2017.07.030

Ikonomidou C, Bittigau P, Ishimaru MJ et al (2000) Ethanol-induced apoptotic neurodegeneration and fetal alcohol syndrome. Science 287:1056–1060. https://doi.org/10.1126/science.287.5455.1056

Ikonomidou C, Bittigau P, Koch C et al (2001) Neurotransmitters and apoptosis in the developing brain. Biochem Pharmacol 62:401–405. https://doi.org/10.1016/s0006-2952(01)00696-7

Irner TB, Teasdale TW, Olofsson M (2011) Cognitive and social development in preschool children born to women using substances. J Addict Dis 31:29–44

Jacks DS, Pendakur K, Shigeoka H (2021) Infant mortality and the repeal of federal prohibition. Econ J 131:2955–2983. https://doi.org/10.1093/EJ/UEAB011

Jaddoe VWV, Bakker R, Hofman A et al (2007) Moderate alcohol consumption during pregnancy and the risk of low birth weight and preterm birth. The generation R study. Ann Epidemiol 17:834–840. https://doi.org/10.1016/J.ANNEPIDEM.2007.04.001

Jarmasz JS, Basalah DA, Chudley AE et al (2017) Human brain abnormalities associated with prenatal alcohol exposure and fetal alcohol spectrum disorder. J Neuropathol Exp Neurol 76:813–833

Jégou S, El Ghazi F, de Lendeu PK et al (2012) Prenatal alcohol exposure affects vasculature development in the neonatal brain. Ann Neurol 72:952–960

Johnson S, Knight R, Marmer DJ et al (1981) Immune deficiency in fetal alcohol syndrome. Pediatr Res 15: 908–911. [PubMed: 7195540]

Jones PJ, Leichter J, Lee M (1981) Placental blood flow in rats fed alcohol before and during gestation. Life Sci 29:1153–1159. https://doi.org/10.1016/0024-3205(81)90204-6

Kaminen-Ahola N, Ahola A, Maga M et al (2010) Maternal ethanol consumption alters the epigenotype and the phenotype of offspring in a mouse model. PLoS Genet 6:e1000811

Karl PI, Kwun R, Slonim A et al (1995) Ethanol elevates fetal serum glutamate levels in the rat. Alcohol Clin Exp Res 19:177–181. https://doi.org/10.1111/j.1530-0277.1995.tb01488.x

Kelly SJ, Mahoney JC, West JR (1990) Changes in brain microvasculature resulting from early postnatal alcohol exposure. Alcohol 7:43–47. https://doi.org/10.1016/0741-8329(90)90059-I

Kennedy LA (1984) Changes in the term mouse placenta associated with maternal alcohol consumption and fetal growth deficits. Am J Obstet Gynecol 149:518–522. https://doi.org/10.1016/0002-9378(84)90028-0

Kim J, Jin H, Park JA et al (2006) Blood-neural barrier: intercellular communication at glio-vascular interface. J Biochem Mol Biol 39:339–345. https://doi.org/10.5483/bmbrep.2006.39.4.339

Kochunov P, Castro C, Davis DM et al (2010) Fetal brain during a binge drinking episode: a dynamic susceptibility contrast MRI fetal brain perfusion study. Neuroreport 21:716–721. https://doi.org/10.1097/WNR.0b013e32833b5047

Konior A, Schramm A, Czesnikiewicz-Guzik M et al (2014) NADPH oxidases in vascular pathology. Antioxid Redox Signal 20:2794–2814. https://doi.org/10.1089/ars.2013.5607

Koop DR (2006) Alcohol metabolism's damaging effects on the cell: a focus on reactive oxygen generation by the enzyme cytochrome P450 2E1. Alcohol Res Health 29:274–280

Lange S (2017) Global prevalence of fetal alcohol spectrum disorder among children and youth: a systematic review and meta-analysis. JAMA Pediatr 171:948–956

Lebel C, Roussotte F, Sowell ER (2011) Imaging the impact of prenatal alcohol exposure on the structure of the developing human brain. Neuropsychol Rev 21: 102–118. [PubMed: 21369875]

Léger C, Dupré N, Aligny C et al (2020) Glutamate controls vessel-associated migration of GABA interneurons from the pial migratory route via NMDA receptors and endothelial protease activation. Cell Mol Life Sci 77:1959–1986. https://doi.org/10.1007/s00018-019-03248-5

Legros H, Launay S, Roussel BD et al (2009) Newborn- and adult-derived brain microvascular endothelial cells show age-related differences in phenotype and glutamate-evoked protease release. J Cereb Blood Flow Metab 29:1146–1158

LeLecuyer M, Laquerrière A, Bekri S et al (2017) PLGF, a placental marker of fetal brain defects after in utero alcohol exposure. Acta Neuropathol Commun 5:44–66

Li Z, Lin H, Zhu Y et al (2001) Disruption of cell cycle kinetics and cyclin-dependent kinase system by ethanol in cultured mcerebellar granule progenitors. Brain Res Dev Brain Res 132:47–58

Liu Y, Balaraman Y, Wang G et al (2009) Alcohol exposure alters DNA methylation profiles in mouse embryos at early neurulation. Epigenetics 4:500–511

Luhmann HJ, Fukuda A, Kilb W (2015) Control of cortical neuronal migration by glutamate and GABA front. Cell Neurosci 9:4–10

Luo J (2014) Autophagy and ethanol neurotoxicity. Autophagy 10:2099–2108. https://doi.org/10.4161/15548627.2014.981916

Lupton C, Burd L, Harwood R (2004) Cost of fetal alcohol spectrum disorders. Am J Med Genet 127:42–50

Lussier AA, Weinberg J, Kobor MS (2017) Epigenetics studies of fetal alcohol Spectrum disorder: where are we now? Epigenomics 9:291–311

Lynch CM, Kinzenbaw DA, Chen X et al (2013) Nox2-derived superoxide contributes to cerebral vascular dysfunction in diet-induced obesity. Stroke 44:3195–3201. https://doi.org/10.1161/STROKEAHA.113.001366

Maier SE, West JR (2001) Drinking patterns and alcohol-related birth defects. Alcohol Res Health 25:168–174

Maier SE, Chen WJA, West JR (1996) Prenatal binge-like alcohol exposure alters neurochemical profiles in fetal rat brain. Pharmacol Biochem Behav 55:521–529. https://doi.org/10.1016/S0091-3057(96)00282-1

Mann LI, Bhakthavathsalan A, Liu M et al (1975) Effect of alcohol on fetal cerebral function and metabolism. Am J Obstet Gynecol 122:845–851. https://doi.org/10.1016/0002-9378(75)90726-7

Manzo-Avalos S, Saavedra-Molina A (2010) Cellular and mitochondrial effects of alcohol consumption. Int J Environ Res Public Health 7:4281–4304. https://doi.org/10.3390/ijerph7124281

Marcussen BL, Goodlett CR, Mahoney JC et al (1994) Developing rat purkinje cells are more vulnerable to alcohol-induced depletion during differentiation than during neurogenesis. Alcohol 11:147–156. https://doi.org/10.1016/0741-8329(94)90056-6

Marx N, Schönbeck U, Lazar MA et al (1998) Peroxisome proliferator-activated receptor gamma activators inhibit gene expression and migration in human vascular smooth muscle cells. Circ Res 83:1097–1103. https://doi.org/10.1161/01.res.83.11.1097

Marx N, Bourcier T, Sukhova GK et al (1999) PPARgamma activation in human endothelial cells increases plasminogen activator inhibitor type-1 expression: PPARgamma as a potential mediator in vascular disease. Arterioscler Thromb Vasc Biol 19: 546–551. https://doi.org/10.1161/01.atv.19.3.546

Mathiisen TM, Lehre KP, Danbolt NC et al (2010) The perivascular astroglial sheath provides a complete covering of the brain microvessels: an electronmicroscopic 3D reconstruction. Glia 58:1094–1103. https://doi.org/10.1002/glia.20990

Mattson SN, Schoenfeld AM, Riley EP (2001) Teratogenic effects of alcohol on brain and behavior. Alcohol Res Health 25:185–191

Mattson SN, Crocker N, Nguyen TT (2011) Fetal alcohol spectrum disorders: neuropsychological and behavioral features. Neuropsychol Rev 21:81–101. [PubMed: 21503685]

May PA, Gossage JP (2011) Maternal risk factors for fetal alcohol spectrum disorders: not as simple as it might seem. Alcohol Res Health 34:15–26

May PA, Gossage JP, Kalberg WO et al (2009) Prevalence and epidemiologic characteristics of FASD from various research methods with an emphasis on recent in-school studies. Dev Disabil Res Rev 15:176–192

May PA, Chambers CD, Kalberg WO et al (2018) Prevalence of fetal alcohol Spectrum disorders in 4 US communities. JAMA 319:474–482. [PubMed: 29411031]

Mayock DE, Ness D, Mondares RL et al (2007) Binge alcohol exposure in the second trimester attenuates fetal cerebral blood flow response to hypoxia. J Appl Physiol 10:972–977. https://doi.org/10.1152/japplphysiol.00956.2006

Mayock DE, Ngai AC, Mondares RL et al (2008) Effects of binge alcohol exposure in the second trimester on intracerebral arteriolar function in third trimester fetal

sheep. Brain Res 1226:111–115. https://doi.org/10.1016/j.brainres.2008.05.077
McCarty JH (2005) Cell biology of the neurovascular unit: implications for drug delivery across the blood-brain barrier. Assay Drug Dev Technol 3:89–95. https://doi.org/10.1089/adt.2005.3.89
McConnell HL, Kersch CN, Woltjer RL et al (2017) The translational significance of the neurovascular unit. J Biol Chem 292:762–770. https://doi.org/10.1074/jbc.R116.760215
McGill J, Meyerholz DK, Edsen-Moore M et al (2009) Fetal exposure to ethanol has long-term effects on the severity of influenza virus infections. J Immunol 182: 7803–7808
McLachlan K, Rasmussen C, Oberlander TF et al (2016) Dysregulation of the cortisol diurnal rhythm following prenatal alcohol exposure and early life adversity. Alcohol 53:9–18
Miller MW (1986) Effects of alcohol on the generation and migration of cerebral cortical neurons. Science 233: 1308–1311. https://doi.org/10.1126/science.3749878
Miller MW (1993) Migration of cortical neurons is altered by gestational exposure to ethanol. Alcohol Clin Exp Res 17:304–314
Miller MW (2003) Expression of transforming growth factor-beta in developing rat cerebral cortex: effects of prenatal exposure to ethanol. J Comp Neurol 460: 410–424. https://doi.org/10.1002/cne.10658
Miller MW, Robertson S (1993) Prenatal exposure to ethanol alters the postnatal development and transformation of radial glia to astrocytes in the cortex. J Comp Neurol 337:253–266. https://doi.org/10.1002/cne.903370206
Miller-Pinsler L, Wells PG (2016) Deficient DNA repair exacerbates ethanolinitiated DNA oxidation and embryopathies in ogg1 knockout mice: gender risk and protection by a free radical spin trapping agent. Arch Toxicol 90:415–425. https://doi.org/10.1007/s00204-014-1397-1
Montesinos J, Pascual M, Pla A et al (2015) TLR4 elimination prevents synaptic and myelin alterations and long-term cognitive dysfunctions in adolescent mice with intermittent ethanol treatment. Brain Behav Immun 45:233–244. https://doi.org/10.1016/j.bbi.2014.11.015
Moore EM, Riley EP (2015) What happens when children with fetal alcohol Spectrum disorders become adults? Curr Dev Disord Rep 2:219–227. https://doi.org/10.1007/s40474-015-0053-7
Mukherjee AB, Hodgen GD (1982) Maternal ethanol exposure induces transient impairment of umbilical circulation and fetal hypoxia in monkeys. Science 218:700–702. https://doi.org/10.1126/science.6890235
Muoio V, Persson PB, Sendeski MM (2014) The neurovascular unit – concept review. Acta Physiol 210:790–798. https://doi.org/10.1111/apha.12250
Murugan S, Zhang C, Mojtahedzadeh S et al (2013) Alcohol exposure in utero increases susceptibility to prostate tumorigenesis in rat offspring. Alcohol Clin Exp Res 37:1901–1909
Nagre NN, Subbanna S, Shivakumar M et al (2015) CB1-receptor knockout neonatal mice are protected against ethanol-induced impairments of DNMT1, DNMT3A and DNA methylation. J Neurochem 132: 429–442
Ngai AC, Mondares RL, Mayock DE et al (2008) Fetal alcohol exposure alters cerebrovascular reactivity to vasoactive intestinal peptide in adult sheep. Neonatology 93:45–51. https://doi.org/10.1159/000105524
Nordestgaard BG, Varbo A (2014) Triglycerides and cardiovascular disease. Lancet 384:626–635. [PubMed: 25131982]
Norman MG, O'Kusky JR (1986) The growth and development of microvasculature in human cerebral cortex. J Neuropathol Exp Neurol 45:222–232. https://doi.org/10.1097/00005072-198605000-00003
North K, Tobiasz A, Sullivan RD et al (2018) Prenatal alcohol exposure, anesthesia, and fetal loss in baboon model of pregnancy. J Drug Alcohol Res 7:236064
O'Leary CM, Jacoby PJ, Bartu A et al (2013) Maternal alcohol use and sudden infant death syndrome and infant mortality excluding SIDS. Pediatrics 131: e770–e778. https://doi.org/10.1542/PEDS.2012-1907
Obermeier B, Daneman R, Ransohoff RM (2013) Development, maintenance and disruption of the blood-brain barrier. Nat Med 19:1584–1596. https://doi.org/10.1038/nm.3407[10-12][6-8/Sequira]
Ogony JW, Malahias E, Vadigepalli R et al (2013) Ethanol alters the balance of Sox2, Oct4, and nanog expression in distinct subpopulations during differentiation of embryonic stem cells. Stem Cells Dev 22:2196–2210
Oleson DR, Magee RM, Donahoe RM et al (1998) Immunity and prenatal alcohol exposure. A pilot study in human adolescents. Adv Exper Med Biol 137:255–264. [PubMed: 9666278]
Ornoy A (2007) Embryonic oxidative stress as a mechanism of teratogenesis with special emphasis on diabetic embryopathy. Reprod Toxicol 24:31–41. https://doi.org/10.1016/j.reprotox.2007.04.004
Otero NKH, Thomas JD, Saski CA et al (2012) Choline supplementation and DNA methylation in the hippocampus and prefrontal cortex of rats exposed to alcohol during development. Alcohol Clin Exp Res 36:1701–1709
Ouellet-Morin I, Dionne G, Lupien SJ et al (2011) Prenatal alcohol exposure and cortisol activity in 19-month-old toddlers: an investigation of the moderating effects of sex and testosterone. Psychopharmacology 214:297–307
Paravicini TM, Chrissobolis S, Drummond GR et al (2004) Increased NADPH-oxidase activity and Nox4 expression during chronic hypertension is associated with enhanced cerebral vasodilatation to NADPH in vivo. Stroke 35:584–589. https://doi.org/10.1161/01.STR.0000112974.37028.58
Parkington HC, Kenna KR, Sozo F et al (2014) Maternal alcohol consumption in pregnancy enhances arterial

stiffness and alters vasodilator function that varies between vascular beds in fetal sheep. J Physiol 592: 2591–2603. https://doi.org/10.1113/jphysiol.2013.262873
Parnell SE, Ramadoss J, Delp MD et al (2007) Chronic ethanol increases fetal cerebral blood flow specific to the ethanol-sensitive cerebellum under normoxaemic, hypercapnic and acidaemic conditions: ovine model. Exp Physiol 92:933–943. https://doi.org/10.1113/expphysiol.2007.038091
Parnell SE, Riley EP, Warren KR et al (2018) The contributions of Dr. Kathleen K. Sulik to fetal alcohol spectrum disorders research and prevention. Alcohol 69:15–24
Pei J, Job J, Kully-Martens K et al (2011) Executive function and memory in children with fetal alcohol spectrum disorder. Child Neuropsychol 17:290–309
Pennington SN, Boyd JW, Kalmus GW et al (1983) The molecular mechanism of fetal alcohol syndrome (FAS). I. Ethanol-induced growth suppression. Neurobehav Toxicol Teratol 5:259–262
Pennington JS, Shuvaeva TI, Pennington SN (2002) Maternal dietary ethanol consumption is associated with hypertriglyceridemia in adult rat offspring. Alcoholism: Clin Exp Res 26:848–855
Perkins A, Lehmann C, Lawrence CR et al (2013) Alcohol exposure during development: impact on the Epigenome. Int J Dev Neurosci 31:391–397
Phillips DE, Krueger SK, Wall KA et al (1997) The development of the blood-brain barrier in alcohol-exposed rats. Alcohol 14:333–343
Pollard I (2007) Neuropharmacology of drugs and alcohol in mother and fetus. Semin Fetal Neonatal Med 12: 106–113. https://doi.org/10.1016/j.siny.2006.12.001
Popova EN (1992) Prenatal moderate effects of alcohol on ultrastructure of cortical capillaries in the offspring. Biull Eksp Biol Med 113:161–164
Porter NA (1984) Chemistry of lipid peroxidation. Methods Enzymol 105:273–282
Radek KA, Matthies AM, Burns AL et al (2005) Acute ethanol exposure impairs angiogenesis and the proliferative phase of wound healing. Am J Physiol Heart Circ Physiol 289:H1084–H1090. https://doi.org/10.1152/ajpheart.00080.2005
Radek KA, Kovacs EJ, Gallo RL et al (2008) Acute ethanol exposure disrupts VEGF receptor cell signaling in endothelial cells. Am J Physiol Heart Circ Physiol 295:H174–H184. https://doi.org/10.1152/ajpheart.00699.2007
Rasmussen C, Soleimani M, Pei J (2011) Executive functioning and working memory deficits on the cantab among children with prenatal alcohol exposure. J Popul Ther Clin Pharmacol 18:e44–e53
Richardson BS, Patrick JE, Bousquet J et al (1985) Cerebral metabolism in fetal lamb after maternal infusion of ethanol. Am J Phys 249:R505–R509. https://doi.org/10.1152/ajpregu.1985.249.5.R505
Riley EP, Mcgee CL (2005) Fetal alcohol spectrum disorders: an overview with emphasis on changes in brain and behavior. Exp Biol Med 230:357–365
Riley EP, Infante MA, Warren KR (2011) Fetal alcohol spectrum disorders: an overview. Neuropsychol Rev 21:73–80. https://doi.org/10.1007/s11065-011-9166-x
Rogic S, Wong A, Pavlidis P (2016) Meta-analysis of gene expression patterns in animal models of prenatal alcohol exposure suggests role for protein synthesis inhibition and chromatin remodeling. Alcohol Clin Exp Res 40:717–724
Rosenberg MJ, Wolff CR, El-Emawy A et al (2010) Effects of moderate drinking during pregnancy on placental gene expression. Alcohol 44:673–690
Saha PS, Kim-Sawtelle KR, Bamberg BN et al (2021a) Rosiglitazone restores nitric oxide synthase-dependent reactivity of cerebral arterioles in rats exposed to prenatal alcohol. Alcohol Clin Exp Res 45:1359–1369. https://doi.org/10.1111/acer.14634
Saha PS, Knecht TM, Arrick DM et al (2021b) Constrictor responses of cerebral resistance arterioles in male and female rats exposed to prenatal alcohol. Physiol Rep 9: e15079. https://doi.org/10.14814/phy2.15079
Saha PS, Knecht TM, Arrick DM et al (2023) Prenatal exposure to alcohol impairs responses of cerebral arterioles to activation of potassium channels: role of oxidative stress. Alcohol Clin Exp Res 47:87–94. https://doi.org/10.1111/acer.14980. Epub 2022 Nov 29. PMID: 36446735; PMCID: PMC9974881
Sanderson JL, Donald Partridge L, Fernando Valenzuela C (2009) Modulation of GABAergic and glutamatergic transmission by ethanol in the developing neocortex: an in vitro test of the excessive inhibition hypothesis of fetal alcohol spectrum disorder. Neuropharmacology 56:541–555. https://doi.org/10.1016/j.neuropharm.2008.10.012
Sarkar DK (2016) Male germline transmits fetal alcohol epigenetic marks for multiple generations: a review. Addict Biol 21:23–34
Seleverstov O, Tobiasz A, Jackson JS et al (2017) Maternal alcohol exposure during mid-pregnancy dilates fetal cerebral arteries via endocannabinoid receptors. Alcohol 61:51–61. https://doi.org/10.1016/j.alcohol.2017.01.014
Simakova M, Tobiasz A, Sullivan RD et al (2019) Gestational age-dependent interplay between endocannabinoid receptors and alcohol in fetal cerebral arteries. J Drug Alcohol Res 8:236068. https://doi.org/10.4303/jdar/236068
Siqueira M, Araujo APB, Gomes FCA et al (2021) Ethanol gestational exposure impairs vascular development and endothelial potential to control BBB-associated astrocyte function in the developing cerebral cortex. Mol Neurobiol 58:1755–1768. https://doi.org/10.1007/s12035-020-02214-8
Siqueira M, Arujko APB, Gomes FCA et al (2022) Ethanol gestational exposure impairs vascular development and endothelial potential to control BBB-associated

astrocyte function in the developing cerebral cortex. Mol Neurobiol 58:1755–1768

Smith SM, Garic A, Flentke GR et al (2014) Neural crest development in fetal alcohol syndrome. Birth Defects Res C Embryo Today 102:210–220

Solonskii AV, Logvinov SV, Kutepova NA (2008) Development of brain vessels in human embryos and fetuses in conditions of prenatal exposure to alcohol. Neurosci Behav Physiol 38:373–376. https://doi.org/10.1007/s11055-008-0053-8

Sowell E, Jernigan T, Mattson S et al (1996) Abnormal development of the cerebellar vermis in children prenatally exposed to alcohol: size reduction in lobules I–V. Alcohol Clin Exp Res 20:31–34

Spong CY, Auth J, Vink J et al (2002) Vasoactive intestinal peptide mRNA and immunoreactivity are decreased in fetal alcohol syndrome model. Regul Pept 108:143–147. https://doi.org/10.1016/s0167-0115(02)00104-0

Stevens S, Majors D, Rovet J et al (2012) Social problem solving in children with fetal alcohol spectrum disorders. J Popul Ther Clin Pharmacol 19:e99–e110

Streissguth AP, Landesman-Dwyer S, Martin JC et al (1980) Teratogenic effects of alcohol in humans and laboratory animals. Science 209:353–361. https://doi.org/10.1126/science.6992275

Streissguth AP, Barr HM, Sampson PD et al (1994) Prenatal alcohol and offspring development: the first fourteen years. Drug Alcohol Depend 36:89–99

Sun T, Hevner RF (2014) Growth and folding of the mammalian cerebral cortex: from molecules to malformations. Nat Rev Neurosci 15:217–232

Tam SJ, Watts RJ (2010) Connecting vascular and nervous system development: angiogenesis and the bloodbrain barrier. Annu Rev Neurosci 33:379–408. https://doi.org/10.1146/annurev-neuro-060909-152829

Thomas JD, Weinert SP, Sharif S et al (1997) MK-801 administration during ethanol withdrawal in neonatal rat pups attenuates ethanol-induced behavioral deficits. Alcohol Clin Exp Res 21:1218–1225. https://doi.org/10.1111/j.1530-0277.1997.tb04441.x

Thomas JD, Warren KR, Hewitt BG (2010) Fetal alcohol spectrum disorders: from research to policy. Alcohol Res Health 33:118–126

Tobiasz AM, Duncan JR, Bursac Z et al (2018) The effect of prenatal alcohol exposure on fetal growth and cardiovascular parameters in a baboon model of pregnancy. Reprod Sci 25:1116–1123. https://doi.org/10.1177/1933719117734317

Tokuda K, Izumi Y, Zorumski CF (2013) Locally-generated acetaldehyde contributes to the effects of ethanol on neurosteroids and long-term potentiation in the hippocampus. Neurol Clin Neurosci 1:138–147. https://doi.org/10.1111/ncn3.39

Topper LA, Baculis BC, Valenzuela CF (2015) Exposure of neonatal rats to alcohol has differential effects on neuroinflammation and neuronal survival in the cerebellum and hippocampus. J Neuroinflammation 12:160–182. https://doi.org/10.1186/s12974-015-0382-9

Trindade P, Hampton B, Manhaes AC et al (2016) Developmental alcohol exposure leads to a persistent change on astrocyte secretome. J Neurochem 137:730–743. https://doi.org/10.1111/jnc.13542

Turcotte LA, Aberle NS, Norby FL et al (2002) Influence of prenatal ethanol exposure on vascular contractile response in rat thoracic aorta. Alcohol 26:75–81. https://doi.org/10.1016/s0741-8329(01)00198-7

Uc A, Vasiliauskas E, Piccoli DA et al (1997) Chronic intestinal pseudoobstruction associated with fetal alcohol syndrome. Dig Dis Sci 42:1163–1167

Ulrich F, Carretero-Ortega J, Menéndez J et al (2016) Reck enables cerebrovascular development by promoting canonical WNT signaling. Development 143:1055–1059. https://doi.org/10.1242/dev.136507

Ungerer M, Knezovich J, Ramsay M (2013) In utero alcohol exposure, epigenetic changes, and their consequences. Alcohol Res Curr Rev 35:37–46

Walchli T, Wacker A, Frei K et al (2015) Wiring the vascular network with neural cues: a CNS perspective. Neuron 87:271–296. https://doi.org/10.1016/j.neuron.2015.06.038

Wang X, Kroenke CD (2015) Utilization of magnetic resonance imaging in research involving animal models of fetal alcohol spectrum disorders. Alcohol Res 37:39–51

Wang LL, Yang AK, He SM et al (2010) Identification of molecular targets associated with ethanol toxicity and implications in drug development. Curr Pharm Des 16:1313–1355. https://doi.org/10.2174/138161210791034030

Wei EP, Kontos HA, Said SI (1980) Mechanism of action of vasoactive intestinal polypeptide on cerebral arterioles. Am J Phys 239:H765–H768. https://doi.org/10.1152/ajpheart.1980.239.6.H765

Welch JH, Mayfield JJ, Leibowitz AL et al (2016) Third trimester-equivalent ethanol exposure causes microhemorrhages in the rat brain. Neuroscience 324:107–118. https://doi.org/10.1016/j.neuroscience.2016.03.004

Wells PG, McCallum GP, Chen CS et al (2009) Oxidative stress in developmental origins of disease: teratogenesis, neurodevelopmental deficits, and cancer. Toxicol Sci 108:4–18. https://doi.org/10.1093/toxsci/kfn263

Wells PG, Bhatia S, Drake DM et al (2016) Fetal oxidative stress mechanisms of neurodevelopmental deficits and exacerbation by ethanol and methamphetamine. Birth Defects Res C Embryo Today Rev 108:108–130. https://doi.org/10.1002/bdrc.21134

West JR (1987) Fetal alcohol-induced brain damage and the problem of determining temporal vulnerability: a review. Alcohol Drug Res 7:423–441

West JR, Kelly SJ, Pierce DR (1987) Severity of alcohol-induced deficits in rats during the third trimester equivalent is determined by the pattern of exposure. Alcohol (Suppl) 1:461–465

Wilhelm CJ, Guizzetti M (2015) Fetal alcohol Spectrum disorders: an overview from the glia perspective. Front

Integr Neurosci 9(11):65. https://doi.org/10.3389/fnint.2015.00065
Williams JK, Baptista PM, Daunais JB et al (2008) The effects of ethanol consumption on vasculogenesis potential in non human primates. Alcohol Clin Exp Res 32:155–161. https://doi.org/10.1111/j.1530-0277.2007.00558.x
Wisborg K, Kesmodel U, Henriksen TB et al (2001) Exposure to tobacco smoke in utero and the risk of stillbirth and death in the first year of life. Am J Epidemiol 154:322–327. https://doi.org/10.1093/AJE/154.4.322
Wisniewski K, Dambska M, Sher J et al (1983) A clinical neuropathological study of the fetal alcohol syndrome. Neuropediatrics 14:197–201
Wolburg H, Noell S, Mack A et al (2009) Brain endothelial cells and the glio-vascular complex. Cell Tissue Res 335:75–96. https://doi.org/10.1007/s00441-008-0658-9
Won C, Lin Z, Kumar TP et al (2013) Autonomous vascular networks synchronize GABA neuron migration in the embryonic forebrain. Nat Commun 4:2149–2154
Wong AW, McCallum GP, Jeng W et al (2008) Oxoguanine glycosylase 1 protects against methamphetamine-enhanced fetal brain oxidative DNA damage and neurodevelopmental deficits. J Neurosci 28:9047–9054. https://doi.org/10.1523/JNEUROSCI.2557-08.20086
Wozniak JR, Muetzel RL (2011) What does diffusion tensor imaging reveal about the brain and cognition in fetal alcohol spectrum disorders? Neuropsychol Rev 21:133–147. [PubMed: 21347880]
Xu G, Broadbelt KG, Haynes RL et al (2011) Late development of the GABAergic system in the human cerebral cortex and white matter. J Neuropathol Exp Neurol 70:841–858
Yang F, Luo J (2015) Endoplasmic reticulum stress and ethanol neurotoxicity. Biomolecules 5:2538–2553. https://doi.org/10.3390/biom5042538
Yang Y, Roussotte F, Kan E et al (2012) Abnormal cortical thickness alterations in fetal alcohol spectrum disorders and their relationships with facial dysmorphology. Cereb Cortex 22:1170–1179
Yang J, Qiu H, Qu P et al (2015) Prenatal alcohol exposure and congenital heart defects: a meta-analysis. PLoS One 10:e0130681
Zeisel SH (2011) What choline metabolism can tell us about the underlying mechanisms of fetal alcohol spectrum disorders. Mol Neurobiol 44:185–191
Zhang X, Lan N, Bach P et al (2012) Prenatal alcohol exposure alters the course and severity of adjuvant-induced arthritis in female rats. Brain Behav Immun 26:439–450
Zhao Y, Ren H, Dwyer DS et al (2015) Different sites of alcohol action in the NMDA receptor GluN2A and GluN2B subunits. Neuropharmacology 97:240–250
Zhou FC, Sari Y, Powrozek TA (2005) Fetal alcohol exposure reduces serotonin innervation and compromises development of the forebrain along the serotonergic pathway. Alcohol Clin Exp Res 29:141–149. https://doi.org/10.1097/01.ALC.0000150636.19677.6F

The Role of the Hedgehog Pathway in Alcohol-Induced Birth Defects

3

Xiaojia Ji, Esraa Salim, Michael Tarpley, Cassandra Duncan, Dina Abu Rabe, Gregory J. Cole, and Kevin P. Williams

Abstract

In this chapter, we review the current literature that focuses on the role of Sonic hedgehog (Shh) signaling, a major morphogenic pathway regulating embryonic development, in the pathology of fetal alcohol spectrum disorder (FASD), caused by prenatal alcohol exposure (PAE). Ethanol exposure disrupts Shh signaling during development across a range of species including in mice, chick, and zebrafish. Ethanol appears to interfere with Shh signaling through multiple mechanisms, both direct and indirect, including reduced Shh ligand production, impaired post-translational processing, and inducing apoptosis in Shh-expressing cells during gastrulation. These disruptions result in a spectrum of developmental defects characteristic of FASD, such as craniofacial abnormalities, brain malformations, and limb deformities. Genetic susceptibility to PAE is linked to mutations in Shh pathway components. Activation of Shh signaling, genetically or pharmacologically, has been effective in mitigating ethanol-induced defects. This chapter also examines the teratogenic effects of cannabinoids (CBs) and ethanol, which synergistically disrupt Shh signaling. CBs directly interact with Smoothened, a key Shh receptor, amplifying developmental defects when combined with ethanol exposure. This chapter details the critical role of Shh signaling in embryogenesis and its vulnerability to environmental teratogens such as ethanol and CBs.

Xiaojia Ji and Esraa Salim have equally contributed to this chapter.

X. Ji · E. Salim · M. Tarpley
Biomanufacturing Research Institute and Technology Enterprise, North Carolina Central University, Durham, NC, USA

C. Duncan
Biomanufacturing Research Institute and Technology Enterprise, North Carolina Central University, Durham, NC, USA

INBS PhD Program, North Carolina Central University, Durham, NC, USA

D. A. Rabe
Bowles Center for Alcohol Studies, University of North Carolina, Chapel Hill, NC, USA

G. J. Cole
Julius L. Chambers Biomedical/Biotechnology Research Institute, North Carolina Central University, Durham, NC, USA

Department of Biological and Biomedical Sciences, North Carolina Central University, Durham, NC, USA

K. P. Williams (✉)
Biomanufacturing Research Institute and Technology Enterprise, North Carolina Central University, Durham, NC, USA

Department of Pharmaceutical Sciences, North Carolina Central University, Durham, NC, USA
e-mail: kpwilliams@nccu.edu

A. N. Bukiya, D. W. Ali (eds.), *Molecular Mechanisms and Lifelong Consequences of Prenatal Exposure to Psychoactive Substances*, Advances in Experimental Medicine and Biology 1500,
https://doi.org/10.1007/978-3-032-12741-9_3

Keywords

Sonic hedgehog · Holoprosencephaly · FASD · Smoothened · Primary cilium · Cannabinoid

3.1 Introduction

Ethanol is known to be teratogenic to vertebrate embryos across a wide range of species (Cohen Jr and Sulik 1992; Parnell and Eberhart 2023). A number of pathophysiological and genetic mechanisms have been reported to explain the impaired growth and morphogenesis observed in fetal alcohol spectrum disorder (FASD) (Beames and Lipinski 2020; Eberhart and Parnell 2016; Everson and Eberhart 2023; Lovely et al. 2017). Prenatal alcohol exposure (PAE) causes teratogenic effects on fetal development, leading to FASD, which has an incidence rate of 1 and 5% among first graders in the USA (May et al. 2018). Fetal alcohol syndrome (FAS) (Jones and Smith 1973; Jones 1986), the most severe form of FASD, has distinctive craniofacial characteristics that are comparable to those in the holoprosencephaly (HPE) spectrum, a severe midline brain malformation (Jones 1986; Sulik 2014; Del Campo and Jones 2017), many of which are recapitulated in animal models of FASD (Godin et al. 2011; Hong and Krauss 2017; O'Leary-Moore et al. 2011; Sulik et al. 1981). Craniofacial features include a small or absent philtrum, a thin upper lip, narrowly spaced eyes, epicanthal folds, short palpebral fissures, microphthalmia, and, to a lesser degree, small lower jaws and a generally flat midface (Del Campo and Jones 2017). In addition to characteristic craniofacial features, individuals with FAS can exhibit limb deformities, impaired brain development, growth restrictions before and after birth, as well as behavioral and cognitive impairments (Jones 1986; Sulik 2014), resulting in intellectual and emotional difficulties (Kelly et al. 2000; Mattson et al. 2011; Streissguth et al. 1991). While PAE causes a range of congenital disabilities, individuals vary in their susceptibility to the teratogenic effects of ethanol (reviewed in (Eberhart and Parnell 2016). Exposure of embryos to ethanol leads to a diverse range of clinical outcomes, from unaffected to severe, that cannot be attributed solely to the level of ethanol, with genetics also playing a role (Parnell and Eberhart 2023; Beames and Lipinski 2020; Eberhart and Parnell 2016; Everson and Eberhart 2023; Lovely et al. 2017; Everson et al. 2020; Smith et al. 2014a; McCarthy and Eberhart 2014). The impact of ethanol on embryonic development has been described in detail elsewhere (Parnell and Eberhart 2023).

This chapter focuses on the substantial published evidence suggesting that Sonic hedgehog (Shh) pathway signaling, a critical morphogenic pathway, is reduced by PAE which contributes to the pathology of FASD. Further, the mechanisms (direct and indirect) by which PAE might cause such a critical decrease in Shh signaling are explored.

3.2 The Sonic Hedgehog Pathway

The *hedgehog* (*Hh*) gene was first identified in drosophila in 1980 as a segment polarity gene (Nüsslein-Volhard and Wieschaus 1980). Using complementary DNA cloning, three Hh homologs were identified in vertebrates: Sonic (Shh), Indian, and Desert (Echelard et al. 1993; Krauss et al. 1993; Riddle et al. 1993; Roelink et al. 1994). All three mammalian Hh ligands bind to the same signaling apparatus and produce comparable biological responses (Pathi et al. 2001). Shh, the most studied, plays an essential role in both embryonic development and the growth of various adult tissues (Ingham and McMahon 2001; Groves et al. 2020; Jing et al. 2023). Shh fulfills a crucial role in developmental processes, particularly during gastrulation and neurulation (Lanoue et al. 1997; Wallis and Muenke 2000). Shh expression in embryos occurs in localized regions of the notochord, floor plate, and posterior region of developing limb buds (reviewed in (Tickle and Towers 2017; Ingham 2022). Shh functions as a morphogen in the patterning of these embryonic tissues, with its activity levels and duration specifying neuronal cell types (see recent review (Ingham 2022). In humans, SHH expression is detected in the notochord and ventral neural tube at 26 days, in the forelimbs at 32 days, and in the hindlimbs at 37 days (Odent et al. 1999). Mutations of SHH observed in human families with HPE (Odent et al. 1999), and mutation of *Shh* in mice (Chiang et al. 1996) confirmed its critical role in central nervous system development and in limb patterning.

The Shh signaling process involves multiple steps and components (Fig. 3.1), ranging from its processing and secretion to its interaction with the responding cell (reviewed in (Groves et al. 2020; Jing et al. 2023; Ingham 2022; Qi and Li 2020;

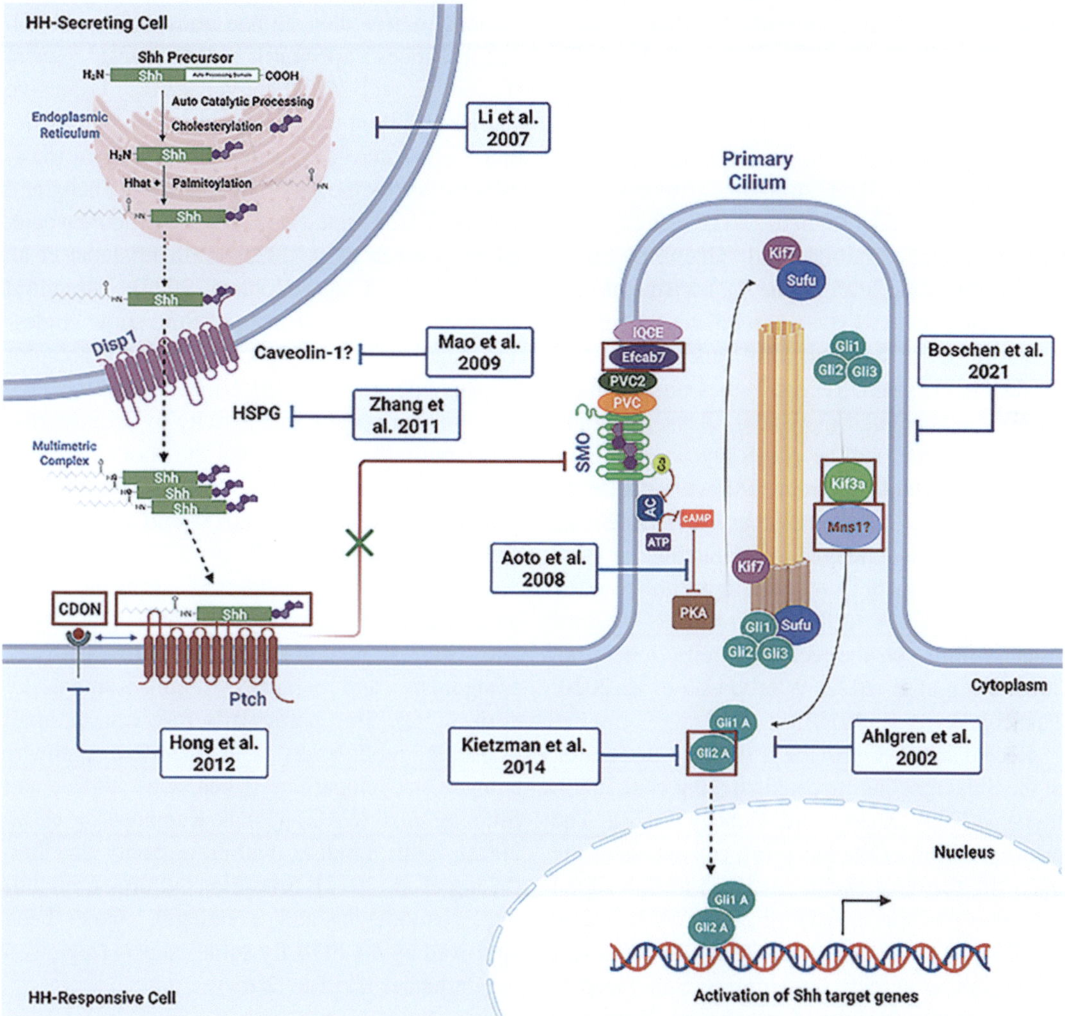

Fig. 3.1 *Sonic hedgehog (Shh) signaling pathway from production to target gene activation highlighting potential mechanisms and genes involved in PAE.* In the HH-secreting cell, Shh undergoes post-translational modifications, including auto-catalytic processing and cholesterol addition, and palmitoylation in the endoplasmic reticulum (ER) before release via Disp1. At the HH-responsive cell, Shh binds to the Patched (Ptch) receptor, relieving inhibition of Smoothened (Smo). This triggers a signaling cascade that activates Gli transcription factors, which then translocate to the nucleus, binding DNA and activating Shh target genes. The primary cilium plays a key role in Shh signaling. Blue citation boxes highlight key research on ethanol's impact on Shh signaling pathway at different regulatory points. Genes shown to affect PAE are highlighted with red boxes

Zhang and Beachy 2023), and refs therein). During its biogenesis, Shh is autocatalytically cleaved yielding an N-terminal product which receives a cholesterol modification at the C-terminus (Porter et al. 1996). Shh is then palmitoylated at the N-terminus (Pepinsky et al. 1998), a process mediated by Hh acyltransferase (Hhat) (Buglino and Resh 2008). It was reported that a loss-of-function mutation of *Hhat* affects Shh processing, leading to HPE and craniofacial defects in a mouse model (Resh 2021; Sasai et al. 2019). Several proposed mechanisms explain the transport of Shh from secreting to receiving/responsive cells over both short and long distances, including cell-derived structures (reviewed in (Jing et al. 2023; Ingham 2022; Zhang and Beachy 2023; Gradilla and Guerrero 2022; Chideriotis et al. 2025)). The 12-transmembrane protein Dispatched-1 (Disp1) mediates the release of Shh from the secreting cell (Burke et al. 1999; Caspary et al. 2002). Recent studies suggest that a series of extracellular molecular relays, including Scube2, heparan sulfate proteoglycans (HSPG), cell-adhesion-molecule-related/downregulated by oncogenes (CDO, also known as CDON), brother of CDO, and hedgehog-interacting protein (HHIP), participate in transporting Shh from the extracellular space to its receptor, to its receptor Patched (Ptch) on the receiving cell (Gude et al. 2023; Tang et al. 2022; Wierbowski et al. 2020; Tukachinsky et al. 2012).

Recent reviews provide a detailed discussion of the Shh signaling mechanism (Jing et al. 2023; Ingham 2022; Zhang and Beachy 2023). The primary cilium of the receiving cell serves as the main site for most events involved in Shh signal reception (reviewed in (Jing et al. 2023; Zhang and Beachy 2023; Mill et al. 2023). In summary, when Shh is absent, the primary Shh receptor Ptch, directly inhibits Smoothened (Smo), a G-protein coupled receptor (GPCR) that functions as the main effector molecule of the Shh pathway. Signaling begins when the Shh ligand binds to Ptch, which relieves Ptch's suppression of Smo, allowing Smo to translocate into the primary cilium and release its inhibitory G-protein (G_i), which then inhibits adenylyl cyclase (AC). This inhibition of AC causes a reduction in ciliary protein kinase A (PKA) levels. High ciliary PKA levels inhibit activation of the main transcription factors of the Shh pathway, glioma-associated homolog 1 and 2 (Gli1 and Gli2). In the inactive state, another protein, Suppressor of fused (Sufu) acts to sequester the Gli proteins (Zhang et al. 2013a). Activation of the Shh pathway lowers ciliary PKA levels, which releases the inhibition of Gli1 and Gli2, allowing them to exit the cilium and move to the nucleus, where they initiate transcription of Shh target genes (primarily cell cycle genes) (Pedersen and Akhmanova 2014). Extensive studies highlight the critical role of sterols, particularly cholesterol, in mediating Shh signal transmission across the plasma membrane (Zhang and Beachy 2023; Huang et al. 2018; Kinnebrew et al. 2019; Nguyen et al. 2022; Radhakrishnan et al. 2020; Siebold and Rohatgi 2023). Structural analyses of the active state of Smo show cholesterol binding in a deep pocket within the receptor (Deshpande et al. 2019; Qi et al. 2019). Ptch appears to suppress Smo activity by sequestering cholesterol, thereby reducing the pool of accessible membrane cholesterol and preventing Smo activation (Zhang et al. 2018) and reviewed in (Zhang and Beachy 2023).

Shh pathway cell-based screens have identified small molecule compounds that modulate Shh signaling, including Shh pathway antagonists and agonists (Frank-Kamenetsky et al. 2002). Smo particularly responds to small molecule modulation with the Shh pathway antagonist cyclopamine (Chen et al. 2002a) and Smo agonist (SAG) (Frank-Kamenetsky et al. 2002), both binding within a cavity in Smo (Wang et al. 2014). Smo-directed drugs, including vismodegib and sonidegib, have been approved by the FDA for some cancers (reviewed in (Carpenter and Ray 2019)).

3.3 Animal Models of FASD

Several animal models have been created to study FASD (Patten et al. 2014), including those using mice (Sulik et al. 1981), chick (Kiecker 2016; Sandor and Elias 1968; Flentke and Smith 2018; Smith 2008), and zebrafish (Blader and Strähle 1998; Loucks and Ahlgren 2012; Manikandan et al. 2022; Fernandes and Lovely 2021). These models replicate the pathological features observed in humans with FASD, such as craniofacial and brain defects (Klem et al. 2025), reduced eye size (Sulik et al. 1981; Zhang et al. 2014), limb abnormalities, smooth philtrum (Sulik and Johnston 1983), various behavioral alterations as well as cognitive and socio-emotional difficulties (Kelly et al. 2000; Mattson et al. 2011; Bailey et al. 2015; Burton et al. 2017; Fernandes et al. 2015; Streissguth and Dehaene 1993). For example, zebrafish embryos exposed to ethanol display FASD characteristics, such as microphthalmia, with the severity of these defects depending on both the amount and timing of ethanol exposure (Zhang et al. 2014; Ali et al. 2011; McCarthy et al. 2013; Swartz et al. 2014). A major advantage of these animal models is that developmental staging can be assessed with precision from the known fertilization time, allowing precise control over ethanol exposure and timing (Parnell and Eberhart 2023). Most ethanol exposure studies in animal models focus on gastrulation through to early nervous system development including neural tube closure, and compared to all of development, these events span a relatively short period. In terms of comparative development timing for gastrulation through to neurulation (Parnell and Eberhart 2023; Gilbert 2000; Hamburger and Hamilton 1951; Kaufman and Kaufman 1992; Kimmel et al. 1995), this spans E16 through E28 in humans, E6.5 to E10 in mice, 6–20 hpf in zebrafish (Fig. 3.2), and corresponds to Hamburger–Hamilton (HH) stages 3–10 in chick embryos.

Depending on the animal model, ethanol is given in different ways. Zebrafish embryos are placed in 0.25–2% ethanol water, reaching internal levels ~25–30% of the bath. Chick embryos receive direct ethanol on the yolk or embryo (e.g., 20 μL of 1% or 125 μL of 20%). In mice, ethanol is given by injection or gavage (2.9–3.9 g/kg), producing blood levels of ~150–300 mg/dL (Kimmel et al. 1995; Godin et al. 2010; Lovely et al. 2014). Although the methods differ, they are designed to model human-like exposures during critical stages of development.

Animal studies have also demonstrated the importance of genetic variations in FASD (reviewed in (Eberhart and Parnell 2016; Ehrhart et al. 2019)). Another chapter in this book describes FASD models in more detail (Reid et al. 2026).

3.4 Link Between Ethanol Teratogenesis and Shh Signaling

Multiple pathways have been identified as molecular targets of ethanol teratogenesis following PAE (Eberhart and Parnell 2016), including differentiation-related pathways such as retinoic acid (RA) (reviewed in (Fainsod et al. 2020; Shabtai and Fainsod 2018)), Shh (Ahlgren et al. 2002), Wnt (Vangipuram and Lyman 2012), mitogen-activated protein kinase (Dou et al. 2013) and glycosylation defects (Binkhorst et al. 2012). Significant literature points to disruption of Shh signaling (Everson et al. 2020; Ahlgren et al. 2002; Aoto et al. 2008; Arenzana et al. 2006; Boa-Amponsem et al. 2020; Fish et al. 2019; Loucks and Ahlgren 2009; Yelin et al. 2007; Zhang et al. 2013b; Smith et al. 2014b; Sidik et al. 2021), a major morphogenic pathway regulating embryonic development, as a key mediator of PAE effects (summarized in Table 3.1). Shh signaling effectors such as the Gli transcription factors have been shown to be downregulated by ethanol during embryogenesis (Ahlgren et al. 2002; Zhang et al. 2013b). Comparable effects have been observed across species with ethanol perturbing Shh activity in chicken (Ahlgren et al. 2002), zebrafish (Loucks and Ahlgren 2009; Li et al. 2007; Zhang et al. 2011), and mouse (Yamada et al. 2005) embryos leading to ethanol-induced birth defects. A computational analysis of publicly available databases also implicated the Shh pathway as a candidate for FASD (Lombard et al. 2007).

Some of the earliest studies assessing a link between Shh and embryonic alcohol used the zebrafish model. Zebrafish embryos treated with ethanol (2.4%) for 3 h up to the early gastrula stage had a high frequency of cyclopia

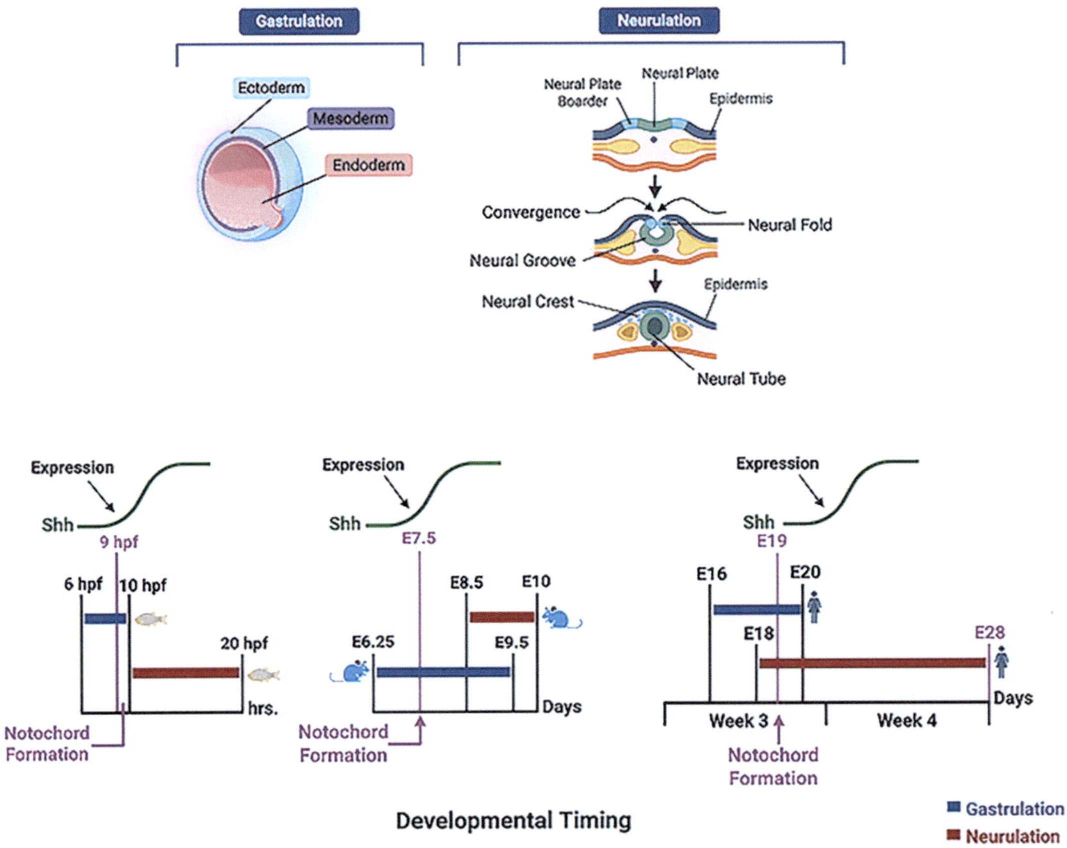

Fig. 3.2 *Developmental timing of Shh expression across three different FASD models and impact of PAE.* Upper: schematics of gastrulation and neurulation. Lower: green curves represent Shh expression relative to developmental events including gastrulation (blue bars), neurulation (red bars), and notochord formation (pink labels). Left panel: zebrafish development measured in hours post-fertilization (hpf). Middle panel: mouse development measured in embryonic days (E). Right panel: human development measured in embryonic days (E). Embryonic timing for zebrafish (Parnell and Eberhart 2023), mouse (Parnell and Eberhart 2023; Bardot and Hadjantonakis 2020; Zohn and Sarkar 2008), and human (Parnell and Eberhart 2023; Odent et al. 1999; de Bree et al. 2018; Muhr and Ackerman 2023)

accompanied by a loss of *shh* expression in the anterior brain (Blader and Strähle 1998). That ethanol can cause cyclopia in fish was observed as far back as 1910 (Stockard 1910), and has been reported in other vertebrates, including humans (Cohen Jr and Sulik 1992). A connection between the effects of PAE and Shh alterations was made due to observations of phenotypic similarities in craniofacial abnormalities resulting from both ethanol exposure and reduced Shh signaling (Ahlgren et al. 2002). In this study by Ahlgren et al. (2002), chick eggs were injected with ethanol and neural cranial cell death was observed. Further, an analysis of regulatory gene expression in chick embryos, 1 day after ethanol treatment at HH stage 9–10, found that in comparison to wingless-related integration site (*Wnt-1*) and fibroblast growth factor-8 (*Fgf-8*), the expression of Shh pathway genes including *Shh*, *Ptch*, and *Gli1-3* were drastically reduced by ethanol, whereas the expression of *Smo* was not impacted by ethanol (Ahlgren et al. 2002). Treatment with Shh-blocking antibody gave a comparable effect to ethanol (Ahlgren et al. 2002), and it was also demonstrated that overexpression of *Shh* (retroviral expression of Chick *Shh* at three-somite stage) could completely prevent the effects of ethanol on cell death (Ahlgren et al. 2002). More recently,

Table 3.1 Studies linking effects of PAE to Shh pathway disruption

Study	Model	Ethanol treatment dose and timing	Phenotype	Impact on Shh pathway	Reference
Ahlgren 2002	Chick	20 μl 1%; early development (HH stage 9–10);	Loss of cranial neural crest cells, reduced frontonasal mass, craniofacial abnormalities, increased apoptosis in neural crest	Reduced *Shh, Ptch, Gli1, Gli2*, and *Gli3* mRNA levels (2–eight fold); disrupted Shh signaling and caused neural crest cell death	Ahlgren et al. (2002)
Chrisman 2004	Mouse	2.9, 3.4, or 3.9 g/kg; E9.3 and E9.5	Dose-dependent limb defects: Apical ectodermal ridge (AER) disorganization, postaxial ectrodactyly, digit loss/fusion, ulna/carpal bone loss, preaxial AER loss at higher doses	Reduced *Shh* expression in the zone of polarizing activity (ZPA) and *Fgf8* in the AER, disrupting AER-ZPA signaling feedback	Chrisman et al. (2004)
Li 2007	Zebrafish	0.25–2.0%; embryo dome stage (4.25 hpf) for 6 h	Dose-dependent developmental defects including growth retardation, HPE, cyclopia, pericardial edema, U-shaped somites, and foreshortened tails	A dose-dependent decrease in Shh target gene expression (*ptc, gli1, nkx2.2*), reduced cholesterol-modified Shh levels, and impaired Hh signaling	Li et al. (2007)
Higashiyama 2007	Mouse	2 × 30 mL/kg (25%); GD 7	Holoprosencephalic malformations, including microcephaly, narrow face, short nose, single nostril, midfacial dysplasia, and missing midline commissural fibers	Down-regulation of *Shh* and *Nkx2.1* transcripts in ethanol-exposed embryos, observed through in situ hybridization	Higashiyama et al. (2007)
Loucks 2007	Zebrafish	1.5% (low) or 2.5% (high) at the dome stage (4 hpf) for 24 h	Cyclopia in 69% of embryos at high-dose exposure, reduced eye size, craniofacial defects, and shortened body length	Reduction of *gli1* expression, suppression of *six3b* and *dlx3b*, and disruption of early prechordal plate migration, leading to failure in eye field separation and neural crest development	Loucks et al. (2007)
Aoto 2008	Mouse	i.p. injections 2 × 25% (2.9 g /kg) on E7.0, 4 h apart	HPE, including severe midline defects, microcephaly, and facial malformations	Impaired *Shh* expression and induced apoptosis in prechordal mesendoderm (PME) cells, activated protein kinase A (PKA), and increased oxidative stress	Aoto et al. (2008)
Mao 2009	Zebrafish	Low levels (0, 0.2, 0.4, 0.6, and 0.8%) during gastrulation	Craniofacial malformations, growth retardation, and defects resembling FAS	Disrupts cholesterol modification of Shh, leading to defective intracellular transport from the Golgi to the plasma membrane. Shh accumulates in the cytoplasm, reducing secretion into the extracellular matrix and impairing hedgehog signaling	Mao et al. (2009)
Loucks 2009	Zebrafish	1.0%–2.5% at dome stage (4.3 hpf)	Dose-dependent reduction in body length, defects in notochord and somites, loss of muscle pioneer cells, axial shortening, cyclopia	Reduction in Shh signaling, affecting notochord and somite formation	Loucks and Ahlgren (2009)

(continued)

Table 3.1 (continued)

Study	Model	Ethanol treatment dose and timing	Phenotype	Impact on Shh pathway	Reference
Zhang 2011	Zebrafish	0.5%–1.5%; 6–24 hpf or 6–48 hpf	Microphthalmia, optic nerve hypoplasia, reduced eye size, and disrupted retinal lamination. Synergistic effects with agrin knockdown enhance severity	Reduced *agrin* expression, affecting *pax6a* and *mbx* expression. Disrupts Shh function, but Shh overexpression rescues microphthalmia	Zhang et al. (2011)
Hong 2012	Mouse	E7.0, 3.48 g/kg ethanol combined with *Cdon* mutation	Synergistic defects in early midline patterning, disruption of SHH signaling in the developing forebrain, and a range of HPE phenotypes	Reduced *Shh* expression in the ventral forebrain from the 14–15 somite stage onward, with reduced expression of Shh target genes (*Ptch1, Gli1, Nkx2.1*) in the ventral telencephalon	Hong and Krauss (2012)
Zhang 2013	Zebrafish	0.5%–2.0%; 6–10 hpf, 10–18 hpf, 6–24 hpf, 24–48 hpf, or 48–72 hpf	Disrupts forebrain and hindbrain development, affecting GABAergic and glutamatergic neurons	Perturbation of Shh signaling and fibroblast growth factor (Fgf) function, affecting neuronal survival and development	Zhang et al. (2013b)
Brennan 2013	Chick	125 μL of 20%; injected into yolk sac at HH stage 7 (peak ~0.294 g/dL)	Microphthalmia, disrupted optic vesicle to optic cup transition, abnormal lens and retina development	No change in *Shh* mRNA, but significant reduction in active Shh-N protein; downstream targets (*Ptch, Gli1, Gli3*) unaffected	Brennan and Giles (2013)
Kietzman 2014	Mouse	2 × 2.9 g/kg, on GD7 (4 h apart) in *Shh+/–* and *Gli2+/–* mutant mice	Exacerbated facial dysmorphology, including midfacial deficiency, exencephaly, median cleft lip, otocephaly, and proboscis; increased severity of HPE	Increased dysmorphology scores in *Shh+/–* and *Gli2+/–* fetuses by 3.2- and 6.6-fold; reduction in Shh and Gli2 function	Kietzman et al. (2014)
Zhang 2015	Zebrafish	0.5%, 6–24 hpf	Microphthalmia; disrupted midbrain–hindbrain boundary (MHB); reduced Pax6a expression in retina	Reduced Shh signaling; subthreshold *shh* morpholino (MO) combined with ethanol caused disrupted MHB formation; *shh* mRNA overexpression unable to rescue ethanol + RA MO-induced eye defects	Zhang et al. (2015)
Burton 2017	Zebrafish	1% and 3%, 8–10 hpf or 24–27 hpf	Microphthalmia, disrupted MHB, and altered anxiety-like behavior (increased risk-taking in novel tank test)	Disrupted Shh-dependent development, especially when combined with *shh* MO; *shh* mRNA rescued both morphology and behavior deficits	Burton et al. (2017)
Kahn 2017	Mouse	2 × 3.48 g/kg; E8.0, 4 h apart	Optic nerve hypoplasia (ONH)	Ethanol exposure and *Cdon–/–* mutation independently reduce Shh signaling in retinal progenitor cells (RPCs), causing decreased Gli1 expression, impaired RPC proliferation, precocious differentiation, and defective optic nerve axon extension	Kahn et al. (2017)

Fish 2019	Mouse	Low (1.4 g/kg) or high (2.8 g/kg), 2x at E8.0 & E8.25 ± cannabinoids (e.g., THC, HU-210, CP55,940)	Microphthalmia, coloboma, median facial defects, HPE-like brain malformations; eye defects worsened with combined EtOH + CBs	Ethanol and cannabinoids both inhibit Shh signaling; CBs act via CB1 receptor, directly suppressing Smo; reduced *Shh* and *Gli1* gene expression	Fish et al. (2019)
	Zebrafish	0.5% or 2% at shield stage (~6 hpf) ± cannabinoids	Cannabinoids exacerbate alcohol-induced eye and brain malformations	CBs and ethanol combined exposure amplify Shh pathway disruption	
	Shh-LIGHT2 cells	CBs ± Shh ligand	Inhibited Shh-induced luciferase activity	CBs suppress Gli-dependent transcription via CB1-Smo interaction	
Boa-Amponsem 2020	Zebrafish	0.5–1.0% at 8–10 hpf or 24–27 hpf; 1–3 mg/L ACEA (CB1R agonist); shh morpholino (0.3 pmol)	Microphthalmia when ethanol is combined with *shh* MO or high-dose ACEA; altered risk-taking behavior (e.g., reduced tank diving)	Ethanol + *shh* MO or ACEA suppress Shh signaling; disrupted Shh–Fgf crosstalk leads to reduced *fgf8* and *gad1* expression; *fgf8* mRNA rescues the defect	Boa-Amponsem et al. (2020)
Sidik 2021	Zebrafish	1% from 6 hpf (shield stage) for 24 h; ± 50 μM cyclopamine; ± 37.5 μM blebbistatin	Ethanol alone causes mild or no defects in wild type; causes cyclopia, midfacial hypoplasia, and severe facial defects in *vangl2* mutants or when combined with cyclopamine or blebbistatin	Ethanol does not directly suppress *shh* transcription, but disrupts convergent extension, leading to mislocalization of *shh* *(shha)* expression, impairing its signaling function during facial midline development	Sidik et al. (2021)
Boschen 2021	Mouse	2.9 g/kg × 2, 4 h apart, at E9.0	HPE, midfacial hypoplasia, hypotelorism, fused upper lip, narrow nostrils, and disrupted craniofacial morphology	Suppressed *Shh* mRNA expression in the ventral forebrain, reduces Shh target gene expression (*Gli1, Ptch1*), and disrupts ventral midline patterning	Boschen et al. (2021a)
Zhang 2023	Zebrafish	0.5–1.5% from 3 to 24 hpf; morpholino knockdown of *agrin* or *shh*; rescue with *shh* mRNA	Cardiac edema, microcephaly, reduced eye size	Disrupted expression of cardiac marker genes (*cmlc2, nkx2.5, vmhc*); loss of Shh signaling can be rescued by *shh* mRNA	Zhang et al. (2023)

zebrafish heterozygous for sonic hedgehog signaling molecule a (*shha*) were found to be more susceptible to ethanol-induced facial defects (Everson et al. 2020). Taken together these results implicated ethanol causing a loss in Shh ligand production.

3.5 PAE Prevents Correct Shh Processing

Ethanol exposure in zebrafish embryos during gastrulation prevents the C-terminal cholesterol esterification of Shh during post-translational processing, resulting in reduced membrane-associated Shh, decreased Shh signaling, and FASD-like phenotypes (e.g., HPE, cyclopia) (Li et al. 2007). In the same study, cholesterol supplementation restored the ethanol-suppressed Shh signaling and prevented the ethanol-induced defects at the molecular, cellular, and developmental stages (Li et al. 2007). In a follow-up study, the same group found that Shh associates with caveolin-1 in the Golgi to form complexes, which are then packaged in vesicles and transported to the plasma membrane within lipid raft microdomains. Ethanol exposure did not significantly impact *shh* mRNA translation or the trafficking of Shh from the ER to the Golgi apparatus. However, ethanol prevented Shh from entering the transport vesicles and specifically reduced the amount of the caveolin-1/Shh complex in lipid rafts. This disruption led to cytoplasmic accumulation of Shh and a deficiency in Shh ligand secretion into the extracellular matrix (Mao et al. 2009). Genetic defects in cholesterol synthesis also share similarities with the effects of PAE, with researchers linking both in part to alterations in Shh signaling (Guizzetti and Costa 2007; Guizzetti and Costa 2008).

3.6 Overlap of PAE and Shh Reduction Phenotypes

Shh signaling plays a crucial role in embryonic neural, craniofacial, and eye development (Cavodeassi et al. 2018; Chen et al. 2018; Cordero et al. 2004; Eberhart et al. 2006; Wang et al. 2013; Brennan and Giles 2014). Shh signaling alteration during development leads to varying effects depending on the extent of pathway interference, with severe cases potentially causing fatal brain developmental disorders like HPE (Arsić et al. 2007; Heyne et al. 2015, 2016; Edison and Muenke 2003; Belloni et al. 1996). The pathogenesis of HPE commonly involves mutations in *SHH* (Odent et al. 1999; Roessler et al. 1996) and its downstream activator *GLI2* (reviewed in (Lo et al. 2021a; Roessler and Muenke 2010; Roessler et al. 2003)), with severe HPE occurring in the absence of both *SHH* alleles (Houschyar et al. 2016; Ming and Muenke 1998). The phenotypic characteristics of FAS compare with those of HPE (Hong and Krauss 2012, 2017; Lipinski et al. 2010a; Sulik 1984; Abramyan 2019; Ronen and Andrews 1991), and children with severe FASD display mild characteristics of HPE (Sulik and Johnston 1983; Lo et al. 2021a).

Ethanol has consistently been shown to disrupt Shh signaling and interfere with the development of the eyes, face, and brain, structures that all originate from the anterior neural tube (Lanoue et al. 1997; Wallis and Muenke 2000; Zhang et al. 2001). Ethanol exposure at the gastrulation-stage strongly inhibits Shh activity (Ahlgren et al. 2002; Zhang et al. 2013b; Hong and Krauss 2012; Kahn et al. 2017; Boschen et al. 2021a), and appears to do this by inducing apoptosis of the cells within the presumptive notochord and ventral neural plate which will later produce Shh (Ahlgren et al. 2002; Dunty Jr et al. 2001; Lipinski et al. 2010b), resulting in the loss of Shh and the development of brain and craniofacial defects.

It is well known in mice, that FASD facial features and the associated forebrain abnormalities resemble those seen in the HPE spectrum (Ahlgren et al. 2002; Sulik and Johnston 1982), and that impaired Shh expression underlies the pathogenesis of ethanol-induced HPE (Aoto et al. 2008; Hong and Krauss 2012). In a mouse model of FASD (Higashiyama et al. 2007), gastrulation-stage (GD7) exposure to ethanol (two doses of ethanol, 30 mg/kg in total) resulted in reduced *Shh* expression at GD8.5 and midline structure defects at GD10.5. In pregnant mice exposed to ethanol at GD7, the severe midline defects seen in embryos at GD10.5 was accompanied by excessive apoptosis in the prechordal mesendoderm (PME, a tissue essential for ventro-median forebrain induction), decreased Shh expression, and increased PKA activity (Aoto et al. 2008). Pre-treatment with a PKA inhibitor (KT5720) blocked this ethanol-induced reduction in Shh protein expression and subsequent apoptosis in the PME (Aoto et al. 2008). Furthermore, administration of anti-oxidants such as vitamin C and E to mouse embryos blocked the reduction in Shh expression caused by ethanol, with vitamin E reducing the incidence of ethanol-induced birth defects in early gestation (Aoto et al. 2008).

Mice with genetic disruptions of Shh pathway components, including *Cdon*, *Ptch2*, and *Gli1/2*, produce embryos with increased susceptibility to the effects of PAE, including increases in HPE and limb defects (Hong and Krauss 2012; Kietzman et al. 2014; Kahn et al. 2017; Heyne et al. 2015; Lo et al. 2021a; Fish et al. 2017a) (summarized in Table 3.2). While mice with single *Gli2* loss were comparable to wild-type, exposure to low-dose ethanol resulted in severe HPE phenotype (Kietzman et al. 2014). In a mouse strain (129S6) previously shown to be resistant to the teratogenic effects of ethanol (Downing et al. 2009), mutating the Shh co-receptor *Cdon*, sensitized the mice to the effects of PAE (given at E7) resulting in HPE-related phenotypes (assessed at E10 to E19) (Hong and Krauss 2012). Interestingly, the *Cdon*$^{-/-}$ mice themselves showed no obvious HPE-like phenotype (Hong and Krauss 2012). Further, the expression levels of *Shh*, *Ptch1*, *Fgf-8*, and *Gli1* were reduced in the ventral forebrains of the PAE-treated *Cdon*$^{-/-}$ embryos compared to controls (Hong and Krauss 2012). In a follow up study, Hong and Krauss (2012) showed that this HPE-induced phenotype in PAE-treated *Cdon*$^{-/-}$ mice could be rescued by reducing *Ptch1* gene dosage (Hong and Krauss 2013). They showed that ethanol exposed *Cdon*$^{-/-}$;*Ptch1*$^{+/-}$ embryos had significantly less HPE phenotypes compared to the *Cdon*$^{-/-}$;*Ptch1*$^{+/+}$ embryos (15% versus 65%) (Hong and Krauss 2013). The ethanol exposed *Cdon*$^{-/-}$;*Ptch1*$^{+/-}$ embryos also had less reduced *Shh* expression (Hong and Krauss 2013). Thus, decreasing the repression of the Shh pathway was able to mitigate the effects of PAE in these *Cdon*$^{-/-}$ mice.

In another mouse strain (C57BL/6 J), loss of both copies of *Gli2* results in embryos with characteristic HPE features including altered ventral forebrain patterning (observed at GD15) (Heyne et al. 2016). Treatment of wild-type mice at GD7.75 with the Smo inhibitor vismodegib (Gould et al. 2014), produced craniofacial and brain defects comparable to those seen in the *Gli2*$^{-/-}$ fetuses (Heyne et al. 2016). The authors suggested that the defects seen in *Gli2*$^{-/-}$ fetuses are due in part to changes in the cells that respond to Shh signaling during early neurulation (Heyne et al. 2016).

Treating pregnant mice with ethanol at GD8 led to defects in optic nerve development (Kahn et al. 2017). The same was seen in the *Cdon*$^{-/-}$ embryos with the conclusion that both effects occur through a comparable pathogenic mechanism involving Shh pathway inhibition (Kahn et al. 2017). In the same study, while *Gli1* expression was disrupted in the developing eye in PAE-treated or *Cdon*$^{-/-}$ embryos, *Shh* was not altered (Kahn et al. 2017). Interestingly, and in contrast to the HPE phenotype seen in ethanol-treated *Cdon*$^{-/-}$ embryos (Hong and Krauss 2012), the optic nerve hypoplasia phenotype was not exacerbated by the effect of PAE in *Cdon*$^{-/-}$ embryos (Kahn et al. 2017). Hong and Krauss (2017) also found that, t-butyl alcohol (which does not impact alcohol dehydrogenase (ADH)), also induces HPE phenotypes in the same *Cdon*$^{-/-}$ PAE model, and hence concluded that ethanol itself rather than a metabolite of ethanol is an HPE-inducing teratogen (Hong and Krauss 2017). This same team found that *Cdon*$^{-/-}$ embryos treated with ethanol had decreased expression of target genes induced by Nodal (Hong et al. 2020), a morphogen that acts upstream of Shh (Robertson 2014; Shen 2007), and indicated that Cdon also regulates Nodal signaling (Hong et al. 2020). Nodal signaling facilitates the development of the prechordal plate (PCP) from the anterior primitive streak (APS) (Robertson 2014; Shen 2007) (the APS

Table 3.2 Shh pathway-related genes shown to modulate the effects of PAE

Study	PAE Model	Gene	Impact on PAE	Impact on Shh pathway	Reference
Hong 2012, 2013, 2016	Mouse	*Cdon*	Combined loss of *Cdon* and ethanol exposure caused severe HPE, including midfacial anomalies, single nostril, hypotelorism, and agnathia, whereas loss of *Cdon* or ethanol alone had little effect	Ethanol-treated *Cdon−/−* embryos showed reduced Shh expression and target gene (*Ptch1, Gli1, Nkx2.1*) levels in the ventral forebrain, leading to defective rostroventral midline patterning and delayed Shh induction	Hong and Krauss (2012 and Hong and Krauss (2013)
Fish 2017	Mouse	*Shh*	Heterozygous *Shh+/−* embryos had a significantly higher incidence and severity of ethanol-induced limb defects, including oligodactyly, interdigital spacing, and missing digits	Ethanol exposure in *Shh+/−* embryos exacerbated forelimb defects, likely by disrupting Shh expression in the zone of polarizing activity (ZPA) during limb development	Fish et al. (2017a)
Fish 2017	Mouse	*Gli2*	Heterozygous *Gli2+/−* embryos exhibited a significantly increased incidence of ethanol-induced forelimb defects, including digit deletions and altered limb morphology	Ethanol exposure in *Gli2+/−* embryos exacerbated limb defects, likely due to impaired *Shh* signaling downstream of *Gli2*	Fish et al. (2017a)
Boschen, 2018	Mouse	*Mns1*	Knockdown of *Mns1* significantly increased susceptibility to ethanol-induced ocular, craniofacial, and CNS defects, including microphthalmia, cleft palate, and holoprosencephaly	Not directly measured; likely disrupted Shh signaling indirectly via defective motile cilia function, affecting morphogen gradients during gastrulation	Boschen et al. (2018)
Everson 2020	Zebrafish	*Shha*	*Shha* heterozygotes developed craniofacial defects (e.g., midfacial cartilage abnormalities) only when exposed to ethanol or PBO; co-exposure caused synergistic increases in defect severity	Ethanol and PBO exposure in shha mutants impaired midline craniofacial development, indicating sensitization to disrupted hedgehog signaling	Everson et al. (2020)
Boschen, 2021	Mouse	*Kif3a*	Partial loss (*Kif3a+/−*) exacerbated behavioral effects of neurulation-stage alcohol exposure (NAE), including increased hyperactivity and reduced habituation in adolescent mice	*Kif3a* knockdown disrupts primary cilia function, impairs Gli processing, and enhances NAE-induced Shh pathway suppression (e.g., reduced *Shh, Gli1*, altered Gli3 ratios)	Boschen et al. (2021a)
Fish, 2024	Mouse	*Efcab7*	Deletion of *Efcab7* significantly increased the severity of alcohol-induced eye and craniofacial malformations, including anophthalmia and midline facial defects	*Efcab7* deletion impaired Smo-mediated Shh signaling; increased sensitivity to the Shh antagonist vismodegib, and reduced responsiveness to SAG	Fish et al. (2024)

emerges at ~E6.5 around the onset of gastrulation). The PCP is the region from which Shh is subsequently produced, leading to patterning events generating the forebrain (Cordero et al. 2004). The same authors using the *Cdon*$^{-/-}$ model (Hong et al. 2020), suggested that the period of sensitivity to ethanol for inducing HPE defects, which is short and ends by E7.5, overlaps with Nodal-induced specification and occurs prior to Shh expression and induction of midline patterning.

3.7 Timing of Shh Pathway Expression During Development and the Impact of PAE

In terms of timing for the development of zebrafish embryos, Shh acts at the end of gastrulation (~10 h post-fertilization, hpf) (Fig. 3.2 shows embryonic Shh expression timing in zebrafish, mice, and humans), with the ventral presumptive brain serving as a crucial source of Shh (Eberhart et al. 2006). The *shh* expression occurs in the notochord (Muller et al. 1999), which forms around 9–10 hpf (Kimmel et al. 1995; Glickman et al. 2003). At the end of gastrulation (10–10.33 hpf), *shh* expression is observed in the ventral neural keel (Krauss et al. 1993; Ekker et al. 1995; Graf et al. 2015; Hammerschmidt et al. 1996a; Okuda et al. 2010), which forms around 8–10 hpf (Van Slyke et al. 2014), in the axis region (Krauss et al. 1993; Cardozo et al. 2014), neural plate and ectoderm (Norton et al. 2005), and presumptive floor plate (Ekker et al. 1995). In this model, the cells of the ventral neural tube would function as the responding cells, and at 10 hpf, *smo* appears in the neural plate and axial mesoderm with higher levels seen in presumptive head and tail regions (Chen et al. 2001). In untreated zebrafish embryos, *shh* expression peaks around 12 hpf and remains strong at 24 hpf (Burton et al. 2022), which aligns with other published findings on the widespread dynamic expression of the Shh pathway during zebrafish development (Eberhart et al. 2006; Bergeron et al. 2008; Karlstrom et al. 2003; Mich et al. 2014; Schwend et al. 2010; Xu et al. 2006; Yu et al. 2006) (Fig. 3.2). Additionally, using a Shh:GFP zebrafish transgenic model (Yu et al. 2006; Albert et al. 2003), it was observed that the expression of *shh* was at 9–10 hpf with a peak around 16–17 hpf, decreasing in the next several hours (Yu et al. 2006), with expression persisting out to 72 hpf (Schwend and Ahlgren 2009). Using a comparable Gli-luciferase reporter model in mice, it was found that Shh pathway activity was measurable at E9.5 while spatially restricted, detectable in somites at E10.5 and at E11.5 strongly expressed in the midbrain and developing limbs (Hernández-García et al. 2019).

In a zebrafish model, ethanol given at 8–10 hpf reduced *shh* mRNA expression for at least 24 h following exposure (Burton et al. 2022). In the same study, Burton et al. (2022) did not observe a significant effect of ethanol exposure on *smo* mRNA expression for the same time period. *Smo* expression in untreated embryos first appeared and peaked around 8 hpf with expression gradually decreasing out to 24 hpf. *Smo* expression in zebrafish is very dynamic during early development (Chen et al. 2001; Varga et al. 2001), with embryonic *smo* mRNA first detectable around 5–6 hpf. Hence, similar to the chick study of Ahlgren et al. (2002) described above (Ahlgren et al. 2002), it was found that ethanol exposure in zebrafish embryos during gastrulation at 8–10 hpf significantly decreases *shh* expression while having much less effect on *smo* expression (Burton et al. 2022), with the implication that ethanol is having a more direct effect on Shh-secreting cells rather than Shh-responding cells.

3.8 Impact of PAE on Limb Development: Disruption of Shh Signaling

As mentioned above, the Shh signaling pathway influences several distinct developing organs, such as the brain (Tichy et al. 2015), and also the limb bud (reviewed in (Tickle and Towers 2017)). Ethanol's impact on limb development is comparable across species. The formation of the limb bud and then digits shares similarities in mice, chick, fish, and humans, involving an RA/Fgf/Shh signaling cascade (Pathi et al. 2001; Mercader 2007; Prykhozhij and Neumann 2008; Ingham 1994). The period of limb bud initiation and digit specification is when the limbs are most vulnerable to the effects of ethanol, and in the mouse, this occurs at early neurulation

(~E9.25-9.75) (Fig. 3.2) (Johnson et al. 2007). Ethanol exposure in pregnant mice at GD9.25 disrupts limb patterning (Kotch et al. 1992) by reducing the expression of *Fgf-8* in the apical ectodermal ridge (AER), and *Shh* in the zone of polarizing activity (ZPA) (Chrisman et al. 2004). RA antagonism causes limb defects that morphologically resemble those caused by ethanol and are comparable to the deficits caused by impaired Shh signaling (Johnson et al. 2007). In mice lacking one copy of *Shh* or the Shh transcription factor *Gli2*, ethanol treatment at GD9.25 caused a higher incidence of limb defects, as compared to wild-type (Fish et al. 2017a). Studies also showed in mice that acute maternal treatment with a Shh pathway activator (Smo agonist, SAG) (Frank-Kamenetsky et al. 2002; Chen et al. 2002a), when administered to dams at GD9.25 of pregnancy, increases Shh signaling and affects limb development (Fish et al. 2017b).

3.9 Currently Identified Mechanisms for How Ethanol Impacts Shh Activity: Direct or Indirect?

Understanding how ethanol causes birth defects presents an obvious challenge in the field, with several questions in a gap analysis review posed (Ehrhart et al. 2019), including in particular: what are the downstream consequences of gene expression changes due to embryonic ethanol exposure, and can genetic or pharmacological approaches mitigate the consequences of ethanol exposure? Embryonic ethanol can cause a systemic downregulation of gene expression impacting protein synthesis and chromatin remodeling (Rogic et al. 2016).

As discussed above, whether ethanol directly or indirectly impacts Shh signaling remains unclear (Eberhart and Parnell 2016). A number of mechanisms have been investigated for how ethanol impacts Shh signaling (reviewed in (Eberhart and Parnell 2016)), including decreased Shh ligand levels due to ethanol preventing C-terminal cholesterol esterification of Shh during post-translational processing (Li et al. 2007), increase of inhibitory mechanisms such as PKA activation (Aoto et al. 2008), and ethanol-induced cell death in cells that express Shh and/or in cells that respond to Shh.

In addition, a number of studies indicate the effects of ethanol on development occur due to inhibition of RA (reviewed in (Fainsod et al. 2020; Shabtai and Fainsod 2018)), a critical morphogen during development (Cunningham and Duester 2015), involved in craniofacial (Wu et al. 2022) and anterior-posterior patterning. RA is necessary for inducing *Shh* expression in the notochord and neural plate (Wilson et al. 2003), and alterations in RA levels can impact Shh signaling (Power et al. 1999). It was proposed by several groups (Yelin et al. 2007; Duester 1991; Pullarkat 1991; Deltour et al. 1996; Kot-Leibovich and Fainsod 2009; Clugston and Blaner 2012) that during development ethanol acts as a competitive inhibitor of ADH, an enzyme involved in converting retinol to RA (reviewed in (Duester 1999)), which results in decreased RA leading to the defects associated with PAE. This ethanol-mediated reduction in RA signaling is significant during late blastula/early gastrulation (Kot-Leibovich and Fainsod 2009), inducing changes in the expression of RA-responsive genes (Yelin et al. 2005), subsequently leading to embryonic dysmorphology.

Studies in zebrafish have implicated a role for the proteoglycan agrin, shh, fgf8/19, and RA in the teratogenicity of ethanol, with expression of the shh pathway marker *gli1* reduced (Zhang et al. 2013b, 2015). Ethanol exposure in zebrafish embryos reduces the expression of agrin (Zhang et al. 2011), a heparan sulfate proteoglycan that binds Fgfs and Shh (Cotman et al. 1999). Reducing agrin expression using morpholinos in combination with ethanol produced a small eye phenotype in embryos that could be rescued by *Shh* mRNA overexpression (Zhang et al. 2011). The authors suggested that ethanol mediated reduction in agrin impacts Shh signaling (Zhang et al. 2011). Disruption of *shh* and *fgf* in zebrafish embryos leads to FASD phenotypes such as microphthalmia and disrupted midbrain-hindbrain boundary (MHB) (Zhang et al. 2013b). In a follow-up study (Zhang et al.

2017), the same group observed that while zebrafish embryos chronically exposed to ethanol (2% from 6 to 24 hpf) or injected with *shh* morpholino (MO) had MHB disruption and reduced paired box protein pax-6 (*pax6a*) expression (a marker of eye and forebrain development as previously seen (Zhang et al. 2011; Zhang et al. 2015)), the expression levels of MHB markers such as *pax2a* and *fgf-8a* remained unchanged (Zhang et al. 2017). The authors suggested that the lack of effect on these markers indicates ethanol may act downstream of these genes (Zhang et al. 2017).

In a number of PAE studies, however, ethanol does not appear to affect Shh pathway readouts such as *Gli1* and *Ptch* (Sidik et al. 2021), suggesting an indirect effect of ethanol (Sidik et al. 2021). In a chick eye model, it was observed that while ethanol affected Shh production, downstream effectors of Shh were unchanged (Brennan and Giles 2013). Sidik et al. (2021) undertook an RNA Seq study on single zebrafish embryos and found that ethanol minimally affects the transcriptome (Sidik et al. 2021). The same authors concluded from their study, including in situ analysis, that ethanol indirectly affects Shh signaling and acts to mis-localize the source of Shh (Sidik et al. 2021).

Several studies have assessed the teratogenic effects of the Shh pathway modulators that directly target Smo (Chiang et al. 1996; Boschen et al. 2021a; Heyne et al. 2015; Lipinski et al. 2010a; Fish et al. 2017b; Lipinski et al. 2014). Small molecule antagonists of the Shh pathway such as the natural product cyclopamine (Chen et al. 2002a; Chen et al. 2002b; Taipale et al. 2000) and the synthetic drug vismodegib that specifically target SMO (Fig. 3.3), have significant detrimental effects when given during mouse development, comparable to that of PAE (Heyne et al. 2015; Lipinski et al. 2014). When given to zebrafish embryos during gastrulation, cyclopamine disrupted Shh signaling and neural crest condensation (Eberhart et al. 2006). As mentioned above, facial and neural phenotypes seen with FAS look like those resulting from disrupted Shh signaling during development, including effects caused by Shh pathway antagonists (Heyne et al. 2015; Lipinski et al. 2010a), again emphasizing a connection between Shh pathway and FASD (Eberhart and Parnell 2016).

Using zebrafish embryos, the effects of a direct Shh inhibitor were compared to an indirect Shh inhibitor forskolin (activates adenylate kinase and PKA, which acts to inhibit Shh signaling (Hammerschmidt et al. 1996b), and to ethanol, with treatments beginning just before gastrulation (4 hpf) and continuing through 24 hpf (Loucks et al. 2007). All these treatments produced cyclopia, and while all three reduced *gli1* expression, the timing and level of inhibition varied. Furthermore, each exposure resulted in a different set of eye and head development-related molecular changes (Loucks et al. 2007).

Using a transgenic zebrafish with a fluorescent Shh reporter (glib:mCherry) in which Hh-responding cells fluoresce red when active, embryos (6 to 24 hpf) were exposed to a Shh inhibitor or ethanol. Significant reductions of glib:mCherry fluorescence appeared at inhibitor concentrations >3.125 μM and at ethanol concentrations of 1.25% and 1.5% (Everson et al. 2023), perhaps suggesting a more direct impact of ethanol on Shh signaling.

In a sea urchin model, an organism with a simpler patterning system than the typical FASD animal models, ethanol exposure to embryos causes skeletal defects comparable to those seen in FASD (Rodríguez-Sastre et al. 2023). While Shh signaling plays a role in skeletal patterning in sea urchins (Walton et al. 2009), Shh activation (by SAG) failed to rescue the ethanol-induced defects in sea urchin embryos, leading the authors to conclude that Shh signaling was not relevant for this effect (Rodríguez-Sastre et al. 2023).

3.10 Some Effects of PAE Can Be Mitigated by Shh Pathway Activation

FASD is considered largely irreversible, as it causes significant damage during embryogenesis, including to essential developmental pathways

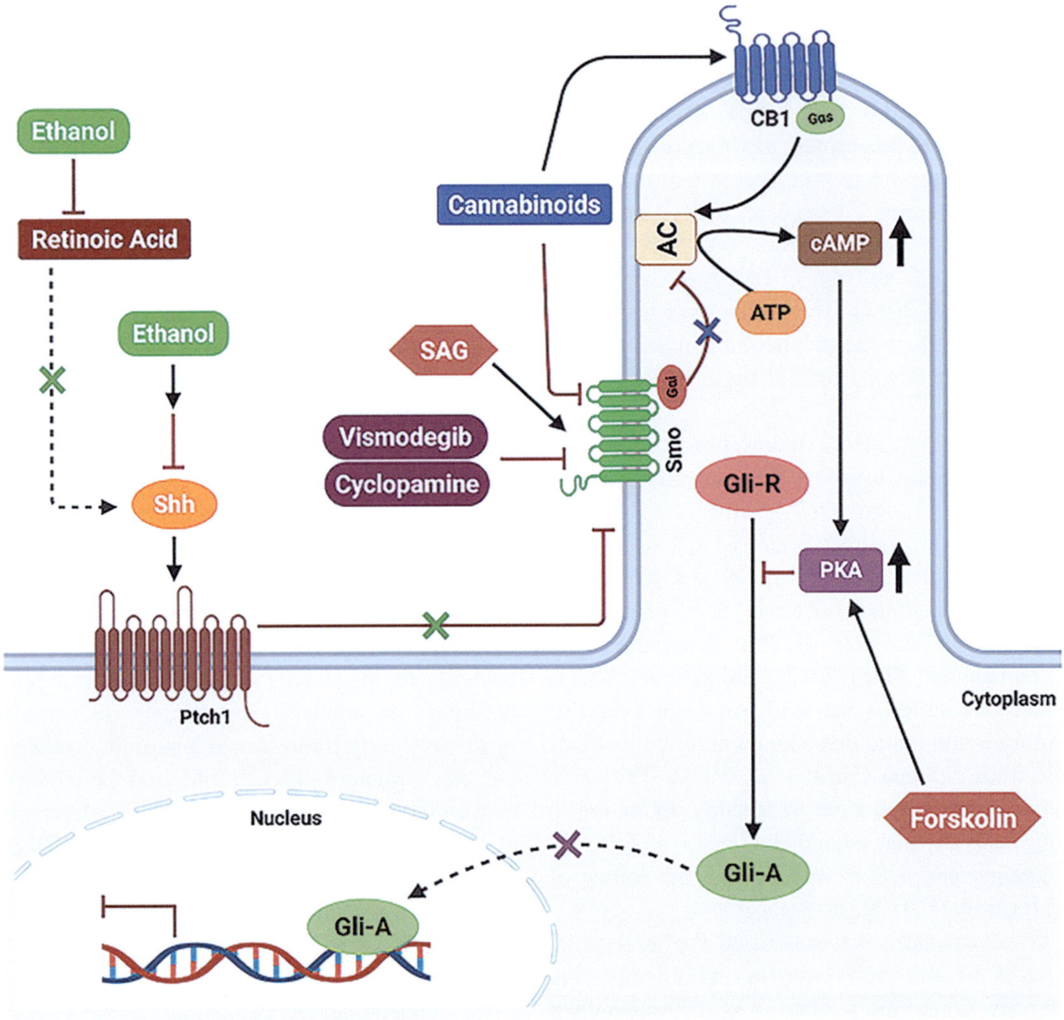

Fig. 3.3 *The teratogenic effects of PAE and Smo inhibitors/cannabinoids occur due to differing effects on developmental Shh signaling.* CB1 receptors are activated via the binding of cannabinoids, modulating cAMP signaling through adenylyl cyclase (AC) and ATP, while ethanol inhibits Shh signaling through Patched1 (Ptch1) receptors. Both pathways converge on Gli transcription factors in the nucleus, with PKA serving as a regulatory intermediate. Pharmacological modulators including vismodegib, cyclopamine, SAG, and forskolin are shown at their respective targets in the signaling cascade

(Ramsay 2010). However, several studies have shown that activating the Shh pathway, either genetically or pharmacologically, can mitigate some of the key effects of PAE. The effects of multiple agonists and regulators of Shh signaling are summarized in Table 3.3 and Fig. 3.4. A number of genes related to the Shh pathway and other growth factors have been identified as either protective or are associated with greater susceptibility to PAE in various FASD models (McCarthy et al. 2013; Hong and Krauss 2012; Kietzman et al. 2014) (see Table 3.2). In zebrafish FASD models, pre-injecting *shh* mRNA at the single-cell stage (Burton et al. 2017; Loucks and Ahlgren 2009; Zhang et al. 2011, 2013b) reversed many morphological and behavioral abnormalities associated with PAE. The observation in zebrafish embryos that overexpression of

Table 3.3 Genetic and pharmacological studies targeting Shh pathway shown to modulate the effects of PAE

Study	PAE model	Treatment	Impact on PAE	Impact on Shh pathway	Reference
Alhgren 2002	Chick	*Shh* overexpression	Rescued cranial neural crest cell survival; restored frontonasal mass size; recovered Shh signaling pathway	Not directly measured at the molecular level; functional rescue of ethanol-induced defects suggests pathway activity was restored	Ahlgren et al. (2002)
Li 2007	Zebrafish	Cholesterol	Prevented FASD-like morphological defects; restored normal phenotype in 94.8% of treated embryos; rescued slow muscle progenitor development	Restored Hh signaling activity; normalized expression of *ptc*, *gli1*, and *nkx2.2*, and recovered Shh membrane localization	Li et al. (2007)
Aoto 2008	Mouse	Vitamin E	Reduced incidence of ethanol-induced HPE from 25% to 5.2%, prevented midline defects, and rescued craniofacial development	Blocked ethanol-induced Shh protein reduction, restored *Shh* expression in prechordal mesendoderm (PME) cells	Aoto et al. (2008)
Aoto 2008	Mouse	PKA inhibitor	Prevented ethanol-induced apoptosis in anterior PME cells, rescued craniofacial development	Blocked ethanol-induced activation of PKA, restored Shh protein expression in PME cells, and prevented ethanol-induced suppression of Shh signaling	Aoto et al. (2008)
Hong 2013	Mouse	Reducing *Ptch1*	Decreased penetrance of ethanol-induced HPE from 65% to 15%, significantly reducing midline defects and craniofacial abnormalities	Restored *Shh* and *Nkx2.1* expression in the ventral forebrain, preventing ethanol-induced suppression of Shh signaling and improving midline patterning	Hong and Krauss (2013)
Loucks and Ahlgren 2009, Zhang, Turton et al. 2011, Zhang, Ojiaku et al. 2013, Burton, Zhang et al. 2017, Zhang, Ezem et al. 2023	Zebrafish	*Shh* mRNA overexpression	Rescued ethanol-induced developmental defects, including craniofacial (cyclopia, microphthalmia), neural (GABAergic and glutamatergic neuron deficits, microcephaly), midbrain-hindbrain boundary (MHB) abnormalities, cardiac defects (cardiac edema, abnormal marker gene expression), and behavioral changes (altered anxiety-like behavior, reduced tank diving)	Restored Shh signaling activity, reversing ethanol-induced disruptions in body axis patterning, CNS development, eye formation, and cardiac gene expression. Prevented ethanol-induced suppression of key Shh target genes (*mbx*, *pax6a*, *gli1*, *fgf19*), ensuring normal neural, cardiac, and behavioral development	Burton et al. (2017, Loucks and Ahlgren (2009), Zhang et al. (2013b), Zhang et al. (2011) and Zhang et al. (2023)

(continued)

Table 3.3 (continued)

Study	PAE model	Treatment	Impact on PAE	Impact on Shh pathway	Reference
Zhang 2013	Zebrafish	Fgf8	Rescued ethanol-induced reduction in GABAergic (*GAD1*) and glutamatergic (*atonal1a*) neuron development in forebrain and cerebellum	Did not directly measure; *fgf8* restored downstream neuronal markers *gad1*, which are partly regulated by Shh signaling	Zhang et al. (2013b)
Muralidharan, Sarmah et al. 2015, Zhang, Anderson et al. 2015	Zebrafish	Retinoic acid	Rescued ethanol-induced retinal and brain defects, including optic nerve hypoplasia, photoreceptor differentiation defects, and midbrain-hindbrain boundary (MHB) disruption. Restored normal retinal morphogenesis, optic nerve width, and prevented microphthalmia	Restored Shh signaling activity, reversing ethanol-induced suppression in retinal and midbrain-hindbrain development. Rescued Shh target gene expression but did not rescue ocular defects caused by direct Shh inhibition, indicating partial pathway interaction	Zhang et al. (2015) and Muralidharan et al. (2015)
Muralidharan, Sarmah et al. 2015, Cadena, Cadena et al. 2020	Zebrafish	Folic acid	Rescued ethanol-induced retinal and morphological defects, including optic nerve hypoplasia, photoreceptor differentiation abnormalities, eye, heart, and swim bladder defects, and improved behavioral outcomes such as sleep, locomotion, thigmotaxis, and visual response	Not directly measured; no evidence of direct Shh pathway modulation	Cadena et al. (2020) and Muralidharan et al. (2015)
Burton 2022	Zebrafish	SAG, purmorphamine	Rescued ethanol-induced microphthalmia, MHB defects, and abnormal risk-taking behavior in juvenile zebrafish	Restored Shh downstream genes *gli1, gli2*, and *pax6a* expression suppressed by ethanol; rescued Shh signaling activity through SMO agonism	Burton et al. (2022)
Fish 2022	Mouse (C57BL/6 J)	Bax−/−	Reduced alcohol-induced eye, facial, and brain defects, including microphthalmia and FAS-like facial dysmorphology; almost complete protection from ethanol-induced apoptosis in the cranial ectoderm	Not directly measured; authors suggest reduced apoptosis may help preserve Shh signaling	Fish et al. (2022)

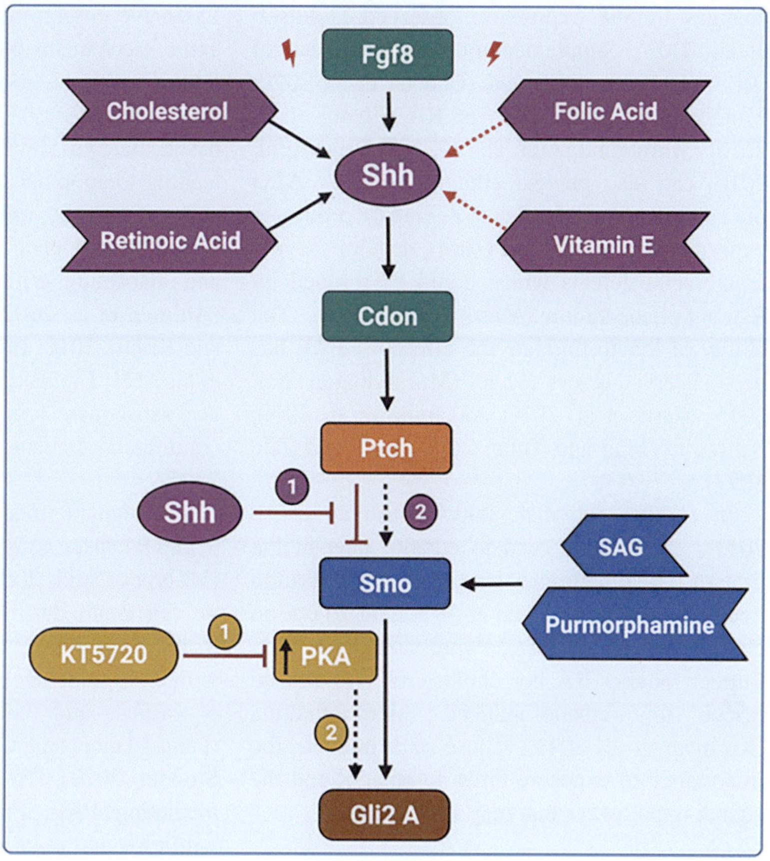

Fig. 3.4 *Treatments that rescue or mitigate the PAE impairment of Shh signaling.* The diagram shows upstream modulators (cholesterol, folic acid, retinoic acid, and vitamin E) that activate Shh, and downstream targets such as Smoothened (Smo), which can be stimulated by SAG and purmorphamine. KT5720 inhibits Protein Kinase A (PKA), potentially restoring pathway activity through Gli2 activation, that mediates the transcriptional response necessary for rescuing Shh pathway function

Shh or fgf-8/fgf-19 rescues FASD phenotypes suggests cross talk between these pathways affected by ethanol (Zhang et al. 2011, 2013b, 2017). Reducing *Ptch1* gene expression rescued the heightened susceptibility of Cdon−/− mice to embryonic ethanol exposure (Hong and Krauss 2013). Similarly, introducing a retrovirus expressing *Shh* into three-somite stage chick embryos before ethanol exposure successfully prevented ethanol-induced neural crest cell death (Ahlgren et al. 2002).

Burton et al. (2022) showed that treatment of zebrafish embryos with small molecule Smo agonists that activate Shh signaling (SAG (Frank-Kamenetsky et al. 2002; Chen et al. 2002a) or purmorphamine (Wu et al. 2002), Fig. 3.3), reduced the severity of ethanol-induced developmental malformations, including changes in eye size and midline brain development. In this model, researchers treated zebrafish embryos with acute ethanol 8–10 hpf and then with SAG before (6–8 hpf) or after ethanol exposure (10–12 hpf) (Burton et al. 2022). This rescue effect depended on dose and occurred primarily when treatment was specifically administered after ethanol exposure. Embryos treated with SAG post-ethanol exposure showed restoration of markers of Shh signaling (*gli1/2*) and eye development (*pax6a*). In juvenile (adolescent) zebrafish, it was shown that embryonic ethanol exposure also produces neurobehavioral impairment (Burton et al. 2017). Embryonic SAG treatment also mitigated ethanol-induced neurodevelop-mental deficits related to anxiety and risk-taking behavior in juvenile fish (Burton et al. 2022). These findings suggested that direct pharmacological activation of canonical Shh signaling at specific developmental stages significantly reduces the severity of alcohol-induced birth defects (Burton et al. 2022).

In mice, RA administration can diminish the ethanol-induced limb defects with appropriate changes in *Shh* expression observed (Johnson et al. 2007). Supplementation with cholesterol (Li et al. 2007), folic acid (Cadena et al. 2020; Muralidharan et al. 2015) or RA (Zhang et al. 2015; Muralidharan et al. 2015; Marrs et al. 2010) can also prevent ethanol-induced FASD phenotypes in zebrafish. Zebrafish embryos exposed to ethanol (3–24 hpf) develop severe craniofacial defects which could be rescued by RA supplementation (Marrs et al. 2010). The ability of RA to mitigate the effects of PAE has been observed across species (Muralidharan et al. 2015; Marrs et al. 2010; Akšamija et al. 2009; Satiroglu-Tufan and Tufan 2004; Twal and Zile 1997).

In another zebrafish study (Kashyap et al. 2011), embryos exposed to ethanol later at the time of retinal neurogenesis (24–48 hpf) develop microphthalmia (analyzed at 48 and 72 h) but no changes in *Shh* or *Ptch2* expression were seen. Further, neither RA nor cholesterol was able to rescue this ethanol-induced microphthalmia (Kashyap et al. 2011). These data indicate the importance of exposure times to ethanol and the signaling pathways that may be impacted.

3.11 Embryonic Ethanol Exposure Causes Cell Death Leading to Reduced Shh Expression

In early development, ethanol exposure triggers apoptotic cell death in specific regions of the embryo, resulting in malformations in adult life (Sulik et al. 1981; Sulik and Johnston 1983; Sulik 1984, 2005). Ethanol exposure at the gastrulation stage initiates pathogenic cascades that lead to the craniofacial and brain dysmorphologies characteristic of FAS, with excessive ectodermal cell death being the first identified pathogenic mechanism (Sulik et al. 1981). During gastrulation, which takes place in the third week of human pregnancy (Fig. 3.2), ethanol impacts the ectoderm, the precursor to the eyes, face, and brain. The loss of midline tissue during this stage contributes to craniofacial dysmorphologies, such as microphthalmia and a smooth philtrum, which are typical features of FAS. Extensive embryonic cell death is a key pathogenic mechanism behind the defects caused by PAE. During the gastrulation stage (GD 17–20 in human pregnancy), PAE targets the ectodermal tissue that will develop into the face and brain, leading to apoptosis (Dunty Jr et al. 2001) of the cells within the presumptive notochord and/or ventral neural plate that will later produce Shh, and disrupting critical cell signaling pathways (Ahlgren et al. 2002; Zhang et al. 2013b; Hong and Krauss 2012; Boschen et al. 2021a; Dunty Jr et al. 2001; Lipinski et al. 2010b). This apoptosis and subsequent loss of Shh results in brain and craniofacial defects characteristic of FAS (Sulik 2005).

In pregnant mice, ethanol exposure at GD7, 8, and 9 causes apoptosis within hours in specific cell types (Sulik 2005). Ethanol-induced apoptotic cell death during the gastrulation stage is a major contributing factor to craniofacial defects with embryonic apoptosis mediated by activation of caspase and the pro-apoptotic effector *Bax* (Peña-Blanco and García-Sáez 2018; Voss and Strasser 2020). To assess the role of *Bax* in mediating PAE, Fish et al. (2022) compared wild-type and mice with full *Bax* deletions (Fish et al. 2022). Pregnant mice were exposed to ethanol at GD7 and embryos assessed 12 h later for apoptotic cell death (Kotch and Sulik 1992) and at GD17 for FAS phenotypes (Fish et al. 2022). In $Bax^{+/+}$ mice, as seen previously (Dunty Jr et al. 2001), ectodermal cell death was observed in embryos indicating a loss of cells that give rise to the forebrain and eyes (Fish et al. 2022).

In particular, they demonstrated that removing both copies of the pro-apoptotic *Bax* gene completely prevented the effects of gastrulation-stage ethanol exposure, including reducing apoptotic cell death and providing nearly complete protection from ethanol-induced eye defects (Fish et al. 2022). With Bax's apoptotic role at the gastrulation stage embryo, the authors speculated whether certain cell phenotypes are either protected from or remain vulnerable to ethanol-induced cell death (Fish et al. 2022). PAE may initiate apoptosis via Tp53 activation (Anthony et al. 2008; Flentke et al. 2019; Huang et al. 2024), and mice with Tp53 genetically knocked-out are protected from PAE (Fish et al. 2021). In the same study by Fish et al. (2022), ribosomal and mitochondrial-related genes were downregulated in the *Bax*$^{-/-}$ embryos compared to *Bax*$^{+/+}$ embryos. Interestingly, genes related to transporting or processing cholesterol and lipids were upregulated in the *Bax*$^{-/-}$ embryos compared to *Bax*$^{+/+}$ embryos (Fish et al. 2022), perhaps linking to impacts on Shh signaling, where, as mentioned previously, cholesterol is critical in Shh synthesis, packaging, and signaling (Siebold and Rohatgi 2023; Briscoe and Thérond 2013).

3.12 FASD Has Been Proposed to Be a Ciliopathy: The Primary Cilium is a Cellular Organ Critical for Shh Function

Ethanol exposure during gastrulation reduces Shh signaling in the anterior neural tube resulting in craniofacial abnormalities within the HPE spectrum (Ahlgren et al. 2002; Yamada et al. 2005). When exposure occurs later during neurulation, it causes milder brain and facial defects (Parnell et al. 2009), still reducing Shh signaling (Boschen et al. 2021a), a process thought to involve primary cilia. Primary cilia are essential for normal development throughout the body, particularly in the neural tube where they transmit extracellular Shh signals into cells (reviewed in (Zhang and Beachy 2023)). Their developmental importance was further emphasized from the discovery of developmental syndromes caused by ciliary gene mutations (ciliopathies) (Brown and Witman 2014; Mahjoub 2013; Valente et al. 2014). PAE disrupts primary cilia function (Boschen et al. 2018, 2020, 2021a), which is necessary for canonical Shh signaling (Breslow et al. 2018; Wheway et al. 2018). Functional primary cilia are crucial for vertebrate development (Goetz and Anderson 2010), including limb patterning (Haycraft and Serra 2008). Some effects of neurulation-stage ethanol exposure resemble those seen in genetic ciliopathies, particularly in brain and facial development (Boschen et al. 2021a; Parnell et al. 2009). Acute ethanol exposure during neurulation appears to impair primary cilia function, altering the expression of numerous cilia-related genes during the exposure period (Boschen et al. 2020, 2021a, b, 2023).

The primary cilium consists of cilia membranes, axoneme, and basal body (Jing et al. 2023; Mahjoub 2013; Cortés et al. 2015). The ciliary membrane separates the cilia from the cytoplasm, and prevents proteins moving to and from the cilium (Stevenson 2023). The basal body secures a ring of microtubules that form the axoneme at the center of the primary cilium. Over 800 proteins have been identified in the primary cilium (Pala et al. 2017), and the movement of Shh signaling proteins through the primary cilium is governed by numerous motor, adaptor, and shuttling proteins (reviewed in (Jing et al. 2023; Zhang and Beachy 2023; Mill et al. 2023; Pala et al. 2017)). Several studies have shown that knocking out key genes important for primary cilia function can exacerbate the effects of ethanol. In mice with reduced expression of the cilia gene meiosis-specific nuclear structural protein 1 (*Mns1*), PAE (given at GD7) significantly increased the rate of craniofacial defects in embryos (assessed at GD17) compared to controls (Boschen et al. 2018). While a role for Mns1 in the primary cilium has not been identified (hence shown with a question mark in Fig. 3.1), it is known to associate with the important cilia component Kif3a, and is expressed in other types of cilia (Lehti et al. 2013). Further, deleting one copy of *Kif3a*, a kinesin II subunit involved in base to tip transport (Jing et al. 2023), increased the effects of ethanol on long-term behavior in mice (Boschen et al. 2021a). Another cilia component gene, EF-hand calcium binding domain7 (*Efcab7*), was identified from comparing the transcriptomes of mice sub-strains either resistant to or sensitive to gastrulation-stage PAE (Boschen et al. 2021b). Deleting one or both copies of *Efcab7*, a gene for a protein that assists in translocating other proteins into and out of the primary cilia, also exacerbated the effects of ethanol in a gene-dosage-dependent manner with effects on eyes, craniofacial parameters and brain (Fish et al. 2024). Interestingly, in the same study (Fish et al. 2024), the mice lacking

Efcab7 also had increased sensitivity to the teratogenic effects of the Smo inhibitor vismodegib and decreased sensitivity to SAG's teratogenic effects, perhaps indicating a disruption in Shh signaling through Smo.

Unbiased RNA-Seq FASD genetic studies have identified numerous candidate genes that modify susceptibility to PAE that would not have been considered otherwise (Swartz et al. 2014; Boschen et al. 2020; 2021b, 2023; Swartz et al. 2020). Likewise, genetic and chemical screens in other studies have also identified genes, pathways, and molecules that interact with ethanol during gastrulation (Engel et al. 2011; Rihel et al. 2010).

3.13 Ethanol and Cannabinoids Have Convergent and Synergistic Effects in Embryos: Both Acting on Shh Signaling

Cannabinoids, both natural and synthetic, can disrupt the development of the brain and face with defects similar to those caused by ethanol (see (Gilbert et al. 2016), and recent reviews (Kovács et al. 2023; Rodrigues et al. 2024; Rouzer et al. 2023)). This section will focus on the role of the Shh pathway in enabling the teratogenic effects of cannabinoids (CB) and interactions with ethanol. Another chapter in this book covers the effect of CBs on development in more detail (Diaz et al. 2026). As with FASD, zebrafish (Lachowicz et al. 2023) and mice have also been used as models in CB studies. In a mouse model, administration of the synthetic CB (sCB) CP-55,940 during early neurulation (GD8) induced defects of the brain, face, and eyes that phenocopy those observed following PAE (Gilbert et al. 2016).

As mentioned previously, Smo is a druggable target within the Shh pathway, with both antagonists and agonists binding in a pocket within Smo (Wang et al. 2014). This druggable site within Smo suggested the existence of an endogenous ligand (Khaliullina et al. 2015). Interestingly, a biochemical analysis identified a pool of endocannabinoids (eCB) as Shh pathway inhibitors, and these eCBs could compete for SAG and bind Smo directly (Khaliullina et al. 2015). Further, the same group demonstrated that phytocannabinoids cannabidiol (CBD) and cannabinol (CBN) could also block Shh signaling and bind directly to Smo (Khaliullina et al. 2015). A number of studies indicate that the teratogenic effects of ethanol and CBs both occur by disrupting the Shh pathway (shown schematically in Fig. 3.3). When ethanol and CBs were administered together, they increased the incidence of brain and craniofacial defects in a synergistic fashion (Fish et al. 2019). In this study in which pregnant mice were exposed to CBs (including delta-9-tetrahydrocannabinol (THC), and sCBs HU-210 and CP 55,940) at GD8, embryos at GD17 showed a range of eye and face malformations comparable to *Shh* mutations (Fish et al. 2019). Combining any of these CBs with low dose ethanol had synergistic effects in causing birth defects in both mice and zebrafish FASD models (Fish et al. 2019). In mice embryos, CP 55,940 exposure at GD8 reduced *Shh* and *Gli1* mRNA levels implicating an effect of CBs on reducing Shh signaling (Fish et al. 2019). These CB-induced effects such as small eye size, could be attenuated by *shh* mRNA injection in the zebrafish model and by a CB1 receptor (CB1R) antagonist in the mice and zebrafish FASD models (Fish et al. 2019). A direct effect of CBs on Smo was implicated by cell line studies in which CBs could compete out SAG induced Shh activation (Fish et al. 2019). In the same study, biochemical crosslinking on mouse GD9.5 embryonic neural tube tissue showed a direct interaction of Smo with CB1 receptors (Fish et al. 2019), while in another study, in contrast, immunoprecipitation of CB1R from E14 mouse embryo tissue did not detect Smo (Lo et al. 2021b).

Using the *Cdon*$^{+/-}$ mouse model discussed earlier (Hong and Krauss 2012; Hong and Krauss 2013), the same group showed that THC, when given at GD7.5 also induces HPE-like phenotypes, including craniofacial midline defects (Lo et al. 2021b), along with decreased expression of *Gli1* and *Shh* (at GD9). THC was able to inhibit *Gli1* expression in *Ptch1*$^{-/-}$ but not in *Sufu*$^{-/-}$ MEFs, indicating THC was acting downstream of Ptch1 and upstream of Sufu, most likely at the level of Smo (Lo et al. 2021b). Direct binding of THC to Smo was also demonstrated by competition studies (Lo et al. 2021b). Further, several experiments in this study, including that the Shh-dependent embryonic ventral neural tube cells that are sensitive to THC have very low levels of CB1R, led to the conclusion that CB1R is not required for inhibition of Shh signaling by THC (Lo et al. 2021b).

In a zebrafish study, increasing the levels of endogenous endocannabinoids (eCB), by inhibiting the enzymes that catabolize eCBs (fatty acid amide hydrolase [FAAH] and monoacylglycerol lipase [MAGL]), resulted in FASD-like pathological and behavioral phenotypes (Boa-Amponsem et al. 2019). Further, these eCB-induced effects could be prevented by *shh* mRNA injection (Boa-Amponsem et al. 2019). In a subsequent zebrafish FASD study, it was shown that ethanol and CBs regulate some aspects of zebrafish neuronal development through a Shh-dependent mechanism (Boa-Amponsem et al. 2020). In this study, ethanol and CB were shown to affect shh and fgf-8 signaling, resulting in behavioral effects in juvenile fish (Boa-Amponsem et al. 2020). These could be prevented by *fgf-8* mRNA overexpression, implicating a role for shh and fgf-8 crosstalk in FASD (Boa-Amponsem et al. 2020). In another zebrafish study looking at early vertebrate motor, embryos were exposed for the first 24 h of development to JZL184 (MAGL inhibitor) or JZL195 (dual MAGL and FAAH inhibitor) and impaired swimming distance was observed at 2 days (Khara and Ali 2023). It was found that co-treatment of the Smo agonist purmorphamine (PUR) with either JZL184 or JZL195 prevented this reduction in swimming distance, implicating an interaction between the eCB system and Shh signaling (Khara and Ali 2023). The teratogenic effects of CBD in a zebrafish embryo model could also be prevented using purmorphamine (Razmara et al. 2025).

Thus, there is significant evidence that the teratogenicity of CBs occurs through their direct inhibition of Hh signaling at the level of Smo (Boa-Amponsem et al. 2020; Fish et al. 2019; Khaliullina et al. 2015; Lo et al. 2021b; Razmara et al. 2025), and that ethanol and CBs can synergize to diminish Shh signaling. While the effects of ethanol are independent of the CB receptor, the observation that CB antagonists can block the effects of ethanol may be due to that they both impact cAMP levels; the net effect of ethanol is to decrease the Smo inhibition of adenyl cyclase (AC) thus increasing cAMP and activating PKA, leading to inhibition of Shh signaling. CB antagonists can attenuate the effects of ethanol by acting to inhibit adenyl cyclase through CB1R (see Fig. 3.3).

In a study looking at heart development in zebrafish, chronic ethanol exposure (1.5% for 3–24 hpf) resulted in gross defects including reduced eye size and heart edema (Zhang et al. 2023). *Shh* mRNA overexpression restored expression of cardiac markers (Zhang et al. 2023). Interestingly, sCBs did not produce this heart edema effect in the zebrafish embryos (Zhang et al. 2023). It was concluded that during early zebrafish development, pathways such as Shh, crucial for heart development, are sensitive to ethanol but not to CBs (Zhang et al. 2023), indicating some differences in teratogenic mechanisms.

In terms of translating these studies into relevance for human health, it is becoming apparent that the co-use of ethanol and CBs amplifies their respective effects (Rouzer et al. 2023) and raises significant safety concerns, especially for pregnant women regarding the risks to the fetus.

3.14 Conclusions

In this chapter, we have described how the Shh pathway occupies a central role in the pathogenesis of ethanol-induced birth defects, mediating ethanol's effects on midline development, neural crest survival, and organ patterning. The Shh signaling pathway is implicated downstream from ethanol in FASD in vertebrate embryos, with significant literature pointing to PAE causing a critical reduction in Shh pathway activity

(Ahlgren et al. 2002; Aoto et al. 2008; Loucks and Ahlgren 2009; Zhang et al. 2011; Boschen et al. 2021b). A large number of studies have shown that PAE impacts the expression of Shh pathway targets (listed in Table 3.1). Genetic studies (listed in Table 3.2) have underscored the importance of gene-environment interactions, where heterozygous mutations in *Shh*, *Gli2*, or *Cdon* lower the threshold for ethanol teratogenicity.

Mechanistically, ethanol appears to disrupt Shh at multiple levels both directly and indirectly, resulting in apoptosis and growth restriction. Several studies have shown a direct impact of ethanol on Shh signaling (see Table 3.1) including impaired cholesterol modification of Shh (Li et al. 2007), disruption of Shh trafficking (Mao et al. 2009), increase of inhibitory mechanisms (Aoto et al. 2008), and disrupted primary cilia function (Boschen et al. 2018, 2020, 2021a), essential for Shh signal transduction.

However, when compared to direct pharmacological inhibition of Shh activity, ethanol seems probably to affect Shh signaling through mechanisms upstream of Shh, as shown by the differing periods during which these agents affect craniofacial development. Embryonic sensitivity to ethanol is highest during early- to mid-gastrulation (mouse GD7), before significant *Shh* expression, while, in contrast, Smo antagonists are most effective during late gastrulation (GD 7.5) and early neurulation (GD8), when *Shh* expression begins to increase (Sulik et al. 1981; Godin et al. 2010; Heyne et al. 2015; Lipinski et al. 2014) (Fig. 3.3). Further, while Sidik et al. (2021) using a LINCS analysis, predicted that a Shh antagonist would mimic the effects of ethanol (Sidik et al. 2021), they observed a strong synergistic interaction between ethanol and cyclopamine (Sidik et al. 2021), suggesting differences in their effects on the embryo.

The studies discussed above suggest that both PAE and Shh pathway disruptions result in a spatiotemporal disruption of Shh signaling (Kahn et al. 2017). Figure 3.5 attempts to summarize this chapter and our current understanding of how ethanol impacts Shh signaling leading to PAE-induced morphological defects. The timing of the ethanol exposure that causes the brain and craniofacial defects characteristic of FAS (Sulik 2005) occurs just before *Shh* expression begins, indicating an indirect effect with PAE causing apoptosis in those cells that will later express *Shh* and disrupting critical pathways (Ahlgren et al. 2002; Zhang et al. 2013b; Hong and Krauss 2012; Boschen et al. 2021a; Dunty Jr et al. 2001; Lipinski et al. 2010b). Whether ethanol prevents the induction of *Shh* expression by disrupting RA or Nodal expression and signaling, or by another mechanism is still uncertain.

Cannabinoids (CB) can exacerbate the effects of ethanol (Fish et al. 2019; Boa-Amponsem et al. 2019), with a direct effect on the Shh pathway implicated (Fish et al. 2019; Khaliullina et al. 2015). The teratogenic effects of CBs are through a non-canonical interaction with Shh signaling and not through canonical CB signaling, with the data suggesting that while ethanol and CBs affect the same developmental pathways, they do so by differing molecular mechanisms.

Emerging strategies to mitigate the effects of PAE, including Smo agonists, RA, and cholesterol supplementation, highlight the potential for pathway-targeted interventions to ameliorate the effects of PAE in animal models. Future research must address the interplay between Shh and other ethanol-sensitive pathways, such as RA and Nodal, to understand their timing and impact on embryonic development.

Acknowledgments The authors acknowledge support from the National Institutes of Health, grant numbers U54AA030451, R01MD017405, R01AA026068, and RCMI U54MD012392. Additional funding was from Golden LEAF Foundation and the BIOIMPACT Initiative of the State of North Carolina through the Biomanufacturing Research Institute & Technology Enterprise (BRITE) Center for Excellence at North Carolina Central University. ChatGPT (version 5, OpenAI) was used to aid in editing and rewriting, to ensure consistency in tone and tense. All figures were created in BioRender. Williams, K. (2025) (Biorender agreement numbers): Fig. 3.1 https://BioRender.com/f8n7w82

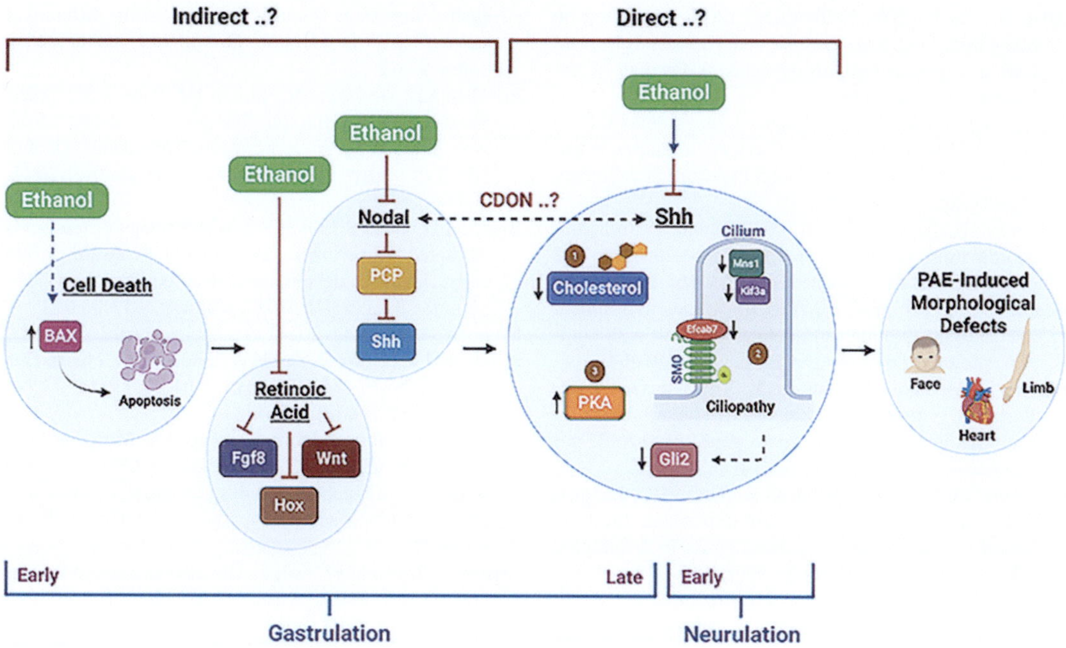

Fig. 3.5 *Proposed direct and indirect mechanisms of ethanol's impact on Shh signaling during embryonic development.* Ethanol's proposed indirect effects are through promoting cell death (e.g., apoptosis), or altering signaling pathways, including Nodal and subsequent Prechordal Plate (PCP), retinoic Acid, and associated signaling molecules (Fgf8, Hox, Wnt). Direct effects of ethanol may include disruption of Sonic hedgehog (Shh) signaling pathways, impacting cholesterol transport, ciliary function, and downstream effectors (Gli2, PKA). Both direct and indirect mechanisms lead to PAE-induced morphological defects in developing structures such as the face, limbs, and heart during gastrulation and early neurulation stages

(DB28UN0QX2); Fig. 3.2 https://BioRender.com/gavgalt (MZ28UN1EUR); Fig. 3.3 https://BioRender.com/05erx2c (ZB28UN1VG4); Fig. 3.4 https://BioRender.com/gheb1vz (GB28UN244R); Fig. 3.5 https://BioRender.com/1bb1ia0 (IU28UN2CFQ).

References

Abramyan J (2019) Hedgehog signaling and embryonic craniofacial disorders. J Dev Biol 7(2):9. https://doi.org/10.3390/jdb7020009

Ahlgren SC, Thakur V, Bronner-Fraser M (2002) Sonic hedgehog rescues cranial neural crest from cell death induced by ethanol exposure. Proc Natl Acad Sci USA 99(16):10476–10481. https://doi.org/10.1073/pnas.162356199

Akšamija A, Habek D, Stanojević M, Ujević B (2009) Fetal malformations associated with the use of Methylphenobarbital and carbamazepine during pregnancy: two case reports and review of the literature. Fetal Diagn Ther 25(1):79–82

Albert S, Müller F, Fischer N, Biellmann D, Neumann C, Blader P et al (2003) Cyclops-independent floor plate differentiation in zebrafish embryos. Dev Dyn 226(1):59–66

Ali S, Champagne DL, Alia A, Richardson MK (2011) Large-scale analysis of acute ethanol exposure in zebrafish development: a critical time window and resilience. PLoS One 6(5):e20037

Anthony B, Zhou FC, Ogawa T, Goodlett CR, Ruiz J (2008) Alcohol exposure alters cell cycle and apoptotic events during early neurulation. Alcohol Alcohol 43(3):261–273

Aoto K, Shikata Y, Higashiyama D, Shiota K, Motoyama J (2008) Fetal ethanol exposure activates protein kinase A and impairs Shh expression in prechordal mesendoderm cells in the pathogenesis of holoprosencephaly. Birth Defects Res A Clin Mol Teratol 82(4):224–231. https://doi.org/10.1002/bdra.20447

Arenzana F, Carvan MJ III, Aijon J, Sanchez-Gonzalez R, Arevalo R, Porteros A (2006) Teratogenic effects of ethanol exposure on zebrafish visual system development. Neurotoxicol Teratol 28(3):342–348

Arsić D, Beasley SW, Sullivan MJ (2007) Switched-on Sonic hedgehog: a gene whose activity extends beyond fetal development–to oncogenesis. J Paediatr Child Health 43(6):421–423

Bailey J, Oliveri A, Zhang C, Frazier J, Mackinnon S, Cole G et al (2015) Long-term behavioral impairment following acute embryonic ethanol exposure in zebrafish. Neurotoxicol Teratol 48:1–8

Bardot ES, Hadjantonakis A-K (2020) Mouse gastrulation: coordination of tissue patterning, specification and diversification of cell fate. Mech Dev 163:103617

Beames TG, Lipinski RJ (2020) Gene-environment interactions: aligning birth defects research with complex etiology. Development 147(21):dev191064

Belloni E, Muenke M, Roessler E, Traverse G, Siegel-Bartelt J, Frumkin A et al (1996) Identification of sonic hedgehog as a candidate gene responsible for holoprosencephaly. Nat Genet 14(3):353–356

Bergeron SA, Milla LA, Villegas R, Shen M-C, Burgess SM, Allende ML et al (2008) Expression profiling identifies novel Hh/Gli-regulated genes in developing zebrafish embryos. Genomics 91(2):165–177

Binkhorst M, Wortmann S, Funke S, Kozicz T, Wevers R, Morava E (2012) Glycosylation defects underlying fetal alcohol spectrum disorder: a novel pathogenetic model: "when the wine goes in, strange things come out"–ST Coleridge, the Piccolomini. J Inherit Metab Dis 35:399–405

Blader P, Strähle U (1998) Ethanol impairs migration of the prechordal plate in the zebrafish embryo. Dev Biol 201(2):185–201. https://doi.org/10.1006/dbio.1998.8995

Boa-Amponsem O, Zhang C, Mukhopadhyay S, Ardrey I, Cole GJ (2019) Ethanol and cannabinoids interact to alter behavior in a zebrafish fetal alcohol spectrum disorder model. Birth Defects Res. 111(12):775–788. https://doi.org/10.1002/bdr2.1458

Boa-Amponsem O, Zhang C, Burton D, Williams KP, Cole GJ (2020) Ethanol and cannabinoids regulate zebrafish GABAergic neuron development and behavior in a sonic hedgehog and fibroblast growth factor-dependent mechanism. Alcohol Clin Exp Res 44(7): 1366–1377. https://doi.org/10.1111/acer.14383

Boschen KE, Gong H, Murdaugh LB, Parnell SE (2018) Knockdown of Mns1 increases susceptibility to craniofacial defects following gastrulation-stage alcohol exposure in mice. Alcohol Clin Exp Res 42(11): 2136–2143

Boschen KE, Ptacek TS, Simon JM, Parnell SE (2020) Transcriptome-wide regulation of key developmental pathways in the mouse neural tube by prenatal alcohol exposure. Alcohol Clin Exp Res 44(8):1540–1550

Boschen KE, Fish EW, Parnell SE (2021a) Prenatal alcohol exposure disrupts sonic hedgehog pathway and primary cilia genes in the mouse neural tube. Reprod Toxicol 105:136–147. https://doi.org/10.1016/j.reprotox.2021.09.002

Boschen KE, Ptacek TS, Berginski ME, Simon JM, Parnell SE (2021b) Transcriptomic analyses of gastrulation-stage mouse embryos with differential susceptibility to alcohol. Dis Model Mech 14(6): dmm049012

Boschen KE, Steensen MC, Simon JM, Parnell SE (2023) Short-term transcriptomic changes in the mouse neural tube induced by an acute alcohol exposure. Alcohol 106:1–9. https://doi.org/10.1016/j.alcohol.2022.09.001

Brennan D, Giles S (2013) Sonic hedgehog expression is disrupted following in ovo ethanol exposure during early chick eye development. Reprod Toxicol 41:49–56. https://doi.org/10.1016/j.reprotox.2013.05.012

Brennan D, Giles S (2014) Ocular involvement in fetal alcohol spectrum disorder: a review. Curr Pharm Des 20(34):5377–5387. https://doi.org/10.2174/1381612820666140205144114

Breslow DK, Hoogendoorn S, Kopp AR, Morgens DW, Vu BK, Kennedy MC et al (2018) A CRISPR-based screen for Hedgehog signaling provides insights into ciliary function and ciliopathies. Nat Genet 50(3): 460–471

Briscoe J, Thérond PP (2013) The mechanisms of hedgehog signalling and its roles in development and disease. Nat Rev Mol Cell Biol 14(7):416–429

Brown JM, Witman GB (2014) Cilia and diseases. Bioscience 64(12):1126–1137

Buglino JA, Resh MD (2008) Hhat is a palmitoylacyltransferase with specificity for N-palmitoylation of sonic hedgehog. J Biol Chem 283(32):22076–22088

Burke R, Nellen D, Bellotto M, Hafen E, Senti K-A, Dickson BJ et al (1999) Dispatched, a novel sterol-sensing domain protein dedicated to the release of cholesterol-modified hedgehog from signaling cells. Cell 99(7):803–815

Burton DF, Zhang C, Boa-Amponsem O, Mackinnon S, Cole GJ (2017) Long-term behavioral change as a result of acute ethanol exposure in zebrafish: evidence for a role for sonic hedgehog but not retinoic acid signaling. Neurotoxicol Teratol 61:66–73. https://doi.org/10.1016/j.ntt.2017.01.006

Burton DF, Boa-Amponsem OM, Dixon MS, Hopkins MJ, Herbin TA, Toney S et al (2022) Pharmacological activation of the Sonic hedgehog pathway with a smoothened small molecule agonist ameliorates the severity of alcohol-induced morphological and behavioral birth defects in a zebrafish model of fetal alcohol spectrum disorder. J Neurosci Res 100(8):1585–1601. https://doi.org/10.1002/jnr.25008

Cadena PG, Cadena MRS, Sarmah S, Marrs JA (2020) Folic acid reduces the ethanol-induced morphological and behavioral defects in embryonic and larval zebrafish (Danio rerio) as a model for fetal alcohol spectrum disorder (FASD). Reprod Toxicol 96:249–257

Cardozo MJ, Sánchez-Arrones L, Sandonis A, Sánchez-Camacho C, Gestri G, Wilson SW et al (2014) Cdon acts as a hedgehog decoy receptor during proximal-distal patterning of the optic vesicle. Nat Commun 5(1):1–13

Carpenter RL, Ray H (2019) Efficacy and safety of sonic hedgehog pathway inhibitors in cancer. Drug Saf 42(2):263

Caspary T, Garcıa-Garcıa MJ, Huangfu D, Eggenschwiler JT, Wyler MR, Rakeman AS et al (2002) Mouse dispatched homolog1 is required for long-range, but not juxtacrine, Hh signaling. Curr Biol 12(18): 1628–1632

Cavodeassi F, Creuzet S, Etchevers HC (2018) The hedgehog pathway and ocular developmental anomalies. Hum Genet 138:1–20

Chen W, Burgess S, Hopkins N (2001) Analysis of the zebrafish smoothened mutant reveals conserved and divergent functions of hedgehog activity. Development 128:2385

Chen JK, Taipale J, Young KE, Maiti T, Beachy PA (2002a) Small molecule modulation of smoothened activity. Proc Natl Acad Sci 99(22):14071–14076

Chen J, Taipale J, Cooper M, Beachy P (2002b) Inhibition of hedgehog signaling by direct binding of cyclopamine to smoothened. Genes Dev 16(21): 2743–2748

Chen S-D, Yang J-L, Hwang W-C, Yang D-I (2018) Emerging roles of sonic hedgehog in adult neurological diseases: neurogenesis and beyond. Int J Mol Sci 19(8):2423

Chiang C, Litingtung Y, Lee E, Young KE, Corden JL, Westphal H et al (1996) Cyclopia and defective axial patterning in mice lacking sonic hedgehog gene function. Nature 383(6599):407–413

Chideriotis S, Anastasiadi AT, Tzounakas VL, Fortis SP, Kriebardis AG, Valsami S (2025) Morphogens and cell-derived structures (exosomes and Cytonemes) as components of the communication between cells. Int J Mol Sci 26(3):881

Chrisman K, Kenney R, Comin J, Thal T, Suchocki L, Yueh YG et al (2004) Gestational ethanol exposure disrupts the expression of FGF8 and sonic hedgehog during limb patterning. Birth Defects Res A Clin Mol Teratol 70(4):163–171. https://doi.org/10.1002/bdra.20019

Clugston R, Blaner W (2012) The adverse effects of alcohol on vitamin a metabolism. Nutrients 4:356–371

Cohen M Jr, Sulik K (1992) Perspectives on holoprosencephaly: part II. Central nervous system, craniofacial anatomy, syndrome commentary, diagnostic approach, and experimental studies. J Craniofac Genet Dev Biol 12(4):196–244

Cordero D, Marcucio R, Hu D, Gaffield W, Tapadia M, Helms JA (2004) Temporal perturbations in sonic hedgehog signaling elicit the spectrum of holoprosencephaly phenotypes. J Clin Invest 114(4): 485–494

Cortés CR, Metzis V, Wicking C (2015) Unmasking the ciliopathies: craniofacial defects and the primary cilium. Wiley Interdiscip Rev Dev Biol 4(6):637–653

Cotman SL, Halfter W, Cole GJ (1999) Identification of extracellular matrix ligands for the heparan sulfate proteoglycan agrin. Exp Cell Res 249(1):54–64

Cunningham TJ, Duester G (2015) Mechanisms of retinoic acid signalling and its roles in organ and limb development. Nat Rev Mol Cell Biol 16(2):110–123

de Bree K, de Bakker BS, Oostra R-J (2018) The development of the human notochord. PLoS One 13(10): e0205752

Del Campo M, Jones KL (2017) A review of the physical features of the fetal alcohol spectrum disorders. Eur J Med Genet 60(1):55–64

Deltour L, Ang HL, Duester G (1996) Ethanol inhibition of retinoic acid synthesis as a potential mechanism for fetal alcohol syndrome. FASEB J 10(9):1050–1057

Deshpande I, Liang J, Hedeen D, Roberts KJ, Zhang Y, Ha B et al (2019) Smoothened stimulation by membrane sterols drives hedgehog pathway activity. Nature 571(7764):284–288

Diaz MR, Varlinskaya EI, Schatz KC (2026) Anxiety, depression, and emotional dysregulation following prenatal substance exposure. In: Bukiya A, Ali DW (eds) Molecular mechanisms and lifelong consequences of prenatal exposure to psychoactive substances. Springer

Dou X, Wilkemeyer MF, Menkari CE, Parnell SE, Sulik KK, Charness ME (2013) Mitogen-activated protein kinase modulates ethanol inhibition of cell adhesion mediated by the L1 neural cell adhesion molecule. Proc Natl Acad Sci 110(14):5683–5688

Downing C, Balderrama-Durbin C, Broncucia H, Gilliam D, Johnson TE (2009) Ethanol teratogenesis in five inbred strains of mice. Alcohol Clin Exp Res 33(7):1238–1245

Duester G (1991) A hypothetical mechanism for fetal alcohol syndrome involving ethanol inhibition of retinoic acid synthesis at the alcohol dehydrogenase step. Alcohol Clin Exp Res 15(3):568–572

Duester G (1999) Function of alcohol dehydrogenase and aldehyde dehydrogenase gene families in retinoid signaling. Adv Exp Med Biol 463:311–319

Dunty WC Jr, Sy C, Zucker RM, Dehart DB, Sulik KK (2001) Selective vulnerability of embryonic cell populations to ethanol-induced apoptosis: implications for alcohol-related birth defects and neurodevelopmental disorder. Alcohol Clin Exp Res 25(10):1523–1535

Eberhart JK, Parnell SE (2016) The genetics of fetal alcohol spectrum disorders. Alcohol Clin Exp Res 40(6): 1154–1165

Eberhart JK, Swartz ME, Crump JG, Kimmel CB (2006) Early hedgehog signaling from neural to oral epithelium organizes anterior craniofacial development. Development 133(6):1069–1077

Echelard Y, Epstein DJ, St-Jacques B, Shen L, Mohler J, McMahon JA et al (1993) Sonic hedgehog, a member of a family of putative signaling molecules, is implicated in the regulation of CNS polarity. Cell 75(7):1417–1430

Edison R, Muenke M (2003) The interplay of genetic and environmental factors in craniofacial morphogenesis: holoprosencephaly and the role of cholesterol. Congenit Anom (Kyoto) 43(1):1–21. https://doi.org/10.1111/j.1741-4520.2003.tb01022.x

Ehrhart F, Roozen S, Verbeek J, Koek G, Kok G, van Kranen H et al (2019) Review and gap analysis: molecular pathways leading to fetal alcohol spectrum disorders. Mol Psychiatry 24(1):10–17

Ekker SC, Ungar AR, Greenstein P, von Kessler DP, Porter JA, Moon RT et al (1995) Patterning activities of vertebrate hedgehog proteins in the developing eye and brain. Curr Biol 5(8):944–955

Engel BD, Ishikawa H, Feldman JL, Wilson CW, Chuang PT, Snedecor J et al (2011) A cell-based screen for inhibitors of flagella-driven motility in Chlamydomonas reveals a novel modulator of ciliary length and retrograde actin flow. Cytoskeleton 68(3): 188–203

Everson JL, Eberhart JK (2023) Gene-alcohol interactions in birth defects. In: Current topics in developmental biology. Elsevier, pp 77–113

Everson JL, Batchu R, Eberhart JK (2020) Multifactorial genetic and environmental hedgehog pathway disruption sensitizes embryos to alcohol-induced craniofacial defects. Alcohol Clin Exp Res 44(10):1988–1996. https://doi.org/10.1111/acer.14427

Everson JL, Tseng YC, Eberhart JK (2023) High-throughput detection of craniofacial defects in fluorescent zebrafish. Birth Defects Res. 115(3):371–389. https://doi.org/10.1002/bdr2.2127

Fainsod A, Bendelac-Kapon L, Shabtai Y (2020) Fetal alcohol spectrum disorder: embryogenesis under reduced retinoic acid signaling conditions. In: The biochemistry of retinoid signaling III: vitamin A and retinoic acid in embryonic development, pp 197–225

Fernandes Y, Lovely CB (2021) Zebrafish models of fetal alcohol spectrum disorders. Genesis 59(11):e23460

Fernandes Y, Rampersad M, Gerlai R (2015) Impairment of social behaviour persists two years after embryonic alcohol exposure in zebrafish: a model of fetal alcohol spectrum disorders. Behav Brain Res 292:102–108

Fish EW, Murdaugh LB, Sulik KK, Williams KP, Parnell SE (2017a) Genetic vulnerabilities to prenatal alcohol exposure: limb defects in sonic hedgehog and GLI2 heterozygous mice. Birth Defects Res 109(11): 860–865. https://doi.org/10.1002/bdr2.1026

Fish EW, Parnell SE, Sulik KK, Baker LK, Murdaugh LB, Lamson D et al (2017b) Preaxial polydactyly following early gestational exposure to the smoothened agonist, SAG, in C57BL/6J mice. Birth Defects Res. 109(1): 49–54. https://doi.org/10.1002/bdra.23571

Fish EW, Murdaugh LB, Zhang C, Boschen KE, Boa-Amponsem O, Mendoza-Romero HN et al (2019) Cannabinoids exacerbate alcohol Teratogenesis by a CB1-hedgehog interaction. Sci Rep 9(1):16057. https://doi.org/10.1038/s41598-019-52336-w

Fish EW, Tucker SK, Peterson RL, Eberhart JK, Parnell SE (2021) Loss of tumor protein 53 protects against alcohol-induced facial malformations in mice and zebrafish. Alcohol Clin Exp Res 45(10):1965–1979

Fish EW, Mendoza-Romero HN, Love CA, Dragicevich CJ, Cannizzo MD, Boschen KE et al (2022) The pro-apoptotic Bax gene modifies susceptibility to craniofacial dysmorphology following gastrulation-stage alcohol exposure. Birth Defects Res 114(19): 1229–1243

Fish EW, Boschen KE, Parnell SE (2024) Efcab7 deletion sensitizes mice to the teratogenic effects of gastrulation-stage alcohol exposure. Reprod Toxicol 130:108729. https://doi.org/10.1016/j.reprotox.2024.108729

Flentke GR, Smith SM (2018) The avian embryo as a model for fetal alcohol spectrum disorder. Biochem Cell Biol 96(2):98–106

Flentke GR, Baulch JW, Berres ME, Garic A, Smith SM (2019) Alcohol-mediated calcium signals dysregulate pro-survival Snai2/PUMA/Bcl2 networks to promote p53-mediated apoptosis in avian neural crest progenitors. Birth Defects Res. 111(12):686–699

Frank-Kamenetsky M, Zhang XM, Bottega S, Guicherit O, Wichterle H, Dudek H et al (2002) Small-molecule modulators of hedgehog signaling: identification and characterization of smoothened agonists and antagonists. J Biol 1(2):10

Gilbert SF (2000) Developmental biology. Sinauer Associates

Gilbert MT, Sulik KK, Fish EW, Baker LK, Dehart DB, Parnell SE (2016) Dose-dependent teratogenicity of the synthetic cannabinoid CP-55,940 in mice. Neurotoxicol Teratol 58:15–22

Glickman NS, Kimmel CB, Jones MA, Adams RJ (2003) Shaping the zebrafish notochord. Development 130(5): 873–887

Godin EA, O'Leary-Moore SK, Khan AA, Parnell SE, Ament JJ, Dehart DB et al (2010) Magnetic resonance microscopy defines ethanol-induced brain abnormalities in prenatal mice: effects of acute insult on gestational day 7. Alcohol Clin Exp Res 34(1): 98–111

Godin EA, Dehart DB, Parnell SE, O'Leary-Moore SK, Sulik KK (2011) Ventromedian forebrain dysgenesis follows early prenatal ethanol exposure in mice. Neurotoxicol Teratol 33(2):231–239

Goetz SC, Anderson KV (2010) The primary cilium: a signalling Centre during vertebrate development. Nat Rev Genet 11(5):331–344

Gould SE, Low JA, Marsters JC Jr, Robarge K, Rubin LL, de Sauvage FJ et al (2014) Discovery and preclinical development of vismodegib. Expert Opin Drug Discov 9(8):969–984

Gradilla A-C, Guerrero I (2022) Hedgehog on track: long-distant signal transport and transfer through direct cell-to-cell contact. In: Curr Top Dev Biol, vol 150, pp 1–24

Graf M, Teo Qi-Wen E-R, Sarusie MV, Rajaei F, Winkler C (2015) Dmrt5 controls corticotrope and gonadotrope differentiation in the zebrafish pituitary. Mol Endocrinol 29(2):187–199

Groves I, Placzek M, Fletcher AG (2020) Of mitogens and morphogens: modelling sonic hedgehog mechanisms in vertebrate development. Philos Trans R Soc Lond B Biol Sci 375(1809):20190660

Gude F, Froese J, Manikowski D, Di Iorio D, Grad J-N, Wegner S et al (2023) Hedgehog is relayed through dynamic heparan sulfate interactions to shape its gradient. Nat Commun 14(1):758

Guizzetti M, Costa LG (2007) Cholesterol homeostasis in the developing brain: a possible new target for ethanol. Hum Exp Toxicol 26(4):355–360

Guizzetti M, Costa LG (2008) Sonic hedgehog in Smith-Lemli-Opitz syndrome and tumor development. J Pediatr Hematol Oncol 30(9):641–642

Hamburger V, Hamilton HL (1951) A series of normal stages in the development of the chick embryo. J Morphol 88(1):49–92

Hammerschmidt M, Pelegri F, Mullins MC, Kane DA, Brand M, Van Eeden F et al (1996a) Mutations affecting morphogenesis during gastrulation and tail formation in the zebrafish, Danio rerio. Development 123(1): 143–151

Hammerschmidt M, Bitgood MJ, McMahon AP (1996b) Protein kinase A is a common negative regulator of hedgehog signaling in the vertebrate embryo. Genes Dev 10(6):647–658

Haycraft CJ, Serra R (2008) Cilia involvement in patterning and maintenance of the skeleton. Curr Top Dev Biol 85:303–332

Hernández-García D, Fuentes-Jiménez D, Rojo-León V, Wood C, García C, Covarrubias L (2019) Hedgehog signaling dynamics in mouse embryos determined by a bioluminiscent reporter. Int J Dev Biol 63:605–613

Heyne GW, Melberg CG, Doroodchi P, Parins KF, Kietzman HW, Everson JL et al (2015) Definition of critical periods for hedgehog pathway antagonist-induced holoprosencephaly, cleft lip, and cleft palate. PLoS One 10(3):e0120517

Heyne GW, Everson JL, Ansen-Wilson LJ, Melberg CG, Fink DM, Parins KF et al (2016) Gli2 gene-environment interactions contribute to the etiological complexity of holoprosencephaly: evidence from a mouse model. Dis Model Mech 9(11):1307–1315

Higashiyama D, Saitsu H, Komada M, Takigawa T, Ishibashi M, Shiota K (2007) Sequential developmental changes in holoprosencephalic mouse embryos exposed to ethanol during the gastrulation period. Birth Defects Res A Clin Mol Teratol 79(7):513–523. https://doi.org/10.1002/bdra.20367

Hong M, Krauss RS (2012) Cdon mutation and fetal ethanol exposure synergize to produce midline signaling defects and holoprosencephaly spectrum disorders in mice. PLoS Genet 8(10):e1002999. https://doi.org/10.1371/journal.pgen.1002999

Hong M, Krauss RS (2013) Rescue of holoprosencephaly in fetal alcohol-exposed Cdon mutant mice by reduced gene dosage of Ptch1. PLoS One 8(11):e79269

Hong M, Krauss RS (2017) Ethanol itself is a holoprosencephaly-inducing teratogen. PLoS One 12(4):e0176440. https://doi.org/10.1371/journal.pone.0176440

Hong M, Christ A, Christa A, Willnow TE, Krauss RS (2020) Cdon mutation and fetal alcohol converge on nodal signaling in a mouse model of holoprosencephaly. elife 9:e60351

Houschyar KS, Smith AA, Helms JA (2016) Shh and holoprosencephaly. In: Epstein's inborn errors of development: the molecular basis of clinical disorders of morphogenesis. Oxford University Press, p 287

Huang P, Zheng S, Wierbowski BM, Kim Y, Nedelcu D, Aravena L et al (2018) Structural basis of smoothened activation in hedgehog signaling. Cell 174(2): 312–24. e16

Huang Y, Flentke GR, Smith SM (2024) Alcohol induces p53-mediated apoptosis in neural crest by stimulating an AMPK-mediated suppression of TORC1, S6K, and ribosomal biogenesis. Reprod Toxicol 130:108747

Ingham PW (1994) Pattern formation: hedgehog points the way. Curr Biol 4(4):347–350

Ingham PW (2022) Hedgehog signaling. Curr Top Dev Biol 149:1–58

Ingham P, McMahon A (2001) Hedgehog signaling in animal development: paradigms and principles. Genes Dev 15(23):3059–3087

Jing J, Wu Z, Wang J, Luo G, Lin H, Fan Y et al (2023) Hedgehog signaling in tissue homeostasis, cancers, and targeted therapies. Signal Transduct Target Ther 8(1):315

Johnson CS, Zucker RM, Hunter ES 3rd, Sulik KK (2007) Perturbation of retinoic acid (RA)-mediated limb development suggests a role for diminished RA signaling in the teratogenesis of ethanol. Birth Defects Res A Clin Mol Teratol 79(9):631–641. https://doi.org/10.1002/bdra.20385

Jones K (1986) Fetal alcohol syndrome. Pediatr Rev 8: 122–125

Jones K, Smith D (1973) Recognition of the fetal alcohol syndrome in early infancy. Lancet 302(7836): 999–1001

Kahn BM, Corman TS, Lovelace K, Hong M, Krauss RS, Epstein DJ (2017) Prenatal ethanol exposure in mice phenocopies Cdon mutation by impeding Shh function in the etiology of optic nerve hypoplasia. Dis Model Mech 10(1):29–37. https://doi.org/10.1242/dmm.026195

Karlstrom RO, Tyurina OV, Kawakami A, Nishioka N, Talbot WS, Sasaki H et al (2003) Genetic analysis of zebrafish gli1 and gli2 reveals divergent requirements for gli genes in vertebrate development. Development 130(8):1549–1564

Kashyap B, Frey RA, Stenkamp DL (2011) Ethanol-induced microphthalmia is not mediated by changes in retinoic acid or sonic hedgehog signaling during retinal neurogenesis. Alcohol Clin Exp Res 35(9): 1644–1661. https://doi.org/10.1111/j.1530-0277.2011.01511.x

Kaufman MH, Kaufman MH (1992) The atlas of mouse development. Academic, London

Kelly SJ, Day N, Streissguth AP (2000) Effects of prenatal alcohol exposure on social behavior in humans and other species. Neurotoxicol Teratol 22(2):143–149

Khaliullina H, Bilgin M, Sampaio JL, Shevchenko A, Eaton S (2015) Endocannabinoids are conserved inhibitors of the Hedgehog pathway. Proc Natl Acad Sci 112(11):3415–3420

Khara LS, Ali DW (2023) The endocannabinoid system's involvement in motor development relies on cannabinoid receptors, TRP channels, and Sonic Hedgehog signaling. Physiol Rep 11(1):e15565

Kiecker C (2016) The chick embryo as a model for the effects of prenatal exposure to alcohol on craniofacial development. Dev Biol 415(2):314–325

Kietzman HW, Everson JL, Sulik KK, Lipinski RJ (2014) The teratogenic effects of prenatal ethanol exposure are exacerbated by Sonic Hedgehog or GLI2 haploinsufficiency in the mouse. PLoS One 9(2): e89448. https://doi.org/10.1371/journal.pone.0089448

Kimmel CB, Ballard WW, Kimmel SR, Ullmann B, Schilling TF (1995) Stages of embryonic development of the zebrafish. Dev Dyn 203(3):253–310

Kinnebrew M, Iverson EJ, Patel BB, Pusapati GV, Kong JH, Johnson KA et al (2019) Cholesterol accessibility at the ciliary membrane controls hedgehog signaling. Elife 8:e50051

Klem JR, Schwantes-An T-H, Abreu M, Suttie M, Gray R, Vo H et al (2025) Mutations in the bone morphogenetic protein signaling pathway sensitize zebrafish and humans to ethanol-induced jaw malformations. Dis Model Mech:dmm. 052223

Kotch LE, Sulik KK (1992) Patterns of ethanol-induced cell death in the developing nervous system of mice; neural fold states through the time of anterior neural tube closure. Int J Dev Neurosci 10(4):273–279

Kotch L, Dehart D, Alles A, Chernoff N, Sulik K (1992) Pathogenesis of ethanol-induced limb reduction defects in mice. Teratology 46(4):323–332

Kot-Leibovich H, Fainsod A (2009) Ethanol induces embryonic malformations by competing for retinaldehyde dehydrogenase activity during vertebrate gastrulation. Dis Model Mech 2(5–6):295–305

Kovács MV, Charchat-Fichman H, Landeira-Fernandez J, Medina AE, Krahe TE (2023) Combined exposure to alcohol and cannabis during development: mechanisms and outcomes. Alcohol 110:1–13. https://doi.org/10.1016/j.alcohol.2023.01.004

Krauss S, Concordet J-P, Ingham PW (1993) A functionally conserved homolog of the drosophila segment polarity gene hh is expressed in tissues with polarizing activity in zebrafish embryos. Cell 75(7):1431–1444

Lachowicz J, Szopa A, Ignatiuk K, Świąder K, Serefko A (2023) Zebrafish as an animal model in cannabinoid research. Int J Mol Sci 24(13):10455

Lanoue L, Dehart DB, Hinsdale ME, Maeda N, Tint GS, Sulik KK (1997) Limb, genital, CNS, and facial malformations result from gene/environment-induced cholesterol deficiency: further evidence for a link to sonic hedgehog. Am J Med Genet 73(1):24–31

Lehti MS, Kotaja N, Sironen A (2013) KIF3A is essential for sperm tail formation and manchette function. Mol Cell Endocrinol 377(1–2):44–55

Li YX, Yang HT, Zdanowicz M, Sicklick JK, Qi Y, Camp TJ et al (2007) Fetal alcohol exposure impairs Hedgehog cholesterol modification and signaling. Lab Investig 87(3):231–240. https://doi.org/10.1038/labinvest.3700516

Lipinski RJ, Song C, Sulik KK, Everson JL, Gipp JJ, Yan D et al (2010a) Cleft lip and palate results from hedgehog signaling antagonism in the mouse: phenotypic characterization and clinical implications. Birth Defects Res A Clin Mol Teratol 88(4):232–240

Lipinski RJ, Godin EA, O'leary-Moore SK, Parnell SE, Sulik KK (2010b) Genesis of teratogen-induced holoprosencephaly in mice. Am J Med Genet C Semin Med Genet 154C(1):29–42

Lipinski RJ, Holloway HT, O'Leary-Moore SK, Ament JJ, Pecevich SJ, Cofer GP et al (2014) Characterization of subtle brain abnormalities in a mouse model of hedgehog pathway antagonist-induced cleft lip and palate. PLoS One 9(7):e102603

Lo HF, Hong M, Krauss RS (2021a) Concepts in multifactorial etiology of developmental disorders: Gene-gene and gene-environment interactions in Holoprosencephaly. Front Cell Dev Biol 9:795194. https://doi.org/10.3389/fcell.2021.795194

Lo H-F, Hong M, Szutorisz H, Hurd YL, Krauss RS (2021b) Δ9-tetrahydrocannabinol inhibits hedgehog-dependent patterning during development. Development 148(19):dev199585

Lombard Z, Tiffin N, Hofmann O, Bajic VB, Hide W, Ramsay M (2007) Computational selection and prioritization of candidate genes for fetal alcohol syndrome. BMC Genomics 8(1):389

Loucks EJ, Ahlgren SC (2009) Deciphering the role of Shh signaling in axial defects produced by ethanol exposure. Birth Defects Res A Clin Mol Teratol 85(6): 556–567. https://doi.org/10.1002/bdra.20564

Loucks E, Ahlgren S (2012) Assessing teratogenic changes in a zebrafish model of fetal alcohol exposure. J Vis Exp: JoVE 61:3704

Loucks EJ, Schwend T, Ahlgren SC (2007) Molecular changes associated with teratogen-induced cyclopia. Birth Defects Res A Clin Mol Teratol 79(9):642–651. https://doi.org/10.1002/bdra.20387

Lovely CB, Nobles RD, Eberhart JK (2014) Developmental age strengthens barriers to ethanol accumulation in zebrafish. Alcohol 48(6):595–602

Lovely C, Rampersad M, Fernandes Y, Eberhart J (2017) Gene–environment interactions in development and disease. Wiley Interdiscip Rev Dev Biol 6(1):e247

Mahjoub MR (2013) The importance of a single primary cilium. Organogenesis 9(2):61–69

Manikandan P, Sarmah S, Marrs JA (2022) Ethanol effects on early developmental stages studied using the

zebrafish. Biomedicine 10(10):2555. https://doi.org/10.3390/biomedicines10102555
Mao H, Diehl AM, Li YX (2009) Sonic hedgehog ligand partners with caveolin-1 for intracellular transport. Lab Investig 89(3):290–300. https://doi.org/10.1038/labinvest.2008.163
Marrs JA, Clendenon SG, Ratcliffe DR, Fielding SM, Liu Q, Bosron WF (2010) Zebrafish fetal alcohol syndrome model: effects of ethanol are rescued by retinoic acid supplement. Alcohol 44(7–8):707–715
Mattson SN, Crocker N, Nguyen TT (2011) Fetal alcohol spectrum disorders: neuropsychological and behavioral features. Neuropsychol Rev 21:81–101
May PA, Chambers CD, Kalberg WO, Zellner J, Feldman H, Buckley D et al (2018) Prevalence of fetal alcohol spectrum disorders in 4 US communities. JAMA 319(5):474–482
McCarthy N, Eberhart JK (2014) Gene–ethanol interactions underlying fetal alcohol spectrum disorders. Cell Mol Life Sci 71(14):2699–2706
McCarthy N, Wetherill L, Lovely CB, Swartz ME, Foroud TM, Eberhart JK (2013) Pdgfra protects against ethanol-induced craniofacial defects in a zebrafish model of FASD. Development 140(15):3254–3265
Mercader N (2007) Early steps of paired fin development in zebrafish compared with tetrapod limb development. Develop Growth Differ 49(6):421–437
Mich JK, Payumo AY, Rack PG, Chen JK (2014) In vivo imaging of Hedgehog pathway activation with a nuclear fluorescent reporter. PLoS One 9(7):e103661
Mill P, Christensen ST, Pedersen LB (2023) Primary cilia as dynamic and diverse signalling hubs in development and disease. Nat Rev Genet 24(7):421–441
Ming JE, Muenke M (1998) Holoprosencephaly: from Homer to hedgehog. Clin Genet 53(3):155–163
Muhr J, Ackerman KM (2023) Embryology, gastrulation. StatPearls [Internet]. StatPearls Publishing
Muller F, Chang B, Albert S, Fischer N, Tora L, Strahle U (1999) Intronic enhancers control expression of zebrafish sonic hedgehog in floor plate and notochord. Development 126(10):2103–2116
Muralidharan P, Sarmah S, Marrs JA (2015) Zebrafish retinal defects induced by ethanol exposure are rescued by retinoic acid and folic acid supplement. Alcohol 49(2):149–163
Nguyen TD, Truong ME, Reiter JF (2022) The intimate connection between lipids and hedgehog signaling. Front Cell Dev Biol 10:876815
Norton WH, Mangoli M, Lele Z, Pogoda H-M, Diamond B, Mercurio S et al (2005) Monorail/Foxa2 regulates floorplate differentiation and specification of oligodendrocytes, serotonergic raphe neurones and cranial motoneurones. Development 132(4):645–658
Nüsslein-Volhard C, Wieschaus E (1980) Mutations affecting segment number and polarity in drosophila. Nature 287(5785):795–801
O'Leary-Moore SK, Parnell SE, Lipinski RJ, Sulik KK (2011) Magnetic resonance-based imaging in animal models of fetal alcohol spectrum disorder. Neuropsychol Rev 21:167–185
Odent S, Attié-Bitach T, Blayau M, Mathieu M, Augé J, Delezoïde A et al (1999) Expression of the sonic hedgehog (SHH) gene during early human development and phenotypic expression of new mutations causing holoprosencephaly. Hum Mol Genet 8(9):1683–1689
Okuda Y, Ogura E, Kondoh H, Kamachi Y (2010) B1 SOX coordinate cell specification with patterning and morphogenesis in the early zebrafish embryo. PLoS Genet 6(5):e1000936
Pala R, Alomari N, Nauli SM (2017) Primary cilium-dependent signaling mechanisms. Int J Mol Sci 18(11):2272
Parnell SE, Eberhart JK (2023) Alcohol and embryology. In: Fetal alcohol spectrum disorders: a multidisciplinary approach. Springer, pp 127–138
Parnell SE, O'Leary-Moore SK, Godin EA, Dehart DB, Johnson BW, Allan Johnson G et al (2009) Magnetic resonance microscopy defines ethanol-induced brain abnormalities in prenatal mice: effects of acute insult on gestational day 8. Alcohol Clin Exp Res 33(6):1001–1011
Pathi S, Pagan-Westphal S, Baker DP, Garber EA, Rayhorn P, Bumcrot D et al (2001) Comparative biological responses to human sonic, Indian, and desert hedgehog. Mech Dev 106(1–2):107–117
Patten AR, Fontaine CJ, Christie BR (2014) A comparison of the different animal models of fetal alcohol spectrum disorders and their use in studying complex behaviors. Front Pediatr 2:93
Pedersen LB, Akhmanova A (2014) Kif7 keeps cilia tips in shape. Nat Cell Biol 16(7):623–625
Peña-Blanco A, García-Sáez AJ (2018) Bax, Bak and beyond—mitochondrial performance in apoptosis. FEBS J 285(3):416–431
Pepinsky R, Zeng C, Wen D, Rayhorn P, Baker D, Williams K et al (1998) Identification of a palmitic acid-modified form of human sonic hedgehog. J Biol Chem 273(22):14037–14045
Porter J, Young K, Beachy P (1996) Cholesterol modification of hedgehog signaling proteins in animal development. Science 274(5285):255–259
Power SC, Lancman J, Smith SM (1999) Retinoic acid is essential for Shh/Hoxd signaling during rat limb outgrowth but not for limb initiation. Dev Dyn 216(4–5):469–480
Prykhozhij SV, Neumann CJ (2008) Distinct roles of Shh and Fgf signaling in regulating cell proliferation during zebrafish pectoral fin development. BMC Dev Biol 8(1):1–11
Pullarkat RK (1991) Hypothesis: prenatal ethanol-induced birth defects and retinoic acid. Alcohol Clin Exp Res 15(3):565–567
Qi X, Li X (2020) Mechanistic insights into the generation and transduction of hedgehog signaling. Trends Biochem Sci 45(5):397–410. https://doi.org/10.1016/j.tibs.2020.01.006

Qi X, Liu H, Thompson B, McDonald J, Zhang C, Li X (2019) Cryo-EM structure of oxysterol-bound human smoothened coupled to a heterotrimeric Gi. Nature 571(7764):279–283

Radhakrishnan A, Rohatgi R, Siebold C (2020) Cholesterol access in cellular membranes controls hedgehog signaling. Nat Chem Biol 16(12):1303–1313

Ramsay M (2010) Genetic and epigenetic insights into fetal alcohol spectrum disorders. Genome Med 2(4):27

Razmara P, Son H-W, Ali DW (2025) Cannabidiol exerts teratogenic effects on developing zebrafish through the sonic hedgehog signaling pathway. Sci Rep 15(1): 14533

Reid HM, Elford H, Till M, Christie BR (2026) Animal models of FASD. In: Bukiya A, Ali DW (eds) Molecular mechanisms and lifelong consequences of prenatal exposure to psychoactive substances. Springer. In press

Resh MD (2021) Palmitoylation of hedgehog proteins by hedgehog acyltransferase: roles in signalling and disease. Open Biol 11(3):200414

Riddle RD, Johnson RL, Laufer E, Tabin C (1993) Sonic hedgehog mediates the polarizing activity of the ZPA. Cell 75(7):1401–1416

Rihel J, Prober DA, Arvanites A, Lam K, Zimmerman S, Jang S et al (2010) Zebrafish behavioral profiling links drugs to biological targets and rest/wake regulation. Science 327(5963):348–351

Robertson EJ (2014) Dose-dependent nodal/Smad signals pattern the early mouse embryo. Semin Cell Dev Biol 32:73–79

Rodrigues RJ, Marques JM, Köfalvi A (2024) Cannabis, endocannabinoids and brain development: from embryogenesis to adolescence. Cells 13(22):1875

Rodríguez-Sastre N, Shapiro N, Hawkins DY, Lion AT, Peyreau M, Correa AE et al (2023) Ethanol exposure perturbs sea urchin development and disrupts developmental timing. Dev Biol 493:89–102. https://doi.org/10.1016/j.ydbio.2022.11.001

Roelink H, Augsburger A, Heemskerk J, Korzh V, Norlin S, i Altaba AR et al (1994) Floor plate and motor neuron induction by vhh-1, a vertebrate homolog of hedgehog expressed by the notochord. Cell 76(4):761–775

Roessler E, Muenke M (2010) The molecular genetics of holoprosencephaly. Am J Med Genet C: Semin Med Genet 154C(1):52–61

Roessler E, Belloni E, Gaudenz K, Jay P, Berta P, Scherer SW et al (1996) Mutations in the human sonic hedgehog gene cause holoprosencephaly. Nat Genet 14(3): 357–360

Roessler E, Du Y-Z, Mullor JL, Casas E, Allen WP, Gillessen-Kaesbach G et al (2003) Loss-of-function mutations in the human GLI2 gene are associated with pituitary anomalies and holoprosencephaly-like features. Proc Natl Acad Sci 100(23):13424–13429

Rogic S, Wong A, Pavlidis P (2016) Meta-analysis of gene expression patterns in animal models of prenatal alcohol exposure suggests role for protein synthesis inhibition and chromatin remodeling. Alcohol Clin Exp Res 40(4):717–727

Ronen GM, Andrews WL (1991) Holoprosencephaly as a possible embryonic alcohol effect. Am J Med Genet 40(2):151–154

Rouzer SK, Gutierrez J, Larin KV, Miranda RC (2023) Alcohol & cannabinoid co-use: implications for impaired fetal brain development following gestational exposure. Exp Neurol 361:114318

Sandor S, Elias S (1968) The influence of aethyl-alcohol on the development of the chick embryo. Rev Roum Embryol Cytol Ser Embryol 5(1):51–76

Sasai N, Toriyama M, Kondo T (2019) Hedgehog signal and genetic disorders. Front Genet 10:1103

Satiroglu-Tufan NL, Tufan AC (2004) Amelioration of ethanol-induced growth retardation by all-trans-retinoic acid and α-tocopherol in shell-less culture of the chick embryo. Reprod Toxicol 18(3):407–412

Schwend T, Ahlgren SC (2009) Zebrafish con/disp1 reveals multiple spatiotemporal requirements for hedgehog-signaling in craniofacial development. BMC Dev Biol 9(1):59

Schwend T, Loucks EJ, Ahlgren SC (2010) Visualization of Gli activity in craniofacial tissues of hedgehog-pathway reporter transgenic zebrafish. PLoS One 5(12):e14396

Shabtai Y, Fainsod A (2018) Competition between ethanol clearance and retinoic acid biosynthesis in the induction of fetal alcohol syndrome. Biochem Cell Biol 96(2):148–160

Shen MM (2007) Nodal signaling: developmental roles and regulation. Development 134:1023

Sidik A, Dixon G, Buckley DM, Kirby HG, Sun S, Eberhart JK (2021) Exposure to ethanol leads to midfacial hypoplasia in a zebrafish model of FASD via indirect interactions with the Shh pathway. BMC Biol 19(1):134. https://doi.org/10.1186/s12915-021-01062-9

Siebold C, Rohatgi R (2023) The inseparable relationship between cholesterol and hedgehog signaling. Annu Rev Biochem 92:273

Smith SM (2008) The avian embryo in fetal alcohol research. In: Alcohol: methods and protocols. Springer, pp 75–84

Smith SM, Garic A, Berres ME, Flentke GR (2014a) Genomic factors that shape craniofacial outcome and neural crest vulnerability in FASD. Front Genet 5:224. https://doi.org/10.3389/fgene.2014.00224

Smith SM, Garic A, Flentke GR, Berres ME (2014b) Neural crest development in fetal alcohol syndrome. Birth Defects Res C Embryo Today 102(3):210–220. https://doi.org/10.1002/bdrc.21078

Stevenson NL (2023) The factory, the antenna and the scaffold: the three-way interplay between the Golgi, cilium and extracellular matrix underlying tissue function. Biol Open 12(2):bio059719

Stockard CR (1910) The influence of alcohol and other anaesthetics on embryonic development. Am J Anat 10:369–392

Streissguth AP, Dehaene P (1993) Fetal alcohol syndrome in twins of alcoholic mothers: concordance of diagnosis and IQ. Am J Med Genet 47(6):857–861

Streissguth AP, Aase JM, Clarren SK, Randels SP, LaDue RA, Smith DF (1991) Fetal alcohol syndrome in adolescents and adults. JAMA 265(15):1961–1967

Sulik KK (1984) Critical periods for alcohol teratogenesis in mice, with special reference to the gastrulation stage of embryogenesis. Ciba Found Symp 105:124–141

Sulik KK (2005) Genesis of alcohol-induced craniofacial dysmorphism. Exp Biol Med (Maywood) 230(6): 366–375. https://doi.org/10.1177/15353702-0323006-04

Sulik KK (2014) Fetal alcohol spectrum disorder: pathogenesis and mechanisms. In: Handbook of clinical neurology. Elsevier, pp 463–475

Sulik K, Johnston M (1982) Embryonic origin of holoprosencephaly: interrelationship of the developing brain and face. Scanning Electron Microsc Pt 1:309–322

Sulik KK, Johnston MC (1983) Sequence of developmental alterations following acute ethanol exposure in mice: craniofacial features of the fetal alcohol syndrome. Am J Anat 166(3):257–269

Sulik KK, Johnston MC, Webb MA (1981) Fetal alcohol syndrome: embryogenesis in a mouse model. Science 214(4523):936–938

Swartz ME, Wells MB, Griffin M, McCarthy N, Lovely CB, McGurk P et al (2014) A screen of zebrafish mutants identifies ethanol-sensitive genetic loci. Alcohol Clin Exp Res 38(3):694–703

Swartz ME, Lovely CB, McCarthy N, Kuka T, Eberhart JK (2020) Novel ethanol-sensitive mutants identified in an F3 forward genetic screen. Alcohol Clin Exp Res 44(1):56–65

Taipale J, Chen JK, Cooper MK, Wang B, Mann RK, Milenkovic L et al (2000) Effects of oncogenic mutations in smoothened and patched can be reversed by cyclopamine. Nature 406(6799):1005–1009

Tang X, Chen R, Mesias VSD, Wang T, Wang Y, Poljak K et al (2022) A SURF4-to-proteoglycan relay mechanism that mediates the sorting and secretion of a tagged variant of sonic hedgehog. Proc Natl Acad Sci U S A 119(11):e2113991119

Tichy J, Zinke J, Bunz B, Meyermann R, Harter PN, Mittelbronn M (2015) Expression profile of sonic hedgehog pathway members in the developing human fetal brain. Biomed Res Int 2015:494269

Tickle C, Towers M (2017) Sonic hedgehog signaling in limb development. Front Cell Dev Biol. 5:14

Tukachinsky H, Kuzmickas RP, Jao CY, Liu J, Salic A (2012) Dispatched and scube mediate the efficient secretion of the cholesterol-modified hedgehog ligand. Cell Rep 2(2):308–320

Twal WO, Zile MH (1997) Retinoic acid reverses ethanol-induced cardiovascular abnormalities in quail embryos. Alcohol Clin Exp Res 21(6):1137–1143

Valente EM, Rosti RO, Gibbs E, Gleeson JG (2014) Primary cilia in neurodevelopmental disorders. Nat Rev Neurol 10(1):27–36

Van Slyke CE, Bradford YM, Westerfield M, Haendel MA (2014) The zebrafish anatomy and stage ontologies: representing the anatomy and development of Danio rerio. Journal of Biomedical Semantics 5(1):1–11

Vangipuram SD, Lyman WD (2012) Ethanol affects differentiation-related pathways and suppresses Wnt signaling protein expression in human neural stem cells. Alcohol Clin Exp Res 36(5):788–797. https://doi.org/10.1111/j.1530-0277.2011.01682.x

Varga ZM, Amores A, Lewis KE, Yan Y-L, Postlethwait JH, Eisen JS et al (2001) Zebrafish smoothened functions in ventral neural tube specification and axon tract formation. Development 128:3497

Voss AK, Strasser A (2020) The essentials of developmental apoptosis. F1000Res 9:9

Wallis D, Muenke M (2000) Mutations in holoprosencephaly. Hum Mutat 16(2):99–108

Walton KD, Warner J, Hertzler PH, McClay DR (2009) Hedgehog signaling patterns mesoderm in the sea urchin. Dev Biol 331(1):26–37

Wang X, Zhao Z, Muller J, Iyu A, Khng AJ, Guccione E et al (2013) Targeted inactivation and identification of targets of the Gli2a transcription factor in the zebrafish. Biology open 2(11):1203–1213

Wang C, Wu H, Evron T, Vardy E, Han GW, Huang X-P et al (2014) Structural basis for smoothened receptor modulation and chemoresistance to anticancer drugs. Nat Commun 5(1):1–11

Wheway G, Nazlamova L, Hancock JT (2018) Signaling through the primary cilium. Front Cell Deve Biol 6:8

Wierbowski BM, Petrov K, Aravena L, Gu G, Xu Y, Salic A (2020) Hedgehog pathway activation requires coreceptor-catalyzed, lipid-dependent relay of the sonic hedgehog ligand. Dev Cell 55(4):450–467. e8

Wilson L, Gale E, Maden M (2003) The role of retinoic acid in the morphogenesis of the neural tube. J Anat 203(4):357–368

Wu X, Ding S, Ding Q, Gray NS, Schultz PG (2002) A small molecule with osteogenesis-inducing activity in multipotent mesenchymal progenitor cells. J Am Chem Soc 124(49):14520–14521

Wu Y, Kurosaka H, Wang Q, Inubushi T, Nakatsugawa K, Kikuchi M et al (2022) Retinoic acid deficiency underlies the etiology of midfacial defects. J Dent Res 101(6):686–694

Xu J, Srinivas BP, Tay SY, Mak A, Yu X, Lee SG et al (2006) Genomewide expression profiling in the zebrafish embryo identifies target genes regulated by Hedgehog signaling during vertebrate development. Genetics 174(2):735–752

Yamada Y, Nagase T, Nagase M, Koshima I (2005) Gene expression changes of sonic hedgehog signaling cascade in a mouse embryonic model of fetal alcohol syndrome. J Craniofac Surg 16(6):1055–1061; discussion 62-3. https://doi.org/10.1097/01.scs.0000183470.31202.c9

Yelin R, Schyr RB-H, Kot H, Zins S, Frumkin A, Pillemer G et al (2005) Ethanol exposure affects gene expression in the embryonic organizer and reduces retinoic acid levels. Dev Biol 279(1):193–204

Yelin R, Kot H, Yelin D, Fainsod A (2007) Early molecular effects of ethanol during vertebrate embryogenesis. Differentiation 75(5):393–403

Yu RM, Lin CC, Chan P, ESH C, Murphy MB, Chan BP et al (2006) Four-dimensional imaging and quantification of gene expression in early developing zebrafish (Danio rerio) embryos. Toxicol Sci 90(2):529–538

Zhang Y, Beachy PA (2023) Cellular and molecular mechanisms of hedgehog signalling. Nat Rev Mol Cell Biol 24:1–20

Zhang XM, Ramalho-Santos M, McMahon AP (2001) Smoothened mutants reveal redundant roles for Shh and Ihh signaling including regulation of L/R asymmetry by the mouse node. Cell 105(6):781–792

Zhang C, Turton QM, Mackinnon S, Sulik KK, Cole GJ (2011) Agrin function associated with ocular development is a target of ethanol exposure in embryonic zebrafish. Birth Defects Res A Clin Mol Teratol 91(3):129–141. https://doi.org/10.1002/bdra.20766

Zhang Y, Fu L, Qi X, Zhang Z, Xia Y, Jia J et al (2013a) Structural insight into the mutual recognition and regulation between suppressor of fused and Gli/ci. Nat Commun 4(1):2608

Zhang C, Ojiaku P, Cole GJ (2013b) Forebrain and hindbrain development in zebrafish is sensitive to ethanol exposure involving agrin, Fgf, and sonic hedgehog function. Birth Defects Res A Clin Mol Teratol 97(1): 8–27. https://doi.org/10.1002/bdra.23099

Zhang C, Frazier JM, Chen H, Liu Y, Lee JA, Cole GJ (2014) Molecular and morphological changes in zebrafish following transient ethanol exposure during defined developmental stages. Neurotoxicol Teratol 44:70–80. https://doi.org/10.1016/j.ntt.2014.06.001

Zhang C, Anderson A, Cole GJ (2015) Analysis of crosstalk between retinoic acid and sonic hedgehog pathways following ethanol exposure in embryonic zebrafish. Birth Defects Res A Clin Mol Teratol 103(12):1046–1057. https://doi.org/10.1002/bdra.23460

Zhang C, Boa-Amponsem O, Cole GJ (2017) Comparison of molecular marker expression in early zebrafish brain development following chronic ethanol or morpholino treatment. Exp Brain Res 235(8):2413–2423. https://doi.org/10.1007/s00221-017-4977-5

Zhang Y, Bulkley DP, Xin Y, Roberts KJ, Asarnow DE, Sharma A et al (2018) Structural basis for cholesterol transport-like activity of the hedgehog receptor patched. Cell 175(5):1352–64. e14

Zhang C, Ezem N, Mackinnon S, Cole GJ (2023) Embryonic ethanol but not cannabinoid exposure affects zebrafish cardiac development via Agrin and sonic hedgehog interaction. Cells 12(9):1327. https://doi.org/10.3390/cells12091327

Zohn IE, Sarkar AA (2008) Modeling neural tube defects in the mouse. Curr Top Dev Biol 84:1–35

4 Prenatal Exposure to Low Alcohol and Alcohol Motivation in the Offspring

Ricardo M. Pautassi, María Carolina Fabio, and Mónica Sanchez

Abstract

Prenatal alcohol exposure (PAE), even at low doses, has been linked to long-term alterations in alcohol-related behaviors, particularly increased alcohol consumption and preference in offspring. This chapter examines how low-dose PAE affects the motivational effects of alcohol, potentially influencing the balance between its rewarding and aversive properties. While high-dose PAE has been extensively studied for its teratogenic effects, the implications of lower, more common exposures remain less understood. Preclinical studies using rodent models suggest that even moderate PAE (1–3 g/kg/day) enhances sensitivity to alcohol's appetitive properties while reducing its aversive effects, promoting future alcohol-seeking behavior. These alterations may be mediated by neurobiological changes, including increased neurogenesis of enkephalin-expressing neurons, disruptions in dopamine and opioid signaling, and modifications in stress-related neural circuits. Behavioral paradigms, such as conditioned place preference and conditioned taste aversion, confirm that PAE enhances the reinforcing effects of ethanol while mitigating its negative consequences. Operant self-administration studies also report greater motivation after PAE. These motivational alterations correlate, albeit with studies not measuring the same variables in the same individual, with increased alcohol consumption in adolescence and adulthood. This chapter further discusses the mechanisms underlying these effects. Understanding the impact of low-dose PAE on alcohol motivation can provide crucial insights into early-life risk factors for problematic drinking and inform preventive interventions.

Keywords

Prenatal alcohol exposure · Ethanol motivation · Reward sensitivity · Conditioned place preference · Operant self-administration · Neurodevelopment

R. M. Pautassi (✉) · M. C. Fabio · M. Sanchez
Instituto de Investigación Médica M. y M. Ferreyra (INIMEC-CONICET-Universidad Nacional de Córdoba), Córdoba, Argentina
e-mail: rpautassi@immf.uncor.edu; mcfabio@immf.uncor.edu; msanchez@immf.uncor.edu

A. N. Bukiya, D. W. Ali (eds.), *Molecular Mechanisms and Lifelong Consequences of Prenatal Exposure to Psychoactive Substances*, Advances in Experimental Medicine and Biology 1500,
https://doi.org/10.1007/978-3-032-12741-9_4

4.1 Introduction

4.1.1 Why Is It Essential to Assess the Effects of Prenatal Alcohol?

Prenatal alcohol exposure (PAE) can lead to a wide range of congenital conditions, collectively known as fetal alcohol spectrum disorders (FASD). Although its exact extent remains a subject of debate PAE is widely prevalent, probably due to many exposures occurring even before the recognition of pregnancy.

Heavy prenatal alcohol exposure (we will also refer to alcohol as ethanol, particularly in the context of preclinical studies) throughout gestation appears to be less common and is more likely to occur in individuals diagnosed with an alcohol use disorder (AUD). A study by Lopez et al. (2017) on pregnant Argentinean women reported an 8.1% prevalence of AUD based on DSM-5 criteria, with 6.4% classified as mild, 0.8% as moderate, and 0.9% as severe. According to the DSM-5, AUD is diagnosed when ≥2 of 11 criteria are met within a 12-month period, with severity classified as mild (2–3 criteria), moderate (4–5 criteria), or severe (≥6 criteria).

However, global studies indicate that the prevalence of (any) alcohol use during pregnancy is alarmingly high. Research conducted in Uruguay showed an increase in alcohol consumption during pregnancy from 2013 to 2016 (Moraes Castro et al. 2019), rising from 24% to 37–40%. These figures, while significant, are still lower than the 48% reported in a meta-analysis of Australian studies (Young et al. 2022). Alcohol consumption during pregnancy is, of course, highly influenced by cultural and economic factors and varies significantly across countries. One study estimated the global prevalence of alcohol use during pregnancy at 9.8% (Popova et al. 2017).

Epidemiological studies have consistently identified PAE as a predictor of increased risk of problematic alcohol use during adolescence and early adulthood. A landmark longitudinal study (Baer et al. 2003, 1998), which began in 1974–75, followed approximately 430 individuals at ages 14 and 21. The results showed that PAE was a stronger predictor of adolescent alcohol use and related problems than a family history of alcoholism, at both time points. Similarly, Alati et al. (2008) reported that exposure to three or more alcoholic drinks during pregnancy was significantly associated with a higher likelihood of alcohol-related problems in early adulthood. These findings suggest that even low to moderate levels of PAE may increase vulnerability to problematic drinking, and effect that may be related to PAE altering the motivational properties of alcohol.

Clinical studies face challenges in assessing the biological mechanisms of PAE and evaluating treatments, mainly due to confounding factors like co-exposure to other drugs, poor nutrition, and inadequate health care access, which often coexist in populations vulnerable to substance use (Konijnenberg 2015). Methodological factors related to sampling and selection bias also affect these studies. For instance, the excellent large-scale study of May et al. (2018) estimated a 1.1–5.0% prevalence of FASD among first-grade children in four U.S. communities. The researchers used active case ascertainment methods, which included in-person physical and neurobehavioral assessments. However, they noted as a limitation that consent rates for screening ranged from 36.9% to 92.5% across the different samples. It is possible that significant differences exist between those who consent and those who do not, with this confound differentially affecting the individual samples.

The use of pre-clinical (rat, mouse) studies reduces the predictive validity of the findings. Still, it helps mitigate these methodological confounders and serves as a critical benchmark for evaluating new hypotheses and treatments. Illustrating this point, the palliative effects of choline supplementation on FASD symptoms were first shown via animal models (Thomas et al. 2007), providing the rationale for subsequent clinical trials (Nguyen et al. 2016). Preclinical studies have also helped address research gaps on the genetic and epigenetic mechanisms of FASD and other developmental disorders, for instance by using the fly species

Drosophila melanogaster as a model system (Morozova et al. 2022; MacPherson et al. 2023). Another emerging line of research is investigating the role of gut microbiota in problematic alcohol use, with increasing evidence linking microbial dysbiosis to altered drinking behaviors. Notably, bacterial extracellular vesicles (bEVs)—critical messengers in host–microbe communication—have been proposed as modulators of addictive behavior (Diaz-Ubilla et al. 2025), although their exact mechanisms remain unclear. A recent study showed that transferring bEVs from high-alcohol-consuming rats (UChB) to alcohol-avoiding Wistar rats significantly increased voluntary alcohol intake (Diaz-Ubilla et al. 2025). This effect, which occurred independently of inflammatory responses, was completely abolished by bilateral vagotomy, implicating the vagus nerve as a key mediator. These findings suggest a novel pathway through which the gut microbiota may influence alcohol consumption (Atukorala et al. 2024). This line of research is also being applied to study PAE mechanisms and potential treatments. A recent study showed that PAE altered bacterial diversity in the gut, specifically taxa relevant for the production of the short-chain fatty butyric acid (Vella et al. 2025). In males PAE seemed to increase the abundance *Faecalibaculum* and Bacilli, at the genera and class levels respectively; whereas PAE females exhibited, compared to controls, increased Prevotellaceae and decreased *Bifidobacterium* (Vella et al. 2025).

One relatively unexplored area has been the preclinical analysis of how prenatal exposure to low doses of ethanol alters postnatal sensitivity to ethanol's motivational effects. Our emphasis on low-dose PAE considers that this is a likely scenario in which PAE takes place. The motivational effects of drugs (i.e., their appetitive, aversive, and negative reinforcing effects) (Pautassi et al. 2009) are key to promoting or deterring subsequent consumption. Therefore, events that tip the balance towards the appetitive impact of a certain drug or lessen its aversive effects are likely to promote engagement with that drug (Edwards and Koob 2010). For instance, it has been demonstrated that adolescent rats appear to be more sensitive to the appetitive effects of ethanol, yet less sensitive to its aversive effects. In Pautassi et al. (2008), the pairing in adolescent rats of a conditioned stimulus with ethanol administration endowed this stimulus with the ability to condition preference for a second conditioned stimulus. This so-called "second-order conditioning" did not occur in adult rats. Others have shown that adolescent rats are less sensitive to ethanol-induced aversion, in paradigms in which a conditioned stimulus is paired with ethanol-induced malaise (Saalfield and Spear 2016). Intriguingly, the apparent greater sensitivity of adolescents to ethanol's appetitive effects, coupled with a blunted response to ethanol-induced aversion is associated with increased ethanol intake in these young rats compared to adults (Vetter et al. 2007).

Preclinical studies examining the impact of PAE on postnatal sensitivity to alcohol often rely on well-established paradigms to assess ethanol-related motivation. One is conditioned place preference (CPP), which measures the association between a specific environment and the rewarding pharmacological effects of ethanol (Tzschentke 2007). During conditioning, the subject is alternately exposed to a context (e.g., a box with black and white stripes and lined with sandpaper) after receiving an ethanol administration and to another context (e.g., a box with a single solid color and a smooth surface) after a neutral treatment. On the test day, usually conducted in a drug-free state, the subject is given free access to both environments. A preference for the ethanol-paired context—evidenced by increased time spent in that environment—indicates that the ethanol's effects were perceived as rewarding. The aversive effects of ethanol, on the other hand, can be measured using the conditioned taste aversion (CTA) paradigm (Fabio et al. 2015a), which involves allowing rats or mice to access a sapid and novel solution (e.g., saccharin, sodium chloride or a lemon-scented solution) while experiencing the post-ingestive effects of ethanol. Subsequent tests, conducted 24 or 48 h after conditioning, typically reveal a decrease in the ingestion of the ethanol-paired solution (Verendeev and Riley 2012). This learned aversion is sometimes accompanied by distinctive orofacial responses (e.g., gaping, passive drips) and behavioral responses (e.g., wall climbing), which are indicative of taste avoidance (Liu et al. 2009). The motivation to ingest ethanol, on the other hand, can be measured via operant self-administration (SA) paradigms, in which a seemingly random behavior (e.g., bar pressing) leads to access to a usually small quantity of ethanol. In general terms, substantial engagement in the behavior is assumed to reflect the underlying motivation for the drug-seeking behavior, driven by its appetite effects. A full description of the range of alcohol drinking models available (e.g., two-bottle choice, intermittent access home-cage drinking, binge-like drinking, operant behavior with fixed or progressive ratio, alcohol reinstatement after deprivation, etc.) cannot be provided in this chapter due to space constraints; however, interested readers can refer to comprehensive reviews such as Tunstall et al. (2020). Together, these paradigms provide complementary benchmarks to assess how a given treatment or condition, for instance PAE, may shape the motivational valence of alcohol later in life, revealing both its rewarding and aversive properties across different behavioral dimensions.

4.1.2 Aim of the Chapter

The central aim of this chapter is to review how low-dose PAE alters the motivational effects of ethanol. The first section will begin by clarifying what is typically meant by low-dose PAE in the preclinical literature. The following sections will examine how PAE modulates ethanol's motivational properties and then address two key questions. The first concerns the neurobiological mechanisms underlying these changes. While considerable behavioral evidence exists, studies on neural correlates—such as patterns of neuronal activation, motivational drives toward alcohol, and synaptic plasticity—are still limited. The second question is whether there is evidence linking altered motivational sensitivity to actual ethanol intake patterns in the offspring. This question is important because consummatory behaviors, such as ethanol intake, do not always exhibit a point-to-point relationship with the appetitive reactivity evoked by the stimulus under analysis.

Most of the literature reviewed in this chapter will focus on preclinical studies, although we may, and already have, refer to clinical work when appropriate. Likewise, within the preclinical field, most studies examining the modulation of PAE on ethanol's motivational effects have been conducted in rats. It should be noted that this is, of course, not an exhaustive review of the literature. We selected studies that seemed most relevant to the specific scope of this chapter.

4.1.3 How Much Low Alcohol Is Low, in the Context of Preclinical PAE Studies?

When we refer to low-dose ethanol in this context, we are talking about a reduced amount of alcohol—either in daily quantity or in the total duration of exposure across gestation—relative to paradigms that use heavy, intoxicating doses throughout most pregnancy. Importantly, "low" doesn't mean "safe." Quite the opposite: the core idea behind this chapter is that even minimal or sporadic ethanol exposure during pregnancy can be enough to trigger significant, long-term consequences in the offspring.

For example, studies that administer 1 g/kg/day of ethanol to pregnant rats via oral gavage during gestational days 17–20 are typically categorized as using low or moderate dose (Popoola et al. 2015). These protocols do not usually produce visible signs of intoxication in the dam and lead to relatively low blood ethanol concentrations compared to moderate or high-exposure models. On the other end of the spectrum, a high-exposure paradigm might involve early postnatal ethanol administration—that is, days 1–10 of the rat or mouse, a developmental window that corresponds to the human third trimester of gestation—where pups receive 5 g/kg/day split into two doses (Marengo et al. 2023). That said, it is not unusual to find studies administering 2 g/kg/day of ethanol to pregnant dams (e.g., during GDs 17–20) and still labeling their exposure as "moderate" PAE (Chotro and

Arias 2003). This is likely because maternal righting reflex remains intact and the observed alterations in maternal care are subtle. When the same authors provided 3 g/kg/day of ethanol to pregnant dams they described that regime as employing a relatively high ethanol dose (Arias and Chotro 2006).

It is also worth noting that in studies focusing specifically on dysmorphology, what is called a "low-dose" ethanol exposure can actually involve doses higher than 2 g/kg/day. For instance, Schambra et al. (2016) examined the effects of PAE in pregnant C57Bl/6 J mice using nasogastric gavage to the dams during gastrulation (gestational day 7, GD7) or neurulation (GD8), with two doses—2.4 or 2.9 g/kg—given 4 h apart. Despite being labeled "low" and "moderate," we consider these doses to be high and overly intoxicating, which is why they are excluded from this chapter.

In contrast, other studies use paradigms that better fit the "low-dose" category, such as providing ethanol to the dams via drinking bottles or liquid diet. When the ethanol concentration is around 6%, and animals have alternating access to alcohol and water, blood alcohol levels (BALs) remain low. For instance, in a protocol originally implemented by Probyn et al. (2012) and later used by Walton et al. (2019), BALs reached just 0.03% -in fact, in some cases, they were undetectable. In the latter study, neither litter size nor birth weight was affected, reinforcing that the model fits well within the parameters of "low alcohol PAE."

On the other hand, when the alcohol concentration is ≥10% and water access is severely restricted, the rat dam can drink around 6–7 g/kg/d (Plaza et al. 2020), thus making these examples of PAE protocols associated with high levels of ethanol stimulation. For instance, Barbier et al. (2009) reported that offspring of PAE dams acquired CPP to ethanol more readily than controls, ingested more ethanol, and displayed greater susceptibility to ethanol-induced locomotor impairment. These results, consistent with the hypothesis of PAE heightening sensitivity to ethanol's rewarding effects and augmenting ethanol intake, were obtained in the offspring of dams continuously exposed to 10% ethanol as the sole fluid before, during, and even a few weeks after gestation. Therefore, results from this study and those of similar studies using PAE protocols will not be considered for discussion in the present chapter.

In sum, while the term 'low-dose' can encompass a range of experimental paradigms, this chapter focuses specifically on those models in which maternal ethanol exposure is limited in both amount and duration, resulting in low levels of intoxication and blood alcohol levels, conditions that allow for the examination of subtle yet potentially impactful effects of mild PAE.

4.2 Does Prenatal Exposure to Low Alcohol Alter the Motivational Effects of Ethanol?

4.2.1 Appetitive Effects

The reinforcing properties of ethanol extend beyond its pharmacological effects, as its orosensory characteristics and the environmental cues associated with its consumption can acquire conditioned stimulus properties. These become predictive of the drug's pharmacological consequences as the fetus experiences ethanol in utero. If ethanol is predominantly perceived as a positive stimulus with appetitive properties, fetuses exposed to the drug should be more likely to exhibit enhanced attraction to ethanol or ethanol-related cues postnatally (Spear and Molina 2005). This increased approach behavior can be observed in their preference for the odor of ethanol or environmental contexts associated with prior exposure, as well as in operant behavior tasks (Miranda-Morales et al. 2014). We will now review some of these studies.

A fundamental model for studying the reinforcing appetitive effects of low-to-moderate PAE has been developed by Juan Carlos Molina's research group. This model has been instrumental in advancing our understanding of how moderate PAE shapes later responses to the drug. It involves the intragastric administration of ethanol at a dose of 1.0 or 2.0 g/kg to pregnant rats during gestational days 17–20, which corresponds to the last week of their gestation yet actually models second-trimester human gestation. Using this approach, it has been demonstrated that fetuses and placentas reach similar BALs than those circulating in the mother's blood and that neonatal rat pups—90–150 min after birth—react differently to alcohol odor compared to control neonates (Dominguez et al. 1996).

In one of the seminal studies conducted using this model, a 2.0 g/kg ethanol solution was given to pregnant Wistar rats on gestational days 17–20, paired with cineole, to analyze whether the motivational effects of ethanol can function as an unconditioned stimulus capable of supporting associative learning in fetuses. When the offspring were 16 days postpartum, the researchers assessed their mouthing behavior, considered an appetitive response, when presented with ethanol or cineole alone, compared to milk. Pups exposed to pairings of ethanol and cineole in utero exhibited heightened mouthing behavior in response to cineol and ethanol compared to controls, a sign of appetitive, ethanol-mediated learning in newborn rats (Abate et al. 2000). Similarly, using the same paradigm, newborns who had experienced ethanol in utero, paired with cineol, showed a heightened suckling response to an artificial nipple in the presence of cineol odor, compared to no odor or a novel odor (Abate et al. 2002). Consistent with these results, PAE (1.0 or 2.0 g/kg on GDs 17–20) enhanced conditioning to alcohol or its gustatory equivalent (sucrose-quinine) in 1-day-old rat pups (March et al. 2009).

The studies just reviewed suggest that low-to-moderate PAE may set the stage for an association between the odor of ethanol and the pharmacological consequences of the drug. It should be noted that, although these findings support this putative pathway, recent comprehensive analyses (Forestell 2024) indicate that such chemosensory learning is a widespread phenomenon, also observed for various non-ethanol compounds in the maternal diet. Ethanol's dual sensory and pharmacological properties, however, may confer it a unique reinforcement value. The pup's apparent increased brain acetaldehyde (ACD) production could promote the association noted (Gaztanaga et al. 2017). ACD is a major metabolite of ethanol, produced primarily in the liver by the enzyme alcohol dehydrogenase and in the brain by catalase. ACD shares alcohol's behavioral effects, and the motivational and motor effects of alcohol in newborn rats appear to be partly modulated by PAE. Notably, catalase inhibition blocked the reinforcing effects of ethanol, assessed a few hours after birth in rats (Nizhnikov et al. 2007); and PAE pups exhibited tolerance to the sedative motor effects of ACD (March et al. 2013).

Moreover, 1.0 g/kg ethanol at GDs 17–20 enhances operant learning for 3% alcohol in 5-day-old pups (Miranda-Morales et al. 2014) but does not alter sucrose-mediated reinforcement (Nizhnikov et al. 2006). In 1-day-old neonates, the same PAE protocol induced reinforcing effects of ethanol at a broader range of doses than in unexposed neonates (Nizhnikov et al. 2006). Specifically, in the latter study the pups were exposed to an artificial nipple shortly before varying doses of ethanol (0.25, 0.5, and 0.75 g/kg) or vehicle. Ninety minutes later, the attachment to the empty surrogate nipple was assessed. Control rats displayed an increased preference for the nipple after only one dose of ethanol, whereas all three doses were equally effective for PAE counterparts (Nizhnikov et al. 2006). PAE also increases response to natural reinforcers (such as sucrose) if this is paired postnatally with ethanol. Infant rats prenatally exposed to 2.0 g/kg of ethanol (GDs 17–20) displayed an increased preference for sucrose when this solution was paired with alcohol and exhibited better resistance to extinction (Culleré et al. 2014). At infancy (postnatal days 14–15, PDs 14–15), this PAE treatment enhanced operant responding for access to ethanol, an effect that was modulated by the opioid system (Miranda-Morales et al. 2010). Altogether, these findings suggest that PAE enhances the reinforcing properties of alcohol, potentially increasing the risk of maladaptive ethanol-seeking behaviors later in life.

PAE pups also exhibited alterations in the motivational properties of ethanol, as assessed through CPP and CTA. As already discussed,

CPP is a paradigm that evaluates the reinforcing effects of a substance by measuring an animal's preference for an environment previously paired with drug administration. CTA, on the other hand, assesses the aversive properties of a substance by associating its consumption with an unpleasant physiological consequence. Pups exposed to 2.0 g/kg on GDs 17–20 (Pautassi et al. 2012) exhibited increased sensitivity to the appetitive reinforcing effects of alcohol, as reflected in heightened CPP. This PAE protocol simultaneously reduced sensitivity to alcohol's aversive effects, as shown by a diminished expression of place aversion without affecting CTA.

In general, there is some agreement that the neural circuits regulating the rewarding effects of different classes of drugs of abuse (e.g., opioids, stimulants, alcohol) partially overlap. Therefore, some lessons for the question we are trying to address in this section can be drawn from PAE studies that have assessed motivational sensitivity in the offspring to drugs other than ethanol. A study exposed dams throughout gestation to ethanol in a fashion that induced, at GD16, 2 h after lights off (thus, presumably, when the dams had drunk the most), mean BALs of 109 mg/dl. This ethanol exposure was associated with increased sensitivity to amphetamine (Uban et al. 2015). The PAE offspring required a lower threshold for sensitization compared to control groups. Behavioral sensitization refers to a progressive increase in drug-induced locomotion, theorized to reflect the transition from a non-addicted to an addicted state (Camarini and Pautassi 2016).

Overall, the findings highlight the lasting impact of PAE on ethanol reinforcement, particularly by enhancing sensitivity to its appetitive effects. This increased responsiveness to ethanol's rewarding properties may contribute to a greater risk of alcohol-seeking behavior later in life.

4.2.2 Aversive Effects

Alcohol is a biphasic motivational drug, not only associated with appetitive effects but also (particularly at high doses or at peak blood ethanol levels) with aversive consequences such as sedation, discomfort, and gastrointestinal malaise. In this section, we will review evidence from animal models suggesting that PAE alters the perception of alcohol's aversive properties, making the offspring less sensitive to these adverse effects. It is worth noting that lower sensitivity to ethanol's effects has been associated, in clinical studies, with greater drinking or alcohol-related negative consequences (Schuckit 1994).

In a study (Gore-Langton and Spear 2019) assessing ethanol-induced CTA after PAE, male and female adolescent Sprague-Dawley rats were given 30-min access to either a polydipsogenic sweet solution ("super saccharin"; 3% sucrose, 0.125% saccharin) (Valenstein et al. 1967) or sodium chloride (NaCl), followed by an intraperitoneal injection of 20% ethanol (0, 1, 1.25, or 1.5 g/kg) across three conditioning sessions. The results showed that PAE attenuated alcohol-induced CTA in males conditioned to SS, whereas no significant effects were observed in females (Gore-Langton and Spear 2019). This reduced sensitivity to ethanol-induced aversive conditioning in PAE animals is consistent with findings from Fabio et al. (2015a), in which a higher dose of ethanol (2.5 g/kg) was used as the unconditional stimulus in the CTA procedure.

Furthermore, a study conducted in infant rats prenatally exposed to 2.0 g/kg of alcohol (GDs 17–20) and administered different alcohol doses on PD13 (0.0, 0.5, or 2.5 g/kg) found that PAE did not alter acute sensitivity to the motor activating effects of alcohol (Arias et al. 2008). In this study (Arias et al. 2008), the rats were tested for spontaneous exploration of an open field (a square-shaped maze), and distance travelled was measured as an index of motor activity. PAE rats exhibited overall (i.e., regardless ethanol or vehicle administration) heightened motor activity (Arias et al. 2008). Similarly, preweaning rats exposed to 2.0 g/kg on GD 10–15 exhibited heightened motor activity in an open field, along with increased anxiety-like responses and greater alcohol intake (Collier et al. 2024).

Altogether, these findings suggest that PAE weakens the ability to associate ethanol with negative consequences, potentially facilitating future alcohol consumption. Moreover, PAE seems to induce, along with blunted sensitivity to ethanol-induced aversion, long-lasting alterations in exploratory and motor behaviors.

4.3 Neurobiological Factors Underlying the PAE-Induced Alterations in the Motivational Effects of Ethanol

PAE has been extensively studied for its behavioral consequences, particularly its role in promoting increased alcohol use during adolescence and adulthood. However, fewer studies have focused on the neurobiological mechanisms underlying these outcomes, in the context of low-dose exposure. In this section, we review evidence pointing to the neural alterations induced by low-PAE that may contribute to long-term changes in alcohol-related motivation and behavior.

While some findings highlight the long-term behavioral impact of low-dose PAE, it is important to note that such exposure often occurs without classic markers of dysmorphology. For instance, the studies using 1–2 g/kg intubations at GD17–20 have, for the most part, revealed no significant alterations in the size or weight of the placenta and umbilical cord, overall body weight of the pups, or the dimensions of the cerebral hemispheres and cerebellum (Abate et al. 2000). Moreover, detection and discrimination of chemosensory stimuli are preserved after this mode of PAE (Dominguez et al. 1996). These findings cement the idea that low-dose PAE may promote early learning about alcohol through the mother's amniotic fluid. This early exposure enables familiarity with ethanol or endows ethanol-related cues with reinforcing properties, making the offspring more likely to consume alcohol later in life, a hypothesis championed by the influential review by Spear and Molina (2005). However, this does not mean that low-dose PAE is devoid of overt neurobiological changes, such as alterations in gene expression or reduced functionality in specific brain areas. We will now review studies on this topic.

Under the framework that PAE may change the perception of alcohol odor and gene expression in the olfactory bulb, Middleton et al. (2009) investigated the impact of prenatal alcohol on adolescent rats. Pregnant rats in this study were given alcohol via a liquid diet from days 11 to 20 of gestation, a critical period for fetal olfactory development. This exposure protocol provided 35% of daily caloric intake via the alcohol solution and resulted in BALs of approximately 150 mg/dL, which the authors defined as modeling moderate ethanol consumption. The adolescent offspring's response to alcohol odor was later assessed, and olfactory bulbs were collected. Microarray analysis, a high-throughput technique used to measure gene expression levels across thousands of genes simultaneously, revealed alterations in the expression of several genes involved in various neurotransmission systems, suggesting a molecular reorganization of the olfactory bulb due to PAE. Changes were observed in genes associated with the glutamatergic, GABAergic, dopaminergic, and serotonergic systems. Specifically, Grin1 and Gria3, which encode subunits of NMDA and AMPA receptors, showed reduced expression, suggesting a decrease in synaptic plasticity and excitatory neurotransmission that could affect alcohol odor perception and susceptibility. In the GABAergic system, the genes Gad1 and Gabrg2, involved in GABA synthesis and function, also exhibited reduced expression, indicating potential alterations in neuronal inhibition within the olfactory bulb. In the dopaminergic system, a reduction in the expression of Drd2, encoding the dopamine D2 receptor, could impact dopaminergic sensitivity and the regulation of reward circuits. Finally, in the serotonergic system, a decrease in the expression of Htr2a, encoding the serotonin 2A receptor, suggests alterations in olfactory perception and emotional behavior in PAE animals. Middleton et al. (2009) concluded that PAE disrupts the expression of genes involved in GABAergic, dopaminergic, and serotonergic neurotransmission in the olfactory bulb, which may contribute to behavioral changes in response to alcohol odor and an increased predisposition to alcohol consumption during adolescence. These findings support the hypothesis that PAE induces changes in olfactory circuits, enhancing the attraction to alcohol in adolescence and promoting greater consumption in later life stages.

A subsequent study (Middleton et al. 2012) examined whether social enrichment could reverse social deficits induced by PAE, and analyzed neurobiological underpinnings of this phenomenon. Female pregnant rats were administered two intraperitoneal doses of alcohol during a critical period of gestation that is essential for early embryonic brain development. This timing allows for the evaluation of both the neurotoxic effects of alcohol on neuronal development and its long-term consequences, including cognitive, behavioral, and developmental deficits in offspring. In this study, social enrichment was defined as housing with unfamiliar conspecifics born to untreated dams from weaning until postnatal day 42. The social interactions of the progeny were evaluated, and gene expression in the amygdala and ventral striatum was subsequently analyzed. Although social enrichment did not affect other social behaviors, it successfully reversed the deficits in social motivation, reducing avoidance in alcohol-exposed rats. Gene expression analysis in the amygdala and ventral striatum revealed that PAE induced alterations in genes related to neurotransmission, vesicular trafficking, and neuronal plasticity during adolescence. These alterations may be linked to the observed increase in social avoidance and the reduction in social motivation in alcohol-exposed animals. Notably, social enrichment exerted restorative effects on the expression of key genes. Specifically, it increased the expression of Galr3, a neuropeptide involved in regulating anxiety and neuronal inhibition, suggesting a possible restoration of the balance of GABAergic transmission and an improvement in social motivation. An increase in Kiss1, a neuropeptide associated with anxiety regulation and social interactions, was also observed, indicating that social enrichment may modulate emotional responses. Furthermore, an interaction between alcohol exposure and social enrichment was identified in the genes Chrna6 and Rabep2, whose expression increased in both groups, though more prominently in animals not exposed to alcohol. This suggests that both prenatal experiences and the postnatal environment can influence neuronal plasticity. These findings suggest that PAE affects key genes involved in neurotransmission and the regulation of social behavior, contributing to the observed deficits. However, social enrichment exerted a compensatory effect by normalizing the expression of genes implicated in anxiety and social motivation.

Another transmitter system heavily involved in the consequences of PAE is the kappa opioid receptor system. This system mediates responses to aversive stimulation, including those triggered by stress and by the negative affective states associated with withdrawal from drugs of abuse. While drugs of abuse often produce acute rewarding effects such as euphoria, their discontinuation after repeated use can induce dysphoria, anxiety, and other aversive states, in which the kappa opioid receptor system plays a key modulatory role. Early reports suggested that PAE may be associated with reduced functionality of the kappa opioid receptor system. Rats exposed to low levels of ethanol in utero (GD 17–20, 1.0 g/kg) exhibited reduced synaptosomal kappa opioid receptor expression in the nucleus accumbens, amygdala, and hippocampus (Nizhnikov et al. 2014). Moreover, in this study, the rats were trained in a conditioned place aversion procedure, using as the unconditional stimulus the effects derived from the administration of an agonist of the kappa opioid receptor system. Control rats exhibit conditioned aversion following kappa stimulation, an effect that was not observed in PAE rats (Nizhnikov et al. 2014). The kappa opioid receptor system functions like a figurative "brake" on the dopaminergic system, especially in key areas related to reward, motivation, and emotion. The dopaminergic system is critically involved in the regulation of reward processes associated with both drugs of abuse and natural stimuli, such as food or social interaction. This prompted the hypothesis that PAE rats could exhibit an exaggerated dopaminergic response to drugs of abuse. The expectation was confirmed. PAE rats given ethanol during adolescence exhibited heightened dopaminergic activity in the ventral tegmental area (VTA), compared to controls reared by vehicle-treated dams (Fabio et al. 2015b).

Subsequent studies (Wille-Bille et al. 2018, 2020) provided, however, a more nuanced picture of the relationships between PAE and the kappa opioid system. This work found several alterations in kappa opioid gene expression induced by PAE. Specifically, they reported a PAE-induced dysregulation of the dynorphin/kappa opioid receptor (PDYN/KOR) system in the VTA, characterized by its upregulation, along with decreased expression of the nociceptine/orphanin FQ receptors in the VTA and reduced PDYN expression in the nucleus accumbens (Wille-Bille et al. 2018). At the VTA, the noted alterations in gene expression were associated with reductions of DNA methylation at the PDYN and at the KOR gene promoter. Interestingly, a follow-up experiment with PAE adolescents raised in an enriched environment reported a reversion of some of these effects (Wille-Bille et al. 2020).

There is evidence of PAE rodents exhibiting heightened an anxiety-prone phenotype, linked to dysregulation of the PDYN/KOR system. Such a profile was evident, for instance, in avoidance of brightly lit areas in the Light-Dark Box test and the Concentric Square Field test, tasks specifically designed to assess anxiety and risk-taking behavior (Wille-Bille et al. 2018). These behavioral alterations after PAE were accompanied by dysregulation of the PDYN/KOR system, which could contribute to increased stress sensitivity and negative emotional states. This can potentially explain why PAE animals in the study (Wille-Bille et al. 2018) showed more anxiety-like behaviors.

More general effects of PAE on neural function have been also reported. In Fabio et al. (2013) the effects of PAE on alcohol consumption and neuronal activity in the adolescent offspring were examined. Pregnant dams received 2.0 g/kg of alcohol via intragastric intubation from GDs 17–20. These offspring doubled their voluntary ethanol intake at adolescence, compared to controls, and exhibit reduced basal neural activity in the infralimbic cortex, a brain region involved in extinction learning and addiction vulnerability. These findings suggest that altered medial prefrontal cortex function may contribute to the predisposition for excessive ethanol consumption after PAE. However, a link between the heightened ethanol intake and ethanol sensitivity was not observed, as PAE did not affect ethanol-induced locomotor activation, which is often considered a proxy for ethanol-induced appetitive effects. PAE also did not affect ultrasonic vocalizations or ethanol metabolism, in the offspring.

Recently, Yao et al. (2023) evaluated the neurobiological effects of PAE by administering 5 g/kg/day of alcohol to pregnant rats from gestational days 7 to 21. This dosing regimen is considered to model chronic and heavy alcohol consumption patterns in humans. Subsequently, they assessed the offspring's predisposition to alcohol intake and susceptibility to post-traumatic stress disorder (PTSD). The PAE males showed a significantly greater preference for alcohol compared to controls and demonstrated greater vulnerability to PTSD. Moreover, PAE altered HCN1 channel function, affecting neuronal activity in the prefrontal cortex and amygdala, which likely favored the greater predisposition to alcohol consumption and increased susceptibility to PTSD in males.

It is interesting to note that, in this chapter, we put our focus on maternal exposure to ethanol during pregnancy. Yet, some researchers have also analyzed the effects of paternal exposure before mating. Although we will not go at length describing these findings or models, it is worth revising neurobiological effects of this type of developmental exposure. For instance, Ceccanti et al. (2016) exposed CD1 male mice to ethanol for 2 months via oral administration in the drinking water, using a protocol that simulates chronic and heavy exposure, with the potential to induce dependence. In that study, after a 10-day habituation period, one group of CD1 male mice received 11% ethanol dissolved in water ad libitum as their only source of liquid for 60 consecutive days. Daily ethanol intake was recorded throughout the entire treatment. At the end of the exposure period, the males were mated with untreated females ($n = 10$) for a period of 2 h, without access to any liquid source. As a control, another group of mice received a sucrose solution with an equivalent caloric intake. A reduction in Nerve Growth Factor (NGF) levels was observed in several brain regions of the offspring of these mice, including the frontal cortex, striatum, and hippocampus. Moreover, compared to controls, these offspring exhibited increased sensitivity to ethanol's rewarding effects, as measured via CPP, at lower doses (0.5 g/kg). Additionally, alterations in neurotrophic receptors were identified, indicating impaired neuroplasticity. These findings reinforce the hypothesis that paternal alcohol exposure can affect pregnancy outcomes, inducing persistent neurobiological modifications in offspring, facilitating a predisposition to alcohol consumption.

Before we close this section, it is worth noting that PAE appears to alter the orexigenic peptides in the hypothalamus that stimulate food intake, a mechanism that may also facilitate ethanol consumption (Cason et al. 2010). One such study (Chang et al. 2012) revealed, in the offspring of dams given intubations of 1.0 or 3 g/kg/day from GD9 to parturition, increased expression of enkephalin, galanin, and orexin in the paraventricular nucleus, nucleus accumbens, and perifornical lateral hypothalamus by PD15. These changes were associated with increased neurogenesis of peptide-expressing neurons at birth and at PD15, as confirmed by BrdU and NeuN markers.

In conclusion, PAE causes significant neurobiological alterations that underlie the behavioral and cognitive deficits observed in individuals affected by this condition. Changes in gene expression, such as alterations in NMDA and AMPA receptor subunits, along with changes in GABA and dopamine receptors, suggest that PAE impacts essential neuronal communication and plasticity processes, which could lead to long-term disruptions in brain function. Furthermore, synaptic dysfunctions in areas such as the olfactory bulb, amygdala, and prefrontal cortex may contribute to altered sensory processing and poor emotional regulation. These findings underscore the importance of neurobiological changes in mediating the effects of PAE and emphasize the need to comprehend the molecular and cellular mechanisms underlying these alterations. Future research into the neurobiological consequences of PAE and potential therapeutic strategies could provide valuable insights into mitigating these effects. A limitation of the present section is that we did not include several important studies demonstrating neurobiological alterations, such as changes in the dopaminergic system, following PAE. However, most of this omitted research involved relatively high doses of ethanol. For example, one study using an intermittent two-bottle choice paradigm found that the offspring exhibited potentiated glutamatergic transmission and increased dendritic complexity in dopamine D1 receptor expressing neurons of the dorsomedial striatum. In this study the maternal ethanol intake initiated before pregnancy, continued during gestation and lasted until postnatal day 10; with ethanol intake reaching or exceeding 15 g/kg/day (Cheng et al. 2018).

4.4 Is There a Relationship Between Prenatal Exposure to Low Alcohol, Altering the Motivational Effects of Ethanol, and Ethanol Intake in the Offspring?

The previous sections provide strong evidence that PAE significantly alters the motivational effects of ethanol by enhancing its appetitive properties while reducing its aversive effects. Additionally, studies have shown that PAE disrupts various neurotransmitter systems, including the GABAergic, dopaminergic, opioidergic and serotonergic systems, as well as synaptic plasticity mechanisms, particularly in brain regions associated with reward, social behavior, and stress responses. Given this background, it follows logically that studies demonstrating such changes in motivational sensitivity should also report increased ethanol intake in offspring exposed to PAE.

A relevant contribution by Chotro and Arias (2003) explored the potential of moderate PAE (1–2 g/kg, GD17–20) to induce an early appetitive motivational memory that enhances ethanol seeking. Although the study did not directly assess ethanol-induced motivation, the findings suggest that PAE may lead to long-lasting behavioral processes biases toward alcohol-related cues. Specifically, they observed that administering naloxone (an opioid antagonist) to pregnant dams or postnatally to PAE pups reduced ethanol intake, which was more pronounced compared to controls, suggesting that in utero exposure conditions may lead to an ethanol preference, possibly mediated by the opioid system in conformity with several of the reports described in previous sections. Perhaps more important, these findings support Spear and Molina's (2005) proposal that fetal learning of ethanol's sensory and reinforcing properties takes place during PAE. Within this framework, it can be hypothesized that postnatal alcohol exposure in PAE-exposed rats—particularly when involving familiar sensory cues like ethanol's flavor or odor—may trigger a conditioned response that enhances the motivational value of alcohol.

The ethanol-induced prenatal conditioned response appears to depend on acetaldehyde, as co-administration of ethanol and D-penicillamine -a compound that sequesters acetaldehyde- blunted both the facilitated acquisition of an operant appetitive conditioned response using ethanol as a reinforcer on PD 5 and the increased consumption of ethanol on PD14 (Gaztañaga et al. 2017). These findings suggest that acetaldehyde plays a key role in the reinforcing effects of PAE and also point to a link between enhanced appetitive motivation for ethanol and increased alcohol intake in the offspring. However, as in previous studies, these variables were assessed in separate experiments, which limits the strength of the conclusions.

Gore-Langton and Spear (2019) used the PAE protocol of 2.0 g/kg/day from GD17 to GD20 and found a noteworthy association: male Sprague-Dawley rats showed reduced ethanol-induced CTA during adolescence and increased ethanol intake in adulthood. However, this increase in intake was not observed during adolescence, nor was it evident in females, which limits the generalizability of the findings. Nonetheless, the study confirms that PAE-induced blunting of ethanol aversion may have enduring effects on alcohol-related behaviors. Supporting this idea, Fabio et al. (2015a) reported that PAE increased ethanol intake in adolescent rats while selectively reducing ethanol-induced -but not lithium chloride-induced- CTA.

Not all findings point in the same direction regarding PAE's effects on alcohol motivation and intake. Blanchard et al. (1993) investigated the impact of PAE on a proxy of ethanol-induced reinforcement, specifically ethanol-induced dopamine release in the nucleus accumbens and striatum of adult male and female rats. While control rats exhibited dopamine release at 0.5 g/kg ethanol, prenatally exposed males showed increased dopamine release only at 1.0 g/kg, and females showed no change in accumbens dopamine levels and a decrease in striatal dopamine release, suggesting sex-specific neurochemical alterations. PAE did not significantly affect alcohol intake.

Further insight into the central questions of this chapter also comes from studies assessing operant responding during adolescence or adulthood following PAE. A seminal study (March et al. 2009) employed an ingenious procedure for assessing operant response. One-day-old neonates were placed supine and secured via a restrictor vest that allowed for head and forepaw movements. These movements activated a sensor, which in turn resulted in the intraoral delivery of ethanol. The researchers reported that one-day-old pups given low-to-moderate PAE (2.0 g/kg, GD 17–20) showed increased operant responding for 3% ethanol or for a solution that mimics the bittersweet orosensory properties of ethanol (i.e., a mixture of sucrose and quinine). A follow-up study by Miranda-Morales et al. (2014), using 5-day-old pups exposed to a lower dose (1 g/kg on GD 17–20), yielded similar results:

PAE-exposed pups, but not controls, exhibited operant learning reinforced by intraoral ethanol.

Not all operant studies have found PAE-specific effects limited to ethanol. For instance, it has been reported (Culleré et al. 2014) that PAE (2.0 g/kg, GDs 17–20) increased nose-poking behavior associated with intraoral sucrose delivery at PD14. These findings suggest that the consequences of PAE are not restricted to ethanol-related stimuli but may also alter responsiveness to other appetitive reinforcers. Notably, this result aligns well with previous studies suggesting an association between sucrose and ethanol preference. Moreover, Cullere's work (2014) still suggested that PAE may enhance ethanol's reinforcing effects. Specifically, at the end of the last sucrose acquisition session, the rats received paired presentations of sucrose with ethanol administration (0.5 g/kg). This procedure, termed a "revaluation" session by the authors, increased the motivational value of sucrose. Notably, only PAE-exposed pups showed greater resistance to extinction following revaluation, suggesting an enhanced sensitivity to the incentive properties conferred by the ethanol-sucrose association.

Taken together, these operant studies illustrate that moderate PAE can heighten the motivational properties of ethanol, even when its reinforcing value is assessed in the presence of orosensory and postabsorptive cues. Although such methodological constraints limit interpretations about pure anticipatory motivation, the consistency of the results across paradigms reinforces the notion that early ethanol exposure leaves a lasting imprint on the neural systems underlying reward-seeking behavior.

4.5 Concluding Comments

The evidence reviewed in this chapter supports the notion that even low-dose PAE can have lasting effects on the motivational properties of ethanol. These effects manifest as increased sensitivity to ethanol's appetitive reinforcing properties (Pautassi et al. 2012; Nizhnikov et al. 2006), reduced sensitivity to its aversive effects (Gore-Langton and Spear 2019), and altered neurobiological mechanisms underlying reward processing (Fabio et al. 2013). More specifically, the preclinical studies reviewed demonstrate that moderate PAE enhances conditioned preference for ethanol-associated cues (Pautassi et al. 2012), facilitates operant responding for ethanol (Miranda-Morales et al. 2014), and increases voluntary ethanol intake (Fabio et al. 2013). These preclinical findings are consistent with epidemiological research suggesting that prenatal alcohol exposure—even at moderate doses—predicts a greater vulnerability to developing alcohol-related problems across the lifespan (Alati et al. 2008).

A key limitation is that it was difficult to find studies that measure both variables (i.e., ethanol-induced motivation and intake) within the same subjects. This is partly because assessing motivational sensitivity to ethanol requires additional ethanol exposure, which can interact with the effects of PAE. Despite this, the lack of such studies precludes a definitive statement as to whether altered reactivity to the motivational properties of ethanol is a causal mechanism leading to greater ethanol intake after PAE. Another limitation, of the studies showing blunted ethanol-mediated aversion, is that PAE may reduce ethanol-induced CTA via a US-preexposure impact (Cole et al. 1996) rather than by altering motivational sensitivity per se. US-preexposure occurs when an organism is exposed to the unconditioned stimulus alone, without any prior pairing with a conditioned stimulus—a phenomenon that can lead to a slower acquisition of the conditioned response.

Another limitation was the scarcity of rodent studies that have specifically examined taste preferences or ethanol acceptance in offspring following low-dose PAE limited to GD 1–7, that is, before gastrulation. Such studies could help determine whether enhanced ethanol intake after PAE also occurs when olfaction is not yet functional. Moreover, despite extensive research, we failed to find studies assessing the anxiolytic effects of ethanol in PAE subjects. Anxiolytic effects are part of the so-called negative reinforcing effects of ethanol that can promote ethanol as a means to cope with negative feelings and discomfort.

Yet another limitation is that the exact cascade of neurotransmitter alterations caused by PAE and leading to greater ethanol intake is still unknown. Earlier hypothesis proposing a simpler downregulation in kappa (Nizhnikov et al. 2014) leading to greater dopaminergic function did not receive complete support. It is likely that multiple converging pathways contribute to the observed phenotype. It is worth noting that, due to space constraints, we did not cover other conspicuous neurobiological alterations, such as PAE-inducing hippocampal neurotoxicity and alterations in neural plasticity (Fontaine et al. 2019), which are also likely contributors to the phenomena under analysis.

Taken together, these findings underscore the importance of considering even moderate PAE as a factor capable of inducing lasting changes in affective and motivational processing, with potential implications for substance use vulnerability later in life. Future studies should seek to simultaneously assess motivational sensitivity and ethanol intake within the same subjects to strengthen causal inferences. Furthermore, research should aim to elucidate how specific neurotransmitter systems, such as the dynorphin/kappa opioid and dopaminergic systems, interact across development following PAE. In this sense, it would be valuable to employ designs with viral-mediated gene transfer (to silence or overexpress kappa opioid receptor signaling). Such technology has been successfully employed to detect mechanisms underlying the regulation of ethanol consumption (Bahi and Dreyer 2017). Last but not least, it is important to mention that the information derived from the reviewed studies supports the notion that public health initiatives should continue to promote abstinence from alcohol during pregnancy to prevent the enduring neurobehavioral effects of PAE.

Declaration of Generative AI and AI-Assisted Technologies in the Writing Process During the preparation of this work, the author(s) used ChatGPT (OpenAI) to refine writing, check grammar, suggest alternative phrasings, and look for primary sources. Additionally, the Grammarly program was used to correct grammatical and spelling errors, thereby improving the clarity and coherence of the text. After using this tool, the author(s) reviewed and edited the content as needed and took full responsibility for the publication's content.

Acknowledgments and Funding Sources Funding was provided by grants PICT 2018–00597 to RMP and SECYT Consolidar 2018 to RMP and MCF.

References

Abate P, Pepino MY, Dominguez HD, Spear NE, Molina JC (2000) Fetal associative learning mediated through maternal alcohol intoxication. Alcohol Clin Exp Res 24(1):39–47

Abate P, Varlinskaya EI, Cheslock SJ, Spear NE, Molina JC (2002) Neonatal activation of alcohol-related prenatal memories: impact on the first suckling response. Alcohol Clin Exp Res 26(10):1512–1522. https://doi.org/10.1097/01.ALC.0000034668.93601.8F

Alati R, Clavarino A, Najman JM, O'Callaghan M, Bor W, Mamun AA, Williams GM (2008) The developmental origin of adolescent alcohol use: findings from the Mater University Study of Pregnancy and its outcomes. Drug Alcohol Depend 98(1–2):136–143

Arias C, Chotro MG (2006) Ethanol-induced preferences or aversions as a function of age in preweanling rats. Behav Neurosci 120(3):710–718. https://doi.org/10.1037/0735-7044.120.3.710

Arias C, Molina JC, Mlewski EC, Pautassi RM, Spear N (2008) Acute sensitivity and acute tolerance to ethanol in preweanling rats with or without prenatal experience with the drug. Pharmacol Biochem Behav 89(4):608–622. https://doi.org/10.1016/j.pbb.2008.02.017

Atukorala I, Hannan N, Hui L (2024) Immersed in a reservoir of potential: amniotic fluid-derived extracellular vesicles. J Transl Med 22(1):348. https://doi.org/10.1186/s12967-024-05154-2

Baer JS, Barr HM, Bookstein FL, Sampson PD, Streissguth AP (1998) Prenatal alcohol exposure and family history of alcoholism in the etiology of adolescent alcohol problems. J Stud Alcohol 59(5):533–543

Baer JS, Sampson PD, Barr HM, Connor PD, Streissguth AP (2003) A 21-year longitudinal analysis of the effects of prenatal alcohol exposure on young adult drinking. Arch Gen Psychiatry 60(4):377–385

Bahi A, Dreyer JL (2017) Viral-mediated overexpression of the Myelin Transcription Factor 1 (MyT1) in the dentate gyrus attenuates anxiety- and ethanol-related behaviors in rats. Psychopharmacology 234(12):

1829–1840. https://doi.org/10.1007/s00213-017-4588-7

Barbier E, Houchi H, Warnault V, Pierrefiche O, Daoust M, Naassila M (2009) Effects of prenatal and postnatal maternal ethanol on offspring response to alcohol and psychostimulants in long evans rats. Neuroscience 161(2):427–440. https://doi.org/10.1016/j.neuroscience.2009.03.076

Blanchard BA, Steindorf S, Wang S, LeFevre R, Mankes RF, Glick SD (1993) Prenatal ethanol exposure alters ethanol-induced dopamine release in nucleus accumbens and striatum in male and female rats. Alcohol Clin Exp Res 17(5):974–981

Camarini R, Pautassi RM (2016) Behavioral sensitization to ethanol: neural basis and factors that influence its acquisition and expression. Brain Res Bull 125:53–78. https://doi.org/10.1016/j.brainresbull.2016.04.006

Cason AM, Smith RJ, Tahsili-Fahadan P, Moorman DE, Sartor GC, Aston-Jones G (2010) Role of orexin/hypocretin in reward-seeking and addiction: implications for obesity. Physiol Behav 100(5):419–428. https://doi.org/10.1016/j.physbeh.2010.03.009

Ceccanti M, Coccurello R, Carito V, Ciafrè S, Ferraguti G, Giacovazzo G, Mancinelli R, Tirassa P, Chaldakov GN, Pascale E, Ceccanti M, Codazzo C, Fiore M (2016) Paternal alcohol exposure in mice alters brain NGF and BDNF and increases ethanol-elicited preference in male offspring. Addict Biol 21(4):776–787. https://doi.org/10.1111/adb.12255

Chang GQ, Karatayev O, Liang SC, Barson JR, Leibowitz SF (2012) Prenatal ethanol exposure stimulates neurogenesis in hypothalamic and limbic peptide systems: possible mechanism for offspring ethanol overconsumption. Neuroscience 222:417–428. https://doi.org/10.1016/j.neuroscience.2012.05.066

Cheng Y, Wang X, Wei X, Xie X, Melo S, Miranda RC, Wang J (2018) Prenatal exposure to alcohol induces functional and structural plasticity in dopamine D1 receptor-expressing neurons of the dorsomedial striatum. Alcohol Clin Exp Res. https://doi.org/10.1111/acer.13806

Chotro MG, Arias C (2003) Prenatal exposure to ethanol increases ethanol consumption: a conditioned response? Alcohol 30(1):19–28. https://doi.org/10.1016/s0741-8329(03)00037-5

Cole KC, VanTilburg D, Burch-Vernon A, Riccio DC (1996) The importance of context in the US preexposure effect in CTA: novel versus latently inhibited contextual stimuli. Learn Motiv 27(4):362–374. https://doi.org/10.1006/lmot.1996.0021

Collier AD, Yasmin N, Karatayev O, Abdulai AR, Yu B, Fam M, Campbell S, Leibowitz SF (2024) Embryonic ethanol exposure and optogenetic activation of hypocretin neurons stimulate similar behaviors early in life associated with later alcohol consumption. Sci Rep 14(1):3021. https://doi.org/10.1038/s41598-024-52465-x

Culleré ME, Spear NE, Molina JC (2014) Prenatal ethanol increases sucrose reinforcement, an effect strengthened by postnatal association of ethanol and sucrose. Alcohol 48(1):25–33. https://doi.org/10.1016/j.alcohol.2013.11.003

Diaz-Ubilla M, Figueroa-Valdes AI, Tobar HE, Quintanilla ME, Diaz E, Morales P, Berrios-Carcamo-P, Santapau D, Gallardo J, de Gregorio C, Ugalde J, Rojas C, Gonzalez-Madrid A, Ezquer M, Israel Y, Alcayaga-Miranda F, Ezquer F (2025) Gut microbiota-derived extracellular vesicles influence alcohol intake preferences in rats. J Extracell Vesicles 14(3):e70059. https://doi.org/10.1002/jev2.70059

Dominguez HD, Lopez MF, Chotro MG, Molina JC (1996) Perinatal responsiveness to alcohol's chemosensory cues as a function of prenatal alcohol administration during gestational days 17-20 in the rat. Neurobiol Learn Mem 65(2):103–112. https://doi.org/10.1006/nlme.1996.0012

Edwards S, Koob GF (2010) Neurobiology of dysregulated motivational systems in drug addiction. Future Neurol 5(3):393–401. https://doi.org/10.2217/fnl.10.14

Fabio MC, March SM, Molina JC, Nizhnikov ME, Spear NE, Pautassi RM (2013) Prenatal ethanol exposure increases ethanol intake and reduces c-Fos expression in infralimbic cortex of adolescent rats. Pharmacol Biochem Behav 103(4):842–852. https://doi.org/10.1016/j.pbb.2012.12.009

Fabio MC, Macchione AF, Nizhnikov ME, Pautassi RM (2015a) Prenatal ethanol increases ethanol intake throughout adolescence, alters ethanol-mediated aversive learning, and affects mu but not delta or kappa opioid receptor mRNA expression. Eur J Neurosci 41(12):1569–1579. https://doi.org/10.1111/ejn.12913

Fabio MC, Vivas LM, Pautassi RM (2015b) Prenatal ethanol exposure alters ethanol-induced Fos immunoreactivity and dopaminergic activity in the mesocorticolimbic pathway of the adolescent brain. Neuroscience 301:221–234. https://doi.org/10.1016/j.neuroscience.2015.06.003

Fontaine CJ, Pinar C, Yang W, Pang AF, Suesser KE, Choi JSJ, Christie BR (2019) Impaired bidirectional synaptic plasticity in juvenile offspring following prenatal ethanol exposure. Alcohol Clin Exp Res 43(10):2153–2166. https://doi.org/10.1111/acer.14170

Forestell CA (2024) Does maternal diet influence future infant taste and odor preferences? A critical analysis. Annu Rev Nutr 44:313–337. https://doi.org/10.1146/annurev-nutr-121222-101404

Gaztanaga M, Angulo-Alcalde A, Spear NE, Chotro MG (2017) The role of acetaldehyde in the increased acceptance of ethanol after prenatal ethanol exposure. Front Behav Neurosci 11:14. https://doi.org/10.3389/fnbeh.2017.00014

Gore-Langton JK, Spear LP (2019) Prenatal ethanol exposure attenuates sensitivity to the aversive effects of ethanol in adolescence and increases adult preference

for a 5% ethanol solution in males, but not females. Alcohol 79:59–69. https://doi.org/10.1016/j.alcohol.2018.12.004
Konijnenberg C (2015) Methodological issues in assessing the impact of prenatal drug exposure. Subst Abuse Res Treat 9(Suppl 2):39–44. https://doi.org/10.4137/sart.S23544
Liu C, Showalter J, Grigson PS (2009) Ethanol-induced conditioned taste avoidance: reward or aversion? Alcohol Clin Exp Res 33(3):522–530. https://doi.org/10.1111/j.1530-0277.2008.00865.x
Lopez MB, Conde K, Cremonte M (2017) Alcohol use disorders in Argentinian girls and women 12 months before delivery: comparison of DSM-IV, DSM-5, and ICD-10 diagnostic criteria. J Addict Med 11(2):106–113. https://doi.org/10.1097/ADM.0000000000000285
MacPherson RA, Shankar V, Anholt RRH, Mackay TFC (2023) Genetic and genomic analyses of Drosophila melanogaster models of chromatin modification disorders. Genetics 224(4). https://doi.org/10.1093/genetics/iyad061
March SM, Abate P, Spear NE, Molina JC (2009) Fetal exposure to moderate ethanol doses: heightened operant responsiveness elicited by ethanol-related reinforcers. Alcohol Clin Exp Res 33(11):1981–1993. https://doi.org/10.1111/j.1530-0277.2009.01037.x
March SM, Abate P, Spear NE, Molina JC (2013) The role of acetaldehyde in ethanol reinforcement assessed by Pavlovian conditioning in newborn rats. Psychopharmacology 226(3):491–499. https://doi.org/10.1007/s00213-012-2920-9
Marengo L, Barey A, Salguero A, Fabio MC, Cendan CM, Moron-Henche I, D'Addario C, Pautassi RM (2023) Neurobehavioral alterations induced by third-trimester gestation-equivalent ethanol exposure are inhibited by folate administration. Dev Psychobiol 65(7):e22426. https://doi.org/10.1002/dev.22426
May PA, Chambers CD, Kalberg WO, Zellner J, Feldman H, Buckley D, Kopald D, Hasken JM, Xu R, Honerkamp-Smith G, Taras H, Manning MA, Robinson LK, Adam MP, Abdul-Rahman O, Vaux K, Jewett T, Elliott AJ, Kable JA, Akshoomoff N, Falk D, Arroyo JA, Hereld D, Riley EP, Charness ME, Coles CD, Warren KR, Jones KL, Hoyme HE (2018) Prevalence of fetal alcohol spectrum disorders in 4 US communities. JAMA 319(5):474–482. https://doi.org/10.1001/jama.2017.21896
Middleton FA, Carrierfenster K, Mooney SM, Youngentob SL (2009) Gestational ethanol exposure alters the behavioral response to ethanol odor and the expression of neurotransmission genes in the olfactory bulb of adolescent rats. Brain Res 1252:105–116
Middleton FA, Varlinskaya EI, Mooney SM (2012) Molecular substrates of social avoidance seen following prenatal ethanol exposure and its reversal by social enrichment. Dev Neurosci 34:115
Miranda-Morales RS, Molina JC, Spear NE, Abate P (2010) Participation of the endogenous opioid system in the acquisition of a prenatal ethanol-related memory: effects on neonatal and preweanling responsiveness to ethanol. Physiol Behav 101(1):153–160. https://doi.org/10.1016/j.physbeh.2010.04.033
Miranda-Morales RS, Nizhnikov ME, Spear NE (2014) Prenatal exposure to ethanol during late gestation facilitates operant self-administration of the drug in 5-day-old rats. Alcohol 48(1):19–23. https://doi.org/10.1016/j.alcohol.2013.11.001
Moraes Castro M, Pinto F, Pereiras C, Fischer Castells A, Vogel Agoglia C, Duarte V, Barceló J, Sosa C, González G (2019) Autodeclaración del consumo de marihuana, tabaco, alcohol y derivados de cocaína en embarazadas en 2013 y 2016, Montevideo, Uruguay. Adicciones 32(3):173–180
Morozova TV, Shankar V, MacPherson RA, Mackay TFC, Anholt RRH (2022) Modulation of the Drosophila transcriptome by developmental exposure to alcohol. BMC Genomics 23(1):347. https://doi.org/10.1186/s12864-022-08559-9
Nguyen TT, Risbud RD, Mattson SN, Chambers CD, Thomas JD (2016) Randomized, double-blind, placebo-controlled clinical trial of choline supplementation in school-aged children with fetal alcohol spectrum disorders. Am J Clin Nutr 104(6):1683–1692. https://doi.org/10.3945/ajcn.116.142075
Nizhnikov ME, Molina JC, Varlinskaya EI, Spear NE (2006) Prenatal ethanol exposure increases ethanol reinforcement in neonatal rats. Alcohol Clin Exp Res 30(1):34–45. https://doi.org/10.1111/j.1530-0277.2006.00009.x
Nizhnikov ME, Molina JC, Spear NE (2007) Central reinforcing effects of ethanol are blocked by catalase inhibition. Alcohol 41(7):525–534. https://doi.org/10.1016/j.alcohol.2007.08.006
Nizhnikov ME, Pautassi RM, Carter JM, Landin JD, Varlinskaya EI, Bordner KA, Werner DF, Spear NE (2014) Brief prenatal ethanol exposure alters behavioral sensitivity to the kappa opioid receptor agonist (U62,066E) and antagonist (Nor-BNI) and reduces kappa opioid receptor expression. Alcohol Clin Exp Res 38(6):1630–1638. https://doi.org/10.1111/acer.12416
Pautassi RM, Myers M, Spear LP, Molina JC, Spear NE (2008) Adolescent but not adult rats exhibit ethanol-mediated appetitive second-order conditioning. Alcohol Clin Exp Res 32(11):2016–2027. https://doi.org/10.1111/j.1530-0277.2008.00789.x
Pautassi RM, Nizhnikov ME, Spear NE (2009) Assessing appetitive, aversive, and negative ethanol-mediated reinforcement through an immature rat model. Neurosci Biobehav Rev 33(6):953–974
Pautassi RM, Nizhnikov ME, Spear NE, Molina JC (2012) Prenatal ethanol exposure leads to greater ethanol-induced appetitive reinforcement. Alcohol 46(6):585–593. https://doi.org/10.1016/j.alcohol.2012.05.004
Plaza W, Gaschino F, Gutierrez C, Santibañez N, Estay-Olmos C, Sotomayor-Zárate R, De la Fuente-Ortega E,

Pautassi RM, Haeger PA (2020) Pre- and postnatal alcohol exposure delays, in female but not in male rats, the extinction of an auditory fear conditioned memory and increases alcohol consumption. Dev Psychobiol 62(4):519–531. https://doi.org/10.1002/dev.21925

Popoola DO, Borrow AP, Sanders JE, Nizhnikov ME, Cameron NM (2015) Can low-level ethanol exposure during pregnancy influence maternal care? An investigation using two strains of rat across two generations. Physiol Behav 148:111–121. https://doi.org/10.1016/j.physbeh.2015.01.001

Popova S, Lange S, Probst C, Gmel G, Rehm J (2017) Estimation of national, regional, and global prevalence of alcohol use during pregnancy and fetal alcohol syndrome: a systematic review and meta-analysis. Lancet Glob Health 5. https://doi.org/10.1016/S2214-109X(17)30021-9

Probyn ME, Zanini S, Ward LC, Bertram JF, Moritz KM (2012) A rodent model of low- to moderate-dose ethanol consumption during pregnancy: patterns of ethanol consumption and effects on fetal and offspring growth. Reprod Fertil Dev 24(6):859–870. https://doi.org/10.1071/RD11200

Saalfield J, Spear L (2016) The ontogeny of ethanol aversion. Physiol Behav 156:164–170. https://doi.org/10.1016/j.physbeh.2016.01.011

Schambra UB, Nunley K, Harrison TA, Lewis CN (2016) Consequences of low or moderate prenatal ethanol exposures during gastrulation or neurulation for open field activity and emotionality in mice. Neurotoxicol Teratol 57:39–53. https://doi.org/10.1016/j.ntt.2016.06.003

Schuckit MA (1994) Alcohol sensitivity and dependence, Experientia, vol 71, pp 341–348. https://doi.org/10.1007/978-3-0348-7330-7_34

Spear NE, Molina JC (2005) Fetal or infantile exposure to ethanol promotes ethanol ingestion in adolescence and adulthood: a theoretical review. Alcohol Clin Exp Res 29(6):909–929

Thomas JD, Biane JS, O'Bryan KA, O'Neill TM, Dominguez HD (2007) Choline supplementation following third-trimester-equivalent alcohol exposure attenuates behavioral alterations in rats. Behav Neurosci 121(1):120–130

Tunstall BJ, Vendruscolo LF, Allen–Worthington K (2020) Chapter 26 - Rat models of alcohol use disorder. In: Suckow MA, Hankenson FC, Wilson RP, Foley PL (eds) The laboratory rat, 3rd edn. Academic Press, pp 967–986. https://doi.org/10.1016/B978-0-12-814338-4.00026-X

Tzschentke TM (2007) Measuring reward with the conditioned place preference (CPP) paradigm: update of the last decade. Addict Biol 12(3–4):227–462

Uban KA, Comeau WL, Bodnar T, Yu WK, Weinberg J, Galea LA (2015) Amphetamine sensitization and cross-sensitization with acute restraint stress: impact of prenatal alcohol exposure in male and female rats. Psychopharmacology 232(10):1705–1716. https://doi.org/10.1007/s00213-014-3804-y

Valenstein ES, Cox VC, Kakolewski JW (1967) Polydipsia elicited by the synergistic action of a saccharin and glucose solution. Science (New York, NY) 157(3788): 552–554. https://doi.org/10.1126/science.157.3788.552

Vella VR, Ainsworth-Cruickshank G, Luft C, Wong KE, Parfrey LW, Vogl AW, Holman PJ, Bodnar TS, Raineki C (2025) Dysregulation of immune system markers, gut microbiota and short-chain fatty acid production following prenatal alcohol exposure: a developmental perspective. Neurochem Int 185:105952. https://doi.org/10.1016/j.neuint.2025.105952

Verendeev A, Riley AL (2012) Conditioned taste aversion and drugs of abuse: history and interpretation. Neurosci Biobehav Rev 36(10):2193–2205. https://doi.org/10.1016/j.neubiorev.2012.08.004

Vetter CS, Doremus-Fitzwater TL, Spear LP (2007) Time course of elevated ethanol intake in adolescent relative to adult rats under continuous, voluntary-access conditions. Alcohol Clin Exp Res 31(7):1159–1168. https://doi.org/10.1111/j.1530-0277.2007.00417.x

Walton SL, Tjongue M, Tare M, Kwok E, Probyn M, Parkington HC, Bertram JF, Moritz KM, Denton KM (2019) Chronic low alcohol intake during pregnancy programs sex-specific cardiovascular deficits in rats. Biol Sex Differ 10(1):21. https://doi.org/10.1186/s13293-019-0235-9

Wille-Bille A, Miranda-Morales RS, Pucci M, Bellia F, D'Addario C, Pautassi RM (2018) Prenatal ethanol induces an anxiety phenotype and alters expression of dynorphin & nociceptin/orphanin FQ genes. Prog Neuro-Psychopharmacol Biol Psychiatry 85:77–88. https://doi.org/10.1016/j.pnpbp.2018.04.005

Wille-Bille A, Bellia F, Jiménez García AM, Miranda-Morales RS, D'Addario C, Pautassi RM (2020) Early exposure to environmental enrichment modulates the effects of prenatal ethanol exposure upon opioid gene expression and adolescent ethanol intake. Neuropharmacology 165:107917. https://doi.org/10.1016/j.neuropharm.2019.107917

Yao H, Wang C, Xia Z (2023) Prenatal alcohol exposure enhanced alcohol preference and susceptibility to PTSD in a sex-dependent manner through the synaptic HCN1 channel. J Affect Disord 324:143–152. https://doi.org/10.1016/j.jad.2022.12.069

Young SL, Steane SE, Kent NL, Reid N, Gallo LA, Moritz KM (2022) Prevalence and patterns of prenatal alcohol exposure in Australian cohort and cross-sectional studies: a systematic review of data collection approaches. Int J Environ Res Public Health 19(20). https://doi.org/10.3390/ijerph192013144

Anxiety, Depression, and Emotional Dysregulation Following Prenatal Substance Exposure

5

Marvin R. Diaz, Elena I. Varlinskaya, and Kelcie C. Schatz

Abstract

Substance use during pregnancy is highly prevalent worldwide leading to a spectrum of lifelong neurobehavioral consequences. One of the most commonly observed effects of prenatal substance use is an increased risk of emotional processing deficits and developing an affective disorder, particularly anxiety and depression, with evidence of symptoms emerging in infancy and both persisting and becoming increasingly exacerbated into adulthood. Among the various substances misused during pregnancy, alcohol, nicotine, cannabis, and opioids have been noted as the most commonly used for a variety of reasons. Despite the legal status of these substances, it is evident that prenatal exposure to alcohol, nicotine, cannabis, and opioids produces a myriad of neurobiological alterations that may underlie the development of negative affective behaviors in the offspring. This chapter discusses the existing clinical and preclinical (using animal models) literature that has identified the spectrum of negative affective behaviors and associated neurobiological alterations across the lifespan resulting from prenatal exposure to these specific substances.

Keywords

Negative affective behavior · Development · Alcohol · Drugs

M. R. Diaz (✉) · E. I. Varlinskaya · K. C. Schatz
Psychology Department, Binghamton University, Binghamton, NY, USA

Center for Development and Behavioral Neuroscience, Binghamton University, Binghamton, NY, USA

Developmental Exposure Alcohol Research Center, Binghamton University, Binghamton, NY, USA
e-mail: mdiaz@binghamton.edu

Substance use during pregnancy is highly prevalent across the world due to a variety of factors (Azeem et al. 2024; Gomez-Ruiz et al. 2022; Health 2022; Pratt Tremblay et al. 2025; Rebbe et al. 2024; Smid et al. 2022). Some of these factors include substance use disorder, lack of knowledge and/or misinformation regarding potential consequences of prenatal substance exposure, and major life events/stressors (Han et al. 2024), in addition to treatment of various psychiatric conditions, including substance use disorder (Azeem et al. 2024). Although there are numerous negative effects of prenatal drug exposure on the developing fetus that are drug specific and which may persist throughout the lifespan (Behnke and Eyler 1993; Chang 2020; Karatayev et al. 2024; Little et al. 2021; Salzwedel et al. 2020), increased negative affective states, including anxiety and depression, have been commonly reported in humans and various preclinical animal

A. N. Bukiya, D. W. Ali (eds.), *Molecular Mechanisms and Lifelong Consequences of Prenatal Exposure to Psychoactive Substances*, Advances in Experimental Medicine and Biology 1500,
https://doi.org/10.1007/978-3-032-12741-9_5

models of prenatal substance exposure (Koponen et al. 2023; Min et al. 2021; Nygaard et al. 2020). Among the various substances that are used and misused by pregnant people, alcohol, nicotine, cannabis, and opioids have been reported to be some of the most commonly used (England et al. 2020). This chapter will discuss the existing clinical and preclinical literature regarding the known effects of prenatal exposure to (1) alcohol, (2) nicotine, (3) cannabis/cannabinoids, and (4) opioids on negative affective behaviors and potential underlying neurobiological mechanisms.

It is crucial to recognize that, regardless of the substance under investigation, several key factors should be considered when comparing clinical human and preclinical animal studies regardless of which substance is being studied. First, the rodent (both mouse and rat) gestational period spans ~20–23 gestational days (G20–23) which is generally considered to be equivalent to the first and second trimesters of human pregnancy, while the first 1–2 postnatal weeks (postnatal days (P) 1–10) are considered equivalent to the third trimester of human pregnancy (Almeida et al. 2020). Thus, drug exposure throughout the entire "gestational-equivalent" period in a rodent includes exposure during both the prenatal and postnatal periods. Second, it is very common in preclinical studies to expose drug-naïve pregnant females with no pre-conception history of drug exposure, which does not appropriately model drug use by pregnant people who do not typically initiate drug use during pregnancy. Another major factor is that various routes of administration are used in animal models, including, but not limited to, injection, voluntary oral, forced intragastric gavage, osmotic minipumps, and inhalation. However, this factor is quite translatable since drugs are administered in a variety of ways by humans. Thus, when comparing clinical and preclinical data, these factors associated with prenatal drug exposure must be considered.

5.1 Prenatal Alcohol Exposure

Alcohol (ethanol) use during pregnancy is highly prevalent globally, with estimated rates ranging from 10% to above 40% in some countries (Keating et al. 2024; Popova et al. 2017, 2018). Given that alcohol readily crosses the placenta and fetal exposure to alcohol may be prolonged relative to maternal exposure due to various factors (Heller and Burd 2014), there are numerous long-term physical, behavioral, and neurobiological consequences of prenatal alcohol exposure (PAE) on the developing fetus collectively termed Fetal Alcohol Spectrum Disorder (FASD), which affect a likely underestimated 2–5% of the general population (Popova et al. 2023). Notably, the frequency, amount, and timing of PAE contribute to the spectrum of alterations observed in FASD (Myrick et al. 2024; O'Leary et al. 2010), which can produce a multitude of potential combinations of effects. Among the various neurobehavioral consequences of PAE, negative affective behaviors, including depression and anxiety, have been recognized as common behavioral impairments, often referred to as secondary disabilities, that can have detrimental long-term effects on quality of life in people with FASD [reviewed by (Burgess and Moritz 2020; Easey et al. 2019; Hellemans et al. 2010; Kelly et al. 2000; O'Connor and Paley 2009; Pei et al. 2011)].

5.1.1 Clinical Studies—Behavioral Alterations

Clinical studies have reported affective impairments as early as infancy, with reduced maternal-infant bonding, increased irritability, and emotional withdrawal in newborns with a history of PAE (Lemola et al. 2009; Molteno et al. 2014; O'Connor et al. 1992), ultimately contributing to higher levels of insecure attachment behaviors throughout childhood [reviewed by (O'Connor and Paley 2009)]. Specifically, one study found that 80% of children with PAE demonstrated attachment insecurity compared to 36% of unexposed children, in addition to higher negative affect measured by intensity and frequency of unhappiness, sadness, and hurt expressed toward the parent while working on a puzzle task (O'Connor et al. 2002). Interestingly, girls, but not boys, from mothers who were high-frequency drinkers showed significantly higher negative affect scores in several measures than those from low-frequency drinking mothers at 5–-7 months of age (Haley et al. 2006), suggesting potential sex differences in the expression of negative affect. In addition to the emergence of negative affect in infancy, another study similarly reported a correlation between infant negative affective behaviors and increased depressive features in early childhood (6-years old) in PAE children (O'Connor 2001). Alcohol exposure during the first trimester was previously reported to increase the odds of childhood anxiety, particularly with moderate and heavy maternal alcohol consumption, whereas exposure during late pregnancy did not show this relationship (O'Leary et al. 2010). A more recent study similarly reported that first trimester PAE was associated with heightened emotional reactivity and a tendency for increased anxious and depressed symptoms at 3 years of age (Lund et al. 2019). Sleep disturbances in children with FASD have also been associated with increased anxiety and depressive symptoms (Dylag et al. 2024). Thus, there is a clear relationship between PAE and negative affective behaviors from infancy through childhood, with various factors that may drive the magnitude of the effects in exposed offspring.

Higher incidence of anxiety and depressive symptoms in individuals with FASD persists throughout the lifetime. A recent meta-analysis identified a higher risk of depression in offspring (age range: 1–18 years) with PAE from mothers with heavy alcohol use during pregnancy (Zhang et al. 2022). Famy and colleagues reported that a large proportion of adult subjects (18 years and older) who met criteria for FASD was diagnosed with depression (Famy et al. 1998). This increased incidence of anxiety and depression in individuals with FASD extends through adult life (age range: 23–71), as the self-reported rates of depression ranged from 33–43% in individuals with PAE/FASD compared to 26.5% in non-exposed adults, with similar elevated rates of anxiety disorder in adults with PAE/FASD (~40%) relative to non-exposed adults (18.4%) (Coles et al. 2022).

5.1.2 Clinical Studies—Neurobiological Mechanisms

Although the mechanisms underlying and/or contributing to the relationship between PAE and increased negative affective behaviors are not fully understood, using diffusion and structural magnetic resonance imaging (MRI) in vivo, human studies have identified some potential neurobiological alterations that have guided the field's understanding of this phenomenon. Reduced volume of the hippocampus, amygdala, and thalamus, structures known to play a role in emotion processing, has been observed in 2–4-week-old infants with PAE (Donald et al. 2016), indicating that these structural changes begin in early development. A recent study also observed reduced amygdala, hippocampus, and thalamus volumes in PAE children (average age: 10 years) relative to unexposed children (Nakhid et al. 2023), suggesting persistent morphological effects of PAE on gross brain volume. Interestingly, this study also identified strong negative correlations between the volume of these structures and scores in tests of anxiety and depression, suggesting that PAE may disrupt the development of some of these brain structures, ultimately contributing to the risk of negative affective behavior. Reductions in the volume of the anterior cingulate cortex, a subregion of the prefrontal cortex involved in emotion regulation, and its connectivity with associated brain structures has also been reported in children with PAE, with a negative correlation between anterior cingulate cortex volume and negative affective behaviors (Andre et al. 2020; Bjorkquist et al. 2010). Reduced caudate volumes were associated with higher levels of anxiety and depression symptoms in children with PAE relative to those without PAE (aged 8–16 years) (Krueger et al. 2020). Ultimately, these human studies have identified the impact of PAE on brain areas involved in regulating affective behaviors at the macroscale, yet a complete understanding of the neurobiological alterations resulting from PAE are still not fully understood.

5.1.3 Animal Models of Prenatal Alcohol Exposure

Animal studies have recapitulated various aspects of negative affective behaviors resulting from PAE. Rodent models of PAE use a variety of routes of ethanol administration, including voluntary ethanol intake, forced consumption (i.e., liquid diet), injections, intragastric gavage, and vapor inhalation across a variety of prenatal periods. Importantly, these different PAE paradigms can produce quite unique dynamics in blood ethanol concentration time-courses (Livy et al. 2003; Pruett et al. 2020) which may ultimately influence offspring outcomes. Regarding PAE, it is worth noting that while it is highly likely that human females consume ethanol at some point before becoming pregnant, in most animal models of PAE, pregnant females experience ethanol for the first time while pregnant which only models the direct effects of ethanol on the developing fetus. Nonetheless, animal models of PAE produce a spectrum of anxiety- and depressive-like behaviors, which can vary depending on the age of assessment and sex.

5.1.4 Animal Studies—Behavioral Alterations

Similar to human infant studies, a nonhuman primate study found that low-dose ethanol exposure via sweetened alcohol beverages (blood ethanol concentrations (BECs): 20–50 mg/dl) during early mid gestation resulted in elevated irritability and emotional reactivity in infant offspring (Coe et al. 2010). In rodents, several studies have shown that PAE at high doses (BECs ~150–250 mg/dl via forced ethanol liquid diet or intragastric gavage) across the entire gestational period and the third trimester-equivalent (ethanol administered to neonatal pups) produce increased immobility in a forced swim test and reduced open arm time in the elevated plus maze, suggestive of increased depressive- and anxiety-like behaviors, respectively, in juvenile Wistar rat (Carneiro et al. 2005), late adolescent/early adult Sprague Dawley rat (Brocardo et al. 2012), and adult Sprague Dawley rat (Dandekar et al. 2019; Wilcoxon et al. 2005) offspring. Similar findings were reported using an ethanol liquid diet from G1–21 in Sprague Dawley rats, with no exposure during the third trimester-equivalent (Hellemans et al. 2008). Exposure to much higher doses of ethanol from G7–20 (BECs ~340 mg/dl) also increased anxiety-like behaviors in the open field, elevated plus maze, and zero maze of adult Sprague Dawley and Wistar male offspring (Dursun et al. 2006; Oubraim et al. 2022; Zhou et al. 2010). Surprisingly, PAE to much lower doses of ethanol (BECs ~30–100 mg/dl) through either only the gestational period or gestational period and third trimester-equivalent via voluntary ethanol consumption in Sprague Dawley rats, C57BL/6J and CD1 mice also increased a variety of anxiety-like behaviors in juvenile, adult and aged offspring (Cullen et al. 2013; Kleiber et al. 2011; Madarnas et al. 2020) as well as depressive-like behaviors in adult C57BL/6J females (Caldwell et al. 2008). These studies indicate that PAE across large gestational periods through multiple daily exposures, regardless of the amount of ethanol exposure (low, high, heavy doses) or the route of administration, can produce negative affective behaviors in offspring at various ages.

Interestingly, several studies have identified specific critical gestational periods during which ethanol exposure can also produce negative affective behaviors. Mooney and Varlinskaya found that PAE via an intraperitoneal injection (BECs >350 mg/dl) on G12, but not G7, produced social anxiety-like behavior in adolescent and adult Long Evans male and female rat offspring (Mooney and Varlinskaya 2011), whereas only adult Long Evans females exhibited social anxiety-like behavior following PAE on G15 (Varlinskaya and Mooney 2014). Identification of G12 as a critical gestational period contributing to the regulation of affective behaviors has been further demonstrated in a different rat strain (Sprague Dawley) via intraperitoneal injections (BECs >300 mg/dl) which similarly increased social anxiety-like behaviors at multiple ages (Diaz et al. 2016; Mooney and Varlinskaya 2018). More recent studies have found that PAE on G12 in Sprague Dawley rats through ethanol vapor inhalation at much lower doses (BECs 60–120 mg/dl) also produced social anxiety-like behaviors at various ages (Przybysz et al. 2023) and non-social anxiety-like behavior in adolescence (Rouzer et al. 2017; Rouzer and Diaz 2022), but only in male offspring. Another potentially critical prenatal period that may regulate the development of affective behavior is the third trimester-equivalent, albeit in an ethanol dose-dependent manner. Specifically, heavy PAE from P3–5 via vapor inhalation (pup BECs ~320 mg/dl) increased anxiety-like behavior on the elevated plus maze in adolescent Sprague Dawley male offspring (Baculis et al. 2015), while heavy PAE from P4–9 increased depressive-like behavior measured by increased immobility time in the forced swim test in adult Wistar rat offspring (Lopatynska-Mazurek et al. 2021). Conversely, a more moderate PAE from P2–12 via vapor inhalation (pup BECs ~100 mg/dl) did not affect anxiety-like behavior in the light/dark box in adolescent Sprague Dawley male offspring (Diaz et al. 2014). This collection of studies highlights critical prenatal periods during which ethanol exposure can dose-dependently enhance the risk of negative affective behaviors in an age- and sex-specific manner.

A surprising observation in some of the animal studies has been a PAE-induced reduction in depressive- and anxiety-like behaviors. For example, Sprague Dawley rat offspring with either G12 moderate or heavy dose PAE showed decreased marble burying in the marble burying task (Rouzer and Diaz 2022) or increased time on the light side of a light/dark box (Diaz et al. 2016), respectively, suggestive of anxiolytic behaviors. A heavy dose G7 PAE via intraperitoneal injection (BECs ~420 mg/dl) reduced anxiety-like behavior in female C57BL/6J mice offspring and reduced immobility time in male offspring, suggestive of reduced depressive-like behaviors (Wieczorek et al. 2015). Similar observations reported greater open arm time on the elevated plus maze in adult Long Evans rat offspring exposed to moderate PAE via voluntary consumption (Acosta et al. 2024). How rodent tests of anxiety and depression directly translate to the human condition remains a critical question in the field, as many of these tests rely on risk-taking and coping behaviors that may be interpreted as something very different than originally considered (Komada et al. 2008; Kraeuter et al. 2019; Molendijk and de Kloet 2015; Reardon 2024; Walf and Frye 2007; Yankelevitch-Yahav et al. 2015)—this must be considered in interpreting assessments of affective behaviors in rodent models. Regardless, these numerous PAE animal studies model various aspects of negative affective behaviors that have been reported in humans with a history of PAE, ultimately providing an important advancement to understanding and discovering the underlying neurobiological mechanisms that contribute to these maladaptive behaviors.

5.1.5 Animal Studies—Neurobiological Mechanisms

Animal studies have significantly expanded our understanding of neurobiological mechanisms that contribute to, or are at least correlated with, PAE-induced negative affective behaviors beyond what human studies have provided. Notably, all of the brain regions related to negative affective behaviors that have been shown to be altered in PAE human studies (i.e., hippocampus, amygdala, and prefrontal cortex) are also affected in animal models of PAE.

In the hippocampus, a moderate dose of PAE across the entire gestation, which increases depressive-like behavior in adult female offspring, also reduced the levels of several isoforms of brain-derived neurotrophic factor (BDNF) mRNA in C57BL/6J mice (Caldwell et al. 2008), whereas PAE from G9–20 decreased BDNF protein in Wistar rats (Yu et al. 2020). Reductions in adult-born neurons was also reported in the hippocampus of adult PAE Wistar offspring (Elibol-Can et al. 2014). Increased markers of oxidative stress within the hippocampus have also been observed in adult Sprague Dawley and Wistar rat offspring that show depressive-like behaviors resulting from PAE during either the entire gestation (Brocardo et al.

2012) or only the third trimester-equivalent (Lopatynska-Mazurek et al. 2021). These studies suggest that PAE disrupts neurogenic processes, including mechanisms involved in cell survival and plasticity, while also enhancing processes that drive cellular damage and death, into adulthood. Interestingly, moderate PAE through all trimester equivalents reduced levels of glial fibrillary acid protein (GFAP), a marker of neurogenesis and astrocytes, in the hippocampus of adolescent Wistar offspring that showed reduced anxiety-like behavior (Brolese et al. 2014), suggesting impairments in either neurogenesis or glial function may also contribute to negative affective behaviors. PAE-induced alterations in specific receptors have also been reported in the hippocampus, including reductions in dopamine D1 and D2 receptors and concomitant increases in muscarinic acetylcholine receptor binding, in juvenile Wistar offspring that showed elevated anxiety- and depressive-like behaviors (Carneiro et al. 2005). Immunoreactivity of cocaine- and amphetamine-regulated transcript peptide (CART), a neuropeptide involved in regulating anxiety and stress, was reduced in the hippocampus of PAE Sprague Dawley offspring that show anxiety- and depressive-like behaviors (Dandekar et al. 2019). PAE also dysregulates gene expression of corticotropin-releasing factor receptor 1 (CRFR1), glucocorticoid receptor (GR), and mineralocorticoid receptor (MR) in a sex-specific manner in various parts of the hippocampus of Sprague Dawley rats (Lam et al. 2018a). How alterations in neuromodulatory systems—such as dopamine, acetylcholine, CART, CRF, GR, and MR—within the hippocampus contribute to negative affective behaviors is not clear; however, activity of these various systems regulates neuronal function and synaptic transmission. In line with this, GABAergic synaptic inhibition, both phasic and tonic, in granule cells within the dentate gyrus of the hippocampus is disrupted in adult PAE Sprague Dawley offspring that exhibit anxiety-like behaviors (Liang et al. 2014). Impairments in hippocampal synaptic plasticity driven, in part, by alterations in GABA function have also been reported in juvenile PAE Sprague Dawley offspring (Fontaine et al. 2019). Collectively, animal studies have shown that PAE disrupts numerous neurobiological mechanisms within the hippocampus that are associated with cell growth, survival, and death, in addition to neuronal and synaptic function and plasticity.

The rodent prefrontal cortex, termed the medial prefrontal cortex, is divided into three major subdivisions: the prelimbic, infralimbic, and anterior cingulate cortex. Moderate PAE throughout the gestational period reduces BDNF protein and various mRNA isoforms across the medial prefrontal cortex of adult C57BL/6J females, which is associated with increased depressive-like behaviors (Caldwell et al. 2008). Markers of oxidative stress were also elevated in the prefrontal cortex of third trimester-equivalent PAE Wistar rat offspring (Lopatynska-Mazurek et al. 2021). Within the anterior cingulate cortex of adult CD1 male mice, PAE was shown to disrupt axonal and dendritic cytoskeletal morphology, in addition to reducing serotonin-positive fibers and serotonin 1A receptor expression, changes related to elevated anxiety-like behavior (Madarnas et al. 2020). GR and CRFR1 mRNA expression was also dysregulated in the infralimbic cortex (Lam et al. 2018a) and in the anterior cingulate cortex (Raineki et al. 2016) of PAE Sprague Dawley offspring in a sex- and stress-dependent manner, which was associated with increased anxiety-like responses. Although it is unclear how these alterations within the prefrontal cortex lead to heightened negative affective behaviors, several studies using a variety of transgenic mouse lines have found that PAE during a relatively narrow gestational period (~G10–20) increases GABA interneuron numbers in a subdivision- and layer-specific manner (Skorput and Yeh 2016) through disruptions in interneuron migration via alterations in L-type calcium channels, and sodium, potassium, chloride cotransporter (NKCC1) function and expression (Cuzon et al. 2008; Lee et al. 2022; Skorput et al. 2019). PAE also shifts the excitatory/inhibitory (glutamate/GABA) synaptic balance in layer 5 pyramidal neurons of the medial prefrontal cortex (Skorput and Yeh 2016). Interestingly, another study reported reduced layer 2/3 pyramidal neuron firing in the prelimbic cortex of adult PAE Sprague Dawley offspring, which was associated with increased social anxiety-like behavior (Przybysz et al. 2023). These studies illustrate a variety of disrupted neurobiological mechanisms resulting from PAE that are correlated with negative affective behaviors. Although no studies have tested a causal relationship between PAE-mediated disruptions in prefrontal cortex activity and negative affective behaviors, Raineki and colleagues showed sex-specific alterations in cFos mRNA depending on the prefrontal cortical subregion resulting from anxiety testing on the elevated plus maze in Sprague Dawley offspring (Raineki et al. 2014).

The amygdala has been considered an epicenter for emotion processing given that its activity is highly associated with affective behaviors. The amygdala is comprised of several nuclei—namely, the basolateral, central, and medial—that each play a unique role in the regulation of affective behaviors. Rodent studies demonstrate that PAE alters all of the amygdala nuclei in various ways. In the basolateral amygdala of Sprague Dawley offspring, PAE throughout gestation increased excitability and the magnitude of long-term potentiation (Zhou et al. 2010), while a relatively brief PAE during the third trimester-equivalent (P3–5) increased spontaneous excitatory glutamatergic transmission (Baculis et al. 2015), suggestive of heightened excitability, in adolescent male offspring that also exhibited elevated anxiety-like behavior. Additionally, third trimester-equivalent PAE (P2–12) disrupted dopamine D1 and D3 receptor regulation of basolateral amygdala inhibitory GABA transmission in Sprague Dawley rats (Diaz et al. 2014). A loss of neurons within the basolateral amygdala has also been reported in adult PAE offspring (PAE through gestation and third trimester-equivalent), which coincided with reduced cannabinoid receptor type 1-positive neurons, serotonin-positive neurons, but elevated serotonin 1A receptor levels in CD1 mice (Madarnas et al. 2020). At the neuronal morphology level, low-dose PAE throughout gestation in Sprague Dawley rats increases dendritic spine numbers and density in basolateral amygdala pyramidal neurons, the main output neurons of this nucleus (Cullen et al. 2013). Finally, CRFR1 mRNA was reduced in adult PAE Sprague Dawley offspring, but not adolescents (Raineki et al. 2016). Given that these neuromodulatory systems regulate synaptic function, neural activity, and plasticity (functional and morphological), it is possible that alterations in these systems (dopamine, cannabinoid, serotonin, and CRF) and overall basolateral amygdala function may contribute, in part, to the elevated anxiety-like behaviors. Within the central amygdala, moderate PAE on G12 alters basal inhibitory GABAergic transmission and neuronal excitability in an age- and sex-dependent manner throughout adolescence in Sprague Dawley offspring (Rouzer and Diaz 2022; Winchester and Diaz 2025). G12 PAE also sex-dependently reduces acute ethanol's enhancing effects on GABA transmission (Winchester and Diaz 2025) and CRFR1-modulation of GABA transmission through alterations in CRFR1 expression (Rouzer and Diaz 2022) in the central amygdala. Interestingly, Rouzer and Diaz showed that PAE-induced anxiety-like behavior was driven, in part, through blunted central amygdala CRFR1 function (Rouzer and Diaz 2022). PAE-induced increases in CRF mRNA were also found in the central amygdala of male Sprague Dawley offspring, but not females (Lan et al. 2015). Additionally, PAE increases markers of neuroinflammation within the amygdala of Wistar offspring, evidenced by elevated interleukin-1β and tumor necrosis factor-α levels (Kokhan et al. 2023). As with the prefrontal cortex, c-Fos mRNA expression was differentially affected by assessment of anxiety-like behavior on the elevated plus maze that was sex- and nucleus-specific in PAE Sprague Dawley offspring (Raineki et al. 2014). These studies illustrate that PAE leads to numerous neurobiological alterations in the amygdala involved in neuronal and cellular function that are either associated with or drive negative affective behaviors.

5.1.6 Prenatal Alcohol Exposure Conclusion

As discussed, animal models of PAE have identified a variety of neural mechanisms and processes that are impacted by PAE throughout the central nervous system. It should also be noted that many other brain areas and mechanisms implicated in various aspects of negative affective behaviors have also been found to be impacted by PAE, including the dorsal raphe nucleus (Eriksen et al. 2000; Kim et al. 2005; Oubraim et al. 2022; Tajuddin and Druse 1999; Zafar et al. 2000) and the hypothalamic-pituitary-adrenal axis (Burgess and Moritz 2020; Hellemans et al. 2008; Lam et al. 2018b, 2019; Wieczorek et al. 2015). Although the FASD field continues to discover more neural targets and mechanisms of PAE involved in negative affective behaviors, new studies are striving to link known mechanisms in order to better treat or improve negative affective behaviors in individuals with FASD.

5.2 Prenatal Nicotine Exposure

Despite immediate and long-term adverse outcomes of prenatal exposure to tobacco smoke, as of 2021, 4.6% of mothers in the United States smoked during pregnancy (Martin et al. 2023). Although epidemiological data on electronic cigarette (e-cigarette)/nicotine vaping use during pregnancy are limited, as many as 2.2–7.0% of individuals have reported using e-cigarettes during pregnancy (Vilcassim et al. 2023).

Cigarette smoke contains over 4000 chemical compounds, and many of them are considered toxic (Talhout et al. 2011), with nicotine being the most important pharmacologically active and pyschoactive compound in tobacco smoke (Thielen et al. 2008). Nicotine is an agonist of nicotinic acetylcholine receptors (nAChRs), a structurally diverse family of ligand-gated ion channels widely expressed in the fetal central nervous system (Dwyer et al. 2008). nAChRs, already detectable in the brain by the first trimester, exhibit a region-specific and temporally regulated pattern of developmental expression and play a prominent role in brain development (Dwyer et al. 2009). Nicotine can alter the normal trajectory of brain development through activation and desensitization of nAChRs (Slotkin 2008; Smith et al. 2010). Nicotine reaches the developing fetus through the placenta, and fetal concentration of nicotine is generally 15% higher than maternal levels (Lambers and Clark 1996). Fetal exposure to nicotine and other compounds in tobacco and e-cigarettes has been shown to be associated with fetal growth restriction as well as higher risks for stillbirth, infant mortality and the incidence of sudden infant death syndrome (Cnattingius 2004; Salihu and Wilson 2007). Long-term effects of prenatal maternal nicotine use include enhanced risk for development of attention-deficit/hyperactivity disorder (ADHD), schizophrenia, anxiety, depression, obesity, and future adolescent substance use (Wells and Lotfipour 2023). In the frame of this chapter, we will focus predominantly on negative affective behaviors, particularly anxiety and depressive disorders, associated with prenatal nicotine exposure.

5.2.1 Clinical Studies—Behavioral Alterations

The association between maternal smoking during pregnancy and childhood anxiety/depressive behaviors has been shown in a large, well-characterized cohort study that included 90,040 mother–child pairs (Moylan et al. 2015). Maternal smoking in early pregnancy and throughout the entire pregnancy was shown to be associated with increased anxiety and depressive behaviors in children at 1.5 and 3 years of age, with higher rates of smoking associated with higher rates of anxiety and depressive behaviors. Prenatal tobacco use also predicted depression and anxiety behaviors in 10-year-old children (Cornelius et al. 2000). Another study that assessed associations between maternal smoking during pregnancy and the risk of depression in offspring during adolescence revealed that this risk was 50% higher for 17-year-old individuals prenatally exposed to nicotine via maternal smoking during the first trimester of pregnancy, with no effects evident for tobacco smoke exposure during the third trimester (Duko et al. 2021). Duko et al. (2022) have also reported that maternal smoking during the third trimester increased risks of experiencing symptoms of anxiety early in adulthood, with a dose response association between prenatal tobacco exposure and increasing anxiety symptoms in offspring (Duko et al. 2022). A similar finding was reported in 22-year-old offspring with a history of prenatal (first, second, and third trimester) cigarette smoking exposure which was associated with higher scores for anxiety and depression in the adult self-report questionnaire (Cornelius et al. 2012). Interestingly, a longitudinal study found that children of light smokers (1–10 cigarettes/day) who quit by the 18th week of gestation scored lower in measures of internalizing behaviors (representative of anxiety and depressive symptoms) in the childhood behavior checklist (CBCL) relative to offspring of heavy smokers (11+ cigarettes/day), suggesting that there exists a dose-response and time of exposure-dependent relationship in risk for emotional disorders (Robinson et al. 2010). Together, these findings suggest that maternal smoking during pregnancy is associated with anxiety and depression in offspring (Wells and Lotfipour 2023), with these internalizing disorders evident during childhood (Cornelius et al. 2000; Moylan et al. 2015), adolescence (Duko et al. 2021), and adulthood (Cornelius et al. 2012; Duko et al. 2022).

5.2.2 Clinical Studies—Neurobiological Mechanisms

Prenatal exposure to nicotine through maternal smoking during pregnancy has been shown to alter normal trajectories of brain development, particularly in areas associated with affective behaviors. Using a standard neuroimaging protocol for preterm infants that included brain repeated ultrasound examinations and magnetic resonance imaging (MRI) at term age, a study revealed that the frontal lobe and cerebellar volumes were significantly smaller in preterm infants prenatally exposed to maternal smoking than in non-exposed preterm infants (Ekblad et al. 2010), with these adverse effects of smoking during pregnancy on brain volumes still evident in 13-year-old adolescents (Ekblad et al. 2022). Similarly, MRI studies revealed that maternal smoking during pregnancy was associated with smaller brain volume, smaller cortical surface area, and less gyrification in 10-year-old children (Zou et al. 2022), smaller caudate nucleus volumes and lower grey-white matter contrast across regions of the frontal, parietal, and temporal lobes in 9- to 12-year-olds (Puga et al. 2024) as well as smaller volume of the amygdala in 13- to 19-year-old adolescents (Haghighi et al. 2013).

Assessments of brain morphology via MRI revealed smaller total brain volumes and smaller cortical grey matter volumes in 6- to 8-year-old children exposed to maternal smoking during the entire pregnancy (El Marroun et al. 2014). Maternal smoking during pregnancy was associated with thinning of the orbitofrontal cortex in 12- to 18-year-old adolescents, and the likelihood of drug experimentation in these adolescents correlated with the degree of thinning (Lotfipour et al. 2009). Thinning of several cortical regions, including the orbitofrontal cortex has also been reported in adolescents prenatally exposed to maternal smoking when compared with non-exposed individuals of the same age, with these differences more pronounced in adolescent females than their male counterparts (Toro et al. 2008).

Together, these MRI studies demonstrate that multiple brain regions, including some involved in regulating affective behaviors, are affected by prenatal nicotine, with the observed alterations lasting into adolescence. These alterations can contribute to a number of adverse consequences of prenatal exposure to nicotine through maternal smoking during pregnancy, including anxiety and depressive disorders evident during childhood and adolescence.

5.2.3 Animal Models of Prenatal Nicotine Exposure

Preclinical models of prenatal nicotine exposure (PNE), allowing for investigation of immediate and lasting into adolescence and/or adulthood behavioral and neurological effects of PNE, have provided valuable information regarding effects of nicotine on the developing brain (Sikic et al. 2022; Smith et al. 2010; Wells and Lotfipour 2023). Unlike nicotine use in humans which is almost exclusively through inhalation, preclinical models of PNE employ different routes of nicotine administration, including subcutaneous injections, osmotic mini pumps, forced consumption in drinking water, and inhalation (Polli and Kohlmeier 2020). Although different modes of PNE are widely used, each mode has certain limitations. For instance, injections given twice a day are associated with a certain level of stress, produce nicotine peaks in plasma, and cause vessel constriction. Osmotic minipumps implanted in pregnant dams do not have these limitations; however, pump implantation is an invasive surgical procedure that requires anesthesia which itself can affect fetal development, and lead to continuous exposure to nicotine. The main disadvantage of nicotine forced consumption is drastic reductions in fluid consumption and body weight of rats (Murrin et al. 1987). Finally, as previously discussed, it is common that nicotine exposure begins during gestation in animal models of PNE, which is not a likely scenario in humans. Thus, since animal models of PNE differ in route and mode of nicotine administration, doses, developmental timing, and strains used, it is rather challenging to compare results from different studies. Nevertheless, animal research has shown long-lasting effects of PNE on brain and behavior, providing insights into mechanisms of nicotine effects on the developing brain (McCarthy et al. 2022).

5.2.4 Animal Studies—Behavioral Alterations

Laboratory rodents of different strains with a history of PNE demonstrate anxiety- and depressive-like behavioral alterations in different behavioral tests. For instance, in Sprague Dawley rats, PNE (G3 through ~P1–3) to a high nicotine dose (6.0 mg/kg/day via osmotic minipumps) resulted in anxiety-like behavioral alterations evident during adolescence (Vaglenova et al. 2004). After the removal of the minipumps, half of the litters were cross-fostered and other litters reared by their dams, yielding four prenatal exposure / postnatal rearing conditions: controls prenatally exposed to saline reared by their dams, nicotine-exposed offspring reared by their dams, nicotine-exposed offspring reared by control dams, and control offspring reared by nicotine-exposed dams. PNE, regardless of rearing conditions, resulted in increased anxiety-like behavior on the elevated plus maze and decreased novelty seeking relative to saline controls reared by their dams. However, saline controls cross-fostered to nicotine-exposed dams also showed increased anxiety and decreased novelty seeking, suggesting alterations in maternal behavior following nicotine exposure and/or nicotine withdrawal. Similar PNE of Sprague Dawley rats (osmotic minipumps, 6 mg/kg/day, G3–21) increased anxiety and depressive-like behavior and impaired spatial memory in offspring when tested in early adolescence, evidenced by reduced ambulation and rearing in the open field, reduced latency to become immobile and longer immobility duration in the forced swim test (Parameshwaran et al. 2012). Adult female CD1 mice prenatally exposed to nicotine (injected with 2 mg/kg nicotine twice daily throughout the entire gestation period) and tested at 6 months of age also showed increased anxiety as well as deficits in sensorimotor integration (Santiago and Huffman 2014).

There is some evidence that effects of prenatal nicotine exposure are sex-dependent. For instance, PNE adolescent female Wistar rat offspring (1.0 mg/kg nicotine twice a day from G9 to G20), but not their male counterparts, showed significantly more immobility in the open field and ingested significantly less sucrose relative to controls, suggesting depression-like behavior in female offspring following PNE (C. Zhang et al. 2019). Conversely, adolescent male NMRI mice (P42–49), but not females with a history of PNE via forced drinking of nicotine solution (300 μg/mL of nicotine detartrate) in 2% saccharin (seven days prior to mating and continued through the entire gestation period) showed anxiety-like behavior in the elevated zero maze and marble burying task, suggesting sex-specific anxiety-like alterations (Polli et al. 2020).

Animal studies using "developmental exposure" (DNE) in which PNE is combined with early postnatal exposure through maternal milk (Polli and Kohlmeier 2020) have also demonstrated alterations in affective behaviors. For instance, DNE in Long Evans rat dams via osmotic minipumps (nicotine solution sufficient to release 0.96 or 2 mg/kg nicotine (free base) per day from G4-P10) resulted in anxiety-like behavior on the elevated plus maze in adult (P72) male and female offspring but not adolescents (P32) (Eppolito et al. 2010). However, Lee and colleagues found that DNE in Sprague Dawley dams via voluntary nicotine intake in sweetened water (0.01% nicotine in water sweetened with 2% saccharin) from G15 to P18 produced adolescent offspring that spent significantly less time in the light compartment than non-exposed controls, indicative of increased anxiety-related behaviors (Lee et al. 2016). Anxiety- and depressive-like behavioral changes have also been reported in young adult C57BL/6J mice following DNE (started two weeks prior to breeding, continued through the entire gestation and up to weaning on P21) (Deng et al. 2023). In that study, only male offspring were assessed for emotional and cognitive alterations in late adolescence/emerging adulthood on P60 using a test battery that included forced swim, sucrose preference, open field, elevated plus maze, light/dark box, object recognition, and Morris water maze. DNE mouse offspring showed depression-like and anxiety-like alterations in almost all behavioral tests, with cognitive impairment also evident in these animals.

Overall, there is clear evidence in preclinical animal models that PNE and DNE can produce a variety of alterations in emotion-related behaviors, with most studies showing increased anxiety- and depressive-like behaviors at various ages. However, as with other prenatal substance exposure, the timing and amount of exposure (and likely the route of administration) influence the magnitude of the effects, and perhaps differentially interact with sex as a biological variable.

5.2.5 Animal Studies—Neurobiological Alterations

Animal studies have shown that PNE can disrupt fetal brain cell maturation and differentiation by activating nAChRs, affecting neural cell proliferation, migration, and synaptic development (Slotkin 2008; Smith et al. 2010). nAChRs are already detectable during the first trimester in humans and during the second prenatal week in rodents, demonstrating transient patterns of expression during early brain development (Smith et al. 2010; Zoli et al. 1995). During PNE, prolonged activation of nAChRs by nicotine leads to desensitization of these receptors, with nAChRs becoming less sensitive to acetylcholine—a neurotransmitter that plays a critical role in the development of the central nervous system (Slotkin 2008). PNE leads to an increase in the number of nAChRs, particularly the α4β2 and α7 subtypes in the fetal brain (Lv et al. 2008), suggesting that nicotine can disrupt the normal balance of nAChR subunits during brain development. Changes in nAChR subunit expression can interfere with normal brain development and function (Smith et al. 2010).

PNE has been shown to decrease cell numbers and/or cell size in several brain regions, including hippocampus (Abdel-Rahman et al. 2005; Roy and Sabherwal 1994), cerebellum (Abdel-Rahman et al. 2005; Abou-Donia et al. 2006), somatosensory cortex (Roy and Sabherwal 1994; Roy et al. 2002) of Sprague Dawley rats, and cingulate cortex of C57BL/6J mice (Zhu et al. 2012). Sex-specific effects of PNE have also been reported. For instance, the number of neurons was significantly lower in the dentate gyrus and CA3 hippocampal subregions of Wistar rat females following PNE relative to controls, with expression of steroidogenic acute regulatory protein in the hippocampus also suppressed in PNE females, but not PNE males (Zhang et al. 2019).

Anxiety- and depression-like alterations evident following PNE are associated with changes in BDNF signaling in brain regions implicated in emotion regulation. Specifically, BDNF gene expression in the hippocampus and PFC was substantially decreased by DNE in C57BL/6 male mice that demonstrated anxiety- and depression-like behavioral alterations (Deng et al. 2023). PNE of ICR mice through cigarette smoke inhalation (G7–16) significantly attenuated BDNF mRNA as well as protein levels in the hippocampus and PFC and enhanced depression-like behaviors in adulthood (Xiao et al. 2016). Given the key role of BDNF in neuronal development, synaptogenesis, and synaptic plasticity, these findings suggest that PNE can alter brain circuits essential for mood regulation and emotional control by affecting BDNF signaling.

Preclinical studies have shown that PNE and DNE also alter various neurotransmitter systems, including serotonin, dopamine, glutamate, and GABA (Blood-Siegfried and Rende 2010), and these alterations may contribute to affective changes associated with prenatal nicotine. For instance, PNE via osmotic minipumps (3 mg/kg/day) upregulated serotonin 5-HT1A and 5-HT2 receptors and the 5-HT transporter in adolescent and adult Sprague Dawley male rats, with downregulation of the 5-HT1A receptor evident in females. Both males and females exhibited presynaptic hyperactivity of serotonin and dopamine pathways, indexed via increased neurotransmitter turnover (Slotkin and Seidler 2010). Furthermore, patterns of sex differences in serotonin receptor alterations associated with PNE have been shown to be region-dependent (Slotkin et al. 2006). Specifically, PNE elicited 5-HT1A receptor binding elevation in the cerebral cortex of male Sprague Dawley rats, with no changes evident in females, as well as some increases in 5-HT2 receptors regardless of sex. In the striatum of males, PNE produced no significant changes in 5-HT1A receptor binding, with females showing reductions of 5-HT1A receptor binding. Prenatal nicotine also enhanced striatal 5-HT2 receptor binding in males and diminished it in females. Whereas 5-HT1A receptors in the brainstem were not affected by prenatal nicotine, 5-HT2 receptors showed overall upregulation regardless of sex.

PNE has been shown to substantially impact the development of the dopamine system, resulting in region-specific and sex-dependent alterations of the dopamine pathway. For instance, PNE via osmotic minipumps (3 or 6 mg/kg/day) decreased dopamine concentration in the ventral tegmental area and striatum of P22 male Sprague Dawley rats, while dopamine concentration in the substantia nigra was increased in these animals. In the striatum, D2 receptor numbers were reduced as well (Richardson and Tizabi 1994). Decreases in dihydroxyphenylacetic acid (DOPAC), a dopamine metabolite, levels in the neocortex of young adult Sprague Dawley male rats have been reported following PNE via nicotine injections of 3 or 6 mg/kg/day (Muneoka et al. 1999). Similarly, PNE via forced drinking resulted in reduced dopamine release in the medial prefrontal cortex evident on P56–63. PNE also reduced the number of tyrosine hydroxylase-positive varicosities in the medial prefrontal cortex and nucleus accumbens (Alkam et al. 2017). Sex-dependent effects of PNE via osmotic minipumps (3 mg/kg/day) on the dopamine system within the corticostriatal circuitry have been shown in adolescent Sprague Dawley rat offspring (Dwyer et al. 2019). In males, PNE decreased Catechol-O-methyl transferase (COMT)-dependent dopamine turnover to homovanillic acid in the prefrontal cortex and increased D2-like receptor G-protein coupling in the ventral striatum and pallidum. In females, PNE decreased dopamine transporter binding in the nucleus accumbens core. PNE increased dopamine content in the prefrontal cortex and dopamine D3 receptor binding in the ventral striatum and pallidum regardless of sex. PNE has also been shown to affect nicotine-stimulated dopamine release in the nucleus accumbens shell of adolescent Lewis rat offspring (Kane et al. 2004). Specifically, dopamine release in response to 0.07 mg/kg nicotine given by intravenous injection was attenuated by PNE in both males and females, while higher doses of

0.105 mg/kg produced comparable effects in PNE animals and controls.

Glutamate signaling in the developing brain is also significantly altered by PNE, primarily by impacting the expression and function of glutamate receptors within multiple brain regions involved in negative affective behaviors, including the PFC and hippocampus. PNE (osmotic mini pump, 6 mg/kg/day) produced persistent alterations in the hippocampal glutamatergic system of postweaning 3-week-old Sprague Dawley rats with reduced synaptic plasticity (LTP), basal synaptic transmission, and AMPA receptor-mediated synaptic currents (Parameshwaran et al. 2012). These deficits in synaptic transmission and plasticity were accompanied by decreased levels of several key synaptic proteins: vesicular glutamate transporter 1 (VGLUT1), synaptophysin, AMPA receptor subunit GluR1, phospho(Ser845) GluR1, and postsynaptic density 95 (PSD-95). Another study found that PNE in Sprague Dawley rats (4 mg/kg/day via osmotic minipumps) affected hippocampal AMPA and NMDA receptors (AMPAR and NMDAR) throughout ontogeny (Wang et al. 2011). On P1, PNE increased AMPAR subunit GluR1 and NMDAR subunits NR1, NR2a, and NR2d. However, these changes were no longer evident on P14. In young adult offspring, PNE resulted in significant downregulation of AMPAR subunit GluR2, NMDAR subunits NR1 and NR2c, as well as reduction of functional AMPARs throughout the hippocampus. These results demonstrate long-lasting effects of PNE on hippocampal glutamatergic signaling, including expression levels and functional distribution of AMPA and NMDA receptors. Furthermore, sex-specific PNE-associated alterations of prefrontal cortex glutamate receptor mRNA have been reported; specifically, PNE of NMRI mice via forced drinking of nicotine solution reduced mRNA expression of GluN1-, GluN2B-, and mGluR2-related genes within the prefrontal cortex of adolescent male offspring, whereas PNE adolescent female offspring had decreased expression of GluA2 mRNA (Polli et al. 2020). Although exact mechanisms of the observed sex-specific effects of PNE are not well understood, it has been suggested that PNE interferes with normal sexual differentiation and can induce long-lasting, sex-dependent alterations in multiple neural systems (Cross et al. 2017).

Prenatal and perinatal nicotine exposure can also alter the development of the GABA system in the brain, leading to potential disruptions in inhibitory function, particularly during adolescence and adulthood. A study using GAD67-GFP knock-in mice to assess effects of DNE (100 or 200 μg/mL in their drinking water, with exposure beginning 3 weeks before breeding until P21) on frontal cortical GABA neuron numbers found a decreased GABA-to-non-GABA neuron ratio across cortical layers II–III, V, and VI of the medial prefrontal cortex in young adult male and female offspring exposed to 200 μg/mL (Martin et al. 2020), indicating a shift in excitatory/inhibitory balance toward excitation.

Effects of DNE on GABAergic and glutamatergic neurotransmission have also been assessed in young adult (P60-P90) Sprague Dawley male rats with a history of daily nicotine exposure (6 mg/kg) during the third trimester-equivalent (P1–7) (Damborsky et al. 2015). Surprisingly, neonatal nicotine exposure had no effects on spontaneous GABAergic neurotransmission measured by spontaneous and miniature inhibitory postsynaptic currents in hippocampal CA1 pyramidal neurons. In contrast, neonatal nicotine exposure enhanced AMPAR-mediated excitatory synaptic transmission, with this effect evident in both evoked and spontaneous activity. Acute nicotine application increased glutamate release regardless of neonatal exposure condition, however, acute nicotine-stimulated GABA release was significantly attenuated in the nicotine-exposed adult rats. Therefore, both systems were affected by neonatal nicotine exposure that persistently increased excitation and reduced the nicotinic modulation of presynaptic GABA release in the adult rat hippocampus.

Together, results from preclinical studies clearly demonstrate that PNE impacts the development of multiple neurotransmitter systems in brain regions that contribute to negative affective behaviors, leading to long-term neurobiological and behavioral consequences evident throughout ontogeny.

5.2.6 Prenatal Nicotine Exposure Conclusion

In summary, clinical and preclinical research has demonstrated that prenatal exposure to nicotine can alter brain regions and neurotransmitter signaling implicated in emotional regulation and may contribute toward the development of anxiety and depression. However, there are numerous factors that may contribute to the magnitude of PNE effects, including timing of exposure, age of assessment, and sex, that require further investigation to fully understand.

5.3 Prenatal Cannabinoid Exposure

The rate of cannabis use among pregnant people has more than doubled between 2002 and 2017, coinciding with the widespread legalization and subsequent increase in availability of regulated cannabis (Brown et al. 2017; Meinhofer et al. 2022; Volkow et al. 2019; Young-Wolff et al. 2017). Legalization has placed cannabis in a unique position among other drugs because this notable shift in public policy has contributed to a growing acceptance of medicinal and recreational cannabis use, as well as a notion that cannabis use is associated with minimal risk, even when used during pregnancy. Indeed, individuals who reported cannabis use during pregnancy expressed an unawareness of its potential risks to the pregnancy and noted that insufficient cautionary advice from healthcare providers also contributed to their use (Weisbeck et al. 2021). In addition to lack of knowledge of possible negative outcomes, there is a perception that cannabis use during pregnancy can alleviate pregnancy symptoms, such as morning sickness, and it has been reported that some cannabis dispensaries even recommend cannabis use to treat morning sickness because of its antiemetic properties (Dickson et al. 2018; Roberson et al. 2014; Westfall et al. 2006). These factors, in combination with a variety of socioeconomic factors such as marital status, paternal cannabis use, and childhood trauma, work synergistically to promote cannabis use during pregnancy (El Marroun et al. 2008; Ko et al. 2020).

Endocannabinoids, and their activity at cannabinoid receptors, the cannabinoid receptor-type 1 (CB1R) and the cannabinoid receptor- type 2 (CB2R), have been shown to play an important role in neurodevelopment (reviewed in (Maccarrone et al. 2014)). CB1R abundance changes dynamically throughout the lifespan, with high levels of gene expression early in development (reviewed in (Bara et al. 2021)). CB1Rs are the most widely expressed G-protein coupled receptor in the brain, and they are present in several brain regions associated with negative affect including the prefrontal cortex and amygdala (Bara et al. 2021; Mackie 2005; Tsou et al. 1998). Given that cannabinoids can readily pass through the placenta, and CB1Rs are present in the developing fetus, maternal cannabis use can influence the neurodevelopmental outcomes of the offspring (Berrendero et al. 1999; Blackard and Tennes 1984). There is ample evidence that prenatal cannabinoid exposure (PCE) can affect the offspring in a wide variety of ways, including altering affective behaviors; however, there is also considerable variability in reports characterizing the precise impact of PCE on neurodevelopment and behavior across the lifespan [reviewed in (Ainiti et al. 2023; Andrade 2024; Bassalov et al. 2024; Cupo et al. 2024; Grant et al. 2020; Nashed et al. 2020)].

5.3.1 Clinical Studies—Behavioral Alterations

Clinical studies conducted to evaluate the impact of PCE on behavioral development have identified some alterations in affective behaviors of the offspring, although the available evidence so far remains variable (Bassalov et al. 2024; Grant et al. 2020; Nashed et al. 2020). As early as infancy, babies with PCE in the third trimester showed decreased scores on the Bayley Scales of Infant Development (BSID), a tool used to assess neurodevelopmental progress (Richardson et al. 1995). However, others detected no differences on the BSID in infants with PCE without a specific trimester reported, suggesting that the precise timing of PCE may play a role in determining the behavioral consequences during infancy (Fried and Watkinson 1988). In young children, one study reported that PCE increased anxiety, aggression, and hyperactivity in exposed offspring (Rompala et al. 2021). Interestingly, these behavioral changes were also associated with an increase in the stress hormone cortisol measured in a hair analysis, as well as altered heart rate variability in children with a history of PCE (Rompala et al. 2021). As part of the Maternal Health Practices and Child Development Project, a longitudinal series of studies that were conducted to better understand how prenatal substance exposure impacts offspring, Gray and colleagues found that 10-year-old children with a history of PCE in the first and third trimester reported higher depressive symptoms on the Child Depressive Inventory (Gray et al. 2005). These depressive symptoms in 10-year-old children predicted subsequent delinquent behavior in the same children when they were 14 years old, as measured by the Self Report Delinquency Scale and the Child Behavior Checklist (Day et al. 2011). Furthermore, a study conducted to identify predictors of anxiety and depression in 10-year-old children found that PCE could significantly predict anxiety and depression (Leech et al. 2006). Taken together, these findings indicate that PCE can negatively impact emotional regulation in exposed offspring. However, it is important to note that there are also several studies [reviewed in (Bassalov et al. 2024)] that did not detect negative affective behavioral changes in offspring with a history of PCE, but did identify altered patterns of other behaviors, such as externalizing behaviors like aggression and hyperactivity (Moore et al. 2023; Murnan et al. 2021; Vishnubhotla et al. 2024).

5.3.2 Clinical Studies—Neurobiological Alterations

The precise PCE-induced neurobiological alterations that may increase vulnerability to affective disorders remain unknown. However, although there is considerable variability in the findings, histology, neuroimaging and functional connectivity analyses have identified several brain regions and connections that are apparent targets of PCE. In the fetal brain, PCE is associated with increased opioid and dopamine receptor gene expression in the amygdala (Wang et al. 2004, 2006). In infancy, in an MRI study, PCE was associated with reduced volume of the dorsal and lateral surfaces of the frontal lobe, another brain region that contributes to negative affective states (Peterson et al. 2020). Interestingly, using fMRI, one study found that infants with PCE had an altered pattern of hippocampal-to-frontocortical connectivity, with weaker hippocampal connectivity with regions including the posterior cingulate cortex and anterior insula; but stronger hippocampal connectivity with regions including the dorsomedial prefrontal cortex and motor cortex (Thomason et al. 2021). Furthermore, the stronger hippocampal connectivity patterns in PCE infants were found to be in regions associated with less favorable cognitive and socioemotional behavioral outcomes at age 5, suggesting that this altered fetal connectivity may relate to negative postnatal outcomes across various behavioral domains. This indicates that PCE can have bidirectional effects on functional connectivity in exposed infants. In young children (age 6–8), PCE did not change global brain volumes, however, PCE did increase frontal cortex thickness measured in an MRI (El Marroun et al. 2016). Using data from the adolescent brain cognitive development (ABCD) study, differences in frontolimbic pathways were assessed using diffusion MRI in children around the age of 10 (Evanski et al. 2024). They discovered that children with a history of PCE had decreased fractional anisotropy in the fornix, a brain region important for emotional processing, indicating that PCE can alter white matter integrity in this region (Evanski et al. 2024). In adolescence, a study by Smith and colleagues used fMRI to evaluate blood flow during a battery of cognitive tasks related to executive function. Adolescents with a history of PCE were able to complete the tasks similarly to the non-exposed controls, but PCE adolescents required increased activity in the postcentral gyrus, the cuneus, the middle occipital gyrus, and the posterior cingulate cortex (A. M. Smith et al. 2016). This differential pattern of activation in PCE adolescents mirrors findings in PCE infants, and highlights the fact that despite there being no differences in task performance, the neurobiological mechanisms that support task completion may be altered due to PCE. This suggests that PCE disrupts typical maturation refinement processes, which in turn could influence neurodevelopmental outcomes for exposed offspring.

5.3.3 Animal Models of Prenatal Cannabis/Cannabinoid Exposure

There are several studies that have sought to characterize the effect of PCE on developing offspring using preclinical models. However, preclinical PCE research differs in several important ways from the previously described clinical studies. The cannabis plant contains hundreds of naturally occurring phytocannabinoids, any of which could influence offspring individually or in combination with others (Blebea et al. 2024). The two phytocannabinoids that are best studied are the two most abundant phytocannabinoids synthesized by the cannabis plant, tetrahydrocannabidiol (THC) and cannabidiol (CBD) (Shahbazi et al. 2020). THC is of particular interest because it is the psychoactive component of cannabis that produces the "high" associated with cannabis use, whereas CBD is non-psychoactive and has been shown to have anti-inflammatory properties, which has led to marketing of CBD products for medicinal purposes (Blebea et al. 2024). Importantly, the amount of THC and the ratio between THC and CBD in cannabis has been steadily increasing in recent years, which could enhance negative outcomes related to THC exposure (Chandra et al. 2019). An important consideration for PCE research is that clinical studies are unable to determine the specific cannabinoid that is responsible for producing an effect in the exposed offspring. Alternatively, preclinical research allows for administration of a specific cannabinoid to pregnant animals in order to determine their individual effect on offspring; however, this also limits the ability to translate findings from preclinical studies because pregnant people typically do not exclusively use individual cannabinoids. Another consideration for PCE research is the routes of cannabis administration, which for humans is typically inhalation via smoking or vaporizing, or orally consumed via cannabis infused foods and drinks (Russell et al. 2018). In preclinical models, there are a variety of routes of administration including vaporized and orally consumed; however, many studies administer cannabis via injection, which also limits translatability. Finally, similar to the other drugs discussed, in preclinical models of PCE, the first exposure of the mother-to-be to the studied cannabinoid occurs during pregnancy. Although in humans it is likely more common for PCE to not be the first experience with a cannabis product, increased advertisements for the nausea-reducing effects of cannabis products (Dickson et al. 2018; Gunn et al. 2024; Madson et al. 2025; Roberson et al. 2014; Westfall et al. 2006) may result in increased first-time use during pregnancy. Despite these limitations, preclinical research has provided an important avenue of investigation into the specific effects of cannabinoids and allows for manipulation of specific neural mechanisms to better understand the impact of PCE on the developing offspring.

5.3.4 Animal Studies—Behavioral Alterations

Given that THC is the psychoactive compound in cannabis, there has been an emphasis on investigating the effects of prenatal THC exposure (PTE) in preclinical studies. Trezza and colleagues gave pregnant Wistar rat dams THC through an oral cannula from G15 through P9, to model moderate perinatal THC exposure (Trezza et al. 2008). They found that PTE increased the number of maternal separation-induced ultrasonic vocalizations emitted by infant male rats, decreased the amount of social play behavior by adolescent male rats, and decreased the percentage of time spent on the open arms of an elevated plus maze in adult male rats, all of which are indicative of an anxiety-like phenotype. Furthermore, these findings demonstrate that PTE can produce persistent increases in anxiety-like behavior that endure throughout the lifespan (Trezza et al. 2008). Interestingly, Wistar male rats exposed to the cannabinoid receptor agonist, WIN 55,212-2 (WIN), emitted fewer maternal separation induced ultrasonic vocalizations, an effect opposite of what was reported by Trezza and colleagues (Antonelli et al. 2005). This could be due to a variety of methodological differences including timing of the exposure and because WIN does not act identically to THC, demonstrating that caution is warranted in interpreting the results of prenatal WIN exposure.

As mentioned above, different routes of administration may produce different patterns of alterations following PCE in offspring. For example, Traccis and colleagues administered THC via daily subcutaneous injection to pregnant Sprague Dawley rat dams from G5 to G20 and did not detect differences in time spent in the center of any open field, social behavior, or in sucrose preference, indicating no differences in anxiety or depressive-like behaviors in juvenile PTE females (Traccis et al. 2021). Using the same exposure model, a separate study found no differences in response to acoustic startle or time spent on the open arms of an elevated plus maze in juvenile PTE males, also indicating no increase in anxiety-like behavior (Frau et al. 2019). A similar finding has been reported in adolescent Wistar rat offspring exposed to subcutaneous THC from G5 to G20 where there was no difference in anxiety-like behavior measured on the elevated plus maze and no difference in depressive-like behavior measured in the sucrose preference test (Castelli et al. 2023). Importantly, subcutaneous THC administration did produce other behavioral and neurobiological effects in offspring in these studies (Castelli et al. 2023; Frau et al. 2019; Traccis et al. 2021). Conversely, adult male Long Evans rat offspring spent less time in the center of an open field, indicating increased anxiety-like behavior; however, they did not show any changes in the forced swim test, suggesting no alteration in depressive-like behavior following subcutaneous THC exposure from G1–22 (Newsom and Kelly 2008). Subcutaneous injection of WIN from G5–20 similarly did not enhance anxiety-like behavior of adult male or female offspring when tested on the elevated plus maze, but it did decrease overall social activity, social play, and social investigation frequencies as well as time spent investigating a conspecific in adult male, but not female Wistar rats (Bara et al. 2018). However, intravenous administration of THC from G5-P2 increased depressive-like behaviors in offspring, as demonstrated by decreased sucrose preference in PTE Long Evans rat offspring (Ellis et al. 2022). In a model using vaporized THC from G5–20 in Sprague Dawley rats, there was no effect of exposure on time spent in the center of the open field in adolescent male or female offspring (Breit et al. 2022). Interestingly, in a study where pregnant Sprague Dawley rat dams were exposed to cannabis smoke from G6–20, male and female offspring displayed more anxiety-like behavior on the open field test, but not in the elevated plus maze (Sandini et al. 2023). This suggests that the route of THC administration plays an important role in how prenatal exposure to THC impacts offspring affective behaviors and should be carefully considered in the interpretation of results.

When both sexes have been included in the experimental design, several studies have uncovered interesting sex-specific effects resulting from PTE. In one study, Wistar rats were treated daily with oral THC beginning 5 days prior to breeding, and THC exposure continued daily until G20. They found that adolescent PTE males had a higher approach latency during a novelty suppressed feeding task, indicating increased anxiety-like behavior, an effect not seen in females (Lallai et al. 2022). Another study found that perinatal THC exposure resulted in increased latency to enter the light zone of a light-dark box test in adult female, but not male Wistar rats (Navarro et al. 1994). Taken together, these studies demonstrate that PTE produces sex-specific effects and further investigation of factors that may confer protection or vulnerability for either sex is warranted.

Preclinical models have also been employed to assess the impact of prenatal exposure to the non-psychoactive cannabinoid, CBD, which has been popularized as a potential treatment for a variety of conditions (Malik et al. 2015). Similar to studies investigating the effects of PTE, studies examining the role of prenatal CBD exposure have produced variable results that depend on sex and exposure paradigm. When CBD was administered to pregnant mice from an Agouti variable yellow colony throughout their entire pregnancy and lactation period, adult female offspring demonstrated an increase in marbles buried, suggesting this exposure increased anxiety-like behavior (Wanner et al. 2021). However, in a study using C57BL/6J mice in a cross-fostering design to disentangle the impact of prenatal and postnatal CBD exposure, adult females exposed to CBD only postnatally (birth through weaning), but not both prenatally and postnatally, showed an increase in marbles buried as well as decreased anxiety-like behavior on the elevated plus maze and the light–dark box test (Compagno et al. 2025). Interestingly, this effect on anxiety-like behavior was only present in adult female offspring, with adult male offspring behavior unaffected by pre- or postnatal CBD exposure (Compagno et al. 2025). The discrepancies in these findings are likely due to several methodological differences between the studies, including the cross-fostering design used by Compagno and colleagues, mouse strain, and drug vehicle.

DeVuono and colleagues assessed the impact of intraperitoneally injected G7–20 prenatal THC, cannabidiol, or the combination of both on Wistar rat offspring development. In both sexes, there were no differences in any of the groups on time spent in the center of the open field. In contrast, there were sex-specific effects of cannabinoid exposure in the elevated plus maze, where adolescent females exposed to CBD or the combination of CBD and THC (CBD + THC) spent less time in the open arms, indicating increased anxiety-like behavior, whereas adolescent males exposed to CBD + THC spent more time in the open arms, indicating decreased anxiety-like behavior (DeVuono et al. 2024). Taken together, these findings demonstrate that different combinations of cannabinoids can produce different effects on negative affective behaviors in exposed offspring.

5.3.5 Animal Studies—Neurobiological Alterations

Findings from preclinical studies align with clinical research regarding the brain regions altered by PCE. Prenatal exposure to cannabinoids can influence negative affective behavioral development through alterations of the endocannabinoid system [reviewed in (Lu and Mackie 2021)] directly, or through alterations of a wide variety of other neural mechanisms. Importantly, the endocannabinoid system plays a role in several neurodevelopmental processes, including neurogenesis and migration [reviewed in (Bara et al. 2021; Maccarrone et al. 2014)], and PCE has been proposed to be a "first hit" to the system that may disrupt neurobiological mechanisms in a manner that promotes subsequent behavioral deficits (K. A. Richardson et al. 2016).

As discussed above, the cortex, and in particular the frontal cortex, is a brain region that is important for affective behaviors and is a well-documented target of PCE in clinical studies. In animal models, PTE is associated with increased cortical apoptosis in neonates, but not in adult rats, suggesting that PTE may influence neurodevelopment at specific time points, rather than global enduring changes (Downer et al. 2007). PCE has been shown to alter differentiation of glutamatergic neurons, migration of GABAergic interneurons, and hinder cortical projections in the developing rat cortex (de Salas-Quiroga et al. 2015; Saez et al. 2014). Studies using Wistar rats have identified altered cortical gene expression profiles in both adolescent and adult offspring following PCE including differences in mRNA for CB1Rs, serotonin receptors, dopamine receptors, NMDA receptor subunits, metabotropic glutamate receptors, and GAD2 (Bara et al. 2018; DeVuono et al. 2024). Prenatal WIN exposure decreased glutamate levels in the cortex of adolescent Wistar rat offspring, which in combination with altered glutamate receptor gene expression, suggest that PCE may influence synaptic plasticity mechanisms (Castaldo et al. 2007). Indeed, prenatal WIN or THC exposure did not alter prefrontal cortex long-term potentiation (LTP) in male or female offspring, but WIN does impair long-term depression (LTD) in adult male Wistar rat offspring, a deficit that can be recovered with positive allosteric modulation of $mGluR_5$ (Bara et al. 2018). In addition to WIN and PTE, prenatal CBD exposure or PTE + prenatal CBD exposure combined in Wistar rats altered pyramidal cell firing and local field potential cortical oscillations in a sex specific manner in the prefrontal cortex of adolescent offspring (DeVuono et al. 2024). This demonstrates that PCE can sex-specifically impair synaptic plasticity mechanisms.

Similar to the clinical findings, PCE impacts the hippocampus of offspring. Wistar rat neonates prenatally exposed to WIN have decreased amounts of baseline and potassium evoked hippocampal glutamate levels measured by microdialysis (Mereu et al. 2003). Studies using Wistar rats have documented altered gene expression profiles in the hippocampus following PCE in adolescent offspring, including differences in NMDA receptor subunits, monoamine receptors, and GAD2 (Castelli et al. 2023; DeVuono et al. 2024). Additionally, PCE impacts synaptic plasticity mechanisms in a manner similar to the previously noted effects in the prefrontal cortex. Prenatal WIN exposure in Wistar rats decreased baseline and potassium-evoked glutamate release in adolescent and adult male offspring (Mereu et al. 2003). Furthermore, using the same exposure paradigm, prenatal WIN exposure disrupted the maintenance, but not induction, of LTP in adolescent male offspring, demonstrating that PCE interferes with hippocampal plasticity (Mereu et al. 2003). In the ventral hippocampus, PTE, prenatal CBD exposure, or both in Wistar rats produced altered cell firing patterns differently in adolescent male and female offspring (DeVuono et al. 2024). Taken together, these studies suggest that PCE results in a complex profile of neurobiological alterations that impact several mechanisms related to synaptic function and plasticity that may synergistically promote negative affective behavior.

Assessment of PCE effects on the amygdala shows that cannabis smoke exposure from G6–20 produced a notable transcriptional change in the amygdala of male Sprague Dawley rat offspring, with over 800 increased and decreased differentially expressed genes (Sandini et al. 2023). Enrichment analyses indicated that receptor signaling differences were seen across several neurotransmitters systems, including opioids, glutamate, and GABA. Furthermore, preproenkephalin is increased in the medial and central subnuclei of the Long Evans rat amygdala following PTE, providing additional evidence that opioid function in the amygdala is a target of PCE (Spano et al. 2007). Together with the human study noted earlier showing that PCE in humans leads to upregulation of mu opioid receptors in the amygdala (Wang et al. 2006), there is growing evidence demonstrating interactions between opioid and cannabinoid systems, particularly during neural development. How overactivation of the endogenous cannabinoid system alters endogenous opioid systems is not well understood; however, given the critical role of mu opioid receptors in driving and guiding myelination, proliferation, and differentiation of neural cells during the gestational period [see review: (Spodnick et al. 2025)], it is imperative to further investigate the relationship between these two critical systems across neurodevelopment.

5.3.6 Prenatal Cannabinoid Exposure Conclusions

Given the rapid rise of cannabis use by pregnant people following the legalization and increase in availability of cannabis, it is essential to better understand how PCE impacts the developmental trajectory of offspring. Current evidence demonstrates that PCE can increase the vulnerability of offspring to develop deficits in emotional regulation mechanisms that may manifest as increased anxiety or depression. However, given the chemical complexity and variability in potency of the cannabis plant, in addition to the increasing availability of synthetic cannabis products, there is a critical need for more clinical and preclinical studies of PCE.

5.4 Prenatal Opioid Exposure

The rates of opioid use during pregnancy have significantly risen over the past 2 decades, in part as a result of the opioid epidemic (Spencer et al. 2024). Current estimates indicate that the rates of maternal opioid use disorder (OUD), including long-term and unspecified use, increased from 3.5 to 8.2 per 1000 delivery hospitalizations (131%) from 2010 to 2017, whereas neonatal opioid withdrawal syndrome (NOWS) rates nearly doubled during this period, increasing from 4.0 to 7.3 per 1000 births (82.5%) (Hirai et al. 2021). These rates are a likely underestimate as 6.6% of people reported prescription opioid use during pregnancy in a 2019 survey (Ko et al. 2020) and 14–22% of pregnant people filled at least one opioid prescription during pregnancy 10+ years ago (Bateman et al. 2014; Desai et al. 2014). Given the recency of escalated rates of prenatal opioid exposure (POE) over the last 10–20 years, our understanding surrounding the potential myriad of effects resulting from POE is relatively limited. An important factor to consider regarding POE is the variety of potential opioid drugs that are available and used/misused by pregnant people that have different pharmacokinetic and pharmacodynamic properties, which further complicates our ability to identify the spectrum of consequences of POE on offspring. Related, POE can result from treatment of a pain disorder, an untreated OUD (i.e. opioid addiction), and treatment of OUD using opioid medications for OUD (MOUDs) (also known as medication-assisted treatment (MAT)). Currently, MOUDs (methadone and buprenorphine) are the standard of care for OUD treatment during pregnancy as a form of harm reduction given notable improved neonatal and maternal outcomes relative to misusing opioids (Byrnes and Vassoler 2018; Caritis and Panigrahy 2019; Haight et al. 2018; Rodriguez and Klie 2019; Taylor et al. 2021; Tran et al. 2017). Despite the clear benefits of MOUDs, these drugs are agonists and/or antagonists at the same opioid receptors as misused opioids (mu, kappa, and/or delta opioid receptors), which introduce safety concerns regarding potential long-term benefits of this form of treatment option. Nevertheless, regardless of the specific opioid used during pregnancy, a growing number of effects on the offspring have been reported in clinical and preclinical studies as a result of POE [see reviews: (Baldacchino et al. 2012, 2014; Byrnes and Vassoler 2018; Farid et al. 2008; Grecco and Atwood 2020; Harder and Murphy 2019; Monnelly et al. 2019; Yazdy et al. 2015; Yeoh et al. 2019)], although the full spectrum of long-term effects remains elusive. In fact, the term "Fetal Fentanyl Syndrome" was recently coined given some of the emerging teratogenic effects that have been observed in fentanyl exposed offspring (Mirnics 2025; Wadman et al. 2023). Among the observed effects of POE, studies have reported increased negative affective behaviors and emotional processing deficits, particularly anxiety- and depressive-like symptoms, at various ages regardless of the specific opioid used.

5.4.1 Clinical Studies—Behavioral Alterations

There are few clinical studies that have specifically investigated the impact of POE on negative affective behavioral changes and emotion processing; however, these maladaptive behavioral impairments have been consistently reported through early adulthood. Notably, infants (5–8 months of age) with a history of prenatal MOUD exposure exhibited impairments in self-regulation during an experimental Still-Face Paradigm (Bakhireva et al. 2019), an effect that was exacerbated in infants with POE + PAE (Beauchamp et al. 2020). Although deficits in self-regulation in infancy can signify numerous neurological and neurobehavioral alterations, findings from these studies suggest that impaired self-regulation is related to affect regulation which can ultimately manifest as elevated negative affective behaviors, such as anxiety and depression. Consistent with this notion, children (2-years-old) born with NOWS were also more likely to be diagnosed with an emotional disorder relative to non-exposed children (Hall et al. 2019), whereas 2-year-old methadone-exposed children showed impaired emotional functioning as measured using the Infant-Toddler Symptom Checklist (Levine et al. 2021). POE and NOWS-diagnosed preschool-aged children are at a higher risk of emotional disturbances compared to non-exposed children (Azeem et al. 2024; Sherman et al. 2019). Similarly, a survey of caregivers of methadone-exposed offspring at late pregnancy/birth, 18 months, 2, 4.5, and 9 years of age using a Strengths and Difficulties Questionnaire (SDQ), which assessed emotional symptoms among other behaviors in offspring, found elevated emotional problems that further increased between 4.5 and 9 years of age, a trajectory not observed in the non-exposed group (Jaekel et al. 2021). Beyond 9 years of age, children (6–13-years-old) of methadone-dependent mothers scored significantly higher for measures of anxiety, aggression, depression, and social withdrawal relative to non-exposed children (de Cubas and Field 1993), while a study of ~20-year-old individuals reported higher odds of major depressive disorder and a slight increase in anxiety disorder in the opioid-exposed group compared to the non-exposed (Nygaard et al. 2020). From this collection of studies, it is quite clear that emotional processing deficits and symptoms of negative affect are apparent from birth that persist and can become anxiety and depression disorders, at least through young adulthood. However, given that the opioid epidemic started relatively recently (only ~20 years ago), information regarding the effects of POE on negative affective behaviors beyond young adulthood is lacking.

5.4.2 Clinical Studies—Neurobiological Alterations

Given the limited number of clinical studies examining the impact of POE on offspring behavior and neurodevelopment, it is not surprising that there are even fewer studies investigating neurobiological mechanisms disrupted by POE that may contribute to neurobehavioral impairment. From the few studies that have been conducted using diffusion, functional, and structural MRI, reductions in brain volume of various structures (Aslaksen et al. 2025; Monnelly et al. 2018; Yuan et al. 2014) and abnormal white matter integrity throughout the brain (Merhar et al. 2019) have been reported in POE infants relative to controls. However, regarding brain regions known to be directly involved in negative affective behavioral changes, a relatively recent study evaluated functional connectivity between the amygdala and other relevant brain structures in infants with a history of POE (Radhakrishnan et al. 2021). It was determined that infants with POE had increased functional connectivity between the amygdala and prefrontal cortex relative to unexposed infants, suggestive of POE-induced disruptions in bottom-up and top-down regulation of brain circuits associated with affective behavior. However, as part of the ABCD longitudinal neuroimaging study, it was found that 9–10 year old children with POE did not show a difference in amygdala, parahippocampal, or hippocampal brain volumes compared to unexposed children (Hartwell et al. 2024), suggesting that either not all brain regions are impacted by POE at the gross morphological level (i.e., reduced brain volume) or that alterations that are apparent in infancy, recover through childhood. In support of the former, reduced volume of the basal ganglia and thalamus, but not global brain volume or cerebral cortical volume, was found in 10–14-year-old children with POE (Sirnes et al. 2017). Another possible interpretation is that functional alterations may not be related to morphological effects, which highlights the limitations in modern human neuroscience techniques. Regardless, although it is not clear from these studies how POE disrupts growth of the fetal brain, a recent study used human induced pluripotent stem cells to generate fetal-like cells to determine how exposure to buprenorphine or oxycodone alters cortical development—the effect of buprenorphine was examined since it is one of the approved

MOUDs for pregnant people, while oxycodone was included given the known neurodevelopmental effects resulting from oxycodone use during pregnancy (Nieto-Estevez et al. 2022). Interestingly, it was found that buprenorphine interrupted interneuron development and migration process by disrupting function of nociception opioid receptors which are found in the developing brain. Additionally, this same study found similar effects in a rat model of prenatal buprenorphine exposure, suggesting a possible mechanism that may contribute to the reductions in brain volume observed in human POE brains.

5.4.3 Animal Models of Prenatal Opioid Exposure

Animal models of POE are essential for understanding the array of neurobehavioral consequences resulting from POE. However, some major limitations of the animal POE models include initiation of opioid administration only during the gestational period, while in humans opioid use precedes and continues through pregnancy. Another factor to consider is that similar to the human situation, there are numerous opioids that have been tested, which creates a complex set of data that is difficult to translate to the clinic given the variability in pharmacokinetics and pharmacodynamics, in addition to the dosing patterns. Finally, the routes of opioid administration vary extensively (injection, voluntary oral, forced intragastric gavage, and osmotic minipumps), which lead to procedurally induced differences in pharmacokinetics [see these reviews for more discussion on these limitations (Byrnes and Vassoler 2018; Ferrante and Blendy 2024)]—albeit, opioids are also administered in a variety of ways by humans. Nevertheless, animal models of POE have been extremely useful not only for understanding potential neurobehavioral alterations resulting from POE, but also for determination of other factors that may contribute to the effects of POE (i.e., stress), allowing the field to forecast potential long-term effects in adulthood and beyond, which the human clinical studies have not yet determined.

5.4.4 Animal Studies—Behavioral Alterations

Not surprisingly, animal research has demonstrated negative affective behaviors in POE offspring, reminiscent to those observed in humans. Given that information regarding the specific opioid used for POE and the patterns and routes of administration are available in animal studies, this section will divide the known effects of POE on negative affective behavior by specific opioid.

Two studies have investigated the impact of prenatal exposure to oxycodone on anxiety- and depression-like behaviors in rodent offspring. In the first study by Flores and colleagues (Flores et al. 2024), oxycodone exposure in Sprague Dawley rats began either before pregnancy and continued through the gestational period or was administered only to the lactating dam until weaning via intragastric infusion. Assessment of offspring showed that only juvenile offspring whose mothers received oxycodone during lactation, but not offspring that were prenatally exposed, had reduced social behavior and marble burying behavior, indicative of impairments in affective behaviors. However, another study found that oxycodone exposure in CF1 mice from pre-pregnancy through the entire gestational period via intraperitoneal injection resulted in reduced social behavior and increased anxiety-like behavior on the elevated plus maze in adulthood (Martin et al. 2021). From these studies, it appears that prenatal oxycodone exposure may produce differential effects depending on developmental time of exposure and age of testing, although negative affective behaviors were generally apparent in exposed offspring.

Data on prenatal morphine's effects on anxiety- and depressive-like behaviors in offspring are rather contradicting. One set of studies administered morphine to pregnant Wistar rats from G11–G18 and found that late adolescent offspring exhibited increased anxiety-like behaviors in two different tests of anxiety (light/dark box and elevated plus maze), but did not show depressive-like behaviors in the forced swim test (Ahmadalipour and Rashidy-Pour 2015; Ahmadalipour et al. 2015). Similarly, morphine exposure from G3 to G20 resulted in increased anxiety-like behavior and reduced social behaviors in young adult Sprague Dawley rats (Chen et al. 2015). Elevated depressive-like behaviors, evidenced by increased immobility time in the forced swim test, were also found in juvenile and adult Wistar rat offspring following maternal morphine exposure through the entire gestational period and the first ~20 postnatal days (Klausz et al. 2011). Although these studies provide clear evidence of enhanced negative affective behaviors following prenatal morphine in offspring at various ages, several studies have shown opposing effects. For example, morphine exposure from G11–19 resulted in decreased anxiety-like behaviors in juvenile and adolescent Sprague Dawley female rats assessed on the elevated plus maze and open field, but not in males. Juvenile females prenatally exposed to morphine also demonstrated decreased immobility time in the forced swim test, suggestive of reduced depressive-like behaviors; however, adolescent females showed increased immobility time (Chen et al. 2022). Reduced anxiety-like responses and impaired fear extinction resulting from contextual fear conditioning in adult Sprague Dawley offspring were also reported following G9–G18 morphine exposure (Tan et al. 2015). Finally, a short morphine exposure from G15 to G17 also decreased anxiety-like behaviors in adult Wistar male, but not female rat offspring (Nakhjiri et al. 2017). These findings suggest that effects of prenatal exposure to morphine on negative affective behaviors can be quite variable depending on various factors, including timing of exposure, offspring sex and age, and behavioral test. Nevertheless, it is important to note that reductions in anxiety- or depressive-like behaviors relative to controls is also a maladaptive behavioral response that can lead to other behavioral issues.

As previously noted, although MOUDs are an important pharmacotherapeutic option for harm reduction associated with OUD, MOUDs are also agonists at opioid receptors which ultimately have the potential to produce long-term effects in opioid-exposed offspring. Unlike discrepant findings from prenatal morphine exposure, prenatal MOUD exposure more consistently increases negative affective behaviors in a variety of ways, yet somewhat dependent on the MOUD being tested and in a sex-dependent manner. For example, prenatal exposure to buprenorphine or methadone between G3–20, through different routes of administration (intraperitoneal or subcutaneous), consistently increased anxiety- and depressive-like behaviors and reduced social interactions in Sprague Dawley adolescents (Hung et al. 2013; Wu et al. 2014, 2017), young adults (Chen et al. 2015), and older adults (Gamble and Diaz 2023; Gamble et al. 2025). However, using an implanted osmotic mini pump that delivers constant amounts of the substance, from pre-conception through the entire gestational period, buprenorphine exposed male and female Sprague Dawley offspring showed increased anxiety-like behaviors in several tests through adolescence, whereas methadone exposure produced opposing effects in males and females (increase in females and decrease in males) (Nyberg et al. 2024). Collectively, consistent with the clinical literature, these animal studies suggest that despite some of the beneficial effects of MOUD use during pregnancy on the mother and offspring, prenatal MOUD exposure does generally increase the expression of negative affective behaviors in offspring beyond childhood, which may present future complications in exposed offspring as they mature into adulthood.

Given the recent spike in fentanyl use in all demographics, particularly in pregnant people, and now widely recognized detrimental consequences of prenatal fentanyl use in neonates and young children, termed "Fetal Fentanyl Syndrome," animal studies have begun to investigate the potential spectrum of prenatal fentanyl exposure effects. Although several studies have examined various neurobehavioral consequences of prenatal fentanyl exposure in C57BL/6J mice and Sprague Dawley rats (Alipio et al. 2021; Crawford et al. 2023; Olusakin et al. 2023), thus far only two studies have assessed negative affective behaviors in fentanyl-exposed offspring. One study gave pregnant C57BL/6J mice voluntary access to fentanyl in the drinking water through the entire gestational period which continued until offspring were weaned from the mother on P21 (Alipio et al. 2021). Interestingly, adolescent males, but not females, with a history of fentanyl exposure displayed increased anxiety-like behaviors on the elevated plus maze whereas adolescent females, but not their male counterparts, showed a depressive-like phenotype measured by reduced grooming after splashing the mice with a sucrose water solution. The second study used a zebrafish model of developmental fentanyl exposure, whereby zebrafish embryos were exposed to varying concentrations of a fentanyl-containing solution (Wang et al. 2022). Embryonic fentanyl-exposed zebrafish displayed elevated thigmotaxis, a proxy for anxiety-like behavior, and impaired social behaviors. While the findings from these two studies using two very distinct vertebrate species are consistent with the general observations that POE increases the incidence of negative affective behaviors and that these effects may likely be sex-dependent (at least in mammals), there is a clear need for additional studies to fully understand the extent of prenatal fentanyl exposure effects on affective behaviors.

5.4.5 Animal Studies—Neurobiological Alterations

Since the effects of prenatal exposure to various opioids have been investigated in animal models, it is not surprising that numerous neurobiological alterations have been observed in exposed offspring. While neurobiological alterations have been shown in brain areas/neural circuits involved in negative affective behaviors, no studies have causally linked POE-induced neurobiological alterations with anxiety- and depressive-like behaviors. Nonetheless, animal models have been extremely useful for identifying neurobiological targets of POE. As in the previous subsection on behavioral alterations, here we will describe the known neurobiological alterations related to negative affective behaviors induced by prenatal exposure to the specific opioid.

The studies that found prenatal oxycodone exposure-associated increases in various negative affective behaviors also found alterations in a variety of differentially expressed genes (DEGs) throughout the brain. Specifically, Flores and colleagues discovered increased expression of genes involved in synaptic function, mitochondrial function and synaptogenesis in the prefrontal cortex of oxycodone-exposed juvenile Sprague Dawley rat offspring (Flores et al. 2024). Martin and colleagues reported sex-specific changes in opioid receptor genes (*OPRD1 and OPRK1*) in the hippocampus, whereas changes in genes encoding the neuropeptide vasopressin (*AVP*) and DNA methyltransferase (*DNMT3a*), an epigenetic regulator, were detected in the hypothalamus in adult CF1 mice offspring (Martin et al. 2021). While these findings do not fully explain how these brain structures function differently in oxycodone-exposed offspring, they highlight that developmental oxycodone exposure disrupts various mechanisms involved in development and regulation of neural function in brain areas that regulate negative affective behaviors.

Studies examining prenatal exposure to morphine have focused more on alterations in the hippocampus, showing reductions in signaling molecules involved in neurogenesis and neuronal survival processes, in addition to synaptic plasticity. Specifically, G11–G18 morphine exposure in Wistar rats decreased hippocampal levels of BDNF in late adolescents that exhibited increased anxiety-like behaviors (Ahmadalipour et al. 2015), suggesting that molecular regulation of synaptic function and plasticity is impaired in exposed offspring. Interestingly, morphine-exposed adult Sprague Dawley offspring (G9–G18) that showed impaired fear extinction and decreased anxiety-like behavior also had reduced LTP in the CA1 region of the hippocampus (Tan et al. 2015). Impairment in hippocampal LTP is a mechanism underlying deficits in learning processes, in this case emotionally-relevant memory processing. Related, as discussed previously, reduced anxiety-like behavior can be maladaptive, particularly in combination with deficits in fear extinction, and deficits in hippocampal plasticity may, in part, contribute to these behavioral alterations. Although not directly related to negative affective behaviors, several other studies have identified similar alterations in BDNF-related mechanisms, cell survival, synaptic function/plasticity, and opioid receptor expression in the hippocampus of morphine-exposed mouse and rat offspring (Ghafari and Golalipour 2014; Golalipour et al. 2013; Lin et al. 2009; Niu et al. 2009; Sarkaki et al. 2023; Slamberova et al. 2003; Villarreal et al. 2008; Yang et al. 2000, 2003), further supporting the contribution of these various mechanisms and processes to negative affective behaviors among other behavioral deficits. Prenatal morphine-related changes in the prefrontal cortex have also been reported, particularly decreased expression of tyrosine hydroxylase (TH) terminals in adolescent Sprague Dawley female, but not male offspring (Chen et al. 2022), sex-dependent changes in microglial activation in B6D2F1/J mice (decreased in males, but increased in females) (Smith et al. 2022), and enhanced pyramidal neuronal excitability in pre-weanling (P14–18) Lister Hooded rats (Alaee et al. 2023). Microglial changes have also been found in the amygdala of morphine exposed offspring (Smith et al. 2022). While some of these findings were found independent of testing for negative affective behaviors, these alterations are known to be involved in regulating emotion processing, including anxiety- and depressive-like behaviors.

As with the other described opioids, prenatal exposure to MOUDs also disrupts mechanisms involved in neurogenesis and measures of synaptic function and plasticity in offspring that demonstrate negative affective behaviors. These studies have found reductions in neuron numbers, BDNF and its receptor (TrkB receptor), synaptic (SNAP and synaptophysin) and plasticity (CREB, ERK, and PKA) markers, while elevating proinflammatory markers (IL-1β, CD68m and NF-κB) in the prefrontal cortex of buprenorphine-exposed adolescent Sprague Dawley offspring (Hung et al. 2013; Wu et al. 2014, 2017). In the hippocampus of adult Sprague Dawley females, prenatal methadone exposure reduced adult neurogenesis, dentate granule cell excitability, and increased GABA inhibition (Gamble and Diaz 2023; Gamble et al. 2022). Numerous other studies have also reported that prenatal MOUD exposure disrupts these various mechanisms in both the hippocampus (Grecco et al. 2022; Kongstorp et al. 2020; Sahid et al. 2025) and prefrontal cortex (Boggess et al. 2021; Lum et al. 2021) of Sprague Dawley rats and C57BL/6J mice. Finally, elevated glutamate transmission and alterations in gene expression of mu opioid and several dopamine receptors was shown in the basolateral amygdala of adult Sprague Dawley females with prenatal methadone exposure (Gamble et al. 2025). Overall, prenatal MOUD exposure leads to molecular, cellular and functional alterations in brain regions involved in regulating negative affective behaviors.

Finally, although research on prenatal fentanyl exposure is still in its infancy, it has already been discovered that fentanyl-exposed offspring show reductions in expression of genes involved in mitochondrial function within the nucleus accumbens, a brain area involved in emotion and reward processing (Calarco et al. 2021). Several alterations in synaptic activity have also been observed in cortical areas, including the anterior cingulate and somatosensory cortex (Alipio et al. 2021). Finally, in the zebrafish model of developmental fentanyl exposure, exposed zebrafish had increased levels of various neurogenic and neurodevelopmental-associated genes, including *BDFN*, *NPAS4a*, *EGR1*, and *VGF* (Wang et al. 2022).

5.4.6 Prenatal Opioid Exposure Conclusion

Both clinical and preclinical studies have demonstrated clear effects of POE on negative affective behaviors, with the general impact leading to increased deficits in emotion regulation, and anxiety and depressive symptoms. Numerous neurobiological alterations have been observed that collectively indicate that POE disrupts neural development by impairing neuronal survival and function, ultimately leading to central nervous system dysfunction, particularly in brain areas that regulate affective behaviors [see review for more information on neurodevelopment of the opioid system (Spodnick et al. 2025)]. However, the variability in opioid drugs, timing of exposure, and age of assessment complicate a clear understanding of the extent of effects. Additionally, sex as a biological factor must be considered, as some of the observations are sex-specific, but not all. Importantly, animal models are instrumental in foreshadowing the potential long-term effects of POE as the generation of individuals with a history of POE due to the opioid epidemic are only now reaching adulthood.

5.5 Conclusions

In light of the high prevalence of drug use during pregnancy, understanding the spectrum of effects on offspring resulting from prenatal substance exposure is critical. While the incidence of affective disorders, including anxiety and depression, is estimated to be ~20% in the general adult population (Terlizzi and Zablotsky 2024), it is clear that prenatal exposure to substances of misuse, particularly alcohol, nicotine, cannabis/cannabinoids, and opioids, significantly increases the risk of developing an affective disorder throughout the lifespan. Since many pregnancies are unplanned, prenatal substance use is underreported, and mental illness often goes undiagnosed in our society, these rates are likely an underestimate of the true impact of prenatal substance exposure on the prevalence of affective disorders. How prenatal exposure to these substances produces negative affective behaviors is not fully understood, but a review of the existing literature has identified numerous similar and yet unique neurobiological alterations in the hippocampus, prefrontal cortex and amygdala that likely contribute to behavioral alterations—a summary of these neurobiological mechanisms is illustrated in Fig. 5.1. However, it is worth noting that since our understanding of the effects of prenatal substance exposure is still in its infancy, studies examining these brain areas have not been conducted in the context of all of the discussed drugs.

It is also essential to consider the multitude of additional factors that likely exacerbate the effects of prenatal substance exposure, including, but not limited to, genetics (Kaminen-Ahola 2020; Knopik et al. 2019; Smith et al. 2020), environment (Schuetze et al. 2021), stress (de Kloet et al. 2005; Willford and Kaufman 2024), and polydrug use (Garrison et al. 2016; Jansson et al. 2012), all of which can occur pre-conception, throughout pregnancy, and during the postnatal period. Although a thorough discussion regarding these additional factors is beyond the focus of this chapter, it is noteworthy that the mother's prior history (i.e. adversity and mental illness) can interact with drug use during pregnancy leading to epigenetic reprogramming during fetal development which can disrupt the neurodevelopmental trajectory of the offspring throughout the lifespan (Boschen et al. 2018; Oberlander et al. 2008; Palma-Gudiel et al. 2015; Roth et al. 2009). Technological advances, such as RNA-sequencing, will be instrumental in furthering our understanding of genetic and epigenetic mechanisms that may drive alterations in emotion processing, among the myriad of other neurobehavioral consequences of prenatal substance exposure. From the evidence presented, it is clear that while we have an understanding of the general impact of substance use during pregnancy on offspring development, we have only begun to scratch the surface regarding the full spectrum of effects.

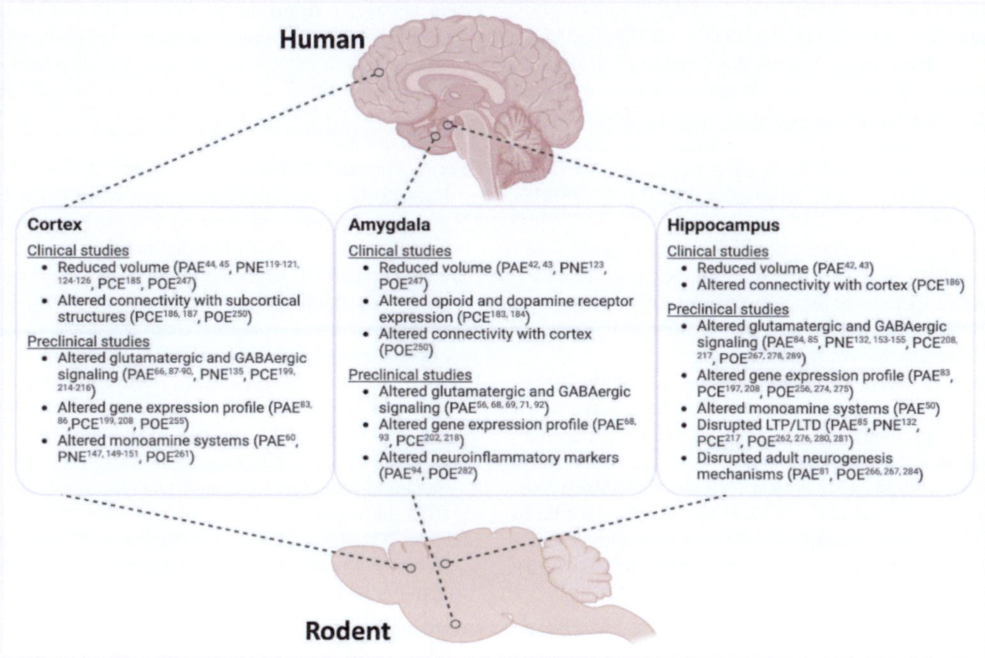

Fig. 5.1 Summary of neurobiological alterations in the hippocampus, prefrontal cortex, and amygdala resulting from prenatal exposures to alcohol, nicotine, cannabinoids, and opioids reported in human clinical and preclinical animal studies. PAE—prenatal alcohol exposure; PNE—prenatal nicotine exposure; PCE—prenatal cannabinoid exposure; POE—prenatal opioid exposure

References

Abdel-Rahman A, Dechkovskaia AM, Sutton JM, Chen WC, Guan X, Khan WA, Abou-Donia MB (2005) Maternal exposure of rats to nicotine via infusion during gestation produces neurobehavioral deficits and elevated expression of glial fibrillary acidic protein in the cerebellum and CA1 subfield in the offspring at puberty. Toxicology 209(3):245–261. https://doi.org/10.1016/j.tox.2004.12.037

Abou-Donia MB, Khan WA, Dechkovskaia AM, Goldstein LB, Bullman SL, Abdel-Rahman A (2006) In utero exposure to nicotine and chlorpyrifos alone, and in combination produces persistent sensorimotor deficits and Purkinje neuron loss in the cerebellum of adult offspring rats. Arch Toxicol 80(9):620–631. https://doi.org/10.1007/s00204-006-0077-1

Acosta G, Rico KT, Madden JT, LaCour A, Wang E, Sanchez LM et al (2024) The effects of moderate prenatal alcohol exposure on performance in hippocampal-sensitive spatial memory and anxiety tasks by adult male and female rat offspring. Alcohol 121:75–86. https://doi.org/10.1016/j.alcohol.2024.08.002

Ahmadalipour A, Rashidy-Pour A (2015) Effects of treadmill running exercise during the adolescent period of life on behavioral deficits in juvenile rats induced by prenatal morphine exposure. Physiol Behav 139:26–33. https://doi.org/10.1016/j.physbeh.2014.10.038

Ahmadalipour A, Sadeghzadeh J, Vafaei AA, Bandegi AR, Mohammadkhani R, Rashidy-Pour A (2015) Effects of environmental enrichment on behavioral deficits and alterations in hippocampal BDNF induced by prenatal exposure to morphine in juvenile rats. Neuroscience 305:372–383. https://doi.org/10.1016/j.neuroscience.2015.08.015

Ainiti DF, Lykeridou A, Nanou C, Deltsidou A (2023) Cannabis use during pregnancy and its effect on the fetus, newborn and later childhood: a systematic review. Eur J Midwifery 7:19. https://doi.org/10.18332/ejm/168727

Alaee E, Pachenari N, Khani F, Semnanian S, Shojaei A, Azizi H (2023) Enhancement of neuronal excitability in the medial prefrontal cortex following prenatal morphine exposure. Brain Res Bull 204:110803. https://doi.org/10.1016/j.brainresbull.2023.110803

Alipio JB, Haga C, Fox ME, Arakawa K, Balaji R, Cramer N et al (2021) Perinatal fentanyl exposure leads to long-lasting impairments in somatosensory circuit function and behavior. J Neurosci 41(15):3400–3417. https://doi.org/10.1523/JNEUROSCI.2470-20.2020

Alkam T, Mamiya T, Kimura N, Yoshida A, Kihara D, Tsunoda Y et al (2017) Prenatal nicotine exposure decreases the release of dopamine in the medial frontal cortex and induces atomoxetine-responsive neurobehavioral deficits in mice. Psychopharmacology 234(12):1853–1869. https://doi.org/10.1007/s00213-017-4591-z

Almeida L, Andreu-Fernandez V, Navarro-Tapia E, Aras-Lopez R, Serra-Delgado M, Martinez L et al (2020) Murine models for the study of Fetal Alcohol Spectrum disorders: an overview. Front Pediatr 8:359. https://doi.org/10.3389/fped.2020.00359

Andrade C (2024) Maternal cannabis use during pregnancy and maternal and neonatal adverse outcomes. J Clin Psychiatry 85(4). https://doi.org/10.4088/JCP.24f15611

Andre QR, McMorris CA, Kar P, Ritter C, Gibbard WB, Tortorelli C, Lebel C (2020) Different brain profiles in children with prenatal alcohol exposure with or without early adverse exposures. Hum Brain Mapp 41(15): 4375–4385. https://doi.org/10.1002/hbm.25130

Antonelli T, Tomasini MC, Tattoli M, Cassano T, Tanganelli S, Finetti S et al (2005) Prenatal exposure to the CB1 receptor agonist WIN 55,212-2 causes learning disruption associated with impaired cortical NMDA receptor function and emotional reactivity changes in rat offspring. Cereb Cortex 15(12): 2013–2020. https://doi.org/10.1093/cercor/bhi076

Aslaksen AK, Bjuland KJ, Hoem ML, Horgen G, Haugen OH, Skranes J, Aukland SM (2025) Children had smaller brain volumes and cortical surface areas after prenatal opioid maintenance therapy exposure. Acta Paediatr 114(2):398–409. https://doi.org/10.1111/apa.17448

Azeem A, Lobel M, Heiselman C, Preis H (2024) Using the PROMOTE screener to identify psychosocial risk factors for prenatal substance use. J Addict Med. https://doi.org/10.1097/ADM.0000000000001427

Baculis BC, Diaz MR, Valenzuela CF (2015) Third trimester-equivalent ethanol exposure increases anxiety-like behavior and glutamatergic transmission in the basolateral amygdala. Pharmacol Biochem Behav 137:78–85. https://doi.org/10.1016/j.pbb.2015.08.009

Bakhireva LN, Holbrook BD, Shrestha S, Leyva Y, Ashley M, Cano S et al (2019) Association between prenatal opioid exposure, neonatal opioid withdrawal syndrome, and neurodevelopmental and behavioral outcomes at 5-8 months of age. Early Hum Dev 128: 69–76. https://doi.org/10.1016/j.earlhumdev.2018.10.010

Baldacchino A, Balfour DJ, Passetti F, Humphris G, Matthews K (2012) Neuropsychological consequences of chronic opioid use: a quantitative review and meta-analysis. Neurosci Biobehav Rev 36(9):2056–2068. https://doi.org/10.1016/j.neubiorev.2012.06.006

Baldacchino A, Arbuckle K, Petrie DJ, McCowan C (2014) Neurobehavioral consequences of chronic intrauterine opioid exposure in infants and preschool children: a systematic review and meta-analysis. BMC Psychiatry 14:104. https://doi.org/10.1186/1471-244X-14-104

Bara A, Manduca A, Bernabeu A, Borsoi M, Serviado M, Lassalle O et al (2018) Sex-dependent effects of in utero cannabinoid exposure on cortical function. elife 7. https://doi.org/10.7554/eLife.36234

Bara A, Ferland JN, Rompala G, Szutorisz H, Hurd YL (2021) Cannabis and synaptic reprogramming of the developing brain. Nat Rev Neurosci 22(7):423–438. https://doi.org/10.1038/s41583-021-00465-5

Bassalov H, Yakirevich-Amir N, Reuveni I, Monk C, Florentin S, Bonne O, Matok I (2024) Prenatal cannabis exposure and the risk for neuropsychiatric anomalies in the offspring: a systematic review and meta-analysis. Am J Obstet Gynecol 231(6):574–588 e578. https://doi.org/10.1016/j.ajog.2024.06.014

Bateman BT, Hernandez-Diaz S, Rathmell JP, Seeger JD, Doherty M, Fischer MA, Huybrechts KF (2014) Patterns of opioid utilization in pregnancy in a large cohort of commercial insurance beneficiaries in the United States. Anesthesiology 120(5):1216–1224. https://doi.org/10.1097/ALN.0000000000000172

Beauchamp, K. G., Lowe, J., Schrader, R. M., Shrestha, S., Aragon, C., Moss, N., ... Bakhireva, L. N. (2020). Self-regulation and emotional reactivity in infants with prenatal exposure to opioids and alcohol. Early Hum Dev, 148, 105119. doi:https://doi.org/10.1016/j.earlhumdev.2020.105119

Behnke M, Eyler FD (1993) The consequences of prenatal substance use for the developing fetus, newborn, and young child. Int J Addict 28(13):1341–1391. https://doi.org/10.3109/10826089309062191

Berrendero F, Sepe N, Ramos JA, Di Marzo V, Fernandez-Ruiz JJ (1999) Analysis of cannabinoid receptor binding and mRNA expression and endogenous cannabinoid contents in the developing rat brain during late gestation and early postnatal period. Synapse 33(3): 181–191. https://doi.org/10.1002/(SICI)1098-2396(19990901)33:3<181::AID-SYN3>3.0.CO;2-R

Bjorkquist OA, Fryer SL, Reiss AL, Mattson SN, Riley EP (2010) Cingulate gyrus morphology in children and adolescents with fetal alcohol spectrum disorders. Psychiatry Res 181(2):101–107. https://doi.org/10.1016/j.pscychresns.2009.10.004

Blackard C, Tennes K (1984) Human placental transfer of cannabinoids. N Engl J Med 311(12):797. https://doi.org/10.1056/NEJM198409203111213

Blebea NM, Pricopie AI, Vlad RA, Hancu G (2024) Phytocannabinoids: exploring pharmacological profiles and their impact on therapeutical use. Int J Mol Sci 25(8). https://doi.org/10.3390/ijms25084204

Blood-Siegfried J, Rende EK (2010) The long-term effects of prenatal nicotine exposure on neurologic development. J Midwifery Womens Health 55(2):143–152. https://doi.org/10.1016/j.jmwh.2009.05.006

Boggess T, Williamson JC, Niebergall EB, Sexton H, Mazur A, Egleton RD et al (2021) Alterations in excitatory and inhibitory synaptic development within the mesolimbic dopamine pathway in a mouse model of prenatal drug exposure. Front Pediatr 9:794544. https://doi.org/10.3389/fped.2021.794544

Boschen KE, Keller SM, Roth TL, Klintsova AY (2018) Epigenetic mechanisms in alcohol- and adversity-induced developmental origins of neurobehavioral functioning. Neurotoxicol Teratol 66:63–79. https://doi.org/10.1016/j.ntt.2017.12.009

Breit KR, Rodriguez CG, Lei A, Hussain S, Thomas JD (2022) Effects of prenatal alcohol and delta-9-tetrahydrocannabinol exposure via electronic cigarettes on motor development. Alcohol Clin Exp Res 46(8): 1408–1422. https://doi.org/10.1111/acer.14892

Brocardo PS, Boehme F, Patten A, Cox A, Gil-Mohapel J, Christie BR (2012) Anxiety- and depression-like behaviors are accompanied by an increase in oxidative stress in a rat model of fetal alcohol spectrum disorders: protective effects of voluntary physical exercise. Neuropharmacology 62(4):1607–1618. https://doi.org/10.1016/j.neuropharm.2011.10.006

Brolese G, Lunardi P, Broetto N, Engelke DS, Lirio F, Batassini C et al (2014) Moderate prenatal alcohol exposure alters behavior and neuroglial parameters in adolescent rats. Behav Brain Res 269:175–184. https://doi.org/10.1016/j.bbr.2014.04.023

Brown QL, Sarvet AL, Shmulewitz D, Martins SS, Wall MM, Hasin DS (2017) Trends in marijuana use among pregnant and nonpregnant reproductive-aged women, 2002–2014. JAMA 317(2):207–209. https://doi.org/10.1001/jama.2016.17383

Burgess DJ, Moritz KM (2020) Prenatal alcohol exposure and developmental programming of mental illness. J Dev Orig Health Dis 11(3):211–221. https://doi.org/10.1017/S2040174420000082

Byrnes EM, Vassoler FM (2018) Modeling prenatal opioid exposure in animals: current findings and future directions. Front Neuroendocrinol 51:1–13. https://doi.org/10.1016/j.yfrne.2017.09.001

Calarco CA, Fox ME, Van Terheyden S, Turner MD, Alipio JB, Chandra R, Lobo MK (2021) Mitochondria-related nuclear gene expression in the nucleus accumbens and blood mitochondrial copy number after developmental fentanyl exposure in adolescent male and female C57BL/6 mice. Front Psych 12:737389. https://doi.org/10.3389/fpsyt.2021.737389

Caldwell KK, Sheema S, Paz RD, Samudio-Ruiz SL, Laughlin MH, Spence NE et al (2008) Fetal alcohol spectrum disorder-associated depression: evidence for reductions in the levels of brain-derived neurotrophic factor in a mouse model. Pharmacol Biochem Behav 90(4):614–624. https://doi.org/10.1016/j.pbb.2008.05.004

Caritis SN, Panigrahy A (2019) Opioids affect the fetal brain: reframing the detoxification debate. Am J Obstet Gynecol. https://doi.org/10.1016/j.ajog.2019.07.022

Carneiro LM, Diogenes JP, Vasconcelos SM, Aragao GF, Noronha EC, Gomes PB, Viana GS (2005) Behavioral and neurochemical effects on rat offspring after prenatal exposure to ethanol. Neurotoxicol Teratol 27(4): 585–592. https://doi.org/10.1016/j.ntt.2005.06.006

Castaldo P, Magi S, Gaetani S, Cassano T, Ferraro L, Antonelli T et al (2007) Prenatal exposure to the cannabinoid receptor agonist WIN 55,212-2 increases glutamate uptake through overexpression of GLT1 and EAAC1 glutamate transporter subtypes in rat frontal cerebral cortex. Neuropharmacology 53(3):369–378. https://doi.org/10.1016/j.neuropharm.2007.05.019

Castelli V, Lavanco G, Feo S, D'Amico C, Micale V, Kuchar M et al (2023) Prenatal exposure to Delta9-tetrahydrocannabinol affects hippocampus-related cognitive functions in the adolescent rat offspring: focus on specific markers of neuroplasticity. Pharmaceutics 15(2). https://doi.org/10.3390/pharmaceutics15020692

Chandra S, Radwan MM, Majumdar CG, Church JC, Freeman TP, ElSohly MA (2019) New trends in cannabis potency in USA and Europe during the last decade (2008-2017). Eur Arch Psychiatry Clin Neurosci 269(1):5–15. https://doi.org/10.1007/s00406-019-00983-5

Chang G (2020) Maternal substance use: consequences, identification, and interventions. Alcohol Res 40(2):06. https://doi.org/10.35946/arcr.v40.2.06

Chen HH, Chiang YC, Yuan ZF, Kuo CC, Lai MD, Hung TW et al (2015) Buprenorphine, methadone, and morphine treatment during pregnancy: behavioral effects on the offspring in rats. Neuropsychiatr Dis Treat 11: 609–618. https://doi.org/10.2147/NDT.S70585

Chen Y, Du M, Kang N, Guan X, Liang B, Chen Z, Zhang J (2022) Prenatal morphine exposure differentially alters addictive and emotional behavior in adolescent and adult rats in a sex-specific manner. Neurochem Res 47(8):2317–2332. https://doi.org/10.1007/s11064-022-03619-8

Cnattingius S (2004) The epidemiology of smoking during pregnancy: smoking prevalence, maternal characteristics, and pregnancy outcomes. Nicotine Tob Res 6(Suppl 2):S125–S140. https://doi.org/10.1080/14622200410001669187

Coe CL, Lubach GR, Crispen HR, Shirtcliff EA, Schneider ML (2010) Challenges to maternal wellbeing during pregnancy impact temperament, attention, and neuromotor responses in the infant rhesus monkey. Dev Psychobiol 52(7):625–637. https://doi.org/10.1002/dev.20489

Coles CD, Grant TM, Kable JA, Stoner SA, Perez A, Collaborative Initiative on Fetal Alcohol Spectrum, D (2022) Prenatal alcohol exposure and mental health at midlife: a preliminary report on two longitudinal cohorts. Alcohol Clin Exp Res 46(2):232–242. https://doi.org/10.1111/acer.14761

Compagno MK, Silver CR, Cox-Holmes A, Basso KB, Bishop C, Bernstein AM et al (2025) Maternal ingestion of cannabidiol (CBD) in mice leads to sex-dependent changes in memory, anxiety, and metabolism in the adult offspring, and causes a decrease in survival to weaning age. Pharmacol Biochem Behav 247:173902. https://doi.org/10.1016/j.pbb.2024.173902

Cornelius MD, Leech SL, Goldschmidt L, Day NL (2000) Prenatal tobacco exposure: is it a risk factor for early tobacco experimentation? Nicotine Tob Res 2(1): 45–52. https://doi.org/10.1080/14622200050011295

Cornelius MD, Goldschmidt L, Day NL (2012) Prenatal cigarette smoking: long-term effects on young adult behavior problems and smoking behavior. Neurotoxicol Teratol 34(6):554–559. https://doi.org/10.1016/j.ntt.2012.09.003

Crawford CA, Taylor JA, Park GI, Rios JW, Bunch J, Greenwood CJ et al (2023) Effects of neonatal fentanyl on late adolescent opioid-mediated behavior. Front Neurosci 17:1094241. https://doi.org/10.3389/fnins.2023.1094241

Cross SJ, Linker KE, Leslie FM (2017) Sex-dependent effects of nicotine on the developing brain. J Neurosci Res 95(1–2):422–436. https://doi.org/10.1002/jnr.23878

Cullen CL, Burne TH, Lavidis NA, Moritz KM (2013) Low dose prenatal ethanol exposure induces anxiety-like behaviour and alters dendritic morphology in the basolateral amygdala of rat offspring. PLoS One 8(1): e54924. https://doi.org/10.1371/journal.pone.0054924

Cupo L, Dominguez-Cancino KA, Nazif-Munoz JI, Chakravarty MM (2024) Prenatal cannabis exposure in the clinic and laboratory: what do we know and where do we need to go? Drug Alcohol Depend Rep 13:100282. https://doi.org/10.1016/j.dadr.2024.100282

Cuzon VC, Yeh PW, Yanagawa Y, Obata K, Yeh HH (2008) Ethanol consumption during early pregnancy alters the disposition of tangentially migrating GABAergic interneurons in the fetal cortex. J Neurosci 28(8):1854–1864. https://doi.org/10.1523/JNEUROSCI.5110-07.2008

Damborsky JC, Griffith WH, Winzer-Serhan UH (2015) Neonatal nicotine exposure increases excitatory synaptic transmission and attenuates nicotine-stimulated GABA release in the adult rat hippocampus. Neuropharmacology 88:187–198. https://doi.org/10.1016/j.neuropharm.2014.06.010

Dandekar MP, Bharne AP, Borkar PD, Subhedar NK, Kokare DM (2019) Maternal ethanol exposure reshapes CART system in the rat brain: correlation with development of anxiety, depression and memory deficits. Neuroscience 406:126–139. https://doi.org/10.1016/j.neuroscience.2019.02.010

Day NL, Leech SL, Goldschmidt L (2011) The effects of prenatal marijuana exposure on delinquent behaviors are mediated by measures of neurocognitive functioning. Neurotoxicol Teratol 33(1):129–136. https://doi.org/10.1016/j.ntt.2010.07.006

de Cubas MM, Field T (1993) Children of methadone-dependent women: developmental outcomes. Am J Orthopsychiatry 63(2):266–276

de Kloet ER, Sibug RM, Helmerhorst FM, Schmidt MV (2005) Stress, genes and the mechanism of programming the brain for later life. Neurosci Biobehav Rev 29(2):271–281. https://doi.org/10.1016/j.neubiorev.2004.10.008

de Salas-Quiroga A, Diaz-Alonso J, Garcia-Rincon D, Remmers F, Vega D, Gomez-Canas M et al (2015) Prenatal exposure to cannabinoids evokes long-lasting functional alterations by targeting CB1 receptors on developing cortical neurons. Proc Natl Acad Sci USA 112(44):13693–13698. https://doi.org/10.1073/pnas.1514962112

Deng L, Wang Q, Lou Y (2023) Maternal nicotine intoxication before pregnancy induces depressive- and anxiety-like behaviors as well as cognitive deficits in male offspring and correlates with neurobiological changes. Brain Behav 13(7):e3052. https://doi.org/10.1002/brb3.3052

Desai RJ, Hernandez-Diaz S, Bateman BT, Huybrechts KF (2014) Increase in prescription opioid use during pregnancy among Medicaid-enrolled women. Obstet Gynecol 123(5):997–1002. https://doi.org/10.1097/AOG.0000000000000208

DeVuono MV, Nashed MG, Sarikahya MH, Kocsis A, Lee K, Vanin SR et al (2024) Prenatal tetrahydrocannabinol and cannabidiol exposure produce sex-specific pathophysiological phenotypes in the adolescent prefrontal cortex and hippocampus. Neurobiol Dis 199: 106588. https://doi.org/10.1016/j.nbd.2024.106588

Diaz MR, Jotty K, Locke JL, Jones SR, Valenzuela CF (2014) Moderate Alcohol exposure during the rat equivalent to the third trimester of human pregnancy alters regulation of GABAA receptor-mediated synaptic transmission by dopamine in the basolateral amygdala. Front Pediatr 2:46. https://doi.org/10.3389/fped.2014.00046

Diaz MR, Mooney SM, Varlinskaya EI (2016) Acute prenatal exposure to ethanol on gestational day 12 elicits opposing deficits in social behaviors and anxiety-like behaviors in Sprague Dawley rats. Behav Brain Res 310:11–19. https://doi.org/10.1016/j.bbr.2016.05.003

Dickson B, Mansfield C, Guiahi M, Allshouse AA, Borgelt LM, Sheeder J et al (2018) Recommendations from cannabis dispensaries about first-trimester cannabis use. Obstet Gynecol 131(6):1031–1038. https://doi.org/10.1097/AOG.0000000000002619

Donald KA, Fouche JP, Roos A, Koen N, Howells FM, Riley EP et al (2016) Alcohol exposure in utero is associated with decreased gray matter volume in neonates. Metab Brain Dis 31(1):81–91. https://doi.org/10.1007/s11011-015-9771-0

Downer EJ, Gowran A, Campbell VA (2007) A comparison of the apoptotic effect of Delta(9)-tetrahydrocannabinol in the neonatal and adult rat cerebral cortex. Brain Res 1175:39–47. https://doi.org/10.1016/j.brainres.2007.07.076

Duko B, Pereira G, Betts K, Tait RJ, Newnham J, Alati R (2021) Prenatal alcohol and tobacco use and the risk of depression in offspring at age of 17 years: findings from the Raine study. J Affect Disord 279:426–433. https://doi.org/10.1016/j.jad.2020.10.030

Duko B, Pereira G, Tait RJ, Betts K, Newnham J, Alati R (2022) Prenatal tobacco and alcohol exposures and the risk of anxiety symptoms in young adulthood: a population-based cohort study. Psychiatry Res 310: 114466. https://doi.org/10.1016/j.psychres.2022.114466

Dursun I, Jakubowska-Dogru E, Uzbay T (2006) Effects of prenatal exposure to alcohol on activity, anxiety, motor coordination, and memory in young adult Wistar rats. Pharmacol Biochem Behav 85(2):345–355. https://doi.org/10.1016/j.pbb.2006.09.001

Dwyer JB, Broide RS, Leslie FM (2008) Nicotine and brain development. Birth Defects Res C Embryo Today 84(1):30–44. https://doi.org/10.1002/bdrc.20118

Dwyer JB, McQuown SC, Leslie FM (2009) The dynamic effects of nicotine on the developing brain. Pharmacol Ther 122(2):125–139. https://doi.org/10.1016/j.pharmthera.2009.02.003

Dwyer JB, Cardenas A, Franke RM, Chen Y, Bai Y, Belluzzi JD et al (2019) Prenatal nicotine sex-dependently alters adolescent dopamine system development. Transl Psychiatry 9(1):304. https://doi.org/10.1038/s41398-019-0640-1

Dylag KA, Wieczorek-Stawinska W, Cichon-Chojnacka-A, Piaskowska A, Jaroszewska K, Wasiak K et al (2024) Anxiety and depression and sleep problems among patients with Fetal Alcohol Spectrum disorders. Children (Basel) 12(1). https://doi.org/10.3390/children12010001

Easey KE, Dyer ML, Timpson NJ, Munafo MR (2019) Prenatal alcohol exposure and offspring mental health: a systematic review. Drug Alcohol Depend 197:344–353. https://doi.org/10.1016/j.drugalcdep.2019.01.007

Ekblad M, Korkeila J, Parkkola R, Lapinleimu H, Haataja L, Lehtonen L, Group, P. S (2010) Maternal smoking during pregnancy and regional brain volumes in preterm infants. J Pediatr 156(2):185–190 e181. https://doi.org/10.1016/j.jpeds.2009.07.061

Ekblad MO, Ngum P, Merisaari H, Saunavaara V, Parkkola R, Setanen S (2022) Maternal smoking during pregnancy negatively affects brain volumes proportional to intracranial volume in adolescents born very preterm. Front Hum Neurosci 16:1085986. https://doi.org/10.3389/fnhum.2022.1085986

El Marroun H, Tiemeier H, Jaddoe VW, Hofman A, Mackenbach JP, Steegers EA et al (2008) Demographic, emotional and social determinants of cannabis use in early pregnancy: the Generation R study. Drug Alcohol Depend 98(3):218–226. https://doi.org/10.1016/j.drugalcdep.2008.05.010

El Marroun H, Schmidt MN, Franken IH, Jaddoe VW, Hofman A, van der Lugt A et al (2014) Prenatal tobacco exposure and brain morphology: a prospective study in young children. Neuropsychopharmacology 39(4):792–800. https://doi.org/10.1038/npp.2013.273

El Marroun H, Tiemeier H, Franken IH, Jaddoe VW, van der Lugt A, Verhulst FC et al (2016) Prenatal cannabis and tobacco exposure in relation to brain morphology: a prospective neuroimaging study in Young children. Biol Psychiatry 79(12):971–979. https://doi.org/10.1016/j.biopsych.2015.08.024

Elibol-Can B, Dursun I, Telkes I, Kilic E, Canan S, Jakubowska-Dogru E (2014) Examination of age-dependent effects of fetal ethanol exposure on behavior, hippocampal cell counts, and doublecortin immunoreactivity in rats. Dev Neurobiol 74(5): 498–513. https://doi.org/10.1002/dneu.22143

Ellis RJ, Bara A, Vargas CA, Frick AL, Loh E, Landry J et al (2022) Prenatal Delta(9)-tetrahydrocannabinol exposure in males leads to motivational disturbances related to striatal epigenetic dysregulation. Biol Psychiatry 92(2):127–138. https://doi.org/10.1016/j.biopsych.2021.09.017

England LJ, Bennett C, Denny CH, Honein MA, Gilboa SM, Kim SY et al (2020) Alcohol use and co-use of other substances among pregnant females aged 12-44 years – United States, 2015-2018. MMWR Morb Mortal Wkly Rep 69(31):1009–1014. https://doi.org/10.15585/mmwr.mm6931a1

Eppolito AK, Bachus SE, McDonald CG, Meador-Woodruff JH, Smith RF (2010) Late emerging effects of prenatal and early postnatal nicotine exposure on the cholinergic system and anxiety-like behavior. Neurotoxicol Teratol 32(3):336–345. https://doi.org/10.1016/j.ntt.2009.12.009

Eriksen JL, Gillespie RA, Druse MJ (2000) Effects of in utero ethanol exposure and maternal treatment with a 5-HT(1A) agonist on S100B-containing glial cells. Brain Res Dev Brain Res 121(2):133–143. https://doi.org/10.1016/s0165-3806(00)00029-8

Evanski JM, Zundel CG, Baglot SL, Desai S, Gowatch LC, Ely SL et al (2024) The first "hit" to the endocannabinoid system? Associations between prenatal cannabis exposure and Frontolimbic White matter pathways in children. Biol Psychiatry Glob Open Sci 4(1):11–18. https://doi.org/10.1016/j.bpsgos.2023.09.005

Famy C, Streissguth AP, Unis AS (1998) Mental illness in adults with fetal alcohol syndrome or fetal alcohol effects. Am J Psychiatry 155(4):552–554. https://doi.org/10.1176/ajp.155.4.552

Farid WO, Dunlop SA, Tait RJ, Hulse GK (2008) The effects of maternally administered methadone, buprenorphine and naltrexone on offspring: review of human and animal data. Curr Neuropharmacol 6(2): 125–150. https://doi.org/10.2174/157015908784533842

Ferrante JR, Blendy JA (2024) Advances in animal models of prenatal opioid exposure. Trends Neurosci 47(5): 367–382. https://doi.org/10.1016/j.tins.2024.03.005

Flores A, Nguyen NM, Devanaboyina M, Sanketh S, Athota P, Jagadesan S et al (2024) Neurobehavioral characterization of perinatal oxycodone-exposed offspring in early adolescence. J Neuroimmune Pharmacol 19(1):29. https://doi.org/10.1007/s11481-024-10129-7

Fontaine CJ, Pinar C, Yang W, Pang AF, Suesser KE, Choi JSJ, Christie BR (2019) Impaired bidirectional synaptic plasticity in juvenile offspring following prenatal ethanol exposure. Alcohol Clin Exp Res 43(10): 2153–2166. https://doi.org/10.1111/acer.14170

Frau R, Miczan V, Traccis F, Aroni S, Pongor CI, Saba P et al (2019) Prenatal THC exposure produces a hyperdopaminergic phenotype rescued by pregnenolone. Nat Neurosci 22(12):1975–1985. https://doi.org/10.1038/s41593-019-0512-2

Fried PA, Watkinson B (1988) 12- and 24-month neurobehavioural follow-up of children prenatally exposed to marihuana, cigarettes and alcohol. Neurotoxicol Teratol 10(4):305–313. https://doi.org/10.1016/0892-0362(88)90032-3

Gamble ME, Diaz MR (2023) Prenatal methadone exposure leads to disruptions in adult-born dentate granule cell survival and female persistent fear responding. Addict Neurosci 8:100120. https://doi.org/10.1016/j.addicn.2023.100120

Gamble ME, Marfatia R, Diaz MR (2022) Prenatal methadone exposure leads to long-term memory impairments and disruptions of dentate granule cell function in a sex-dependent manner. Addict Biol 27(5). https://doi.org/10.1111/adb.13215

Gamble ME, Montero M, Silberstein DN, Deak T, Varlinskaya EI, Diaz MR (2025) Prenatal methadone exposure produces functional and molecular alterations in the basolateral amygdala and decreased voluntary ethanol intake in female, but not male offspring. Front Behav Neurosci 19:1570951. https://doi.org/10.3389/fnbeh.2025.1570951

Garrison L, Leeman L, Savich RD, Gutierrez H, Rayburn WF, Bakhireva LN (2016) Fetal growth outcomes in a cohort of Polydrug- and opioid-dependent patients. J Reprod Med 61(7–8):311–319

Ghafari S, Golalipour MJ (2014) Prenatal morphine exposure reduces pyramidal neurons in CA1, CA2 and CA3 subfields of mice hippocampus. Iran J Basic Med Sci 17(3):155–161

Golalipour MJ, Ghafari S, Kafshgiri SK, Moghadam MH, Moharri AR (2013) Effect of maternal morphine sulfate exposure on neuronal plasticity of dentate gyrus in Balb/c mice offspring. Pak J Biol Sci 16(6):281–286. https://doi.org/10.3923/pjbs.2013.281.286

Gomez-Ruiz LM, Marchei E, Rotolo MC, Brunetti P, Mannocchi G, Acosta-Lopez A et al (2022) Prevalence of licit and illicit drugs use during pregnancy in Mexican women. Pharmaceuticals (Basel) 15(3). https://doi.org/10.3390/ph15030382

Grant KS, Conover E, Chambers CD (2020) Update on the developmental consequences of cannabis use during pregnancy and lactation. Birth Defects Res 112(15): 1126–1138. https://doi.org/10.1002/bdr2.1766

Gray KA, Day NL, Leech S, Richardson GA (2005) Prenatal marijuana exposure: effect on child depressive symptoms at ten years of age. Neurotoxicol Teratol 27(3):439–448. https://doi.org/10.1016/j.ntt.2005.03.010

Grecco GG, Atwood BK (2020) Prenatal opioid exposure enhances responsiveness to future drug reward and alters sensitivity to pain: a review of preclinical models and contributing mechanisms. eNeuro 7(6). https://doi.org/10.1523/ENEURO.0393-20.2020

Grecco GG, Shahid SS, Atwood BK, Wu YC (2022) Alterations of brain microstructures in a mouse model of prenatal opioid exposure detected by diffusion MRI. Sci Rep 12(1):17085. https://doi.org/10.1038/s41598-022-21416-9

Gunn RL, Aston ER, Artis L, Nesi J, Pedersen ER, Micalizzi L (2024) Use of cannabis to manage symptoms of mental and physical health conditions during pregnancy: analysis of a pro-cannabis pregnancy forum. Front Psych 15:1478505. https://doi.org/10.3389/fpsyt.2024.1478505

Haghighi A, Schwartz DH, Abrahamowicz M, Leonard GT, Perron M, Richer L et al (2013) Prenatal exposure to maternal cigarette smoking, amygdala volume, and fat intake in adolescence. JAMA Psychiatry 70(1): 98–105. https://doi.org/10.1001/archgenpsychiatry.2012.1101

Haight SC, Ko JY, Tong VT, Bohm MK, Callaghan WM (2018) Opioid use disorder documented at delivery hospitalization – United States, 1999–2014. MMWR Morb Mortal Wkly Rep 67(31):845–849. https://doi.org/10.15585/mmwr.mm6731a1

Haley DW, Handmaker NS, Lowe J (2006) Infant stress reactivity and prenatal alcohol exposure. Alcohol Clin Exp Res 30(12):2055–2064. https://doi.org/10.1111/j.1530-0277.2006.00251.x

Hall ES, McAllister JM, Wexelblatt SL (2019) Developmental disorders and medical complications among infants with subclinical intrauterine opioid exposures. Popul Health Manag 22(1):19–24. https://doi.org/10.1089/pop.2018.0016

Han B, Compton WM, Einstein EB, Elder E, Volkow ND (2024) Pregnancy and postpartum drug overdose deaths in the US before and during the COVID-19 pandemic. JAMA Psychiatry 81(3):270–283. https://doi.org/10.1001/jamapsychiatry.2023.4523

Harder HJ, Murphy AZ (2019) Early life opioid exposure and potential long-term effects. Neurobiol Stress 10: 100156. https://doi.org/10.1016/j.ynstr.2019.100156

Hartwell M, Bloom M, Elenwo C, Gooch T, Dunn K, Breslin F, Croff JM (2024) Association of prenatal substance exposure and the development of the amygdala, hippocampus, and parahippocampus. J Osteopath Med 124(11):499–508. https://doi.org/10.1515/jom-2023-0277

Health NSoDUa (2022) National Survey on Drug Use and Health—detailed tables; Table 8.27B, types of illicit drug, tobacco product, and alcohol use in past month: among females aged 15 to 44; by pregnancy status. Substance Abuse and Mental Health Services Administration

Hellemans KG, Verma P, Yoon E, Yu W, Weinberg J (2008) Prenatal alcohol exposure increases vulnerability to stress and anxiety-like disorders in adulthood. Ann N Y Acad Sci 1144:154–175. https://doi.org/10.1196/annals.1418.016

Hellemans KG, Sliwowska JH, Verma P, Weinberg J (2010) Prenatal alcohol exposure: fetal programming and later life vulnerability to stress, depression and anxiety disorders. Neurosci Biobehav Rev 34(6): 791–807. https://doi.org/10.1016/j.neubiorev.2009.06.004

Heller M, Burd L (2014) Review of ethanol dispersion, distribution, and elimination from the fetal compartment. Birth Defects Res A Clin Mol Teratol 100(4): 277–283. https://doi.org/10.1002/bdra.23232

Hirai AH, Ko JY, Owens PL, Stocks C, Patrick SW (2021) Neonatal abstinence syndrome and maternal opioid-related diagnoses in the US, 2010–2017. JAMA 325(2):146–155. https://doi.org/10.1001/jama.2020.24991

Hung CJ, Wu CC, Chen WY, Chang CY, Kuan YH, Pan HC et al (2013) Depression-like effect of prenatal buprenorphine exposure in rats. PLoS One 8(12): e82262. https://doi.org/10.1371/journal.pone.0082262

Jaekel J, Kim HM, Lee SJ, Schwartz A, Henderson JMT, Woodward LJ (2021) Emotional and behavioral trajectories of 2 to 9 years old children born to opioid-dependent mothers. Res Child Adolesc Psychopathol 49(4):443–457. https://doi.org/10.1007/s10802-020-00766-w

Jansson LM, Di Pietro JA, Elko A, Williams EL, Milio L, Velez M (2012) Pregnancies exposed to methadone, methadone and other illicit substances, and poly-drugs without methadone: a comparison of fetal neurobehaviors and infant outcomes. Drug Alcohol Depend 122(3):213–219. https://doi.org/10.1016/j.drugalcdep.2011.10.003

Kaminen-Ahola N (2020) Fetal alcohol spectrum disorders: genetic and epigenetic mechanisms. Prenat Diagn 40(9):1185–1192. https://doi.org/10.1002/pd.5731

Kane VB, Fu Y, Matta SG, Sharp BM (2004) Gestational nicotine exposure attenuates nicotine-stimulated dopamine release in the nucleus accumbens shell of adolescent Lewis rats. J Pharmacol Exp Ther 308(2): 521–528. https://doi.org/10.1124/jpet.103.059899

Karatayev O, Collier AD, Targoff SR, Leibowitz SF (2024) Neurological disorders induced by drug use: effects of adolescent and embryonic drug exposure on behavioral neurodevelopment. Int J Mol Sci 25(15). https://doi.org/10.3390/ijms25158341

Keating O, Brown RH, Kuenssberg R, Driscoll S, McDougall S, O'Rourke S (2024) The international prevalence of prenatal alcohol use obtained via meconium biomarkers: a systematic literature review. Alcohol Clin Exp Res (Hoboken) 48(9):1657–1676. https://doi.org/10.1111/acer.15410

Kelly SJ, Day N, Streissguth AP (2000) Effects of prenatal alcohol exposure on social behavior in humans and other species. Neurotoxicol Teratol 22(2):143–149. https://doi.org/10.1016/s0892-0362(99)00073-2

Kim EK, Lee MH, Kim H, Sim YJ, Shin MS, Lee SJ et al (2005) Maternal ethanol administration inhibits 5-hydroxytryptamine synthesis and tryptophan hydroxylase expression in the dorsal raphe of rat offspring. Brain Dev 27(7):472–476. https://doi.org/10.1016/j.braindev.2004.11.008

Klausz B, Pinter O, Sobor M, Gyarmati Z, Furst Z, Timar J, Zelena D (2011) Changes in adaptability following perinatal morphine exposure in juvenile and adult rats. Eur J Pharmacol 654(2):166–172. https://doi.org/10.1016/j.ejphar.2010.11.025

Kleiber ML, Wright E, Singh SM (2011) Maternal voluntary drinking in C57BL/6J mice: advancing a model for fetal alcohol spectrum disorders. Behav Brain Res 223(2):376–387. https://doi.org/10.1016/j.bbr.2011.05.005

Knopik VS, Marceau K, Bidwell LC, Rolan E (2019) Prenatal substance exposure and offspring development: does DNA methylation play a role? Neurotoxicol Teratol 71:50–63. https://doi.org/10.1016/j.ntt.2018.01.009

Ko JY, D'Angelo DV, Haight SC, Morrow B, Cox S, von Essen BS et al (2020) Vital signs: prescription opioid pain reliever use during pregnancy — 34 U.-S. Jurisdictions, 2019. MMWR Morb Mortal Wkly Rep *69*(28):897–903. https://doi.org/10.15585/mmwr.mm6928a1

Kokhan VS, Anokhin PK, Proskuryakova TV, Shokhonova VA, Ageldinov RA, Shamakina IY (2023) Interleukin-1beta and TNF-alpha are elevated in the amygdala of adult rats prenatally exposed to ethanol. Biomed Khim 69(5):300–306. https://doi.org/10.18097/PBMC20236905300

Komada M, Takao K, Miyakawa T (2008) Elevated plus maze for mice. J Vis Exp 22. https://doi.org/10.3791/1088

Kongstorp M, Bogen IL, Steinsland S, Nerem E, Salih TW, Stiris T, Andersen JM (2020) Prenatal exposure to methadone or buprenorphine alters micro-opioid receptor binding and downstream signaling in the rat brain. Int J Dev Neurosci 80(5):443–453. https://doi.org/10.1002/jdn.10043

Koponen AM, Nissinen NM, Gissler M, Autti-Ramo I, Kahila H, Sarkola T (2023) Adverse childhood experiences and neurodevelopmental disorders among youth with and without prenatal substance exposure: a longitudinal matched register-based cohort study. Nordisk Alkohol Nark 40(2):176–198. https://doi.org/10.1177/14550725221110190

Kraeuter AK, Guest PC, Sarnyai Z (2019) The elevated plus maze test for measuring anxiety-like behavior in

rodents. Methods Mol Biol 1916:69–74. https://doi.org/10.1007/978-1-4939-8994-2_4
Krueger AM, Roediger DJ, Mueller BA, Boys CA, Hendrickson TJ, Schumacher MJ et al (2020) Paralimbic structural abnormalities are associated with internalizing symptoms in children with prenatal alcohol exposure. Alcohol Clin Exp Res 44(8):1598–1608. https://doi.org/10.1111/acer.14390
Lallai V, Manca L, Sherafat Y, Fowler CD (2022) Effects of prenatal nicotine, THC, or co-exposure on cognitive behaviors in adolescent male and female rats. Nicotine Tob Res 24(8):1150–1160. https://doi.org/10.1093/ntr/ntac018
Lam VYY, Raineki C, Ellis L, Yu W, Weinberg J (2018a) Interactive effects of prenatal alcohol exposure and chronic stress in adulthood on anxiety-like behavior and central stress-related receptor mRNA expression: sex- and time-dependent effects. Psychoneuroendocrinology 97:8–19. https://doi.org/10.1016/j.psyneuen.2018.06.018
Lam VYY, Raineki C, Takeuchi LE, Ellis L, Woodward TS, Weinberg J (2018b) Chronic stress alters behavior in the forced swim test and underlying neural activity in animals exposed to Alcohol prenatally: sex- and time-dependent effects. Front Behav Neurosci 12:42. https://doi.org/10.3389/fnbeh.2018.00042
Lam VYY, Raineki C, Wang LY, Chiu M, Lee G, Ellis L et al (2019) Role of corticosterone in anxiety- and depressive-like behavior and HPA regulation following prenatal alcohol exposure. Prog Neuro-Psychopharmacol Biol Psychiatry 90:1–15. https://doi.org/10.1016/j.pnpbp.2018.10.008
Lambers DS, Clark KE (1996) The maternal and fetal physiologic effects of nicotine. Semin Perinatol 20(2):115–126. https://doi.org/10.1016/s0146-0005(96)80079-6
Lan N, Hellemans KG, Ellis L, Weinberg J (2015) Exposure to chronic mild stress differentially alters Corticotropin-releasing hormone and arginine vasopressin mRNA expression in the stress-responsive Neurocircuitry of male and female rats prenatally exposed to alcohol. Alcohol Clin Exp Res 39(12):2414–2421. https://doi.org/10.1111/acer.12916
Lee H, Chung S, Noh J (2016) Maternal nicotine exposure during late gestation and lactation increases anxiety-like and impulsive decision-making behavior in adolescent offspring of rat. Toxicol Res 32(4):275–280. https://doi.org/10.5487/TR.2016.32.4.275
Lee SM, Yeh PWL, Yeh HH (2022) L-type calcium channels contribute to ethanol-induced aberrant tangential migration of primordial cortical GABAergic interneurons in the embryonic medial prefrontal cortex. eNeuro 9(1). https://doi.org/10.1523/ENEURO.0359-21.2021
Leech SL, Larkby CA, Day R, Day NL (2006) Predictors and correlates of high levels of depression and anxiety symptoms among children at age 10. J Am Acad Child Adolesc Psychiatry 45(2):223–230. https://doi.org/10.1097/01.chi.0000184930.18552.4d
Lemola S, Stadlmayr W, Grob A (2009) Infant irritability: the impact of fetal alcohol exposure, maternal depressive symptoms, and low emotional support from the husband. Infant Ment Health J 30(1):57–81. https://doi.org/10.1002/imhj.20203
Levine TA, Davie-Gray A, Kim HM, Lee SJ, Woodward LJ (2021) Prenatal methadone exposure and child developmental outcomes in 2-year-old children. Dev Med Child Neurol. https://doi.org/10.1111/dmcn.14808
Liang J, Shen Y, Shao XM, Scott MB, Ly E, Wong S et al (2014) Dihydromyricetin prevents fetal alcohol exposure-induced behavioral and physiological deficits: the roles of GABAA receptors in adolescence. Neurochem Res 39(6):1147–1161. https://doi.org/10.1007/s11064-014-1291-5
Lin CS, Tao PL, Jong YJ, Chen WF, Yang CH, Huang LT et al (2009) Prenatal morphine alters the synaptic complex of postsynaptic density 95 with N-methyl-D-aspartate receptor subunit in hippocampal CA1 subregion of rat offspring leading to long-term cognitive deficits. Neuroscience 158(4):1326–1337. https://doi.org/10.1016/j.neuroscience.2008.11.007
Little B, Sud N, Nobile Z, Bhattacharya D (2021) Teratogenic effects of maternal drug abuse on developing brain and underlying neurotransmitter mechanisms. Neurotoxicology 86:172–179. https://doi.org/10.1016/j.neuro.2021.08.007
Livy DJ, Parnell SE, West JR (2003) Blood ethanol concentration profiles: a comparison between rats and mice. Alcohol 29(3):165–171. https://doi.org/10.1016/s0741-8329(03)00025-9
Lopatynska-Mazurek M, Komsta L, Gibula-Tarlowska E, Kotlinska JH (2021) Aversive learning deficits and depressive-like behaviors are accompanied by an increase in oxidative stress in a rat model of Fetal Alcohol Spectrum disorders: the protective effect of rapamycin. Int J Mol Sci 22(13). https://doi.org/10.3390/ijms22137083
Lotfipour S, Ferguson E, Leonard G, Perron M, Pike B, Richer L et al (2009) Orbitofrontal cortex and drug use during adolescence: role of prenatal exposure to maternal smoking and BDNF genotype. Arch Gen Psychiatry 66(11):1244–1252. https://doi.org/10.1001/archgenpsychiatry.2009.124
Lu HC, Mackie K (2021) Review of the endocannabinoid system. Biol Psychiatry Cogn Neurosci Neuroimaging 6(6):607–615. https://doi.org/10.1016/j.bpsc.2020.07.016
Lum JS, Bird KM, Wilkie J, Millard SJ, Pallimulla S, Newell KA, Wright IM (2021) Prenatal methadone exposure impairs adolescent cognition and GABAergic neurodevelopment in a novel rat model of maternal methadone treatment. Prog Neuro-Psychopharmacol Biol Psychiatry 110:110281. https://doi.org/10.1016/j.pnpbp.2021.110281
Lund IO, Moen Eilertsen E, Gjerde LC, Roysamb E, Wood M, Reichborn-Kjennerud T, Ystrom E (2019) Is the association between maternal alcohol

consumption in pregnancy and pre-school child behavioural and emotional problems causal? Multiple approaches for controlling unmeasured confounding. Addiction 114(6):1004–1014. https://doi.org/10.1111/add.14573

Lv J, Mao C, Zhu L, Zhang H, Pengpeng H, Xu F et al (2008) The effect of prenatal nicotine on expression of nicotine receptor subunits in the fetal brain. Neurotoxicology 29(4):722–726. https://doi.org/10.1016/j.neuro.2008.04.015

Maccarrone M, Guzman M, Mackie K, Doherty P, Harkany T (2014) Programming of neural cells by (endo)cannabinoids: from physiological rules to emerging therapies. Nat Rev Neurosci 15(12): 786–801. https://doi.org/10.1038/nrn3846

Mackie K (2005) Distribution of cannabinoid receptors in the central and peripheral nervous system. Handb Exp Pharmacol 168:299–325. https://doi.org/10.1007/3-540-26573-2_10

Madarnas C, Villalba NM, Soriano D, Brusco A (2020) Anxious behavior of adult CD1 mice perinatally exposed to low concentrations of ethanol correlates with morphological changes in cingulate cortex and amygdala. Front Behav Neurosci 14:92. https://doi.org/10.3389/fnbeh.2020.00092

Madson MJ, Srivastava U, Gade Y (2025) Recommendations from Arizona budtenders to mystery callers regarding morning sickness. J Obstet Gynecol Neonatal Nurs. https://doi.org/10.1016/j.jogn.2025.02.001

Malik Z, Baik D, Schey R (2015) The role of cannabinoids in regulation of nausea and vomiting, and visceral pain. Curr Gastroenterol Rep 17(2):429. https://doi.org/10.1007/s11894-015-0429-1

Martin MM, McCarthy DM, Schatschneider C, Trupiano MX, Jones SK, Kalluri A, Bhide PG (2020) Effects of developmental nicotine exposure on frontal cortical GABA-to-non-GABA neuron ratio and novelty-seeking behavior. Cereb Cortex 30(3):1830–1842. https://doi.org/10.1093/cercor/bhz207

Martin RE, Green MT, Kinkade JA, Schmidt RR, Willemse TE, Schenk AK et al (2021) Maternal oxycodone treatment results in neurobehavioral disruptions in mice offspring. eNeuro 8(4). https://doi.org/10.1523/ENEURO.0150-21.2021

Martin JA, Osterman MJK, Driscoll AK (2023) Declines in cigarette smoking during pregnancy in the United States, 2016–2021. NCHS Data Brief 458:1–8

McCarthy DM, Zhang L, Wilkes BJ, Vaillancourt DE, Biederman J, Bhide PG (2022) Nicotine and the developing brain: insights from preclinical models. Pharmacol Biochem Behav 214:173355. https://doi.org/10.1016/j.pbb.2022.173355

Meinhofer A, Hinde JM, Keyes KM, Lugo-Candelas C (2022) Association of comorbid behavioral and medical conditions with cannabis use disorder in pregnancy. JAMA Psychiatry 79(1):50–58. https://doi.org/10.1001/jamapsychiatry.2021.3193

Mereu G, Fa M, Ferraro L, Cagiano R, Antonelli T, Tattoli M et al (2003) Prenatal exposure to a cannabinoid agonist produces memory deficits linked to dysfunction in hippocampal long-term potentiation and glutamate release. Proc Natl Acad Sci USA 100(8): 4915–4920. https://doi.org/10.1073/pnas.0537849100

Merhar SL, Parikh NA, Braimah A, Poindexter BB, Tkach J, Kline-Fath B (2019) White matter injury and structural anomalies in infants with prenatal opioid exposure. AJNR Am J Neuroradiol 40(12): 2161–2165. https://doi.org/10.3174/ajnr.A6282

Min MO, Albert JM, Lorincz-Comi N, Minnes S, Lester B, Momotaz H et al (2021) Prenatal substance exposure and developmental trajectories of internalizing symptoms: toddlerhood to preadolescence. Drug Alcohol Depend 218:108411. https://doi.org/10.1016/j.drugalcdep.2020.108411

Mirnics K (2025) Fetal fentanyl syndrome – only the "tip of the iceberg"? Eur Neuropsychopharmacol 90:69–70. https://doi.org/10.1016/j.euroneuro.2024.10.011

Molendijk ML, de Kloet ER (2015) Immobility in the forced swim test is adaptive and does not reflect depression. Psychoneuroendocrinology 62:389–391. https://doi.org/10.1016/j.psyneuen.2015.08.028

Molteno CD, Jacobson JL, Carter RC, Dodge NC, Jacobson SW (2014) Infant emotional withdrawal: a precursor of affective and cognitive disturbance in fetal alcohol spectrum disorders. Alcohol Clin Exp Res 38(2):479–488. https://doi.org/10.1111/acer.12240

Monnelly VJ, Anblagan D, Quigley A, Cabez MB, Cooper ES, Mactier H et al (2018) Prenatal methadone exposure is associated with altered neonatal brain development. Neuroimage Clin 18:9–14. https://doi.org/10.1016/j.nicl.2017.12.033

Monnelly VJ, Hamilton R, Chappell FM, Mactier H, Boardman JP (2019) Childhood neurodevelopment after prescription of maintenance methadone for opioid dependency in pregnancy: a systematic review and meta-analysis. Dev Med Child Neurol 61(7):750–760. https://doi.org/10.1111/dmcn.14117

Mooney SM, Varlinskaya EI (2011) Acute prenatal exposure to ethanol and social behavior: effects of age, sex, and timing of exposure. Behav Brain Res 216(1): 358–364. https://doi.org/10.1016/j.bbr.2010.08.014

Mooney SM, Varlinskaya EI (2018) Enhanced sensitivity to socially facilitating and anxiolytic effects of ethanol in adolescent Sprague Dawley rats following acute prenatal ethanol exposure. Alcohol 69:25–32. https://doi.org/10.1016/j.alcohol.2017.11.002

Moore BF, Salmons KA, Hoyt AT, Swenson KS, Bates EA, Sauder KA et al (2023) Associations between prenatal and postnatal exposure to cannabis with cognition and behavior at age 5 years: the healthy start study. Int J Environ Res Public Health 20(6). https://doi.org/10.3390/ijerph20064880

Moylan S, Gustavson K, Overland S, Karevold EB, Jacka FN, Pasco JA, Berk M (2015) The impact of maternal smoking during pregnancy on depressive and anxiety behaviors in children: the Norwegian Mother and Child Cohort Study. BMC Med 13:24. https://doi.org/10.1186/s12916-014-0257-4

Muneoka K, Nakatsu T, Fuji J, Ogawa T, Takigawa M (1999) Prenatal administration of nicotine results in dopaminergic alterations in the neocortex. Neurotoxicol Teratol 21(5):603–609. https://doi.org/10.1016/s0892-0362(99)00028-8

Murnan AW, Keim SA, Yeates KO, Boone KM, Sheppard KW, Klebanoff MA (2021) Behavioral and cognitive differences in early childhood related to prenatal marijuana exposure. J Appl Dev Psychol 77. https://doi.org/10.1016/j.appdev.2021.101348

Murrin LC, Ferrer JR, Zeng WY, Haley NJ (1987) Nicotine administration to rats: methodological considerations. Life Sci 40(17):1699–1708. https://doi.org/10.1016/0024-3205(87)90020-8

Myrick A, Jimenez D, Jacquez B, Sun MS, Noor S, Milligan ED et al (2024) Maternal alcohol drinking patterns predict offspring neurobehavioral outcomes. Neuropharmacology 257:110044. https://doi.org/10.1016/j.neuropharm.2024.110044

Nakhid D, Patel D, McMorris CA, Gibbard WB, Tortorelli C, Pei J, Lebel C (2023) Limbic brain subregions associated with mental health symptoms in youth with and without prenatal alcohol exposure. Alcohol Clin Exp Res (Hoboken) 47(11):2033–2044. https://doi.org/10.1111/acer.15181

Nakhjiri E, Saboory E, Roshan-Milani S, Rasmi Y, Khalafkhani D (2017) Effect of prenatal restraint stress and morphine co-administration on plasma vasopressin concentration and anxiety behaviors in adult rat offspring. Stress 20(2):205–211. https://doi.org/10.1080/10253890.2017.1306053

Nashed MG, Hardy DB, Laviolette SR (2020) Prenatal cannabinoid exposure: emerging evidence of physiological and neuropsychiatric abnormalities. Front Psych 11:624275. https://doi.org/10.3389/fpsyt.2020.624275

Navarro M, Rubio P, Rodriguez de Fonseca F (1994) Sex-dimorphic psychomotor activation after perinatal exposure to (−)-delta 9-tetrahydrocannabinol. An ontogenic study in Wistar rats. Psychopharmacology 116(4):414–422. https://doi.org/10.1007/BF02247471

Newsom RJ, Kelly SJ (2008) Perinatal delta-9-tetrahydrocannabinol exposure disrupts social and open field behavior in adult male rats. Neurotoxicol Teratol 30(3):213–219. https://doi.org/10.1016/j.ntt.2007.12.007

Nieto-Estevez V, Donegan JJ, McMahon CL, Elam HB, Chavera TA, Varma P et al (2022) Buprenorphine exposure alters the development and migration of interneurons in the cortex. Front Mol Neurosci 15:889922. https://doi.org/10.3389/fnmol.2022.889922

Niu L, Cao B, Zhu H, Mei B, Wang M, Yang Y, Zhou Y (2009) Impaired in vivo synaptic plasticity in dentate gyrus and spatial memory in juvenile rats induced by prenatal morphine exposure. Hippocampus 19(7):649–657. https://doi.org/10.1002/hipo.20540

Nyberg H, Bogen IL, Nygaard E, Andersen JM (2024) Effects of prenatal exposure to methadone or buprenorphine and maternal separation on anxiety-like behavior in rats. Drug Alcohol Depend 262:111367. https://doi.org/10.1016/j.drugalcdep.2024.111367

Nygaard E, Slinning K, Moe V, Fjell A, Walhovd KB (2020) Mental health in youth prenatally exposed to opioids and poly-drugs and raised in permanent foster/adoptive homes: a prospective longitudinal study. Early Hum Dev 140:104910. https://doi.org/10.1016/j.earlhumdev.2019.104910

O'Connor MJ, Sigma M, Kasari C (1992) Attachment behavior of infants exposed prenatally to alcohol: mediating effects of infant affect and mother-infant interaction. Dev Psychopathol 4(2):243–256. https://doi.org/10.1017/S0954579400000122

O'Leary CM, Bower C, Zubrick SR, Geelhoed E, Kurinczuk JJ, Nassar N (2010) A new method of prenatal alcohol classification accounting for dose, pattern and timing of exposure: improving our ability to examine fetal effects from low to moderate alcohol. J Epidemiol Community Health 64(11):956–962. https://doi.org/10.1136/jech.2009.091785

Oberlander TF, Weinberg J, Papsdorf M, Grunau R, Misri S, Devlin AM (2008) Prenatal exposure to maternal depression, neonatal methylation of human glucocorticoid receptor gene (NR3C1) and infant cortisol stress responses. Epigenetics 3(2):97–106. https://doi.org/10.4161/epi.3.2.6034

O'Connor MJ (2001) Prenatal alcohol exposure and infant negative affect as precursors of depressive features in children. Infant Ment Health J 22(3):271–430. https://doi.org/10.1002/imhj.1002

O'Connor MJ, Paley B (2009) Psychiatric conditions associated with prenatal alcohol exposure. Dev Disabil Res Rev 15(3):225–234. https://doi.org/10.1002/ddrr.74

O'Connor MJ, Kogan N, Findlay R (2002) Prenatal alcohol exposure and attachment behavior in children. Alcohol Clin Exp Res 26(10):1592–1602. https://doi.org/10.1097/01.ALC.0000034665.79909.F0

Olusakin J, Kumar G, Basu M, Calarco CA, Fox ME, Alipio JB et al (2023) Transcriptomic profiling of reward and sensory brain areas in perinatal fentanyl exposed juvenile mice. Neuropsychopharmacology 48(12):1724–1734. https://doi.org/10.1038/s41386-023-01639-8

Oubraim S, Wang R, Hausknecht K, Kaczocha M, Shen RY, Haj-Dahmane S (2022) Prenatal ethanol exposure causes anxiety-like phenotype and alters synaptic nitric oxide and endocannabinoid signaling in dorsal raphe nucleus of adult male rats. Transl Psychiatry 12(1):440. https://doi.org/10.1038/s41398-022-02210-7

Palma-Gudiel H, Cordova-Palomera A, Eixarch E, Deuschle M, Fananas L (2015) Maternal psychosocial stress during pregnancy alters the epigenetic signature of the glucocorticoid receptor gene promoter in their offspring: a meta-analysis. Epigenetics 10(10):

893–902. https://doi.org/10.1080/15592294.2015.1088630

Parameshwaran K, Buabeid MA, Karuppagounder SS, Uthayathas S, Thiruchelvam K, Shonesy B et al (2012) Developmental nicotine exposure induced alterations in behavior and glutamate receptor function in hippocampus. Cell Mol Life Sci 69(5):829–841. https://doi.org/10.1007/s00018-011-0805-4

Pei J, Denys K, Hughes J, Rasmussen C (2011) Mental health issues in fetal alcohol spectrum disorder. J Ment Health 20(5):438–448. https://doi.org/10.3109/09638237.2011.577113

Peterson BS, Rosen T, Dingman S, Toth ZR, Sawardekar S, Hao X et al (2020) Associations of maternal prenatal drug abuse with measures of newborn brain structure, tissue organization, and metabolite concentrations. JAMA Pediatr 174(9):831–842. https://doi.org/10.1001/jamapediatrics.2020.1622

Polli FS, Kohlmeier KA (2020) Prenatal nicotine exposure in rodents: why are there so many variations in behavioral outcomes? Nicotine Tob Res 22(10):1694–1710. https://doi.org/10.1093/ntr/ntz196

Polli FS, Scharff MB, Ipsen TH, Aznar S, Kohlmeier KA, Andreasen JT (2020) Prenatal nicotine exposure in mice induces sex-dependent anxiety-like behavior, cognitive deficits, hyperactivity, and changes in the expression of glutamate receptor associated-genes in the prefrontal cortex. Pharmacol Biochem Behav 195: 172951. https://doi.org/10.1016/j.pbb.2020.172951

Popova S, Lange S, Probst C, Gmel G, Rehm J (2017) Estimation of national, regional, and global prevalence of alcohol use during pregnancy and fetal alcohol syndrome: a systematic review and meta-analysis. Lancet Glob Health 5(3):e290–e299. https://doi.org/10.1016/S2214-109X(17)30021-9

Popova S, Lange S, Probst C, Gmel G, Rehm J (2018) Global prevalence of alcohol use and binge drinking during pregnancy, and fetal alcohol spectrum disorder. Biochem Cell Biol 96(2):237–240. https://doi.org/10.1139/bcb-2017-0077

Popova S, Charness ME, Burd L, Crawford A, Hoyme HE, Mukherjee RAS et al (2023) Fetal alcohol spectrum disorders. Nat Rev Dis Primers 9(1):11. https://doi.org/10.1038/s41572-023-00420-x

Pratt Tremblay G, Dimanlig-Cruz S, Dion A, Corsi DJ (2025) Trends in prenatal substance use across Ontario, Canada. JAMA Netw Open 8(1):e2455310. https://doi.org/10.1001/jamanetworkopen.2024.55310

Pruett S, Tan W, Howell GE 3rd, Nanduri B (2020) Dosage scaling of alcohol in binge exposure models in mice: an empirical assessment of the relationship between dose, alcohol exposure, and peak blood concentrations in humans and mice. Alcohol 89:9–17. https://doi.org/10.1016/j.alcohol.2020.03.011

Przybysz KR, Spodnick MB, Johnson JM, Varlinskaya EI, Diaz MR (2023) Moderate prenatal alcohol exposure produces sex-specific social impairments and attenuates prelimbic excitability and amygdala-cortex modulation of adult social behaviour. Addict Biol 28(1):e13252. https://doi.org/10.1111/adb.13252

Puga TB, Doucet GE, Thiel GE, Theye E, Dai HD (2024) Prenatal tobacco exposure, brain subcortical volumes, and Gray-White matter contrast. JAMA Netw Open 7(12):e2451786. https://doi.org/10.1001/jamanetworkopen.2024.51786

Radhakrishnan R, Elsaid NMH, Sadhasivam S, Reher TA, Hines AC, Yoder KK et al (2021) Resting state functional MRI in infants with prenatal opioid exposure-a pilot study. Neuroradiology 63(4):585–591. https://doi.org/10.1007/s00234-020-02552-3

Raineki C, Hellemans KG, Bodnar T, Lavigne KM, Ellis L, Woodward TS, Weinberg J (2014) Neurocircuitry underlying stress and emotional regulation in animals prenatally exposed to alcohol and subjected to chronic mild stress in adulthood. Front Endocrinol (Lausanne) 5:5. https://doi.org/10.3389/fendo.2014.00005

Raineki C, Chew L, Mok P, Ellis L, Weinberg J (2016) Short- and long-term effects of stress during adolescence on emotionality and HPA function of animals exposed to alcohol prenatally. Psychoneuroendocrinology 74:13–23. https://doi.org/10.1016/j.psyneuen.2016.08.015

Reardon S (2024) Pressue grows to ditch controversial forced swim test in rodent studies of depression. Science 383(6689). https://doi.org/10.1126/science.zrf1p5t

Rebbe R, Sieger ML, Reddy J, Prindle J (2024) U.S. State rates of newborns reported to child protection at birth for prenatal substance exposure. Int J Drug Policy 130: 104527. https://doi.org/10.1016/j.drugpo.2024.104527

Richardson SA, Tizabi Y (1994) Hyperactivity in the offspring of nicotine-treated rats: role of the mesolimbic and nigrostriatal dopaminergic pathways. Pharmacol Biochem Behav 47(2):331–337. https://doi.org/10.1016/0091-3057(94)90018-3

Richardson GA, Day NL, Goldschmidt L (1995) Prenatal alcohol, marijuana, and tobacco use: infant mental and motor development. Neurotoxicol Teratol 17(4): 479–487. https://doi.org/10.1016/0892-0362(95)00006-d

Richardson KA, Hester AK, McLemore GL (2016) Prenatal cannabis exposure – the "first hit" to the endocannabinoid system. Neurotoxicol Teratol 58:5–14. https://doi.org/10.1016/j.ntt.2016.08.003

Roberson EK, Patrick WK, Hurwitz EL (2014) Marijuana use and maternal experiences of severe nausea during pregnancy in Hawai'i. Hawaii J Med Public Health 73(9):283–287

Robinson M, McLean NJ, Oddy WH, Mattes E, Bulsara M, Li J et al (2010) Smoking cessation in pregnancy and the risk of child behavioural problems: a longitudinal prospective cohort study. J Epidemiol Community Health 64(7):622–629. https://doi.org/10.1136/jech.2009.088658

Rodriguez CE, Klie KA (2019) Pharmacological treatment of opioid use disorder in pregnancy. Semin Perinatol 43(3):141–148. https://doi.org/10.1053/j.semperi.2019.01.003

Rompala G, Nomura Y, Hurd YL (2021) Maternal cannabis use is associated with suppression of immune gene networks in placenta and increased anxiety phenotypes in offspring. Proc Natl Acad Sci USA 118(47). https://doi.org/10.1073/pnas.2106115118

Roth TL, Lubin FD, Funk AJ, Sweatt JD (2009) Lasting epigenetic influence of early-life adversity on the BDNF gene. Biol Psychiatry 65(9):760–769. https://doi.org/10.1016/j.biopsych.2008.11.028

Rouzer SK, Diaz MR (2022) Moderate prenatal alcohol exposure modifies sex-specific CRFR1 activity in the central amygdala and anxiety-like behavior in adolescent offspring. Neuropsychopharmacology 47(12):2140–2149. https://doi.org/10.1038/s41386-022-01327-z

Rouzer SK, Cole JM, Johnson JM, Varlinskaya EI, Diaz MR (2017) Moderate maternal Alcohol exposure on gestational Day 12 impacts anxiety-like behavior in offspring. Front Behav Neurosci 11:183. https://doi.org/10.3389/fnbeh.2017.00183

Roy TS, Sabherwal U (1994) Effects of prenatal nicotine exposure on the morphogenesis of somatosensory cortex. Neurotoxicol Teratol 16(4):411–421. https://doi.org/10.1016/0892-0362(94)90030-2

Roy TS, Seidler FJ, Slotkin TA (2002) Prenatal nicotine exposure evokes alterations of cell structure in hippocampus and somatosensory cortex. J Pharmacol Exp Ther 300(1):124–133. https://doi.org/10.1124/jpet.300.1.124

Russell C, Rueda S, Room R, Tyndall M, Fischer B (2018) Routes of administration for cannabis use – basic prevalence and related health outcomes: a scoping review and synthesis. Int J Drug Policy 52:87–96. https://doi.org/10.1016/j.drugpo.2017.11.008

Saez TM, Aronne MP, Caltana L, Brusco AH (2014) Prenatal exposure to the CB1 and CB2 cannabinoid receptor agonist WIN 55,212-2 alters migration of early-born glutamatergic neurons and GABAergic interneurons in the rat cerebral cortex. J Neurochem 129(4):637–648. https://doi.org/10.1111/jnc.12636

Sahid AS, Bebbington MJ, Marcus A, Baracz SJ, Zimmermann KS, Oei J et al (2025) Perinatal exposure to methadone or buprenorphine impairs hippocampal-dependent cognition and brain development in juvenile rats. Prog Neuro-Psychopharmacol Biol Psychiatry 137:111255. https://doi.org/10.1016/j.pnpbp.2025.111255

Salihu HM, Wilson RE (2007) Epidemiology of prenatal smoking and perinatal outcomes. Early Hum Dev 83(11):713–720. https://doi.org/10.1016/j.earlhumdev.2007.08.002

Salzwedel A, Chen G, Chen Y, Grewen K, Gao W (2020) Functional dissection of prenatal drug effects on baby brain and behavioral development. Hum Brain Mapp 41(17):4789–4803. https://doi.org/10.1002/hbm.25158

Sandini TM, Onofrychuk TJ, Roebuck AJ, Hammond SA, Udenze D, Hayat S et al (2023) Repeated exposure to high-THC cannabis smoke during gestation alters sex ratio, behavior, and amygdala gene expression of sprague dawley rat offspring. eNeuro 10(11). https://doi.org/10.1523/ENEURO.0100-23.2023

Santiago SE, Huffman KJ (2014) Prenatal nicotine exposure increases anxiety and modifies sensorimotor integration behaviors in adult female mice. Neurosci Res 79:41–51. https://doi.org/10.1016/j.neures.2013.10.006

Sarkaki A, Mard SA, Bakhtiari N, Yazdanfar N (2023) Sex-specific effects of developmental morphine exposure and rearing environments on hippocampal spatial memory. Int J Dev Neurosci 83(2):178–190. https://doi.org/10.1002/jdn.10245

Schuetze P, Godleski S, Sassaman J (2021) Prenatal exposure to opioids: associations between the caregiving environment and externalizing behaviors. Neurotoxicol Teratol 87:107019. https://doi.org/10.1016/j.ntt.2021.107019

Shahbazi F, Grandi V, Banerjee A, Trant JF (2020) Cannabinoids and cannabinoid receptors: the story so far. iScience 23(7):101301. https://doi.org/10.1016/j.isci.2020.101301

Sherman LJ, Ali MM, Mutter R, Larson J (2019) Mental disorders among children born with neonatal abstinence syndrome. Psychiatr Serv 70(2):151. https://doi.org/10.1176/appi.ps.201800341

Sikic A, Frie JA, Khokhar JY, Murray JE (2022) Sex differences in the Behavioural outcomes of prenatal nicotine and tobacco exposure. Front Neurosci 16:921429. https://doi.org/10.3389/fnins.2022.921429

Sirnes E, Oltedal L, Bartsch H, Eide GE, Elgen IB, Aukland SM (2017) Brain morphology in school-aged children with prenatal opioid exposure: a structural MRI study. Early Hum Dev 106–107:33–39. https://doi.org/10.1016/j.earlhumdev.2017.01.009

Skorput AG, Yeh HH (2016) Chronic gestational exposure to ethanol leads to enduring aberrances in cortical form and function in the medial prefrontal cortex. Alcohol Clin Exp Res 40(7):1479–1488. https://doi.org/10.1111/acer.13107

Skorput AG, Lee SM, Yeh PW, Yeh HH (2019) The NKCC1 antagonist bumetanide mitigates interneuronopathy associated with ethanol exposure in utero. elife 8. https://doi.org/10.7554/eLife.48648

Slamberova R, Rimanoczy A, Bar N, Schindler CJ, Vathy I (2003) Density of mu-opioid receptors in the hippocampus of adult male and female rats is altered by prenatal morphine exposure and gonadal hormone treatment. Hippocampus 13(4):461–471. https://doi.org/10.1002/hipo.10076

Slotkin TA (2008) If nicotine is a developmental neurotoxicant in animal studies, dare we recommend nicotine replacement therapy in pregnant women and adolescents? Neurotoxicol Teratol 30(1):1–19. https://doi.org/10.1016/j.ntt.2007.09.002

Slotkin TA, Seidler FJ (2010) Mimicking maternal smoking and pharmacotherapy of preterm labor: interactions of fetal nicotine and dexamethasone on serotonin and dopamine synaptic function in adolescence and adulthood. Brain Res Bull 82(1–2):124–134. https://doi.org/10.1016/j.brainresbull.2010.02.015

Slotkin TA, Tate CA, Cousins MM, Seidler FJ (2006) Prenatal nicotine exposure alters the responses to subsequent nicotine administration and withdrawal in adolescence: serotonin receptors and cell signaling. Neuropsychopharmacology 31(11):2462–2475. https://doi.org/10.1038/sj.npp.1300988

Smid MC, Allshouse AA, McMillin GA, Nunez K, Cavin T, Worden J et al (2022) Umbilical cord collection and drug testing to estimate prenatal substance exposure in Utah. Obstet Gynecol 140(2):153–162. https://doi.org/10.1097/AOG.0000000000004868

Smith AM, Dwoskin LP, Pauly JR (2010) Early exposure to nicotine during critical periods of brain development: mechanisms and consequences. J Pediatr Biochem 1(2):125–141. https://doi.org/10.3233/JPB-2010-0012

Smith AM, Mioduszewski O, Hatchard T, Byron-Alhassan A, Fall C, Fried PA (2016) Prenatal marijuana exposure impacts executive functioning into young adulthood: an fMRI study. Neurotoxicol Teratol 58:53–59. https://doi.org/10.1016/j.ntt.2016.05.010

Smith A, Kaufman F, Sandy MS, Cardenas A (2020) Cannabis exposure during critical windows of development: epigenetic and molecular pathways implicated in neuropsychiatric disease. Curr Environ Health Rep 7(3):325–342. https://doi.org/10.1007/s40572-020-00275-4

Smith BL, Guzman TA, Brendle AH, Laaker CJ, Ford A, Hiltz AR et al (2022) Perinatal morphine exposure leads to sex-dependent executive function deficits and microglial changes in mice. eNeuro 9(5). https://doi.org/10.1523/ENEURO.0238-22.2022

Spano MS, Ellgren M, Wang X, Hurd YL (2007) Prenatal cannabis exposure increases heroin seeking with allostatic changes in limbic enkephalin systems in adulthood. Biol Psychiatry 61(4):554–563. https://doi.org/10.1016/j.biopsych.2006.03.073

Spencer MR, Garnett MF, Minino AM (2024) Drug overdose deaths in the united sates, 2002–2022. National Center for Health Statistics

Spodnick MB, McElderry SC, Diaz MR (2025) Opioid receptor signaling throughout ontogeny: shaping neural and behavioral trajectories. Neurosci Biobehav Rev 170:106033. https://doi.org/10.1016/j.neubiorev.2025.106033

Tajuddin NF, Druse MJ (1999) In utero ethanol exposure decreased the density of serotonin neurons. Maternal ipsapirone treatment exerted a protective effect. Brain Res Dev Brain Res 117(1):91–97. https://doi.org/10.1016/s0165-3806(99)00102-9

Talhout R, Schulz T, Florek E, van Benthem J, Wester P, Opperhuizen A (2011) Hazardous compounds in tobacco smoke. Int J Environ Res Public Health 8(2):613–628. https://doi.org/10.3390/ijerph8020613

Tan JW, Duan TT, Zhou QX, Ding ZY, Jing L, Cao J et al (2015) Impaired contextual fear extinction and hippocampal synaptic plasticity in adult rats induced by prenatal morphine exposure. Addict Biol 20(4):652–662. https://doi.org/10.1111/adb.12158

Taylor JL, Johnson S, Cruz R, Gray JR, Schiff D, Bagley SM (2021) Integrating harm reduction into outpatient opioid use disorder treatment settings: harm reduction in outpatient addiction treatment. J Gen Intern Med 36(12):3810–3819. https://doi.org/10.1007/s11606-021-06904-4

Terlizzi EP, Zablotsky B (2024) Symptoms of anxiety and depression among adults: United States, 2019 and 2022. Natl Health Stat Report 213. https://doi.org/10.15620/cdc/64018

Thielen A, Klus H, Muller L (2008) Tobacco smoke: unraveling a controversial subject. Exp Toxicol Pathol 60(2–3):141–156. https://doi.org/10.1016/j.etp.2008.01.014

Thomason ME, Palopoli AC, Jariwala NN, Werchan DM, Chen A, Adhikari S et al (2021) Miswiring the brain: human prenatal Delta9-tetrahydrocannabinol use associated with altered fetal hippocampal brain network connectivity. Dev Cogn Neurosci 51:101000. https://doi.org/10.1016/j.dcn.2021.101000

Toro R, Leonard G, Lerner JV, Lerner RM, Perron M, Pike GB et al (2008) Prenatal exposure to maternal cigarette smoking and the adolescent cerebral cortex. Neuropsychopharmacology 33(5):1019–1027. https://doi.org/10.1038/sj.npp.1301484

Traccis F, Serra V, Sagheddu C, Congiu M, Saba P, Giua G et al (2021) Prenatal THC does not affect female mesolimbic dopaminergic system in preadolescent rats. Int J Mol Sci 22(4). https://doi.org/10.3390/ijms22041666

Tran BX, Boggiano VL, Nguyen CT, Nguyen LH, Le Nguyen AT, Latkin CA (2017) Barriers to accessing and using health insurance cards among methadone maintenance treatment patients in northern Vietnam. Subst Abuse Treat Prev Policy 12(1):35. https://doi.org/10.1186/s13011-017-0119-0

Trezza V, Campolongo P, Cassano T, Macheda T, Dipasquale P, Carratu MR et al (2008) Effects of perinatal exposure to delta-9-tetrahydrocannabinol on the emotional reactivity of the offspring: a longitudinal behavioral study in Wistar rats. Psychopharmacology 198(4):529–537. https://doi.org/10.1007/s00213-008-1162-3

Tsou K, Brown S, Sanudo-Pena MC, Mackie K, Walker JM (1998) Immunohistochemical distribution of cannabinoid CB1 receptors in the rat central nervous system. Neuroscience 83(2):393–411. https://doi.org/10.1016/s0306-4522(97)00436-3

Vaglenova J, Birru S, Pandiella NM, Breese CR (2004) An assessment of the long-term developmental and behavioral teratogenicity of prenatal nicotine exposure. Behav Brain Res 150(1–2):159–170. https://doi.org/10.1016/j.bbr.2003.07.005

Varlinskaya EI, Mooney SM (2014) Acute exposure to ethanol on gestational day 15 affects social motivation of female offspring. Behav Brain Res 261:106–109. https://doi.org/10.1016/j.bbr.2013.12.016

Vilcassim MJR, Stowe S, Majumder R, Subramaniam A, Sinkey RG (2023) Electronic cigarette use during pregnancy: is it harmful? Toxics 11(3). https://doi.org/10.3390/toxics11030278

Villarreal DM, Derrick B, Vathy I (2008) Prenatal morphine exposure attenuates the maintenance of late LTP in lateral perforant path projections to the dentate gyrus and the CA3 region in vivo. J Neurophysiol 99(3): 1235–1242. https://doi.org/10.1152/jn.00981.2007

Vishnubhotla RV, Ahmad ST, Zhao Y, Radhakrishnan R (2024) Impact of prenatal marijuana exposure on adolescent brain structural and functional connectivity and behavioural outcomes. Brain Commun 6(2):fcae001. https://doi.org/10.1093/braincomms/fcae001

Volkow ND, Han B, Compton WM, McCance-Katz EF (2019) Self-reported medical and nonmedical cannabis use among pregnant women in the United States. JAMA 322(2):167–169. https://doi.org/10.1001/jama.2019.7982

Wadman E, Fernandes E, Muss C, Powell-Hamilton N, Wojcik MH, Madden JA et al (2023) A novel syndrome associated with prenatal fentanyl exposure. Genet Med Open 1(1):100834. https://doi.org/10.1016/j.gimo.2023.100834

Walf AA, Frye CA (2007) The use of the elevated plus maze as an assay of anxiety-related behavior in rodents. Nat Protoc 2(2):322–328. https://doi.org/10.1038/nprot.2007.44

Wang X, Dow-Edwards D, Anderson V, Minkoff H, Hurd YL (2004) In utero marijuana exposure associated with abnormal amygdala dopamine D2 gene expression in the human fetus. Biol Psychiatry 56(12):909–915. https://doi.org/10.1016/j.biopsych.2004.10.015

Wang X, Dow-Edwards D, Anderson V, Minkoff H, Hurd YL (2006) Discrete opioid gene expression impairment in the human fetal brain associated with maternal marijuana use. Pharmacogenomics J 6(4):255–264. https://doi.org/10.1038/sj.tpj.6500375

Wang H, Davila-Garcia MI, Yarl W, Gondre-Lewis MC (2011) Gestational nicotine exposure regulates expression of AMPA and NMDA receptors and their signaling apparatus in developing and adult rat hippocampus. Neuroscience 188:168–181. https://doi.org/10.1016/j.neuroscience.2011.04.069

Wang B, Chen J, Sheng Z, Lian W, Wu Y, Liu M (2022) Embryonic exposure to fentanyl induces behavioral changes and neurotoxicity in zebrafish larvae. PeerJ 10:e14524. https://doi.org/10.7717/peerj.14524

Wanner NM, Colwell M, Drown C, Faulk C (2021) Developmental cannabidiol exposure increases anxiety and modifies genome-wide brain DNA methylation in adult female mice. Clin Epigenetics 13(1):4. https://doi.org/10.1186/s13148-020-00993-4

Weisbeck SJ, Bright KS, Ginn CS, Smith JM, Hayden KA, Ringham C (2021) Perceptions about cannabis use during pregnancy: a rapid best-framework qualitative synthesis. Can J Public Health 112(1):49–59. https://doi.org/10.17269/s41997-020-00346-x

Wells AC, Lotfipour S (2023) Prenatal nicotine exposure during pregnancy results in adverse neurodevelopmental alterations and neurobehavioral deficits. Adv Drug Alcohol Res 3:11628. https://doi.org/10.3389/adar.2023.11628

Westfall RE, Janssen PA, Lucas P, Capler R (2006) Survey of medicinal cannabis use among childbearing women: patterns of its use in pregnancy and retroactive self-assessment of its efficacy against 'morning sickness'. Complement Ther Clin Pract 12(1):27–33. https://doi.org/10.1016/j.ctcp.2005.09.006

Wieczorek L, Fish EW, O'Leary-Moore SK, Parnell SE, Sulik KK (2015) Hypothalamic-pituitary-adrenal axis and behavioral dysfunction following early binge-like prenatal alcohol exposure in mice. Alcohol 49(3): 207–217. https://doi.org/10.1016/j.alcohol.2015.01.005

Wilcoxon JS, Kuo AG, Disterhoft JF, Redei EE (2005) Behavioral deficits associated with fetal alcohol exposure are reversed by prenatal thyroid hormone treatment: a role for maternal thyroid hormone deficiency in FAE. Mol Psychiatry 10(10):961–971. https://doi.org/10.1038/sj.mp.4001694

Willford JA, Kaufman JM (2024) Through a teratological lens: a narrative review of exposure to stress and drugs of abuse during pregnancy on neurodevelopment. Neurotoxicol Teratol 105:107384. https://doi.org/10.1016/j.ntt.2024.107384

Winchester SE, Diaz MR (2025) Moderate prenatal alcohol exposure alters GABAergic transmission and the actions of acute alcohol in the medial central amygdala of adolescent rats. Neuropharmacology 266:110283. https://doi.org/10.1016/j.neuropharm.2024.110283

Wu CC, Hung CJ, Shen CH, Chen WY, Chang CY, Pan HC et al (2014) Prenatal buprenorphine exposure decreases neurogenesis in rats. Toxicol Lett 225(1): 92–101. https://doi.org/10.1016/j.toxlet.2013.12.001

Wu CC, Hung CJ, Lin SY, Wang YY, Chang CY, Chen WY et al (2017) Treadmill exercise alleviated prenatal buprenorphine exposure-induced depression in rats. Neurochem Int 110:91–100. https://doi.org/10.1016/j.neuint.2017.09.012

Xiao L, Kish VL, Benders KM, Wu ZX (2016) Prenatal and early postnatal exposure to cigarette smoke decreases BDNF/TrkB signaling and increases abnormal behaviors later in life. Int J Neuropsychopharmacol 19(5). https://doi.org/10.1093/ijnp/pyv117

Yang SN, Yang JM, Wu JN, Kao YH, Hsieh WY, Chao CC, Tao PL (2000) Prenatal exposure to morphine alters kinetic properties of NMDA receptor-mediated synaptic currents in the hippocampus of rat offspring. Hippocampus 10(6):654–662. https://doi.org/10.1002/1098-1063(2000)10:6<654::AID-HIPO1003>3.0.CO;2-T

Yang SN, Huang LT, Wang CL, Chen WF, Yang CH, Lin SZ et al (2003) Prenatal administration of morphine decreases CREBSerine-133 phosphorylation and synaptic plasticity range mediated by glutamatergic transmission in the hippocampal CA1 area of cognitive-deficient rat offspring. Hippocampus 13(8): 915–921. https://doi.org/10.1002/hipo.10137

Yankelevitch-Yahav R, Franko M, Huly A, Doron R (2015) The forced swim test as a model of depressive-like behavior. J Vis Exp 97. https://doi.org/10.3791/52587

Yazdy MM, Desai RJ, Brogly SB (2015) Prescription opioids in pregnancy and birth outcomes: a review of the literature. J Pediatr Genet 4(2):56–70. https://doi.org/10.1055/s-0035-1556740

Yeoh SL, Eastwood J, Wright IM, Morton R, Melhuish E, Ward M, Oei JL (2019) Cognitive and motor outcomes of children with prenatal opioid exposure: a systematic review and meta-analysis. JAMA Netw Open 2(7): e197025. https://doi.org/10.1001/jamanetworkopen.2019.7025

Young-Wolff KC, Tucker LY, Alexeeff S, Armstrong MA, Conway A, Weisner C, Goler N (2017) Trends in self-reported and biochemically tested marijuana use among pregnant females in California from 2009-2016. JAMA 318(24):2490–2491. https://doi.org/10.1001/jama.2017.17225

Yu Y, Shi Z, Xu D, Li Y, Qin J, Zhang Z, Wang H (2020) Prenatal ethanol exposure increases susceptibility to depression- and anxiety-like behavior in adult female offspring and its underlying mechanism. Reprod Toxicol 96:36–46. https://doi.org/10.1016/j.reprotox.2020.05.015

Yuan Q, Rubic M, Seah J, Rae C, Wright IM, Kaltenbach K et al (2014) Do maternal opioids reduce neonatal regional brain volumes? A pilot study. J Perinatol 34(12):909–913. https://doi.org/10.1038/jp.2014.111

Zafar H, Shelat SG, Redei E, Tejani-Butt S (2000) Fetal alcohol exposure alters serotonin transporter sites in rat brain. Brain Res 856(1–2):184–192. https://doi.org/10.1016/s0006-8993(99)02350-1

Zhang C, Fan SJ, Sun AB, Liu ZZ, Liu L (2019) Prenatal nicotine exposure induces depression-like behavior in adolescent female rats via modulating neurosteroid in the hippocampus. Mol Med Rep 19(5):4185–4194. https://doi.org/10.3892/mmr.2019.10105

Zhang X, Liu Y, Li J, Li B, Yang X, Sun Q et al (2022) Prenatal Alcohol exposure and the risk of depression in offspring: a meta-analysis. Int J Clin Pract 2022: 5458611. https://doi.org/10.1155/2022/5458611

Zhou R, Wang S, Zhu X (2010) Prenatal ethanol exposure attenuates GABAergic inhibition in basolateral amygdala leading to neuronal hyperexcitability and anxiety-like behavior of adult rat offspring. Neuroscience 170(3):749–757. https://doi.org/10.1016/j.neuroscience.2010.07.055

Zhu J, Zhang X, Xu Y, Spencer TJ, Biederman J, Bhide PG (2012) Prenatal nicotine exposure mouse model showing hyperactivity, reduced cingulate cortex volume, reduced dopamine turnover, and responsiveness to oral methylphenidate treatment. J Neurosci 32(27): 9410–9418. https://doi.org/10.1523/JNEUROSCI.1041-12.2012

Zoli M, Le Novere N, Hill JA Jr, Changeux JP (1995) Developmental regulation of nicotinic ACh receptor subunit mRNAs in the rat central and peripheral nervous systems. J Neurosci 15(3 Pt 1):1912–1939. https://doi.org/10.1523/JNEUROSCI.15-03-01912.1995

Zou R, Boer OD, Felix JF, Muetzel RL, Franken IHA, Cecil CAM, El Marroun H (2022) Association of maternal tobacco use during pregnancy with preadolescent brain morphology among offspring. JAMA Netw Open 5(8):e2224701. https://doi.org/10.1001/jamanetworkopen.2022.24701

Impact of Prenatal Alcohol Exposure on Cerebral Cortex Development

6

L. Oskera, M. Charlet-Briart, S. Tielens, L. Nguyen, and S. Laguesse

Abstract

Fetal alcohol spectrum disorders (FASD) represent a significant global health concern and are the leading cause of preventable birth defects, intellectual disabilities, and persistent behavioral deficits. The neurodevelopmental mechanisms underlying FASD are not yet fully understood, but there is growing interest in the role of cortical development in the manifestation of these disorders. The cerebral cortex serves as the master regulator of higher-order functions, including sensory perception, motor planning, decision-making, and general intelligence—processes that are all adversely affected by prenatal alcohol exposure (PAE). Higher-level functions emerge from a complex and intricately interconnected neuronal network that develops through a series of delicate and sequential stages involving neuronal and glial cell generation, proliferation, migration, differentiation, and maturation. Recent evidence suggests that PAE disrupts these developmental processes, leading to impaired cortical structure, altered connectivity, and ultimately, to the neurobehavioral deficits observed in individuals with FASD. Rodent models, along with *in vitro* approaches, have proven invaluable for elucidating the consequences of PAE on cortical development and the underlying mechanisms associated with PAE-related disorders. Although gaps in knowledge remain, advancing our understanding of the neurodevelopmental basis of FASD is essential for identifying potential therapeutic targets and enhancing early intervention strategies for those affected by FASD in the future.

Keywords

Prenatal alcohol exposure · Cerebral cortex · Fetal alcohol spectrum disorders

6.1 Introduction

Prenatal alcohol exposure (PAE)-associated defects were first recognized by the medical community in 1973 and introduced under the term "Fetal Alcohol Syndrome (FAS)" (Jones and Smith 1973). Over the years, the definition of FAS has evolved to include a broader range of alcohol-related disorders, now commonly referred to as "Fetal Alcohol Spectrum Disorders (FASD)" (Mattson et al. 2011). Today, PAE is a major public health concern, as FASD is the

L. Oskera · M. Charlet-Briart · S. Tielens · L. Nguyen · S. Laguesse (✉)
Laboratory of Molecular Regulation of Neurogenesis, GIGA Institute, University of Liège, Liège, Belgium
e-mail: slaguesse@uliege.be

A. N. Bukiya, D. W. Ali (eds.), *Molecular Mechanisms and Lifelong Consequences of Prenatal Exposure to Psychoactive Substances*, Advances in Experimental Medicine and Biology 1500,
https://doi.org/10.1007/978-3-032-12741-9_6

leading cause of preventable birth defects, intellectual disabilities and developmental disorders (Alcoholism 2023). Despite the well-established harmful effects of alcohol on the brain, alcohol remains the most commonly used recreational drug and is widely socially accepted. A recent report indicated that approximately 10% of women worldwide acknowledge drinking alcohol during pregnancy, with rates ranging from 0.2% in the Eastern Mediterranean Region to 25.2% in the European Region (Popova et al. 2017). Among the 10% of pregnancies exposed to alcohol, one in every 13 results in FASD in childhood, leading to an estimated 0.7% of the global population being affected (Popova et al. 2017). The global economic burden of FASD is significant, with the annual costs of healthcare, social assistance, and special education for affected individuals estimated to range from $22,810 to $24,308 per year per person (Greenmyer et al. 2018). However, these figures likely represent a substantial underestimation due to widespread underdiagnosis, limited awareness and training among healthcare professionals, and the lack of universally accepted diagnostic guidelines encompassing the full spectrum of FASD (Popova and Dozet 2023). Although progress has been made over the past decade, a comprehensive understanding of the exact mechanisms underlying PAE-related brain alterations remains essential.

During embryogenesis, the brain undergoes complex developmental processes that lay the foundation for cognitive, intellectual and behavioral abilities. These key developmental stages make the brain particularly vulnerable to alcohol exposure, with the cerebral cortex being among the most affected structures (Donald et al. 2015). Following maternal consumption, alcohol easily crosses the placenta and reaches the developing fetus which has a very limited ability to metabolize it (Burd et al. 2012). During development, the cerebral cortex undergoes highly regulated, sequential stages of neuronal generation, proliferation, migration, differentiation, and maturation, which are essential for establishing its complex and interconnected neuronal network (Agirman et al. 2017). PAE can affect cortical development throughout the entire duration of pregnancy (Williams and Smith 2015). Animal models and neuroimaging studies in humans have provided valuable insights into the structural and functional consequences of PAE, highlighting disruptions in key neurodevelopmental pathways. The cortical abnormalities observed in individuals with PAE include impairments in neuronal proliferation, migration, and differentiation, leading to altered cortical thickness, impaired connectivity, and cognitive deficits. However, the precise pathophysiological mechanisms underlying these anomalies during cortical development remain poorly understood. In this chapter, we aim to provide a comprehensive understanding of how prenatal alcohol exposure shapes cortical architecture.

6.2 Cerebral Cortex Development in Health

The cerebral cortex is one of the most complex and evolved structures in the brain, comprising 16 billion neurons that communicate within a vast, intricate, and highly interconnected network. It serves as the primary hub for higher-order cognitive functions, including consciousness, sensory perception, decision-making, communication, language, memory, and motor planning (Cadwell et al. 2019). The cerebral cortex is subdivided into distinct functional areas and is mainly organized into six horizontal layers: layer I, supragranular layer II/III, granular layer IV, and infragranular layers V and VI—with layer I being the most superficial one. This organization is broadly conserved across mammalian species and cortical regions (Cadwell et al. 2019). At the cellular level, the cortex is composed of a huge diversity of neurons and glial cells that are precisely distributed across these layers. Neuronal populations are broadly categorized into glutamatergic excitatory neurons (~70–80%), which establish long-range connections, and GABAergic inhibitory neurons (~20–30%), which predominantly form local circuits. To date, over fifty subtypes of projection neurons and more than 20 subtypes of interneurons have been identified (reviewed in Greig et al. 2013; Lim et al. 2018). Understanding how these neuronal populations emerge, differentiate, and integrate to support complex human behaviors remains a major focus of neuroscience research (Villalba et al. 2021).

6.2.1 Projection Neurons

6.2.1.1 Generation

Cortical projection neurons (PN) originate from neural progenitors localized in the dorsal telencephalon within the proliferative zones lining the lateral ventricles, known as ventricular (VZ) and subventricular zones (SVZ) (Greig et al. 2013). Three main types of progenitors contribute to neurogenesis: neuroepithelial cells (NECs), radial glial cells (RGCs—also called apical progenitors (APs)) and intermediate progenitors (IPs). Before the onset of neurogenesis, neuroepithelial cells (NECs) form a pseudostratified epithelial layer that constitutes the VZ and undergo symmetrical divisions to expand the progenitor pool. After few cycles of cell divisions, NECs transition into radial glial cells (RGC) (Villalba et al. 2021). This transition involves remodelling of epithelial features, including downregulation of tight junctions (Aaku-Saraste et al. 1996). RGCs first divide symmetrically to amplify their pool and, as neurogenesis begins—around embryonic day (E) 10.5 in mice and gestational week (GW) 5 in humans—start to divide asymmetrically to generate one RGC and either a neuron or a third type of cortical progenitors called intermediate progenitors (IPs). IPs are initially generated in the apical VZ and migrate basally to the SVZ, where they mostly divide asymmetrically to produce a pair of neurons (Villalba et al. 2021). NECs and RGCs exhibit apico-basal polarity, extending processes from the ventricular surface to the pial surface, enabling interkinetic nuclear migration (INM) and apical mitosis (Takahashi et al. 1993; Taverna and Huttner 2010). In contrast, IPs exhibit multipolar morphology and divide basally within the SVZ (Haubensak et al. 2004) (Fig. 6.1a). The generation of neurons directly from RGCs is called direct neurogenesis and produces all major projection neuron classes, while the production of neurons from IPs is called indirect neurogenesis and amplifies and diversifies each class of PN (Huilgol et al. 2023; Laguesse et al. 2015). Indirect neurogenesis represents the predominant mode of cortical neurons generation in mammals, producing approximately 80% of projection neurons (Villalba et al. 2021). Cortical neurogenesis concludes around E18.5 in mice and GW20 in humans.

Importantly, additional progenitor cell types have been described in the developing cerebral cortex, such as apical Short Neural Precursors (SNPs), Subapical Progenitors (SAPs), and Basal Radial Glial Cells (bRGCs) (Arai and Taverna 2017). While some of these progenitors are sparse and mostly neurogenic in rodents (i.e., SAPs and bRGCs), they are more diverse and abundant in humans, contributing to the increased cortical thickness and complexity associated with advanced cognitive functions (Arai and Taverna 2017).

6.2.1.2 Migration of Projection Neurons

Following neurogenesis, post-mitotic projection neurons migrate radially from the proliferative zones to settle into the cortical plate (CP). Neuronal migration takes place between E11 and E17 in mice and GW9 to GW20 in humans (Fig. 6.1a) (Cadwell et al. 2019). Projection neurons migrate in an inside-out manner, meaning that early born neurons occupy deeper layers and later-born neurons settle in more superficial layers (Takahashi et al. 1999). Around E11 in rodents, the first wave of neurons forms the transient preplate (PP), which is later split into the superficial marginal zone (MZ) and the deeper subplate (SP) as subsequent neuronal cohorts migrate and establish the different layers of the CP (Saito et al. 2019). The regulation of migration is orchestrated by a balanced interplay between cell-autonomous and cell non-autonomous mechanisms (reviewed in Hansen and Hippenmeyer 2020).

Radial migration of projection neurons is a multistep process which can be divided into two distinct modes: somal translocation and glia-guided locomotion (Nadarajah et al. 2001).

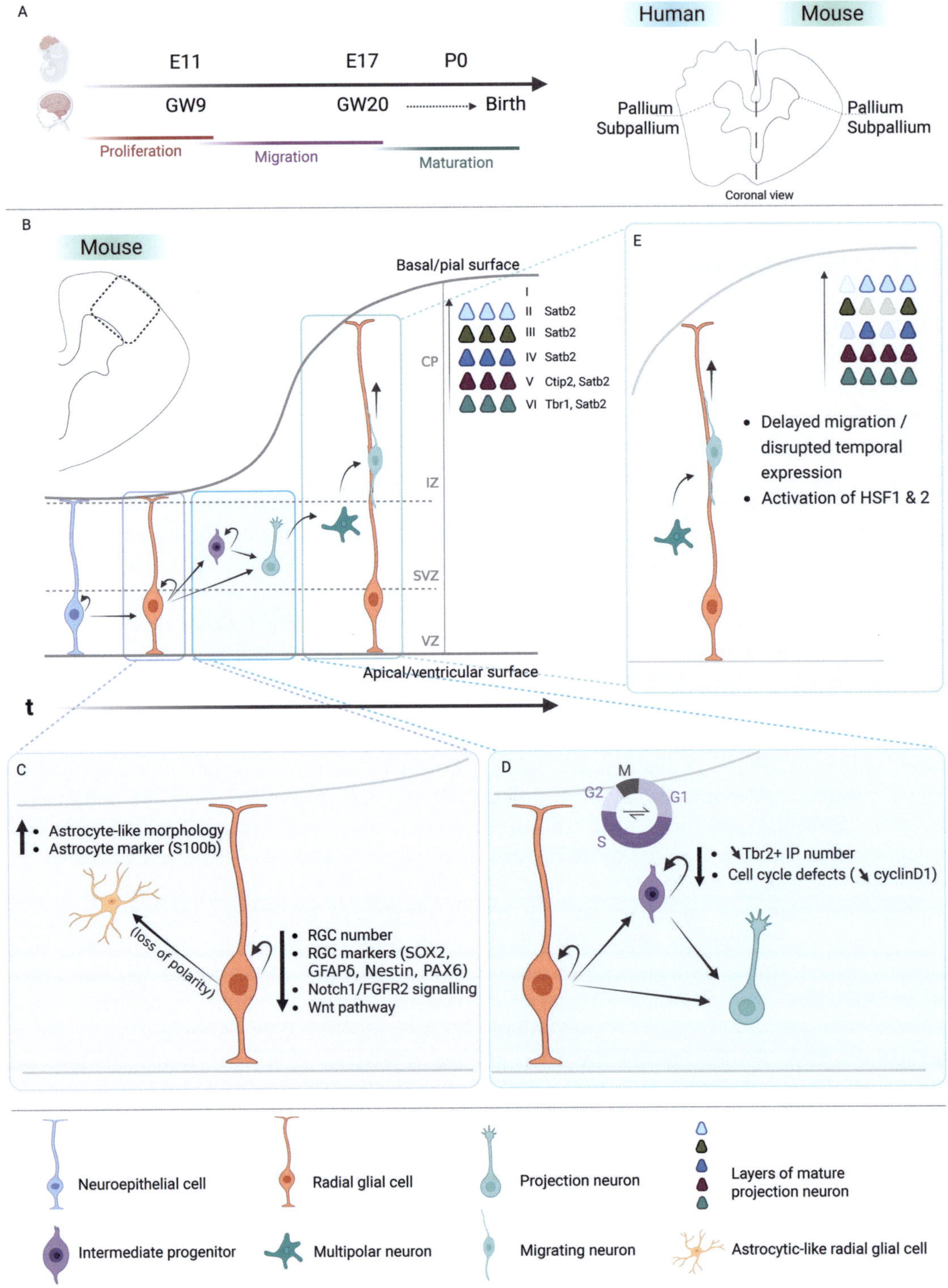

Fig. 6.1 Overview of PAE-induced defects in projection neuron generation and migration during cortical development. (**a**) Scheme depicting the developmental timeline of corticogenesis in mouse and human brain. (**b**) Cortical development in the dorsal telencephalon in mice. During early embryogenesis, NECs mostly divide symmetrically to expand the pool of progenitors in the VZ. As corticogenesis proceeds, they differentiate into RGCs, which divide either symmetrically to amplify their pool or asymmetrically to generate neurons or IPs. IPs

During early corticogenesis, when the cortical wall is relatively thin, neurons migrate via somal translocation. At that time, newborn neurons located in the VZ extend a long, radially oriented leading process toward the pial surface and pull their soma upward by progressively shortening their basal process attached to the pial surface (Nadarajah et al. 2001). At later stages of corticogenesis, when the cortical wall thickens and migration distance increases, neurons switch to a locomotion mode in which they migrate in a glia-guided manner (Nadarajah et al. 2001; Rakic 1972). Once generated in the proliferative zone, newborn bipolar-shaped neurons move toward the SVZ and lower IZ, where they undergo a bipolar-to-multipolar transition. These multipolar-shaped neurons dynamically extend and retract their processes in response to directional cues in their environment, frequently changing migration direction over short distances (Tabata and Nakajima 2003). Upon sensing appropriate environmental cues, they undergo a multipolar-to-bipolar transition, which establishes their polarization. Neurons extend an axonal-like trailing process toward the ventricular surface and a pial-oriented leading process before exiting the IZ to adhere to radial glia fibers, initiating glia-guided radial migration (Fig. 6.1b). The locomotion of projection neurons along glia fibers follows a saltatory pattern, involving cell adhesion molecules and dynamic cytoskeletal remodeling (Noctor et al. 2004; Borrell 2019). For a detailed explanation of the mechanisms underlying neuronal migration, please refer to (Stoufflet et al. 2023; Silva et al. 2018; Heng et al. 2010).

6.2.1.3 Projection Neurons Maturation

Cortical projection neurons form together with interneurons an extensive interconnected network that underlies higher-order functions. Neuronal networks underlying cortical functions are established through neuronal arborization, as neurons are structurally and functionally polarized, defined by two distinct compartments, the axon and dendrites. These structures enable proper information transmission in the brain through synapses, with dendrites receiving neuronal inputs and axons projecting to distal targets. During late embryogenesis and the early postnatal period in mice, dendrites and axons develop through elongation, branching, pathfinding, and synaptic connections (Hasegawa and Kuwako 2022). Once neurons have reached their final position, dendritic outgrowth begins, a shift regulated by the reduction of Sox11 expression (Hoshiba et al. 2016). During this process, projection neurons extend short basal dendrites mostly restricted to the same layer as their soma, while apical dendrites extend across multiple layers toward the pial surface, where they branch extensively (McFarlane 2000). In parallel, after axon specification during neuronal migration, axonal elongation continues at its distal tip, the neuronal growth cone. Dendritic and axonal outgrowth are finely regulated by intrinsic and extrinsic factors, including transcription factors, neurotrophins, cytoskeletal element, cell surface receptors (e.g., Reelin, Notch), secreted factors (e.g., Semaphorins, Wnt family) and cell adhesion molecules (reviewed in Ma and Tymanskyj 2020; Arikkath 2012).

Fig. 6.1 (continued) predominantly undergo neurogenic symmetric divisions in the SVZ. Newborn neurons begin migration along radial glia fibers to reach the CP, following an inside-out pattern. At the end of corticogenesis, RGCs transition to gliogenesis and differentiate into astrocytes. (**c**) PAE decreases RGC proliferation and may promote their differentiation into astrocytes. Reduced RGC proliferative activity leads to a decrease in RGC number, and both Notch1/FGFR2 and Wnt signaling may be involved. (**d**) PAE also decreases IP proliferation by disturbing cell cycle dynamics. PAE reduces CyclinD1 expression specifically in Tbr2+ IPs, suggesting either premature cell cycle exit or delayed cellular growth. (**e**) PAE delays the generation and migration of cPN with more pronounced effects on later-born neurons. *NEC* neuroepithelial cell, *RGC* radial glial cell, *IP* intermediate progenitor, *VZ* ventricular zone, *SVZ* subventricular zone, *cPN* cortical projection neuron, *FGFR2* fibroblast growth factor receptor 2, *Tbr2* T-box brain gene 2

Projection neurons are subdivided in distinct classes based on their axonal targets, molecular identity and laminar location. Classically, three main classes are distinguished. The corticothalamic (CT) neurons—localized in layer VI—project ipsilaterally to the thalamus and express the transcription factor T-Box Brain Transcription Factor 1 (TBR1). The Pyramidal tract (PT) neurons—enriched in layer V—connect to the spinal cord, the ipsilateral cortex, and some subcortical structures (i.e., thalamus, striatum, and midbrain), and express COUP-TF-interacting protein 2 (CTIP2) and FEZ Family Zinc Finger 2 (FEZF2). The last class consists in IntraTelencephalic (IT) neurons—located in layers II–VI—which establish connections with the neocortex, striatum and corticoid structures (e.g., amygdala and claustrum), and express Special AT-rich sequence-binding protein 2 (Satb2) (Fig. 6.1b) (Kamigaki 2019). These neuronal populations cross the midline, primarily through the corpus callosum (CC) and, to a lesser extent, the anterior commissure. The establishment of axonal projections follows a temporally regulated pattern, mirroring the inside-out gradient of cortex layering (Greig et al. 2013; Harris and Shepherd 2015; Di Bella et al. 2024; Pal et al. 2024).

6.2.2 Interneurons

6.2.2.1 Interneuron Generation

Interneurons are derived from the proliferative zone of the ventral subpallium in the telencephalon. The majority (~60%) of cortical interneurons originate from the medial ganglionic eminence (MGE), while others arise from the caudal ganglionic eminence (CGE) and the preoptic area (POA) (Lim et al. 2018; Llorca and Deogracias 2022). Interneurons can be classified into dozens of cortical interneuron subtypes based on the expression of different transcripts, such as somatostatin (SST), parvalbumin (PV), vasointestinal peptide (VIP), and 5-Hydroxytryptamine Receptor 3A (5HT3aR) (Mayer et al. 2018; Yu et al. 2021). Interestingly, recent evidence suggests that the lateral ganglionic eminence (LGE) and cortical progenitors could also give rise to cortical interneurons in the human fetal brain, providing new insights into the origins of cortical interneurons diversity (Delgado et al. 2022; Feng et al. 2025). The specification of GABAergic interneurons relies on a regulatory network of transcription factors expressed by progenitors, including Distal-less homeobox 1 and 2 (Dlx1, Dlx2), Achaete-scute homolog 1 (Ascl1), and Glycogen synthase kinase 1 and 2 (Gsk1, Gsx2) (Long et al. 2009; Wang et al. 2013). Following the expression of this core set of genes, interneurons diversification is initiated.

A long-debated question is whether cortical interneuron diversity is acquired at the original sites during progenitor states or after migration in response to local environment. Recent single-cell and single-nuclei sequencing studies have shed light on this question, showing that part of this diversity already emerges at precursor stages, directly after cells become postmitotic (Mayer et al. 2018; Mi et al. 2018; Bandler et al. 2022). Indeed, these studies report distinct transcriptional signatures between the CGE, medial and dorsal MGE as well as between apical and intermediate progenitors (Mayer et al. 2018; Feng et al. 2025; Li et al. 2022). Transcriptional signature diversity increases during development, leading to temporally and spatially regulated generation of a diverse array of interneurons that later populate the cortex (Mayer et al. 2018; Butt et al. 2005). Beyond these intrinsically encoded diversities, additional layers of transcriptional heterogeneity arise in response to interactions between migrating cortical interneurons and the environment of their distant destinations (Quattrocolo et al. 2017). Together, these findings suggest a model in which genetic identity and GABAergic cell fate are partly defined at the progenitor level and expand during development through a combination of intrinsic and extrinsic mechanisms.

6.2.2.2 Interneuron Migration

Around E12-13, newly postmitotic cortical interneurons leave the proliferative zone in response to repulsive guidance cues expressed in the VZ and SVZ, initiating their tangential migration toward the cortex (Zhu et al. 1999; Marín and Rubenstein 2001). Interneurons migrate to the pallium along two primary migratory streams: a superficial migratory stream (SMS) bordering the MZ and a deep migratory stream (DMS) within the SVZ, running around the presumptive striatum. Around E15-16, interneurons form a third migratory stream, which borders the SP between the SMS and DMS (Toudji et al. 2023). The confinement of interneurons to these migratory routes depends on the chemokine C-X-C Motif Chemokine Ligand 12 (Cxcl12), which is expressed by cells located along the streams (Lepiemme et al. 2022). While interneurons do not appear to distribute randomly across these migratory paths, it remains unclear whether this distribution is dictated by their pre-established identity or local environmental cues.

At the cellular level, newly generated interneurons are highly polarized, characterized by a leading and trailing process. Their tangential migration follows a cyclic process consisting of three steps, during which interneurons change morphology in a saltatory fashion through dynamic cytoskeleton remodeling (Toudji et al. 2023; Tielens et al. 2016). First, they elongate their leading process and extend branches in response to surrounding environmental cues until a branch stabilizes in a specific direction. Next, a centrosome- and Golgi-containing cytoplasmic swelling forms at the leading process, followed by nucleokinesis. Finally, interneurons retract their trailing process (Lepiemme et al. 2022; Bellion et al. 2005). Proper tangential migration depends on the balanced interplay of numerous extrinsic and intrinsic factors, including chemokines, ephrins (Eph), semaphorins (Sema), transcription factors, cytoskeletal elements and RhoGTPases (reviewed in Silva et al. 2018; Toudji et al. 2023). For example, the repulsive cues Sema3A/3F and EphA3, expressed in cells of the presumptive striatum, bind to Neuropilin 1/2 (Nrp1/2) and EphA4 on interneurons, respectively, preventing them from entering that region and guiding their migration towards the developing cortex (Marín et al. 2001; Rudolph et al. 2010).

In addition, blood vessels provide a key source of guidance cues and serves as scaffold for migrating interneurons due to the spatial proximity of developing vascular networks to the migratory streams. Interneuron migration along blood vessels peropheries enriched in Cxcl12 is regulated by ventral oligodendrocytes precursors cells (OPCs) which prevent interneurons from aggregating onto blood vessels through a mechanism known as unilateral contact repulsion (UCoRe) (Stoufflet et al. 2023; Lepiemme et al. 2022).

Once interneurons reach the developing cortex, they switch from tangential to radial migration, moving toward their appropriate cortical layer. This transition is regulated by the loss of responsiveness to Cxcl12 and the expression of the chemoattractant Neuregulin-3 (Nrg3) by cortical projection neurons (Bartolini et al. 2017). After settling into their designated cortical layers during the first postnatal weeks, interneurons terminate migration, influenced by the upregulation of Potassium Chloride Cotransporter 2 (KCC2) and other molecular cues (Bortone and Polleux 2009; Zavalin et al. 2022).

6.2.2.3 Interneuron Specification

For a long time, the classification of cortical interneurons was based on their molecular, electrophysiological and morphological features. The classical view distinguishes three cardinal types of interneurons: PV+, SST+, and 5HT3aR + interneurons. PV+ interneurons form the largest class and include chandelier cells, basket cells, and translaminar interneurons. These fast-spiking neurons are distributed across all cortical layers and predominantly target proximal dendrites. SST+ interneurons include Martinotti and non-Martinotti cells, which are abundant in layers V–VI and preferentially target dendrites. 5HT3aR + interneurons comprise a more heterogenous group and can be further subdivided into disinhibitory VIP+ interneurons (e.g., CR+ bipolar and CCK+ multipolar cells), CCK+/VIP- basket cells, neurogliaform cells, and single-bouquet cells. 5HT3aR+ interneurons are abundantly located in supragranular layers and account for approximately 30% of all cortical interneurons (reviewed in Lim et al. 2018). Recent transcriptomic studies have challenged this classical classification, relying instead on whole-cell transcriptome analysis to identify and categorize interneurons. These studies classify cortical GABAergic cells into five cardinal types: PV+, SST+, VIP+, Lamp5 (5HT3aR+/VIP-), and Sncg (VIP+/CCK+) cells (Tasic et al. 2018; Gouwens et al. 2020; Paul et al. 2017). These five classes are further subdivided into several dozens' GABAergic transcriptomic types, and emerging in-depth analysis are beginning to correlate these transcriptionally defined classes with distinct electrophysiological, morphological, and synaptic connectivity properties. Notably, Paul et al. identified transcriptional signatures within these cardinal GABAergic types that encode synaptic communication pattern and physiological input–output connectivity (Paul et al. 2017). This transcriptomic framework consists of six functional categories: cell-adhesion molecules, neurotransmitters, and modulators receptors, voltage-gated ion channels, regulatory signaling proteins, neuropeptides, vesicle release machinery, and transcription factors (Paul et al. 2017). In addition, Gouwens et al. identified 60 GABAergic transcriptomic types in the mouse visual cortex, each belonging to one of the five cardinal classes (Gouwens et al. 2020). Among these, they defined 28 morphoelectric and transcriptomic types, which exhibit congruent morphological, electrophysiological, and transcriptomic properties and are distinguished by their layer-specific axonal innervation profiles (Gouwens et al. 2020).

6.2.2.4 Integration of Projection Neurons and Interneurons in Cortical Circuits

After migrating toward the cortex, interneurons integrate into their respective cortical layers. This laminar allocation is partially dependent on specific guidance cues secreted by already integrated projection neurons as well as other populations of cortical interneurons. It is believed that cortical projection neurons specifically attract interneurons that would typically target them (Limoni et al. 2021; Lodato et al. 2011). Resident projection neurons also play a crucial role in the proper settling of interneurons into cortical circuits by modulating their number within cortical layers.

Between the end of the first postnatal week and the second postnatal week, more than 30% of GABAergic cells undergo programmed cell death across the entire mouse cerebral cortex (Southwell et al. 2012). This extensive apoptosis affects all interneuron classes and appears to be neuronal activity-dependent (Priya et al. 2018; Denaxa et al. 2018; Wong et al. 2018). Notably, programmed cell death occurs when interneurons begin integrating into nascent cortical circuits, suggesting that interneuron excitability, driven by neuronal inputs from projection neurons, is a key factor in this process (Wong et al. 2018). Interestingly, the rate of neuronal apoptosis is not uniform across neocortical areas (Blanquie et al. 2017), which may explain regional differences in the density of specific interneuron subtypes and inhibitory connectivity patterns. These regional variations could contribute to the functional specialization of different cortical areas.

Once interneurons are properly integrated into cortical layers, they become essential for the maturation of brain circuits. This creates a dynamic interplay between cortical interneurons and projection neurons, which underpins cortical processing. Early in development, interneurons primarily regulate the formation of synaptic connections and the establishment of functional patterns within projection neuron networks (Le Magueresse and Monyer 2013; Douglas and Martin 2004). For example, feedforward inhibition is essential for the proper integration of thalamocortical inputs involved in sensory information processing. In the mature brain, thalamic inputs densely innervate layer IV PV+ interneurons, which in turn target projection neurons to fine-tune responses following sensory information integration (Le Magueresse and Monyer 2013; Douglas and Martin 2004). However, the connectivity of layer IV PV+ interneurons is not fully developed during the first postnatal weeks (Chittajallu and Isaac 2010). During this period, layer V SST+

interneurons bridge the gap by receiving transient thalamic inputs and innervating deep layer projection neurons as well as immature PV+ interneurons (Marques-Smith et al. 2016). Thus, SST+ interneurons emerge as key players in the maturation of deep-layer intracortical circuits and sensory-evoked activity during early postnatal development.

As development progresses, the strength, timing, and specificity of interneuron-projection neuron interactions are refined through activity-dependent processes. In summary, the integration of projection neurons and interneurons within cortical circuits is critical for the precise regulation of neuronal activity and the proper functioning of the cortex. Projection neurons, which transmit signals over long distances within the brain, are crucial for cortical output and communication with other brain regions. In contrast, interneurons—through their local inhibitory functions—regulate the excitability of the cortical network by controlling the timing and balance of excitatory signals. This balance between excitation and inhibition is essential for maintaining the stability and flexibility of cortical circuits, ensuring processes such as sensory perception, motor coordination, and cognition (Harris and Shepherd 2015).

6.2.3 Glial Cells

Alongside the neuronal population, glial cells play an essential role in cortical development. Among them, astrocytes, oligodendrocytes, and microglia contribute to the formation and maintenance of cortical circuits, supporting neuronal development and ensuring proper cortical function throughout life.

6.2.3.1 Astrocytes

Astrocytes are the most abundant type of glial cells in the brain. In the mouse, they primarily originate from RGCs around E18, once RGCs lose their neurogenic potential (Clavreul et al. 2022). Astrocytes are generated through two pathways: direct gliogenesis, where RGCs directly differentiate into astrocyte precursors, and indirect gliogenesis, where RGCs first generate multipotent IPs, expressing markers such as Epidermal Growth Factor Receptor (EGFR), Oligodendrocyte transcription factor 2 (Olig2), Antigen Kiel 67 (MKI67) and Ascl1, which then differentiate into astrocytes (Li et al. 2021a). These precursors migrate to various cortical regions, where they establish their roles in supporting neuronal networks (Clarke and Barres 2013).

During development, astrocytes regulate neurites outgrowth and neuronal migration by secreting extracellular matrix proteins and trophic factors (Guizzetti et al. 2008). Once mature, astrocytes play a crucial role in maintaining the extracellular environment around synapses. They provide metabolic support to neurons, they maintain the blood-brain barrier and regulate cerebral blood flow, ensuring proper delivery of nutrients and waste removal. They also remove excess neurotransmitters, such as glutamate, preventing excitotoxicity. In adult cortical circuits, astrocytes sustain synaptic function, maintain homeostasis, and support plasticity in response to learning and environmental changes (reviewed in Kimelberg and Nedergaard 2010).

6.2.3.2 Oligodendrocytes

Oligodendrocytes are responsible for the formation of myelin in the central nervous system, while this function is dedicated to Schwann cells in the peripheral nervous system. Myelin is a lipid-rich substance that insulates neuronal axons and facilitates the rapid transmission of electrical signals (Simons and Nave 2015). Oligodendrocytes arise from oligodendrocyte progenitor cells (OPCs), which originate from NECs lining the ventricles, and to a lesser extent, from RGCs. OPCs are generated in waves following a highly regulated spatiotemporal pattern. In mice, the two first waves (at E12.5 and E15.5, respectively) originate in the ventral ganglionic eminences and migrate toward the cortex, while the third wave (around E21/P0) arises locally from the dorsal SVZ (van Tilborg et al. 2018). Although first wave OPCs are largely replaced postnatally, they play a crucial role in interneuron migration (Lepiemme et al. 2022; Kessaris et al.

2006). Oligodendrocytes continue myelinating axons into postnatal development and adulthood, facilitating efficient neuronal communication and cortical circuit function (Simons and Nave 2015).

6.2.3.3 Microglia

Microglia are the resident macrophages of the central nervous system. Unlike other glial cells, microglia originate from primitive macrophages in the yolk sac, which migrate into the neuroepithelium via the developing bloodstream around E9 in mice. These precursors then colonize the developing cortex and give rise to embryonic microglia (Ginhoux and Prinz 2015). In the adult brain, microglia can also arise from transdifferentiation of circulating monocytes under certain pathological conditions (Mildner et al. 2007). Microglia are highly dynamic cells, with motile processes that allow them to monitor the neural environment. In the developing brain, microglia are crucial for shaping neural circuits by continuously surveying synapses and other structures, helping prune excess synaptic connections and promoting neurite outgrowth through the production of numerous neuronal protective and trophic factors such as insulin-like growth factor 1 (IGF1) and brain-derived neurotrophic factor (BDNF) (Harry and Kraft 2012). Microglia also play a critical role in maintaining homeostasis of the developing cortex by phagocytizing neural progenitor cells, thus regulating the size of the neural precursor cells pool (Cunningham et al. 2013). As the cortex matures, microglia become more specialized in their functions, contributing to synaptic plasticity, immune surveillance and injury or infection responses.

Throughout development, glial cells are indispensable for the proper formation, maturation, and function of cortical circuits. Astrocytes, oligodendrocytes, and microglia work in concert with neurons to ensure that the network of connections in the cortex is both functional and adaptable. Astrocytes regulate the extracellular environment and support synaptic transmission, oligodendrocytes myelinate axons to ensure efficient signal propagation, and microglia refine the network by pruning excess synapses and maintaining homeostasis.

6.3 Impact of Prenatal Alcohol Exposure on Cerebral Cortex Development

FASD includes four main diagnostic categories: FAS, partial fetal alcohol syndrome (PFAS), alcohol-related neurodevelopmental disorder (ARND), and alcohol-related birth defects (ARBD). This classification is based on facial abnormalities (i.e., short palpebral fissures, a smooth philtrum, a thin upper vermillion border), prenatal and/or postnatal growth disturbance, and CNS deficiencies including abnormal brain growth and cognitive and neurobehavioral impairments (Alcoholism 2023; Riley et al. 2011). These neurological impairments encompass deficits in general intelligence, sensory perception, motor skills, attention, executive function (e.g., inhibition, problem solving, planning), working memory and verbal fluency (Mattson et al. 2019; Carr et al. 2010; Long et al. 2018). Children with FASD may also exhibit impairments in language, learning and memory, vision, and adaptive functioning. These defects are often associated with co-morbidities, such as mental health disorders, epileptic episodes, and sleep disturbances, which complicate their ability to live independently and integrate properly into society (Mattson et al. 2019). Importantly, the cerebral cortex plays a key role in these cognitive and neurobehavioral disabilities due to its fundamental involvement in higher-order functions. Although neuroimaging studies highlight the general consequences of prenatal alcohol exposure on cortical structure, connectivity and related cognitive behaviors, rodent models are invaluable for investigating the impact of PAE on neuronal generation, migration, and specification.

6.3.1 Consequences of PAE on Cortical Development: Generalities

6.3.1.1 Human Studies

Cortical anomalies associated with prenatal alcohol exposure (PAE) have been reported in numerous cross-sectional studies, including smaller total brain volume (Astley et al. 2009; Chen et al. 2012), reduced cortical surface area (Astley et al. 2009; Archibald et al. 2001), decreased cortical gyrification (De Guio et al. 2014; Infante et al. 2015; Hendrickson et al. 2017), variations in cortical thickness (Sowell et al. 2008; Yang et al. 2012; Rajaprakash et al. 2014; Zhou et al. 2011), reduced white matter integrity (Fryer et al. 2009) and altered functional connectivity (Little et al. 2018). While total brain volume is consistently reduced across all FASD cohorts and studies, findings on cortical thickness variations remain inconsistent. Some studies have reported thinner cortices in several frontal, temporal and parietal regions in children with FASD (Rajaprakash et al. 2014; Zhou et al. 2011), whereas others have described increased cortical thickness in the same regions (Sowell et al. 2008; Yang et al. 2012). Quantitative magnetic resonance imaging (MRI) has revealed more significant cortical thickness reductions in males than in females, particularly in some frontal, temporal and occipital regions (Chen et al. 2012; Treit et al. 2017). A longitudinal study further reported regional age-by-diagnosis differences in cortical thickness, volume and gyrification in FASD children aged between 6 and 17 (Hendrickson et al. 2018). These findings must be interpreted in the context of the physiological changes in cortical thickness occurring during childhood and adolescence. Indeed, changes in cortical grey matter volume across ages are physiologically characterized by a prolonged pattern of volume increases during early childhood, followed by consistent decreases until late adolescence, following a U-shaped variation pattern (Lebel et al. 2012). In children and adolescents with PAE, these changes were characterized by volume loss following a more liner decline in most cortical areas, suggesting reduced brain plasticity and premature pruning of neuronal connections (Lebel et al. 2012). Moreover, another study has shown an inverse correlation between the amount of alcohol consumed per occasion during pregnancy and cortical thickness (Robertson et al. 2016). Collectively, these findings suggest that variations in cortical development may be influenced by several factors such as sex, age, and the severity of PAE.

In terms of functional connectivity, global abnormalities have been reported in children with FASD, particularly within cognition- and attention-related brain networks (Wozniak et al. 2013; Sundermann et al. 2023). Resting-state functional MRI studies have shown reduced intra-cortical connectivity in different cortical regions (Fan et al. 2017; Ware et al. 2021), including within prefrontal tracts (Aghamohammadi-Sereshki et al. 2025), as well as reduced inter-cortical connectivity, particularly within the frontal-parietal (Little et al. 2018) and sensorimotor networks (Long et al. 2018). Besides, inter-hemispheric connectivity within the somatosensory cortex has been found to be altered in FASD teenagers (Gao et al. 2019). PAE affects the corpus callosum, leading to alterations in its shape, a reduction in surface area, and compromised integrity of callosal fibers (Treit et al. 2013; Bookstein et al. 2002; Fraize et al. 2023). Interestingly, the severity of brain network defects appears to be linked to the extent of PAE: one study reported widespread brain network alterations in children prenatally exposed to ethanol between the second and third trimesters, whereas no significant alterations were observed in those exposed only during the first trimester (Liang et al. 2024). Findings from super-resolution fetal MRI align with these observations, demonstrating that fetuses exposed to alcohol in the second and third trimester exhibit a significant larger corpus callosum and a smaller periventricular zone, even in cases of minor PAE. Given that the corpus callosum volume is reduced in childhood, the transient increase in fetal callosal size suggests a delay in synaptic pruning, abnormal axon guidance and subsequent disruptions in neuronal connectivity (Stuempflen et al. 2023).

6.3.1.2 Rodent Studies

Consistently, cortical malformations have been observed in rodent models of FASD. While several studies report no significant change in total brain volume following PAE (Fish et al. 2016; Zhang et al. 2019), others have observed reduced brain volume in prenatally exposed rats (Leigland et al. 2013; Coleman Jr et al. 2012; Smiley et al.

2015). Interestingly, most studies reporting reduced brain volume used a perinatal drinking model, which corresponds to third trimester exposure in human. This suggests that alcohol exposure during neuronal growth and maturation can induce widespread apoptosis in the developing brain (Ikonomidou et al. 2000). Several studies have demonstrated persistent reductions in cortical thickness volume and surface area in both young and adult rats, especially in frontal and sensorimotor areas (Leigland et al. 2013; Norton et al. 1988; Miller and Dow-Edwards 1988). In addition, MRI studies using a single acute dose of alcohol in mice have reported facial abnormalities, including a long upper lip, a narrow snout with closely apposed nostrils, and a small mandible (Godin et al. 2011). These physical anomalies were dependent on the timing of alcohol exposure (Parnell et al. 2009; Godin et al. 2010; O'Leary-Moore et al. 2010; Parnell et al. 2013). Similar to humans, PAE also affects functional connectivity in rodents by altering intracortical network and disrupting cortical-subcortical connectivity (Rodriguez et al. 2016; Tang et al. 2019; El Shawa et al. 2013; Miller 1987). Interhemispheric connectivity, mediated by the corpus callosum, is also altered by PAE (Qiang et al. 2002; Altounian et al. 2023). Milbocker et al. have shown that neonatal alcohol exposure delays the trajectory of corpus callosum growth and myelination in adolescent rats, with males exhibiting greater vulnerability (Milbocker et al. 2022). Importantly, rodent models of FASD exhibit behavioral impairments similar to those observed in human patients. These include deficits in neonatal orienting, attention and motor maturity, as well as impairments in activity level, executive function, response inhibition, and sensory processing later in life (Schneider et al. 2011; Gursky et al. 2021).

Cortical anomalies observed in FASD suggest underlying defects in neuronal and glial development. The following sections will explore current knowledge on the effects of PAE on cortical neurogenesis, neuronal migration, specification, and glial cell development using rodent models, *ex vivo* human fetal tissue, *ex vivo* mouse brain slices, *in vitro* human organoids and rodent cell cultures. It is important to note that the findings presented in this chapter come from studies using different models to investigate FASD. Variations in animal models, timing of alcohol exposure, routes of administration, levels of intoxication and timing of analysis may contribute to discrepancies between studies. This challenge in FASD research is discussed later in the chapter, and Table 6.1 outlines key differences between studies to aid readers in interpreting the findings. Furthermore, it is worth mentioning that in this chapter, discussed gestational timepoints are mostly aligned to rodent developmental timeline, which can be translated into human developmental timeline as the following: E11, E13.5, and PND4 approximately correspond to GW6, GW8 and GW21, respectively (Charvet 2020).

6.3.2 Consequences of PAE on Cortical Projection Neurons

6.3.2.1 Progenitor Proliferation and Neurogenesis

Rodent Models

Following proliferative phases of symmetrical divisions, RGCs and IPs generate neurons in the VZ and SVZ, respectively, before giving rise to astrocytes and oligodendrocytes in later stages of neurogenesis. Several *in vivo* models have reported that ethanol exposure during embryogenesis reduces the pool of RGCs by decreasing their proliferative potential and/or affecting the generation of neurons and astrocytes (Li et al. 2021b; Rubert et al. 2006; Santillano et al. 2005). Specifically, thymidine analog 5′-bromo-2′-deoxyuridine (BrdU) incorporation experiments in ethanol-exposed rat embryos have shown that PAE decreases the number of proliferating BrdU+ cells in the dorsal and medial portions of the intermediate telencephalon, which may contribute to the observed reduction in cortical thickness (Rubert et al. 2006). This decreased proliferation was accompanied by reduced expression of the neuronal marker β3-tubulin and the glial fibrillary acidic protein (GFAP) at E14 and E21, suggesting a reduction in the

Table 6.1 Summary of rodent model, route of alcohol administration, timing of exposure, mean blood alcohol concentration, and main conclusions of the study

Rodent model	Route of administration	Timing of exposure	BAC	Main results	References
General consequences of PAE					
Mouse	2 IP injections (2.8 kg/kg; 4 h apart)	E8	380 mg/dl	No change in brain volume	Fish et al. (2016)
Mouse	Voluntary 10% ethanol drinking	E0.5-E8.5	NS	No change in brain volume	Zhang et al. (2019)
Rat	Gavage (4.5 g/kg)	E1-E20		↓ brain volume, cortical volume, thickness and surface area	Leigland et al. (2013)
Mouse	2 SC injections (2.5 g/kg; 2 h apart)	E7	>200 mg/dl	↓ brain volume	Coleman Jr et al. (2012) and Smiley et al. (2015)
Rat	2 SC injections (2.5 g/kg; 2 h apart)	E7	>200 mg/dl	Massive apoptotic neurodegeneration in the forebrain	Ikonomidou et al. (2000)
Rat	Voluntary 2–6% ethanol liquid diet	E5-E10	NS	↓ thickness in frontal cortex	Norton et al. (1988)
Rat	Voluntary 35% ethanol liquid diet	E6-E21	115–130 mg/dl	↓ thickness in motor and somatosensory cortices	Miller and Dow-Edwards (1988)
Mouse	Two IP injections (2.9 g/kg)	E7	440 mg/dl	Facial abnormalities	Parnell et al. (2009)
Rat	Voluntary 5% ethanol drinking	All gestation	60.8 mg/dl	Altered functional cortical connectivity	Rodriguez et al. (2016)
Rat	Voluntary 2.1–6.46% ethanol liquid diet	E6-E21	120 mg/dl	Altered functional PFC connectivity	Tang et al. (2019)
Consequences of PAE on projection neurons					
Mouse	Voluntary 4.8% ethanol liquid diet	E6-E7	178.4 mg/dl	↓ RGC proliferation ↓ SOX2 and Nestin expression ↑ S100β expression	Li et al. (2021a, b)
Rat	Voluntary 5% ethanol liquid diet	E0-sacrifice (E12, E15, E21)	Mum: 103.6 mg/dl Fetus: 107.3 mg/dl	↓ RGC proliferation ↓ cortical thickness ↓ β3-tub and GFAP expression Notch1/FGFR2 signaling	Rubert et al. (2006)
Rat	Daily IP injections (3.5 g/kg)	E10-E18	230 mg/dL (119 to >300 mg/dL)	↓ PAX6 expression ↓ cortical thickness	Aronne et al. (2008)
Rat	Voluntary 5.9% ethanol liquid diet	E0-sacrifice (E12, E14, E16, E18, P3)	89.34 mg/dl	↓ PAX6 expression ↓ cortical thickness ↓ distance between SVZ and DCX+ PN	Aronne et al. (2011)
Mouse	Daily IP injections (2.5 g/kg)	E8.5-E13.5	150 - 200 mg/dl	↓ RGC pool Wnt pathway	Sambo et al. (2022)
Rat	Voluntary 6.7% ethanol liquid diet	4 days E6-E9 E12-E15 E18-E21	E6-E9: 132 mg/dl E12-E15: 148 mg/dl E18-E21: 135 mg/dl	↓ proliferative activity in the VZ ↑ proliferative activity in the SVZ	Miller (1996)
Rat	Voluntary 6.7% ethanol liquid diet	E5-E21	158 mg/dl	Disturbed cell cycle dynamic in VZ and SVZ	Miller and Nowakowski (1991)

(continued)

Table 6.1 (continued)

Rodent model	Route of administration	Timing of exposure	BAC	Main results	References
Rat	Gavage (3.5 g/kg), (12 h intervals)	E15-E18	NS	↓ number of Tbr2+ IPs ↓ cyclin-D1 expression	Riar et al. (2016)
Mouse	Voluntary 5% ethanol liquid diet	E13.5-E16.5	80 mg/dL	Aberrant distribution of Tbr1+ PN in the SP ↓ number of Cux1+ PN in the CP ↓ number of Tbr2+ PN in the upper SVZ	Delatour et al. (2019)
Rat	Voluntary 6.7% ethanol liquid diet	E6-E21	171 mg/dl	↑ time window of neuronal generation and migration Ectopic locations of PN in deep layers	Miller (1986, 1993)
Mouse	Model 1: two daily IP injections (1.5 mg/kg) Model 2: 2% ethanol-containing diet Model 3: daily gavage (3 mg/kg)	E7.5-E18.5	Model 1: 450 mg/dl Model 2: 390–800 mg/dl Model 3: NS	HSF1-HSF2 heterotrimers formation ↓ p35 and MAP genes expression	El Fatimy et al. (2014)
Rat	Voluntary 5% ethanol liquid diet	E10-E21	147.5 mg/dl	Heterotopia	Komatsu et al. (2001)
Rat	Gavage (5.25 g/kg)	P4-P9	333.5 mg/dl	Layer II/III PFC (P26-P30): ↓ complexity and length of proximal basal dendrites ↑ mature spines density in basal dendrites ↓ spine density in apical dendrites	Hamilton et al. (2010) and Whitcher and Klintsova (2008)
Rat	Gavage (4.5 g/kg for dams and 3.0 g/kg for pups)	E1-E22; P2-P10	289.36 mg/dl	Layer II/III PFC (P21): ↓ complexity in apical dendrites Unchanged complexity in basal dendrites	Lawrence et al. (2012)
Mouse	Gavage (E10-E11: 2 g/kg; E12-E18: 4 g/kg/d; P4-P5: 1.5 g/kg; P6-P14: 3 g/kg)	E10-E18; P4-P14	234.8 mg/dl Pup: 255.2 mg/dl	Adult PFC (P90): ↑ diameter and size of dendritic trees in layers II/III No defect in layer V ↑ length and ↓ complexity in long apical dendrites in layer VI	Louth et al. (2018)
Rat	Voluntary 25% ethanol liquid diet	All gestation	NS	Layer V somatosensory cortex (P15): transient ↓ spines density with predominance of immature spines in apical dendrites	Galofré et al. (1987)
Mouse	Voluntary 5% ethanol liquid diet	E13.5-E16.5	80 mg/dL	Layer V somatosensory cortex: P6-P8: transient ↓ dendritic tree complexity P28-P32: persistent ↑ spines density in proximal apical dendrites in favour to immature spines	Delatour et al. (2019, 2020)
Rat	Voluntary 25% ethanol liquid diet	All gestation and lactation	NS	Sensorimotor cortex (P21/P30): Delayed neuronal maturation ↓ basal dendrites complexity and spines density	Popova (2004)

(continued)

Table 6.1 (continued)

Rodent model	Route of administration	Timing of exposure	BAC	Main results	References
Mouse	Gavage (2 or 4 g/kg)	E5-birth	2 g/kg: 150–300 mg/dl 4 g/kg: 300–500 mg/dl	Layer V/VI visual cortex (P0-P30): Persistent ↓ spines density and ↑ mean spine length Synaptic ultrastructural defects	Cui et al. (2010)
Rat	Gavage (1.2–6 g/kg)	E11-E20	Min: 65.7 mg/dl Max: 327.4 mg/dl	Corpus callosum: ↑ number and length of dendritic branches	Qiang et al. (2002)
Rat	Voluntary 6.7% ethanol liquid diet	E6-E21	150 mg/dl (estimated)	Somatosensory cortex (P90) ↑ density of CPN originating from layers V/VI ↓ CPN density in layers II/III	Miller (1997)
Rat	Voluntary ethanol liquid diet (1.5; 2.25; 4; 6 g/kg)	E1-E20	NS	Visual cortex: disrupted axonal pruning of CPN projections	Livy and Elberger (2008)
Mouse	Daily IP injections (2 g/kg)	E15.5-E18.5	<100 mg/dL over a 4-day period	Upper layer somatosensory CPN: P8: ectopic terminations of P60: disrupted homotopic connectivity	Altounian et al. (2023)
Mouse	Voluntary 25% ethanol liquid diet	E0.5-E19.5	138.77 mg/dl	P0: Aberrant visual and somatosensory connectivity Disrupted cortical gene expression gradients	El Shawa et al. (2013)
Rat	Voluntary 6.7% ethanol liquid diet	E6-E21	NS	↑ number of corticospinal neurons during gestation No change in their distribution, axonal patterning or myelination in adult rats	Miller (1987, 2017)
Rat	Gavage (5.2 g/kg)	P4-P9	250.075 mg/dL	P70: ↓ cumulative mPFC-originating axon terminal length in the thalamic nucleus reuniens in females	Smith et al. (2022)
Consequences of PAE on interneurons					
Mouse	Voluntary 1% ethanol liquid diet	E0.5-E14.5	12.7 mg/dl	↓ number of BrdU+ cells in all proliferative zones (E14.5)	Cuzon et al. (2008)
Mouse	Two IP injections (2.9 g/kg; 4 h apart)	E7	440 mg/dl	E12.5: Loss of MGE and POA tissues Dysmorphic lateral ventricles	Godin et al. (2011)
Mouse	Voluntary 2% ethanol liquid diet	E9.5-birth	~30 mg/dL	E12.5: ↑ number of BrdU+ cells in the MGE	Skorput and Yeh (2016)
Mouse	Voluntary 1% ethanol liquid diet	E0.5-E14.5	12.7 mg/dl	↑ number of migrating GABAergic cells ↑ migration speed ↑ number of MGE-derived IN in E14.5 cortex ↑ GABAergic cells density in embryonic cortex ↑ $GABA_AR$ expression and ambient GABA levels in the MGE-CSJ regions and cortical IZ	Cuzon et al. (2008)

(continued)

Table 6.1 (continued)

Rodent model	Route of administration	Timing of exposure	BAC	Main results	References
Mouse	Voluntary 5% ethanol liquid diet	E13.5-E16.5	80 mg/dl	↑ number of Nkx2.1+ IN in E16.5 mPFC ↑ $GABA_A$R-dependant tangential migration ↑ number of PV+ IN in P70 layer V PFC	Cuzon et al. (2008), Lee et al. (2022) and Skorput et al. (2019)
Mouse	Daily SC injection (3 g/kg)	E15-E20	150 mg/dl	↑ activation of endothelial NMDA/tPA/MMP9 pathway IN mispositioning (P15)	Leger et al. (2020)
Mouse	Voluntary 5% ethanol liquid diet	E13.5-E16.5	80 mg/dl	↑ GABAergic cells density in embryonic cortex ↑ PV+ interneuron density in layer V PFC (P70)	Skorput et al. (2015)
Mouse	Daily SC injection (3 g/kg)	E15-E20	150 mg/dl	P15: Ectopic localization of GAD67+ neurons in layer IV ↑ spine density	Leger et al. (2020)
Rat	Voluntary 35% ethanol liquid diet	E0-E21	161 mg/dl	P60: ↓ PV+ cell density in the anterior cingulate cortex	Moore et al. (1998)
Mouse	Voluntary 10% ethanol drinking (4 h/day)	All gestation	30 mg/dl	Adult mice: ↓ PV+ cell density in the posterior parietal cortex No change in CR+ and SST+ IN numbers	Licheri et al. (2023)
Mouse	Voluntary 10% ethanol drinking (4 h/day)	All gestation	80 mg/dl	Adult mice: ↑ density of CR+ IN in the orbitofrontal cortex	Kenton et al. (2020)
Guinea pigs	Oral administration (4 g/kg)	All gestation	328 mg/dl	P60: ↓ IN density in somatosensory cortical layers II/III	Bailey et al. (2004)
Mouse	2 SC injections (2.5 g/kg; 2 h apart)	E7	>200 mg/dl	P82: ↓ density of PV+ IN in frontal cortex P25-P30: ↓ density of PV+ and CR+ IN	Coleman Jr et al. (2012) and Smiley et al. (2015)
Mouse	Vapor chamber (8–9 g/dl; 4 h)	P7	360 mg/dl	E7: apoptosis in layers II-V of the retrosplenial cortex	Bird et al. (2020)
Rat	Vapor chamber	P2-P7	165–252 mg/dl	Somatosensory and motor cortices: ↑ number and ectopic localization of CR+ IN in deep layers ↑ number of calbindin IN in all layers	Granato (2006)
Consequences of PAE on E/I balance					
Mouse	Voluntary 2% ethanol liquid diet	E9.5-birth	~30 mg/dL	P20: ↓ frequency and amplitude of sEPSC in layer V mPFC PN and ↓ extrasynaptically mediated GABAergic tone	Skorput and Yeh (2016)
Mouse	Voluntary 5% ethanol liquid diet	E13.5-E16.5	80 mg/dl	Adult mice: ↓ frequency of sEPSC and ↑ frequency of sIPSCs and mIPSCs in layer V mPFC PN	Skorput et al. (2015)

(continued)

Table 6.1 (continued)

Rodent model	Route of administration	Timing of exposure	BAC	Main results	References
Mouse	Vapor chamber (8–9 g/dl; 4 h)	P7	368.56 mg/dl	P40-P60: ↑ peak amplitude, current density, asynchronous activity and total charge of oIPSC in RSC layer V PN in response to stimulation of layer V PV+ IN	Bird et al. (2021)
Mouse	Voluntary 10% drinking of ethanol (4 h/day)	All gestation	80 mg/dl	Adult mice: ↑ amplitude of $GABA_A$ receptors-mediated sIPSCs in deep layer PN	Kenton et al. (2020)
Consequences of PAE on glial cells					
Mouse	Voluntary ethanol liquid diet feeding	E6-E7	178.4 mg/dl	Accelerated RGC to astrocyte transformation	Li et al. (2021a, b)
Rat	Gavage	P4-P10	Min: 39 mg/dl Max: 301 mg/dl	Disturbed GFAP expression	Goodlett et al. (1993, 1997)
Rat	Voluntary 6.7% ethanol liquid diet	E6-birth	149 mg/dl	↓ number of glial cells in somatosensory cortex	Miller and Potempa (1990)
Mouse	Gavage (2, 4, or 6 g/kg)	P4-P7	125, 321, and 462 mg/dl	↑ cortical levels of ABCA1	Guizzetti et al. (2007)
Mouse	Gradual 36% ethanol diet	E6-E21	206.85 mg/dl	Upregulation of ABCA1 and ABCG1 transporters expression	Zhou et al. (2014)
Rat	Gavage (5.25 g/kg)	P4-P9	321 mg/dL	Delayed myelination in the CC	Milbocker et al. (2022)
Mouse	Vapor chamber with gradual concentrations (4.9 to 7.1 g/dl)	P3-P15	128.2–185.6 mg/dl	↓ mature oligodendrocytes number and ↑ proliferating OPCs number in the CC	Newville et al. (2017)
Mouse	Voluntary 20% drinking (4 h/day)	E4-E21 E4-P21	81.57 mg/dl	↓ expression of MAG, PLP, MBP	Cantacorps et al. (2017)
Mouse	SC injections (3 g/kg)	P0-P1	150 mg/dl	P15: Transient ↓ superficial/deep cortical layers ratio of Olig2+ cells ↑ expression of CNPase and MBP levels in layers V–VI ↓ myelinated axon density and myelin sheath thickness Motor impairments	Brosolo et al. (2022)
Mouse	Gavage (4 g/kg)	P4-P9	401 mg/dl	↑ ILβ and TNFα mRNA levels Shift toward activation-like shaped microglia	Drew et al. (2015)
Mouse	Gavage twice a day (1 or 2 g/kg)	E6-E18	317 mg/dl	↑ Iba1+ amoeboid-type microglia in the dorsal telencephalon (E15.5) and PFC (P3) ↑ M1/M2 ratio Altered cytokine profiles Abnormal neuronal distribution, layer formation, and dopaminergic neuronal projections in the neocortex ameliorated with pioglitazone	Komada et al. (2017)

IP intra-peritoneal, *SC* sub-cutaneous, *BAC* blood alcohol concentration, *NS* not specified, *E* embryonic day, *P* postnatal day, *PN* projection neuron, *IN* interneuron, *PFC* prefrontal cortex, *CC* corpus callosum, *CPN* callosal projection neurons, *RGC* radial glial cell, *IPs* intermediate progenitors, *VZ* ventricular zone, *SVZ* subventricular zone, *E/I* excitatory/inhibitory generation of both neurons and astrocytes (Rubert et al. 2006). In addition, PAE decreased the expression of the RGC markers SRY-Box Transcription Factor 2 (SOX2) and Nestin in the fetal rat cortex, and this reduction was associated with increased levels of the astrocytic marker S100β and a morphological shift in RGCs toward an astrocytic-like appearance in the SVZ (Li et al. 2021b).

Other studies have shown that PAE leads to a reduction in the expression of the RGC marker Paired Box 6 (PAX6) in embryonic rat cortex, which correlates with decreased cortical thickness (Aronne et al. 2008, 2011). Rubert et al. proposed that progenitor defects may arise from disruption of the Notch1/FGFR2 signaling pathway, which is critical for the maintenance of progenitor state. Indeed, levels of Notch1 and FGFR2 were found to be reduced in the cortex of alcohol-exposed rat embryos at E12 and E21 (Rubert et al. 2006). Another proposed mechanism, suggested by Sambo et al., involves the Wnt signaling pathway, which plays a key role in promoting proliferation and preventing differentiation during early development. Single nucleus RNA sequencing of brain tissue in a mouse model revealed that PAE reduces the pool of RGCs expressing Wnt pathway genes (Sambo et al. 2022). In line with these findings, Miller et al. described a BrdU-injected rat model, in which ethanol treatment reduced proliferation in progenitor cells in the VZ while increasing proliferative activity in the SVZ (Miller 1996). The reduced proliferation in the VZ was associated with a longer total cell cycle, whereas the increase in the SVZ was linked to a greater growth fraction (Miller and Nowakowski 1991). These differences between the VZ and SVZ suggest that alcohol may differentially affect apical RGCs and basal IPs. In contrast, further investigating the impact of PAE on cortical IPs, Riar et al. showed that alcohol exposure in rat embryos reduces the number of cells expressing the IP marker Tbr2, which also exhibit decreased expression of cyclin-D1 (Riar et al. 2016). Given the crucial role of cyclin-D1 in the G1-to-S phase transition, these findings suggest that PAE impairs IP proliferation by disrupting cyclin-D1-associated cell cycle events (Riar et al. 2016).

In Vitro Models

Rodent-derived cell culture and forebrain organoids derived from human embryonic stem cells (hESC) have provided further insights into the effects of PAE. Like rodent models, RGCs cultures derived from rat embryos exposed to ethanol *in vivo* displayed a reduced number of Nestin+/BrdU+ cells following *in vitro* BrdU pulse treatment (Rubert et al. 2006). Differentiation assays in telencephalic cultures also revealed a reduced number of β3-tubulin+ clones. Several studies using human forebrain organoids exposed to ethanol *in vitro* have been consistent with these findings (Lu et al. 2023; Adams et al. 2023; Taléns-Visconti et al. 2011). For example, Lu et al. have demonstrated that alcohol exposure decreases the number of Nestin+/BrdU+ RGCs on day 21 and HOP homeobox (HOPX)+/Edu+ outer RGCs (oRGCs) on day 56 following *in vitro* BrdU/Edu pulse treatment (Lu et al. 2023). In addition, ethanol exposure reduced the number of proliferating Ki67+ cells, which were less likely to be in the S and G2/M phases, suggesting premature cell cycle exit due to differentiation or cell death (Adams et al. 2023). These defects were associated with enhanced astrocytic maturation and disrupted RGC morphology, as evidenced by increased GFAP+ and S100β+ astrocytes on day 84, as well as reduced levels of RG process-associated proteins. The loss of polarity in RGCs following alcohol treatment further supported these findings (Lu et al. 2023). Conflicting findings were reported by Talens-Visconti et al., who found that alcohol exposure inhibited the downregulation of SOX2 and PAX6, while also reducing the upregulation of GFAP, which normally occurs during progenitor differentiation (Taléns-Visconti et al. 2011). Despite these discrepancies, the latter studies consistently reported ethanol-induced apoptosis in cortical progenitors, as indicated by increased cleaved caspase-3 (cCasp3) activity (Lu et al. 2023; Adams et al. 2023; Taléns-Visconti et al. 2011).

A more recent study demonstrated that PAE induces nucleolar stress in mouse neural stem cells (NSCs) and late-term fetal brains, activating P53 through MDM2-dependent stabilization, which suppresses proliferation and triggers apoptosis (Huang et al. 2024). This was confirmed by a decreased percentage of proliferating NSCs and a corresponding increase in apoptotic NSCs following alcohol exposure (Huang et al. 2024). Interestingly, the Notch/FGFR2 signaling was also disrupted in telencephalic cultures derived from ethanol-exposed rat embryos, as evidenced by decreased levels of activated Notch1 and FGFR2 (Rubert et al. 2006). Moreover, the PAE-mediated decrease in IPs proliferation observed in rodent models by Riar et al. was confirmed in mouse cell cultures. Following ethanol treatment *in vitro*, BrdU pulse experiment showed a reduced number of Tbr2+/BrdU+ cells, with a decreased proportion of cells in the S-phase and an increased proportion in the G0-G1 phase (Riar et al. 2016). Further analysis indicated that PAE impairs cell cycle dynamics by reducing cyclin D1 levels and retinoblastoma protein (Rb) phosphorylation, both of which are essential for the G1-to-S phase transition in IPs (Riar et al. 2016).

Despite some discrepancies, the overall findings from these studies suggest that PAE leads to reduced or delayed progenitor proliferation. Early ethanol exposure appears to inhibit RGCs proliferation through mechanisms involving the Notch/FGFR2 and Wnt pathways, possibly in conjunction with p53-mediated apoptosis, ultimately disrupting their differentiation into astrocytes (Fig. 6.1c). Additionally, PAE may impair IPs proliferation by altering cell cycle dynamics, leading to either premature cell cycle exit or delayed cellular growth (Fig. 6.1d).

6.3.2.2 Projection Neurons Migration

Rodent Models

Emerging evidence suggests that PAE may also impact the radial migration of projection neurons. Delatour et al. used a mouse model of FASD and observed an aberrant distribution of Tbr1+ projection neurons (deep layers) in the subplate at E16.5, along with a reduced number of Cux1+ cells (superficial layers) in the cortical plate, and fewer Tbr2+ cells in the upper SVZ of the developing somatosensory cortex. They concluded that PAE may delay projection neuron migration or disrupt their temporal expression pattern (Delatour et al. 2019). Another study reported a decreased distance of DCX+ cells from the VZ at E14 in ethanol-exposed rat embryos, which was associated with reduced cortical thickness (Aronne et al. 2011). Consistent with these findings, Miller et al. have reported that PAE prolongs the period of neuronal generation and migration, with more pronounced effects on later-born neurons ending up in deep layers rather than superficial layers, thereby disturbing the inside-out pattern of neurons generation (Miller 1986, 1993). Interestingly, Fatimy et al. proposed a mechanism involving the stress-response regulator Heat Shock Factor 2 (HSF2) as a key player in PAE-induced migration defects. They reported that PAE induces the formation of HSF1-HSF2 heterotrimers due to altered post-translational modifications. The resulting permanent activation of HSF1 and HSF2 led to reduced expression of the cyclin dependent kinase 5 (CDK5) activator p35 and microtubule-associated protein (MAP) genes (e.g., Dcx and Dclx1), both crucial for radial migration (El Fatimy et al. 2014). Finally, PAE has also been associated with cortical heterotopia, characterized by neuronal masses in abnormal locations within the rat cerebral cortex (Mooney et al. 2004; Komatsu et al. 2001).

Collectively, these findings suggest that PAE may interfere with the inside-out formation of cortical projection neurons by delaying the generation and migration of later-born neurons, leading to abnormal layer distribution, with a greater proportion of projection neurons integrating into deep layers rather than superficial ones (Fig. 6.1e).

Human Models

A combined RNA-sequencing analysis of fetal human and mouse cerebral cortex exposed to ethanol identified common signaling pathways and dysregulated genes. The study revealed that ethanol exposure disrupts the expression of genes involved in Transforming growth factor beta (TGF-β), phosphoinositide 3-kinase (PI3K) and Notch signaling, as well as genes related to neuronal migration including Disabled homolog 1 (DAB1), Neuropilin1 and Heat Shock proteins (HSP) (Hashimoto-Torii et al. 2011). In addition, previously reported morphological defects and loss of polarity of RGCs may contribute to migration abnormalities, as RG fibers serve as scaffold for radial migration (Lu et al. 2023).

6.3.2.3 Projection Neurons Maturation

Rodent Models

Dendritic Branching Defects

Dendrite branching defects following PAE have been mostly studied in the prefrontal cortex (PFC), the somatosensory cortex (SSC), and the visual cortex. In layers II/III of the PFC, Hamilton et al. reported that third-trimester alcohol exposure reduced the complexity and length of proximal basal dendritic arborization, together with an increased density of mature spines (Hamilton et al. 2010). In another study, the same group reported a persistent decrease in spine density in the apical dendritic tree of ethanol-exposed rats, without affecting dendritic and spines morphology (Whitcher and Klintsova 2008). Opposing findings were observed by Lawrence et al., who reported decreased complexity in apical dendrites but not in basal dendrites at P21 (Lawrence et al. 2012). They also noted a reduction in spine density across the entire dendritic tree following PAE (Lawrence et al. 2012). These conflicting results may be explained by differences in the timing of alcohol exposure: In the first study, rat pups were exposed from P4 to P9, whereas in the second study, exposure occurred from E1 to E22, followed by a second exposure from P2 to P10.

PAE also appears to alter PFC morphology in a layer-specific manner. Indeed, Louth et al. analyzed projection neurons morphology across different layers of the adult mouse PFC following alcohol exposure during embryogenesis and the early postnatal period. They found that PAE increased the diameter of dendritic trees and the size of apical dendrites in layers II/III, but did not affect layer V neurons. In layer VI, neurons with long apical dendrites exhibited increased length and reduced complexity, whereas neurons with short apical dendrites had an overall decrease in tree size (Louth et al. 2018).

Dendritic branching defects have also been described in the SSC. A transient decrease in spine density, along with a predominance of immature-shaped long spines were reported in apical dendrites of layer V projection neurons in young rats prenatally exposed to ethanol (Galofré et al. 1987). Similarly, Delatour et al. found transient morphological defects in SSC layer V projection neurons, with PAE leading to a short-term reduction in dendritic tree complexity at P6-8 but not at P9-11 (Delatour et al. 2019). These defects were associated with persistent alterations in synaptic function lasting until P28-P32, as reflected by long-term increase in the frequency of excitatory and inhibitory postsynaptic currents (Delatour et al. 2019, 2020). Although dendritic morphological defects disappeared at later ages, PAE still increased spines density in proximal apical dendrites, favoring a greater proportion of immature spines throughout the apical tree (Delatour et al. 2020). The resurgence of spine plasticity beyond the peak of synaptogenesis may suggest delayed cortical circuitry development (Delatour et al. 2020). This hypothesis is further supported by studies reporting delayed neuronal maturation in the cortical sensorimotor area of adolescent PAE rats, including delayed cytological maturation of the cortex and decreased complexity of basal dendrites and spines density (Popova 2004).

Finally, in the mouse visual cortex, diolistic labeling of layers V/VI pyramidal cells from P0 to P30 revealed that PAE induced a persistent decrease in dendritic spines density, with increased mean spine length. This effect was more pronounced at higher ethanol doses (4 g/kg vs. 2 g/kg) (Cui et al. 2010). Transmission electron microscopy further revealed PAE-induced synaptic ultrastructural defects, including thickened postsynaptic densities, narrowed synaptic clefts and reduced synaptic vesicles numbers—all indicators of immature synapses, suggesting delayed dendritic spine and

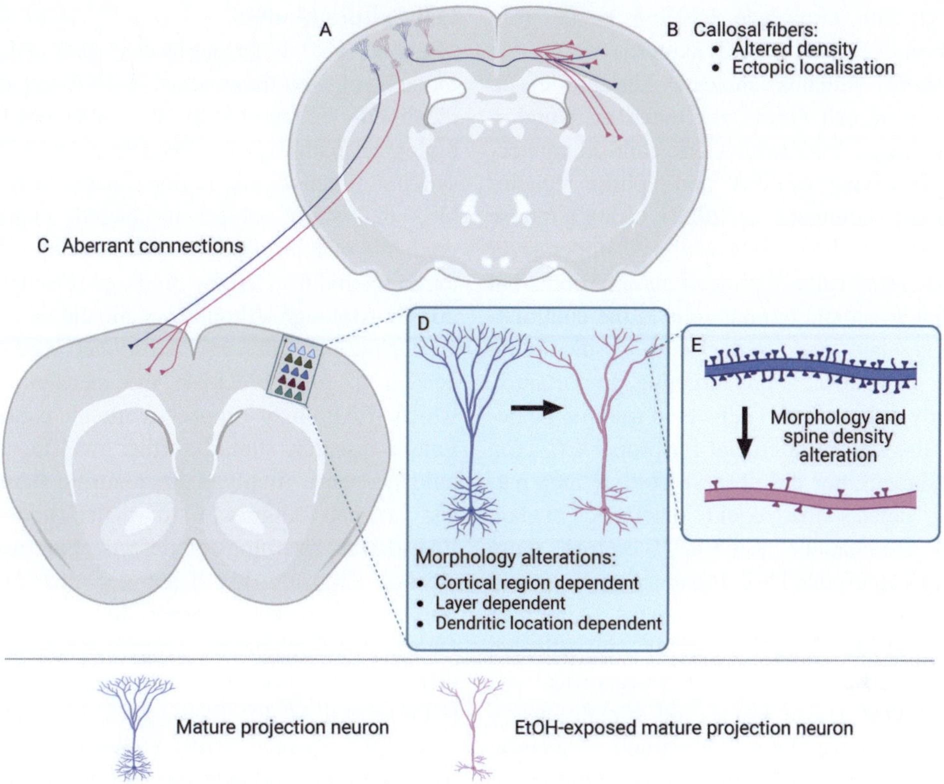

Fig. 6.2 PAE-induced defects in dendritic branching and axonal outgrowth of cortical projection neurons. (**a**–**c**) PAE interferes with intracortical, interhemispheric and cortical-subcortical connectivity of projection neurons through altered density and ectopic localization of projections, as well as aberrant connections. These defects contribute to overall circuit abnormalities within the cortex and subcortical regions, leading to functional deficits. (**d** and **e**) PAE impairs the morphology of dendritic arborizations and spines in projection neurons across different cortical regions. These defects are dependent on cortical area, specific layer and dendritic location

synapse development (Cui et al. 2010). Another study found that PAE increased the number and length of apical and basal dendritic branches in corpus callosum projection neurons in a dose-dependent manner (Qiang et al. 2002). PAE-induced dendritic branching defects are illustrated in Fig. 6.2.

Axonal Growth Defects

Using retrograde labeling techniques, several studies have demonstrated that PAE alters the connectivity pattern of intratelencephalic (IT), corticothalamic (CT), and pyramidal tract (PT) neurons. IT neurons, which project to the neocortex, striatum, and corticoid structures, establish contralateral connections primarily via the corpus callosum (CC). Increasing evidence suggests significant impairments in callosal projection neurons (CPN) across different cortical regions following PAE. Miller et al. reported that PAE increases the density of CPN originating from layers V/VI but decreases CPN density in layers II/III in the SSC of adult rats, leading to an overall increase in total callosal neurons density (Miller 1997). Another study in the rat visual cortex showed that PAE disrupted the temporally regulated axonal pruning of visual CPN projections in a dose-dependent manner. The authors suggested that high doses of ethanol could delay CPN development and/or disrupt axonal pruning timing (Livy and Elberger 2008). However, whether CPN density defects detected with retrograde labeling result from migration deficits or axonal outgrowth impairments remains unclear. Altounia et al. recently proposed a molecular mechanism underlying improper interhemispheric callosal connectivity, involving miRNA and ephrin receptor signaling (Altounian et al. 2023). Using a mouse model of mild PAE, they analyzed upper layer somatosensory callosal projections and found that PAE led to ectopic terminations in the contralateral cingulate and motor cortex, disrupting homotopic callosal axons targeting. Importantly, the study did not report defects in midline guidepost cells, which are crucial for proper CC axon establishment, nor did observe cortical area patterning defects that could otherwise explain ectopic terminations of CPN. Therefore, these findings suggest that PAE impairs intrinsic axonal growth and navigation mechanisms (Altounian et al. 2023). Another study investigated PAE-induced alterations in intraneocortical circuitry within mouse visual and somatosensory cortices. Researchers identified aberrant connections from the visual cortex to the motor cortex, and from the SSC to abnormally caudal cortical regions. In addition, ethanol disrupted medial-lateral gene expression gradients of RorB, Cad8, and Id2 in the caudal frontal cortex and rostral parietal cortex, suggesting potential cortical patterning defects (El Shawa et al. 2013). Miller et al. also investigated PAE effects on the maturation of PT neurons in rats, focusing on corticospinal axons. Retrograde labeling revealed an increased number of corticospinal neurons but no significant impact on their distribution, axonal patterning, or myelination in adult rats. These findings suggest that PAE predominantly affects early developmental events rather than axonal growth and maturation of PT neurons (Miller 1987, 2017). Furthermore, viral tracer injections into layer V of the mPFC of adult rats exposed to third-trimester alcohol exposure revealed sex-specific effects. Ethanol-exposed females—but not males—exhibited reduced cumulative mPFC-originating axon terminal length in the thalamic nucleus reuniens, an essential relay for PFC-hippocampus connectivity (Smith et al. 2022).

Cell Culture Models

In an *in vitro* human pluripotent stem cell-based model of corticogenesis, RNA-sequencing identified ethanol-induced alterations in biological pathways involved in axon guidance, synaptic function, and regional patterning. Notably, the study observed altered expression gradients of transcripts involved in regional patterning, similar to *in vivo* findings (Fischer et al. 2021). Although Altounia et al. did not detect area patterning defects, additional studies are needed to fully elucidate the mechanisms by which PAE may impact cortical patterning. Future research should further investigate key guidance cues involved in dendritic branching and axonal outgrowth to better understand PAE-driven neurological defects. For instance, alcohol exposure has been reported to alter semaphorin receptor expression and disrupt Netrin-1/DCC signaling, both of which are crucial for CC formation and axonal attraction (Kleiber et al. 2013; Tsai et al. 2014; Sepulveda et al. 2011; Xu et al. 2019). However, the precise role of these guidance cues in the context of FASD remains largely unexplored.

In summary, PAE-related impairments in dendritic branching, axonal growth and connectivity are highly diverse and complex. Beyond differences in PAE models, these defects vary depending on cortical area, neuronal subtype and axonal target region (Fig. 6.2).

6.3.3 Consequences of PAE on Cortical Interneurons

6.3.3.1 Interneuron Generation

Little is known about the impact of PAE on interneuron proliferation and neurogenesis. Cuzon et al. reported a reduced number of BrdU + cells in all proliferative zones at E14.5 following mild PAE in mouse embryos (Cuzon et al. 2008). Similarly, Nkx2.1 *in situ* hybridization showed a loss of MGE and POA tissues, along with dysmorphic lateral ventricles and structural anomalies in the GEs at E12.5 (Godin et al. 2011), suggesting decreased proliferative activity after PAE. Conversely, another study found that PAE increased the number of BrdU+ cells in the MGE of E12.5 mouse embryos, while the total area remained unchanged (Skorput and Yeh 2016). These defects were associated with a specific long-lasting increase in PV+ interneurons density in the mPFC of adult mice, indicating that PAE may differently affect distinct progenitor pools (Fig. 6.3) (Skorput and Yeh 2016).

6.3.3.2 Interneurons Migration

PAE significantly impacts the tangential migration of cortical interneurons. Several studies have shown that ethanol consumption during early pregnancy increases the number of Nkx2.1+ migrating interneurons throughout their migratory path, away from the cortico-striatal junction (Cuzon et al. 2008; Lee et al. 2022; Skorput et al. 2019). PAE also enhances their migration speed, leading to increased incorporation of MGE-derived differentiated interneurons in the neocortex (Cuzon et al. 2008; Lee et al. 2022; Skorput et al. 2019). Given the reduced proliferative activity observed by Cuzon et al., these findings suggest that PAE promotes premature tangential migration of interneurons into the cortical plate (Cuzon et al. 2008). Using an *in vitro* model, researchers also demonstrated that PAE increases the expression of $GABA_A$ receptors and elevates ambient GABA levels in the MGE-CSJ regions and cortical IZ, inducing premature responsiveness in primordial interneurons to GABA (Cuzon et al. 2008). Notably, a previous study found that ambient GABA promotes tangential migration via $GABA_A$ receptors activation (Cuzon et al. 2006), potentially explaining the observed migratory defects. Activation of $GABA_A$ receptors in immature interneurons leads to membrane depolarization due to the high expression of the Cl- importer NKCC1 and the low expression of the Cl- exporter KCC2, causing excessive Cl- extrusion following receptor activation. Skorput et al. showed that ethanol potentiates this depolarizing effect by acting as a $GABA_A$ receptor positive allosteric modulator, thereby increasing Cl- efflux and amplifying GABA-induced responses (Skorput et al. 2019). Consistently, blocking NKCC1 with bumetanide normalized these effects (Skorput et al. 2019). In another study, the authors reported long-term increase in PV+ interneurons density in layer V of the PFC and behavioral flexibility defects in adult mice following PAE, both of which were prevented by bumetanide (Skorput et al. 2015). Furthermore, blocking L-Type Calcium Channels (LTCC) with nifedipine abolished the migratory defects, as ethanol exposure increased LTCC activation in migrating cortical interneurons in E16.5 PFC slices (Lee et al. 2022). These findings indicate that calcium and chloride signaling are key players in ethanol-induced aberrant tangential migration of cortical interneurons.

Several studies have demonstrated that ethanol may also act on blood vessels by impairing cortical angiogenesis, leading to perinatal vascular disorganization (Jégou et al. 2012; Lecuyer et al. 2017; Brosolo et al. 2022). At a molecular level, Leger et al. showed that alcohol can act through the endothelial NMDA/tPA/MMP9 pathway (Leger et al. 2020). In response to glutamate binding to endothelial N-methyl-D-aspartate (NMDA) receptors, recruitment of tissue plasminogen activator (tPA) activates Matrix Metallopeptidase 9 (MMP9), which enhances interneuron migration speed along the perineural vascular plexus and radial micro vessels in the mouse cortex (Léger et al. 2020). In a chronic PAE mouse model (E15 to E20), alcohol potentiated glutamate-induced MMP9 activation in P2 cortical slices. This study also reported mispositioning of GAD67+ interneurons in deep layers of P15 mice, along with an increased density of CR+ interneurons in deep layers at the expense of superficial layers in FAE human tissue (Leger et al. 2020).

6.3.3.3 Interneurons Maturation

PAE also disturbs interneuron integration into cortical circuits, with variable effects on neuronal density and distribution, depending on exposure timing, drinking pattern, cortical region and layer (Fig. 6.3). Early exposure (first and second trimesters in humans) increased GABAergic cell density across all cortical layers in E14.5 and E16.5 mouse embryos following alcohol

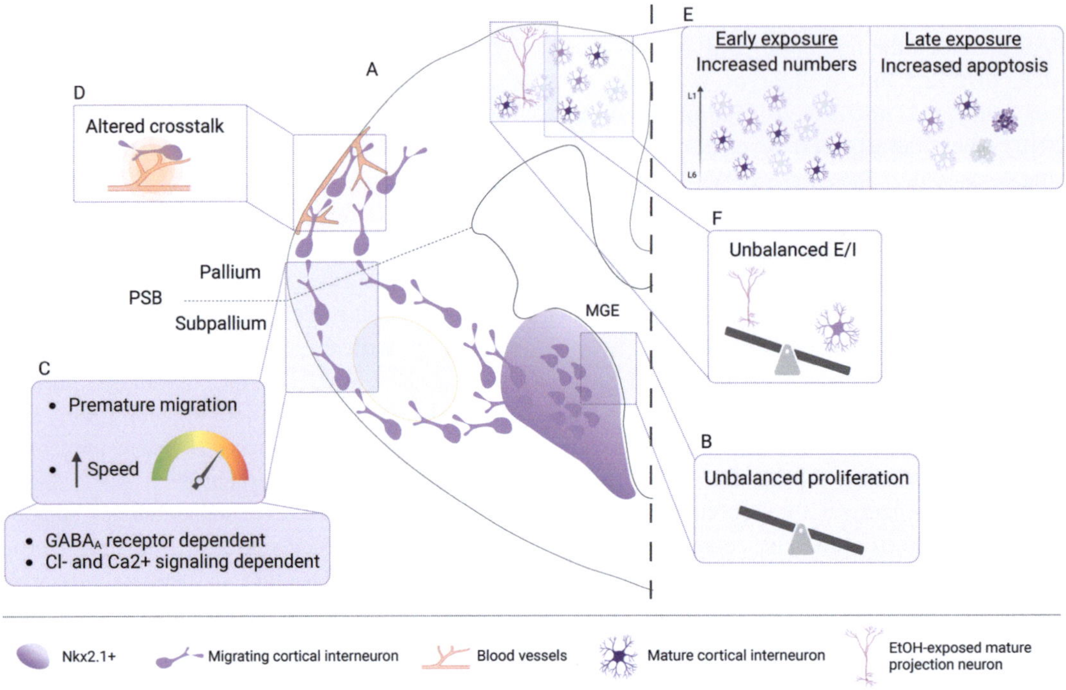

Fig. 6.3 Overview of PAE-induced defects in interneuron generation, migration and layering during cortical development. (**a**) Following generation in the GEs of the ventral telencephalon, INs migrate tangentially to reach and integrate into the cortex in response to extrinsic and intrinsic guidance cues. (**b** and **c**) PAE interferes with IN proliferation in the MGE and promotes migration by increasing migration speed through increased $GABA_A$ receptor activation, which indirectly promotes Cl^- and Ca^{2+} signaling and IN polarization. (**d**) IN migration depends on proper communication between INs and BVs which is impaired by PAE through disruption of the endothelial NMDA/tPA/MMP9 pathway. (**e** and **f**) PAE impairs proper integration of INs in the CP. Early PAE increases IN numbers and promotes ectopic IN integration into deep layers, while late PAE induces IN apoptosis, disturbing the precise balance between excitation and inhibition. *MGE* medial ganglionic eminence, *IN* interneuron, *PAE* prenatal alcohol exposure, *BV* blood vessels, *CP* cortical plate, *NMDA* N-methyl-D-aspartate, *tPA* Tissue plasminogen activator, *MMP9* Matrix Metallopeptidase 9

treatment, without affecting their cortical distribution (Cuzon et al. 2008; Skorput et al. 2015). Postnatally, findings have been inconsistent across different interneuron subtypes. Leger et al. showed that PAE induces ectopic localization of GAD67+ neurons in layer IV and increases spines density in P15 mice (Leger et al. 2020). While Skorput et al. reported an increased PV+ interneuron density in layer V of the entire PFC (Skorput et al. 2015), other studies found decreased PV+ density in the anterior cingulate cortex (Moore et al. 1998) and the posterior parietal cortex (Licheri et al. 2023), with no change in CR+ and SST+ interneurons (Licheri et al. 2023). In contrast, an increased density of CR+ interneurons was reported in the orbitofrontal cortex (Kenton et al. 2020). Chronic PAE in adult guinea pigs decreased interneurons density in layers II-III of the SSC (Bailey et al. 2004) while increasing $GABA_A$ receptor expression (Bailey et al. 2001).

Studies investigating postnatal exposure to ethanol found that acute P7 exposure decreased PV+ and CR+ interneurons densities in adult mice (Coleman Jr et al. 2012; Smiley et al. 2015), and induced apoptosis in layers II–V of the retrosplenial cortex (RSC) (Bird et al. 2020). These apoptotic events may be linked to NMDA receptors inhibition by ethanol, reducing neuronal excitability. Interestingly, the RSC, crucial for navigation, spatial learning and memory, is implicated in FASD-related cognitive deficits (Bird et al. 2020). Another model of chronic PAE from P2 to P7 increased CR+ interneurons, which were abnormally distributed in deep cortical layers, while calbindin interneurons were more concentrated in layers II–III, layer V and deep layer VI in the somatosensory and motor cortices (Granato 2006).

Human studies indicate that PAE delays CR+ interneurons generation in the GE during the first two trimesters, followed by an excessive incorporation into the frontal cortex after birth, often in ectopic positions in deep layers instead of superficial layers (Leger et al. 2020; Marguet et al. 2020). Similarly to mouse models, PAE disrupts the vascular migration of CR+ interneurons in the cortical plate (Marguet et al. 2020). In addition, a study using human pluripotent stem cells exposed to ethanol *in vitro* reported decreased expression of interneuron precursors markers GSX2, Dlx1/2/5/6 and Vgat, while SST and NPY expression increased, suggesting aberrant interneuron differentiation despite normal overall numbers (Larsen et al. 2016).

While findings on interneuron progenitor proliferation are inconsistent between studies, the overarching pattern suggests that PAE-induced premature migration leads to disturbed interneuron integration into cortical layers, with a tendency toward ectopic positions in deep layers (Fig. 6.3). This altered migration profile is characterized by increased migration speed due to impaired GABA-mediated interneuron polarization and disrupted blood vessels-interneurons signaling. Interestingly, early versus late gestational alcohol exposure appears to differentially affect cortical interneuron populations, with early exposure tending to increase interneuron numbers and late exposure leading to apoptosis.

6.3.4 Consequences of PAE on E/I Balance

The excitation/inhibition (E/I) balance is essential for the proper establishment of higher-order functions. This balance is fine-tuned through precise communication between projection neurons and interneurons. In several FASD mouse models, alterations in neuron density and positioning have been associated with impaired electrical properties of specific neuronal populations. For example, in the study by Skorput et al., the PAE-induced increase in PV+ interneurons density in the PFC had long-term consequences on the post-synaptic currents (PSC) of both cortical interneurons and projection neurons (Skorput and Yeh 2016; Skorput et al. 2015). In P20 mice, PAE reduced the frequency and amplitude of spontaneous excitatory PSCs (sEPSCs) in layer V mPFC projection neurons and decreased the extrasynaptically mediated GABAergic tone (Skorput and Yeh 2016). Interestingly, the reduced frequency—but not the amplitude—of sEPSCs persisted into adulthood and was associated with an increased frequency of spontaneous and miniature inhibitory PSCs (sIPSCs and mIPSCs) in layer V projection neurons (Skorput et al. 2015). One possible explanation for the reduced sEPSCs in layer V pyramidal neurons is an increased inhibitory input from PV+ interneurons in other cortical layers. Indeed, layer II/III pyramidal neurons targeted by PV+ interneurons constitute the main presynaptic source of sEPSCs recorded in layer V. Meanwhile, the increased frequency of IPSCs with unchanged amplitude suggest a presynaptic mechanism, in which PAE enhances inhibitory synapse formation onto layer V projection neurons (Skorput et al. 2015). Additional findings by Bird et al. further supported this conclusion. Their study analysed optically evoked IPSCs (oIPSCs) in layer V projection neurons in response to stimulation of layer V PV+ interneurons in the RSC of adolescent mice following acute ethanol exposure at P7 (Bird et al. 2021). They reported increased peak amplitude, current density, asynchronous activity and total charge of oIPSC in ethanol-exposed mice, indicating that PAE leads to long-lasting changes in synapses between projection neurons and PV+ interneurons (Bird et al. 2021). Similar findings by Kenton et al. showed that an increased density of CR+ interneurons in the OFC of adult PAE mice was associated with an increased amplitude of $GABA_A$ receptors-mediated sIPSCs in deep layer pyramidal neurons. This suggests postsynaptic mechanisms in which PAE enhances the density of $GABA_A$ receptors at perisomatic synapses without altering their subunits composition, as indicated by the unmodified decay time (Kenton et al. 2020).

Together, these results underscore the disruption of E/I balance caused by PAE—most often shifting the balance toward inhibition, depending on the cortical region and neuronal populations analyzed. Importantly, E/I imbalance severely disrupts neuronal networks underlying cognitive and sensory processing, potentially explaining the behavioral deficits observed in FASD patients.

6.3.5 Consequences of PAE on Glial Cells

6.3.5.1 Astrocytes

Cortical astrocytes are generated around birth from radial glial cells following the neurogenesis period. *In vitro* studies suggest that PAE reduces RGCs proliferation and survival, limiting their differentiation into astrocytes (Rubert et al. 2006; Taléns-Visconti et al. 2011; Nash et al. 2012; Vemuri and Chetty 2005). However, Li et al. reported an accelerated transformation of RGCs into astrocytes in a mouse model of PAE (Li et al. 2021b). Beyond effects on astrocyte progenitors, several studies have indicated that ethanol disrupts astrocytic properties, impairing neuronal growth and health through oxidative stress induction (Montoliu et al. 1995; Blanco et al. 2004), impaired neurite outgrowth (Pascual and Guerri 2007; Yanni et al. 2002; Chen and Charness 2008; Paul and Medina 2012; Tomás et al. 2005), and disrupted brain lipid homeostasis (Guizzetti et al. 2007; Zhou et al. 2014). Ethanol strongly affects GFAP expression in the cortex, with variations depending on the PAE model used (Goodlett et al. 1993, 1997). In addition, ethanol inhibits astrocyte proliferation (Kötter and Klein 1999; Guizzetti and Costa 1996), aligning with findings of reduced glial cell numbers in an *in vivo* FASD model of the rat SSC (Miller and Potempa 1990) (Fig. 6.4). Given the abundance of glial cells in the brain, this reduction may contribute to ethanol-induced microcephaly. Co-culture experiments have shown that alcohol alters the production and release of neurotrophic factors and neurite outgrowth inhibitors, impairing neuritogenesis and neuronal survival (Pascual and Guerri 2007; Yanni et al. 2002; Chen and Charness 2008; Paul and Medina 2012; Tomás et al. 2005). Further research should explore the role of glial cells as midline guideposts for callosal fiber development, given the significant impact of PAE on corpus callosum formation.

In vitro studies have also demonstrated that ethanol induces reactive species production and inflammatory signaling in astrocytes (Montoliu et al. 1995; Blanco et al. 2004). Astrocyte-mediated oxidative stress may contribute to neuronal death, potentially explaining the apoptotic events and reduced cortical size observed after PAE. Furthermore, ethanol disrupts brain cholesterol homeostasis by increasing lipoprotein release from astrocytes (Guizzetti et al. 2007; Zhou et al. 2014). Proper cholesterol levels are essential for cell proliferation and neuronal survival, and astrocyte-produced lipoproteins regulate cholesterol clearance in the brain (Zhang and Liu 2015). Guizzetti et al. found that neonatal alcohol exposure in mice increases cortical levels of ABCA1, a key astrocytic lipoprotein transporter (Guizzetti et al. 2007). Similarly, studies have reported that PAE upregulates ABCA1 and ABCG1 transporters expression, reducing cortical cholesterol levels in young female mice (Zhou et al. 2014).

6.3.5.2 Oligodendrocytes

Since myelination mainly occurs postnatally, PAE might not be expected to significantly impair this process. However, studies have highlighted white matter abnormalities following PAE (Lancaster 1994), including delayed myelination in the corpus callosum (Milbocker et al. 2022) and reduced intracortical myelination (Kilpatrick et al. 2022). Growing evidence suggests that PAE permanently disrupts OPCs programming, impairing their maturation into oligodendrocytes (Fig. 6.4).

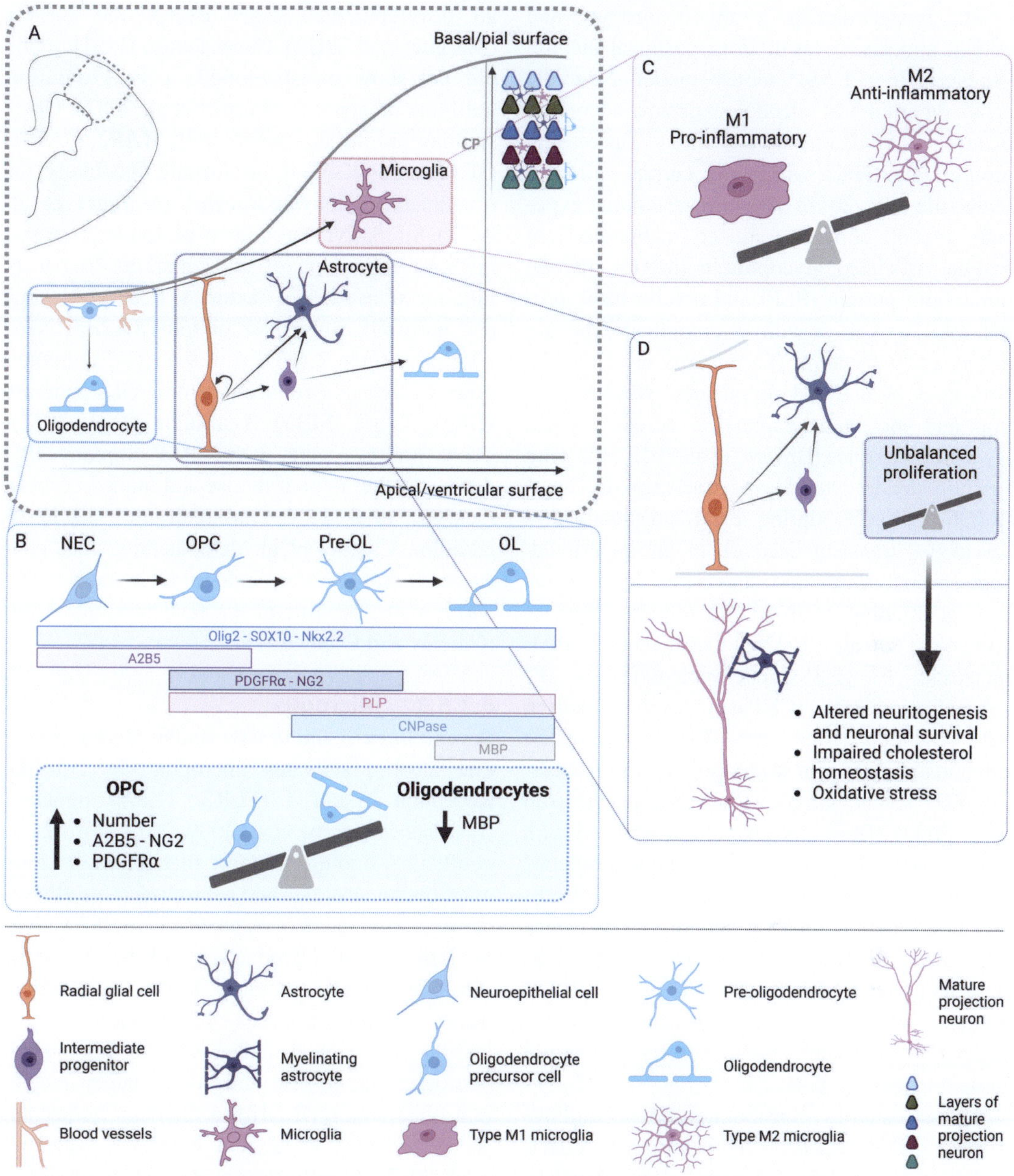

Fig. 6.4 Overview of PAE-induced defects in cortical glial cells. (**a**) Generation of astrocytes, oligodendrocytes and microglia in the cerebral cortex. Astrocytes originate either directly from RGCs or indirectly from IPs, which also generate oligodendrocytes to a lesser extent. OLs mainly arise from OPCs migrating in waves from the ventral GE and locally within the cortex as gliogenesis proceeds. Microglia mostly originate from primitive macrophages in the yolk sac, which migrate into the neuroepithelium via the developing bloodstream. (**b**) PAE dampens the differentiation of OPCs into oligodendrocytes, as indicated by increased expression of proliferation markers and decreased expression of myelin-associated proteins. (**c**) PAE increases the number of activated amoeboid-shaped and M1 microglia, at the expense of quiescent, ramified-shaped and M2 microglia. (**d**) PAE interferes with progenitor differentiation and astrocytes proliferation, thus impacting astrocytic properties. This results in altered signaling between astrocytes and neurons, inducing oxidative stress and impairing neuritogenesis, neuronal survival and cholesterol homeostasis. *OL* oligodendrocyte, *OPC* oligodendrocyte progenitor cell, *RGC* radial glial cell, *IP* intermediate progenitor, *GE* ganglionic eminence

The greatest damage to oligodendrocytes and myelin appears to result from postnatal alcohol exposure. In a FASD mouse model, Newville et al. reported that alcohol exposure decreased mature oligodendrocytes while increasing proliferating OPCs within the corpus callosum (Newville et al. 2017). Another gestational exposure model showed reduced expression of myelin-associated glycoprotein (MAG), myelin proteolipid protein (PLP) and myelin basic protein (MBP), with or without continued exposure during early lactation (Cantacorps et al. 2017). Brosolo et al. analysed oligodendrocytes localization and molecular expression across cortical layers in PAE mice (Brosolo et al. 2022). Staining for oligodendrocyte lineage transcription factor 2 (Olig2)+ cells during early postnatal days revealed a transient decrease in the superficial/deep cortical layers ratio, suggesting delayed cortical positioning of migrating oligodendrocytes (Brosolo et al. 2022). Consistently, PAE increased 2′,3′-Cyclic-nucleotide 3′--phosphodiesterase (CNPase) levels—marking the transition from pre-OLs to immature oligodendrocytes—in layers V–VI, while reducing MBP levels in layer VI in P15 mice (Brosolo et al. 2022). These defects were associated with long-term myelin impairments, including reduced myelinated axon density, thinner myelin sheaths and motor deficits in P15 alcohol-exposed mice (Brosolo et al. 2022). Collectively, these findings indicate that PAE delays oligodendrocytes differentiation, particularly in deep cortical layers, leading to persistent myelin defects and motor impairments (Fig. 6.4).

Human studies corroborate rodent findings regarding PAE-induced oligodendrocytes differentiation impairments. During early development, neural stem cell-derived OPCs expressing platelet-derived growth factor receptor-α (PDGFR-α) differentiate into immature pre-OLs, which mature into OLs expressing MBP and producing myelin. While PDGFR-α is rapidly downregulated as OPCs differentiate, Olig2 remains expressed in OPCs, pre-OLs and OLs (Marguet et al. 2020). Marguet et al. reported significantly increased PDGFR-α expression in the GE and CP of human FASD brain tissues at all developmental stages except the earliest (Marguet et al. 2022). Consistently, FASD brains did not show massive olig2+ cells generation until late pregnancy (Marguet et al. 2022). Olig2 staining did not co-express with MAP2, GABA, GFAP, or PDGFR-α, confirming specificity for (pre-)mature oligodendrocytes (Marguet et al. 2022). Similarly, Darbinian et al. found increased mRNAs expression of OPC markers (octamer-binding transcription factor 4 (Oct4), Nanog) and early OL progenitor proteins (A2B5, Neural/glial antigen 2 (NG2)) in fetal FASD human brains, alongside reduced mature OLs markers (Olig1, Olig2, MBP) (Darbinian et al. 2021). These findings suggest that PAE impairs OPC differentiation in both mouse and human cortices (Marguet et al. 2022; Darbinian et al. 2021). In addition, Creeley et al. demonstrated that late-stage alcohol exposure induces OLs apoptosis in white matter regions of the fetal macaque brain (Creeley and Olney 2013).

6.3.5.3 Microglia

Several *in vitro* and *in vivo* studies have reported that alcohol activates microglia via Toll-like Receptors 2 and 4 (TLR2, TLR4) signaling (Fernandez-Lizarbe et al. 2009, 2013). However, conflicting findings suggest that microglia may exert both neurotoxic and neuroprotective effects. On one hand, alcohol-induced microglial activation triggers ROS production and the release of pro-inflammatory cytokines, leading to neuronal death (Alfonso-Loeches and Guerri 2011; Padilla-Valdez et al. 2024). On the other hand, microglia can release anti-inflammatory factors (e.g., Interleukin (IL)-10) to maintain homeostasis in response to alcohol exposure (Marshall et al. 2013). In a third trimester mouse model of FASD, PAE increased ILβ and TNFα mRNA levels and altered microglia morphology, shifting toward an activated profile in the cerebral cortex (Drew et al. 2015). These defects were prevented by treatment with the anti-inflammatory drugs pioglitazone and hydrogen sulfide (Drew et al. 2015; Mohseni et al. 2020). In another FASD mouse model (E6 to E18), Komada et al. found that PAE disrupts microglial activation and differentiation (Komada et al. 2017). Under normal conditions, activated microglia exhibit a globular, amoeboid-like morphology, while quiescent, ramified microglia display numerous processes. M1 microglia are pro-inflammatory and essential for pathogen defense, whereas M2 microglia are anti-inflammatory and promote tissue repair (Komada et al. 2017). PAE increased the presence of Allograft inflammatory factor 1 (Iba1)+ amoeboid microglia in the dorsal telencephalon of E15.5 embryos and in the PFC of P3 pups, while reducing the population of ramified microglia (Komada et al. 2017). This shift corresponded with an increased M1/M2 ratio and altered cytokine profiles, indicating aberrant microglial activation (Komada et al. 2017). Interestingly, this study also revealed abnormalities in neuronal distribution, cortical layer formation, and dopaminergic neuronal projections in the neocortex of alcohol-exposed mice. These defects were ameliorated following treatment with pioglitazone (Komada et al. 2017). In summary, the mechanisms underlying PAE-induced microglial dysfunction remain unclear, but they likely involve an imbalance between neurotoxic pro-inflammatory effects and residual neuroprotective functions (Fig. 6.4).

6.4 Sex Differences in FASD

Although sex differences have not been extensively discussed in this chapter, sexual dimorphism has been reported in certain traits among individuals with FASD. Research indicates a higher prevalence of FASD in young boys compared to girls; however, this sex difference is no longer observed when children are diagnosed later in life (Thanh et al. 2014). Similarly, boys with FASD show lower viability at birth and reduced overall survival compared to their female counterparts (May et al. 2017). While major sex differences are not evident in the presentation of FASD symptoms, variability exists in the prevalence of mental health outcomes. Males with PAE exhibit higher rates of ADHD, conduct disorder, oppositional defiant disorder, as well as impairments in motor function, memory, attention, executive functioning, and adaptive behavior. In contrast, females are more prone to anxiety and mood disorders, display more severe dysmorphia and perform worse in non-verbal IQ tasks (May et al. 2017; Flannigan et al. 2023).

Consistent with these behavioral differences, structural variabilities have also been observed. Neuroimaging studies indicate that males with FASD experience more pronounced reductions in total brain volume and cortical thickness, particularly in frontal, temporal, and occipital regions (Treit et al. 2017). A longitudinal study of children aged 3 to 8 found that males with PAE show greater age-related changes in grey matter volumes than females (Long et al. 2024). Similarly, diffusion tensor imaging studies have shown that males exhibit higher fractional anisotropy (FA)—a measure of fiber density, axonal diameter, and myelination in white matter—in specific regions of the corpus callosum and corticospinal tract (Treit et al. 2017). Several factors may contribute to these sex differences, including fetal sex-specific placental functions, sex hormones, and differences in alcohol metabolism. First, maternal cytokine levels vary depending on fetal sex (Bake et al. 2023), and studies have linked altered regional brain activity and connectivity to maternal proinflammatory cytokine levels (Goldstein et al. 2021). Second, sex differences exist in placental gene expression and upstream epigenetic regulation (Bake et al. 2023). Transcriptomic analyses of the placenta have identified differentially expressed genes involved in cell adhesion, cell-cell interaction, and mTOR and PPAR signaling—key pathways in cortical development (Braun et al. 2022). Third, sex hormones play a critical role in neurodevelopment by regulating synapse formation, GABAergic activity, neuropeptide expression and neurotransmitter receptors distribution via sex hormone receptors expressed in neurons both in nuclei and at synaptic sites (McEwen and Milner 2017). Estrogens, in particular, influence neuronal migration, directly targeting GABAergic neurons and promoting the release of brain-derived neurotrophic factor (BDNF) from specific cell types (Tobet et al. 2009). Studies have shown that estrogens affect dendritic and spines morphology in the PFC of both rats and monkeys (McEwen and Milner 2017; Tobet et al. 2009), suggesting that some morphological abnormalities observed in FASD mays be estrogen-dependent. Importantly, beyond maternal hormones exposure, the human fetus begins producing testosterone and estrogen around GW8-9, with testosterone levels already significantly higher in males than in females by GW12. This early hormonal differentiation influences brain development and may interact with PAE-related neurodevelopmental effects (Scott et al. 2009). Research in animal models indicates that PAE decreases testosterone levels in male fetuses, newborns and adult rodents, while it reduces luteinizing hormone (LH) levels in adolescent female rodents (Gabriel et al. 1998). Alcohol can also indirectly affect the fetus by altering maternal hormonal balance and placental function (Gabriel et al. 1998). Finally, while sex differences in alcohol metabolism are well documented—mainly due to lower activity of hepatic and gastric alcohol dehydrogenase (ADH) in women (Baraona et al. 2001)—it remains unclear whether the fetus' limited ability to metabolize alcohol contributes to sex differences in FASD outcomes (Zelner and Koren 2013).

6.5 Discrepancies Between Studies

The review of the literature highlights numerous discrepancies between studies modelling FASD, emphasizing the vast complexity of these disorders and the plethora of facets to explore. When modelling FASD, results must therefore be interpreted based on the level of intoxication achieved, the specific period of brain development targeted, the pattern of administration (chronic or acute), the route of administration (ingestion, injection, or inhalation) and the timing of analysis. Rodent models have proven to be valuable tools for studying FASD, providing most of the results discussed in this chapter (Patten et al. 2014).

6.5.1 Developmental Period of Exposure

In humans, the first trimester (E1-10 in rodents) corresponds to the formation of the neural tube and gastrulation, followed by cell proliferation and migration in the second trimester (E10-20 in rodents). The third trimester (PND 1-10 in rodents) marks a "brain growth spurt," with neuronal maturation, neurite outgrowth and synaptogenesis. Typically, first trimester-equivalent alcohol exposure is associated with the facial dysmorphology typical of FAS (Parnell et al. 2009, 2013; Godin et al. 2010; O'Leary-Moore et al. 2010), while second- and third-trimester PAE usually induce long-term defects in neuronal circuitry (Miller 1993, 1996) and massive apoptosis (Ikonomidou et al. 2000), respectively. Corticogenesis follows a precise temporally regulated pattern, with neural cells subpopulations generated at different times from distinct progenitor pools. Thus, the exact time window of PAE must be carefully monitored depending on the targeted stage and specific cell population analyzed to avoid discrepancies between studies.

6.5.2 Blood Alcohol Concentration (BAC)

Most studies use a BAC of 80 mg/dl which is considered legally intoxicated, and some report a direct correlation between BAC and the severity of the FASD phenotype (Maier and West 2001), cortical thickness (Robertson et al. 2016) and neuronal maturation defects (Cui et al. 2010). However, the severity of reported defects also depends on the length of the gestation period covered by PAE. A single acute dose during pregnancy would not induce the same defects as chronic PAE throughout the entire gestation period. Nevertheless, both continuous low-level exposure and single high-level exposure have been reported to induce structural damages, reinforcing the consensus that there is no "safe" amount of alcohol or time window during pregnancy.

6.5.3 Route of Administration

The pharmacokinetics of ethanol differ between oral gavage, intraperitoneal injection (IP) or vapor administration. Injection and inhalation allow a faster increase in BAC, leading to higher values that do not mimic the route of intake in humans. For example, an equivalent ethanol dose results in a higher incidence of malformation when administered via IP injection compared to gavage. In addition, both injections and gavage induce significant stress, and numerous studies have shown that stress alters dendritic spines morphology in the cortex (Radley et al. 2008; Leuner and Shors 2013), making stress a confounding factor in analyzing PAE-induced neuronal maturation defects.

Beyond animal models, cell culture and human organoids are emerging as valuable tools to decipher the mechanisms by which alcohol impacts cortical development. Some *in vitro* models use cells derived from animals exposed to ethanol *in vivo*, while others employ cell culture and brain organoids directly exposed to ethanol *in vitro*. However, direct exposure to ethanol has been shown to induce apoptosis and premature differentiation, effects not typically found in most *in vivo* models (Adams et al. 2023; Sarieva and Mayer 2021). This raises the question of whether these findings reflect real consequences of ethanol exposure or are artifacts of the model due to poor metabolization of ethanol, leading to reduced amount of acetaldehyde and acetate. Moreover, cell culture models do not allow exposure to the metabolites found in the blood after excessive alcohol consumption, highlighting additional limitations of *in vitro* models for studying FASD.

6.6 Conclusions

In summary, cortical development forms the foundation for higher-order cognitive abilities, including sensory perception, reasoning, decision-making, and motor control. The cerebral cortex is composed of a complex neuronal network that emerges through finely coordinated neurodevelopmental processes, making it particularly vulnerable to pharmacological disruptions such as PAE. Alcohol exposure during pregnancy significantly impacts all stages of cortical development, from neuronal proliferation to gliogenesis, ultimately impairing proper communication between cortical neurons. These disruptions lead to altered cortical circuitry, resulting in the persistent cognitive and behavioral deficits characteristic of FASD, which remains the most common preventable cause of birth defects, intellectual disabilities, and developmental disorders. While the severity of FASD symptoms varies depending on factors like dosage, timing of exposure, and genetic predisposition, the risks are unequivocal. Given the enduring consequences of PAE, public health initiatives must emphasize awareness, prevention, and early intervention to safeguard fetal brain development and reduce FASD prevalence. Although this chapter highlights growing insights into the effects of PAE on cortical development, further research is crucial to uncover the exact pathological mechanisms involved in FASD and to develop targeted therapies to mitigate its impact.

References

Aaku-Saraste E, Hellwig A, Huttner WB (1996) Loss of occludin and functional tight junctions, but not ZO-1, during neural tube closure – remodeling of the neuroepithelium prior to neurogenesis. Dev Biol 180(2):664–679

Adams JW et al (2023) Impact of alcohol exposure on neural development and network formation in human cortical organoids. Mol Psychiatry 28(4):1571–1584

Aghamohammadi-Sereshki A et al (2025) Properties of the prefrontal tracts and cingulum bundle in children with prenatal alcohol exposure. J Affect Disord 369:164–173

Agirman G, Broix L, Nguyen L (2017) Cerebral cortex development: an outside-in perspective. FEBS Lett 591(24):3978–3992

Alcoholism, N.I.o.A.A.a. Fetal Alcohol Spectrum Disorders (2023) Available from: https://www.niaaa.nih.gov/research/fetal-alcohol-spectrum-disorders

Alfonso-Loeches S, Guerri C (2011) Molecular and behavioral aspects of the actions of alcohol on the adult and developing brain. Crit Rev Clin Lab Sci 48(1):19–47

Altounian M, Bellon A, Mann F (2023) Neuronal miR-17-5p contributes to interhemispheric cortical connectivity defects induced by prenatal alcohol exposure. Cell Rep 42(9):113020

Arai Y, Taverna E (2017) Neural progenitor cell polarity and cortical development. Front Cell Neurosci 11:384

Archibald SL et al (2001) Brain dysmorphology in individuals with severe prenatal alcohol exposure. Dev Med Child Neurol 43(3):148–154

Arikkath J (2012) Molecular mechanisms of dendrite morphogenesis. Front Cell Neurosci 6:61

Aronne MP et al (2008) Prenatal ethanol exposure reduces the expression of the transcriptional factor Pax6 in the developing rat brain. Ann N Y Acad Sci 1139:478–498

Aronne MP et al (2011) Effects of prenatal ethanol exposure on rat brain radial glia and neuroblast migration. Exp Neurol 229(2):364–371

Astley SJ et al (2009) Magnetic resonance imaging outcomes from a comprehensive magnetic resonance study of children with fetal alcohol spectrum disorders. Alcohol Clin Exp Res 33(10):1671–1689

Bailey CD, Brien JF, Reynolds JN (2001) Chronic prenatal ethanol exposure increases GABA(A) receptor subunit protein expression in the adult guinea pig cerebral cortex. J Neurosci 21(12):4381–4389

Bailey CD, Brien JF, Reynolds JN (2004) Chronic prenatal ethanol exposure alters the proportion of GABAergic neurons in layers II/III of the adult guinea pig somatosensory cortex. Neurotoxicol Teratol 26(1):59–63

Bake S et al (2023) The interaction of genetic sex and prenatal alcohol exposure on health across the lifespan. Front Neuroendocrinol 71:101103

Bandler RC et al (2022) Single-cell delineation of lineage and genetic identity in the mouse brain. Nature 601(7893):404–409

Baraona E et al (2001) Gender differences in pharmacokinetics of alcohol. Alcohol Clin Exp Res 25(4):502–507

Bartolini G et al (2017) Neuregulin 3 mediates cortical plate invasion and laminar allocation of GABAergic interneurons. Cell Rep 18(5):1157–1170

Bellion A et al (2005) Nucleokinesis in tangentially migrating neurons comprises two alternating phases: forward migration of the Golgi/centrosome associated with centrosome splitting and myosin contraction at the rear. J Neurosci 25(24):5691–5699

Bird CW et al (2020) Neonatal ethanol exposure triggers apoptosis in the murine retrosplenial cortex: role of inhibition of NMDA receptor-driven action potential firing. Neuropharmacology 162:107837

Bird CW et al (2021) Enhancement of parvalbumin interneuron-mediated neurotransmission in the retrosplenial cortex of adolescent mice following third trimester-equivalent ethanol exposure. Sci Rep 11(1):1716

Blanco AM et al (2004) Ethanol-induced iNOS and COX-2 expression in cultured astrocytes via NF-kappa B. Neuroreport 15(4):681–685

Blanquie O et al (2017) Electrical activity controls area-specific expression of neuronal apoptosis in the mouse developing cerebral cortex. Elife:6

Bookstein FL et al (2002) Corpus callosum shape and neuropsychological deficits in adult males with heavy fetal alcohol exposure. Neuroimage 15(1):233–251

Borrell V (2019) Recent advances in understanding neocortical development. F1000Res:8

Bortone D, Polleux F (2009) KCC2 expression promotes the termination of cortical interneuron migration in a voltage-sensitive calcium-dependent manner. Neuron 62(1):53–71

Braun AE et al (2022) Sex at the interface: the origin and impact of sex differences in the developing human placenta. Biol Sex Differ 13(1):50

Brosolo M et al (2022) In utero alcohol exposure impairs vessel-associated positioning and differentiation of oligodendrocytes in the developing neocortex. Neurobiol Dis 171:105791

Burd L, Blair J, Dropps K (2012) Prenatal alcohol exposure, blood alcohol concentrations and alcohol elimination rates for the mother, fetus and newborn. J Perinatol 32(9):652–659

Butt SJ et al (2005) The temporal and spatial origins of cortical interneurons predict their physiological subtype. Neuron 48(4):591–604

Cadwell CR et al (2019) Development and arealization of the cerebral cortex. Neuron 103(6):980–1004

Cantacorps L et al (2017) Maternal alcohol binge drinking induces persistent neuroinflammation associated with myelin damage and behavioural dysfunctions in offspring mice. Neuropharmacology 123:368–384

Carr JL, Agnihotri S, Keightley M (2010) Sensory processing and adaptive behavior deficits of children across the fetal alcohol spectrum disorder continuum. Alcohol Clin Exp Res 34(6):1022–1032

Charvet CJ (2020) Closing the gap from transcription to the structural connectome enhances the study of connections in the human brain. Dev Dyn 249(9):1047–1061

Chen S, Charness ME (2008) Ethanol inhibits neuronal differentiation by disrupting activity-dependent neuroprotective protein signaling. Proc Natl Acad Sci U S A 105(50):19962–19967

Chen X et al (2012) Understanding specific effects of prenatal alcohol exposure on brain structure in young adults. Hum Brain Mapp 33(7):1663–1676

Chittajallu R, Isaac JT (2010) Emergence of cortical inhibition by coordinated sensory-driven plasticity at distinct synaptic loci. Nat Neurosci 13(10):1240–1248

Clarke LE, Barres BA (2013) Emerging roles of astrocytes in neural circuit development. Nat Rev Neurosci 14(5):311–321

Clavreul S, Dumas L, Loulier K (2022) Astrocyte development in the cerebral cortex: complexity of their origin, genesis, and maturation. Front Neurosci 16: 916055

Coleman LG Jr et al (2012) Postnatal day 7 ethanol treatment causes persistent reductions in adult mouse brain volume and cortical neurons with sex specific effects on neurogenesis. Alcohol 46(6):603–612

Creeley CE, Olney JW (2013) Drug-induced apoptosis: mechanism by which alcohol and many other drugs can disrupt brain development. Brain Sci 3(3): 1153–1181

Cui ZJ et al (2010) Prenatal alcohol exposure induces long-term changes in dendritic spines and synapses in the mouse visual cortex. Alcohol Alcohol 45(4): 312–319

Cunningham CL, Martínez-Cerdeño V, Noctor SC (2013) Microglia regulate the number of neural precursor cells in the developing cerebral cortex. J Neurosci 33(10): 4216–4233

Cuzon VC et al (2006) Ambient GABA promotes cortical entry of tangentially migrating cells derived from the medial ganglionic eminence. Cereb Cortex 16(10): 1377–1388

Cuzon VC et al (2008) Ethanol consumption during early pregnancy alters the disposition of tangentially migrating GABAergic interneurons in the fetal cortex. J Neurosci 28(8):1854–1864

Darbinian N et al (2021) Ethanol-mediated alterations in oligodendrocyte differentiation in the developing brain. Neurobiol Dis 148:105181

De Guio F et al (2014) A study of cortical morphology in children with fetal alcohol spectrum disorders. Hum Brain Mapp 35(5):2285–2296

Delatour LC, Yeh PW, Yeh HH (2019) Ethanol exposure in utero disrupts radial migration and pyramidal cell development in the somatosensory cortex. Cereb Cortex 29(5):2125–2139

Delatour LC, Yeh PWL, Yeh HH (2020) Prenatal exposure to ethanol alters synaptic activity in layer V/VI pyramidal neurons of the somatosensory cortex. Cereb Cortex 30(3):1735–1751

Delgado RN et al (2022) Individual human cortical progenitors can produce excitatory and inhibitory neurons. Nature 601(7893):397–403

Denaxa M et al (2018) Modulation of apoptosis controls inhibitory interneuron number in the cortex. Cell Rep 22(7):1710–1721

Di Bella DJ et al (2024) Making Ramon y Cajal proud: development of cell identity and diversity in the cerebral cortex. Neuron 112(13):2091–2111

Donald KA et al (2015) Neuroimaging effects of prenatal alcohol exposure on the developing human brain: a magnetic resonance imaging review. Acta Neuropsychiatr 27(5):251–269

Douglas RJ, Martin KA (2004) Neuronal circuits of the neocortex. Annu Rev Neurosci 27:419–451

Drew PD et al (2015) Pioglitazone blocks ethanol induction of microglial activation and immune responses in the hippocampus, cerebellum, and cerebral cortex in a mouse model of fetal alcohol spectrum disorders. Alcohol Clin Exp Res 39(3):445–454

El Fatimy R et al (2014) Heat shock factor 2 is a stress-responsive mediator of neuronal migration defects in models of fetal alcohol syndrome. EMBO Mol Med 6(8):1043–1061

El Shawa H, Abbott CW 3rd, Huffman KJ (2013) Prenatal ethanol exposure disrupts intraneocortical circuitry, cortical gene expression, and behavior in a mouse model of FASD. J Neurosci 33(48):18893–18905

Fan J et al (2017) Localized reductions in resting-state functional connectivity in children with prenatal alcohol exposure. Hum Brain Mapp 38(10):5217–5233

Feng X et al (2025) Cortical arealization of interneurons defines shared and distinct molecular programs in developing human and macaque brains. Nat Commun 16(1):672

Fernandez-Lizarbe S, Pascual M, Guerri C (2009) Critical role of TLR4 response in the activation of microglia induced by ethanol. J Immunol 183(7):4733–4744

Fernandez-Lizarbe S, Montesinos J, Guerri C (2013) Ethanol induces TLR4/TLR2 association, triggering an inflammatory response in microglial cells. J Neurochem 126(2):261–273

Fischer M et al (2021) Transcriptomic changes due to early, chronic intermittent alcohol exposure during forebrain development implicate WNT signaling, cell-type specification, and cortical regionalization as primary determinants of fetal alcohol syndrome. Alcohol Clin Exp Res 45(5):979–995

Fish EW et al (2016) Acute alcohol exposure during neurulation: behavioral and brain structural consequences in adolescent C57BL/6J mice. Behav Brain Res 311: 70–80

Flannigan K et al (2023) Sex-related differences among individuals assessed for fetal alcohol spectrum disorder in Canada. Alcohol Clin Exp Res (Hoboken) 47(3): 613–623

Fraize J et al (2023) Mapping corpus callosum surface reduction in fetal alcohol spectrum disorders with sulci and connectivity-based parcellation. Front Neurosci 17:1188367

Fryer SL et al (2009) Characterization of white matter microstructure in fetal alcohol spectrum disorders. Alcohol Clin Exp Res 33(3):514–521

Gabriel K et al (1998) The hormonal effects of alcohol use on the mother and fetus. Alcohol Health Res World 22(3):170–177

Galofré E et al (1987) Effects of prenatal ethanol exposure on dendritic spines of layer V pyramidal neurons in the somatosensory cortex of the rat. J Neurol Sci 81(2-3): 185–195

Gao L et al (2019) Quantitative assessment of cerebral connectivity deficiency and cognitive impairment in children with prenatal alcohol exposure. Chaos 29(4): 041101

Ginhoux F, Prinz M (2015) Origin of microglia: current concepts and past controversies. Cold Spring Harb Perspect Biol 7(8):a020537

Godin EA et al (2010) Magnetic resonance microscopy defines ethanol-induced brain abnormalities in prenatal mice: effects of acute insult on gestational day 7. Alcohol Clin Exp Res 34(1):98–111

Godin EA et al (2011) Ventromedian forebrain dysgenesis follows early prenatal ethanol exposure in mice. Neurotoxicol Teratol 33(2):231–239

Goldstein JM et al (2021) Impact of prenatal maternal cytokine exposure on sex differences in brain circuitry regulating stress in offspring 45 years later. Proc Natl Acad Sci U S A 118(15)

Goodlett CR et al (1993) Transient cortical astrogliosis induced by alcohol exposure during the neonatal brain growth spurt in rats. Brain Res Dev Brain Res 72(1):85–97

Goodlett CR et al (1997) Binge-like alcohol exposure of neonatal rats via intragastric intubation induces both Purkinje cell loss and cortical astrogliosis. Alcohol Clin Exp Res 21(6):1010–1017

Gouwens NW et al (2020) Integrated morphoelectric and transcriptomic classification of cortical GABAergic cells. Cell 183(4):935–953.e19

Granato A (2006) Altered organization of cortical interneurons in rats exposed to ethanol during neonatal life. Brain Res 1069(1):23–30

Greenmyer JR et al (2018) A multicountry updated assessment of the economic impact of fetal alcohol spectrum disorder: costs for children and adults. J Addict Med 12(6):466–473

Greig LC et al (2013) Molecular logic of neocortical projection neuron specification, development and diversity. Nat Rev Neurosci 14(11):755–769

Guizzetti M, Costa LG (1996) Inhibition of muscarinic receptor-stimulated glial cell proliferation by ethanol. J Neurochem 67(6):2236–2245

Guizzetti M et al (2007) Ethanol induces cholesterol efflux and up-regulates ATP-binding cassette cholesterol transporters in fetal astrocytes. J Biol Chem 282(26): 18740–18749

Guizzetti M et al (2008) Modulation of neuritogenesis by astrocyte muscarinic receptors. J Biol Chem 283(46): 31884–31897

Gursky ZH, Savage LM, Klintsova AY (2021) Executive functioning-specific behavioral impairments in a rat model of human third trimester binge drinking implicate prefrontal-thalamo-hippocampal circuitry in Fetal Alcohol Spectrum Disorders. Behav Brain Res 405: 113208

Hamilton GF, Whitcher LT, Klintsova AY (2010) Postnatal binge-like alcohol exposure decreases dendritic complexity while increasing the density of mature spines in mPFC Layer II/III pyramidal neurons. Synapse 64(2):127–135

Hansen AH, Hippenmeyer S (2020) Non-cell-autonomous mechanisms in radial projection neuron migration in the developing cerebral cortex. Front Cell Dev Biol 8: 574382

Harris KD, Shepherd GM (2015) The neocortical circuit: themes and variations. Nat Neurosci 18(2):170–181

Harry GJ, Kraft AD (2012) Microglia in the developing brain: a potential target with lifetime effects. Neurotoxicology 33(2):191–206

Hasegawa K, Kuwako KI (2022) Molecular mechanisms regulating the spatial configuration of neurites. Semin Cell Dev Biol 129:103–114

Hashimoto-Torii K et al (2011) Combined transcriptome analysis of fetal human and mouse cerebral cortex exposed to alcohol. Proc Natl Acad Sci U S A 108(10):4212–4217

Haubensak W et al (2004) Neurons arise in the basal neuroepithelium of the early mammalian telencephalon: a major site of neurogenesis. Proc Natl Acad Sci U S A 101(9):3196–3201

Hendrickson TJ et al (2017) Cortical gyrification is abnormal in children with prenatal alcohol exposure. Neuroimage Clin 15:391–400

Hendrickson TJ et al (2018) Two-year cortical trajectories are abnormal in children and adolescents with prenatal alcohol exposure. Dev Cogn Neurosci 30:123–133

Heng JI, Chariot A, Nguyen L (2010) Molecular layers underlying cytoskeletal remodelling during cortical development. Trends Neurosci 33(1):38–47

Hoshiba Y et al (2016) Sox11 balances dendritic morphogenesis with neuronal migration in the developing cerebral cortex. J Neurosci 36(21):5775–5784

Huang Y et al (2024) Alcohol exposure induces nucleolar stress and apoptosis in mouse neural stem cells and late-term fetal brain. Cells 13(5)

Huilgol D et al (2023) Direct and indirect neurogenesis generate a mosaic of distinct glutamatergic projection neuron types in cerebral cortex. Neuron 111(16): 2557–2569 e4

Ikonomidou C et al (2000) Ethanol-induced apoptotic neurodegeneration and fetal alcohol syndrome. Science 287(5455):1056–1060

Infante MA et al (2015) Atypical cortical gyrification in adolescents with histories of heavy prenatal alcohol exposure. Brain Res 1624:446–454

Jégou S et al (2012) Prenatal alcohol exposure affects vasculature development in the neonatal brain. Ann Neurol 72(6):952–960

Jones KL, Smith DW (1973) Recognition of the fetal alcohol syndrome in early infancy. Lancet 302(7836): 999–1001

Kamigaki T (2019) Dissecting executive control circuits with neuron types. Neurosci Res 141:13–22

Kenton JA et al (2020) Moderate prenatal alcohol exposure alters the number and function of GABAergic interneurons in the murine orbitofrontal cortex. Alcohol 88:33–41

Kessaris N et al (2006) Competing waves of oligodendrocytes in the forebrain and postnatal elimination of an embryonic lineage. Nat Neurosci 9(2): 173–179

Kilpatrick LA et al (2022) Impact of prenatal alcohol exposure on intracortical myelination and deep white matter in children with attention deficit hyperactivity disorder. Neuroimage Rep 2(1)

Kimelberg HK, Nedergaard M (2010) Functions of astrocytes and their potential as therapeutic targets. Neurotherapeutics 7(4):338–353
Kleiber ML et al (2013) Neurodevelopmental alcohol exposure elicits long-term changes to gene expression that alter distinct molecular pathways dependent on timing of exposure. J Neurodev Disord 5(1):6
Komada M et al (2017) Mechanisms underlying neuroinflammation and neurodevelopmental toxicity in the mouse neocortex following prenatal exposure to ethanol. Sci Rep 7(1):4934
Komatsu S et al (2001) Prenatal exposure to ethanol induces leptomeningeal heterotopia in the cerebral cortex of the rat fetus. Acta Neuropathol 101(1):22–26
Kötter K, Klein J (1999) Ethanol inhibits astroglial cell proliferation by disruption of phospholipase D-mediated signaling. J Neurochem 73(6):2517–2523
Laguesse S, Peyre E, Nguyen L (2015) Progenitor genealogy in the developing cerebral cortex. Cell Tissue Res 359(1):17–32
Lancaster FE (1994) Alcohol and white matter development – a review. Alcohol Clin Exp Res 18(3): 644–647
Larsen ZH et al (2016) Effects of ethanol on cellular composition and network excitability of human pluripotent stem cell-derived neurons. Alcohol Clin Exp Res 40(11):2339–2350
Lawrence RC, Otero NK, Kelly SJ (2012) Selective effects of perinatal ethanol exposure in medial prefrontal cortex and nucleus accumbens. Neurotoxicol Teratol 34(1):128–135
Le Magueresse C, Monyer H (2013) GABAergic interneurons shape the functional maturation of the cortex. Neuron 77(3):388–405
Lebel C et al (2012) A longitudinal study of the long-term consequences of drinking during pregnancy: heavy in utero alcohol exposure disrupts the normal processes of brain development. J Neurosci 32(44):15243–15251
Lecuyer M et al (2017) PLGF, a placental marker of fetal brain defects after in utero alcohol exposure. Acta Neuropathol Commun 5(1):44
Lee SM, Yeh PWL, Yeh HH (2022) L-type calcium channels contribute to ethanol-induced aberrant tangential migration of primordial cortical GABAergic interneurons in the embryonic medial prefrontal cortex. eNeuro 9(1)
Leger C et al (2020) In utero alcohol exposure exacerbates endothelial protease activity from pial microvessels and impairs GABA interneuron positioning. Neurobiol Dis 145:105074
Léger C et al (2020) Glutamate controls vessel-associated migration of GABA interneurons from the pial migratory route via NMDA receptors and endothelial protease activation. Cell Mol Life Sci 77(10):1959–1986
Leigland LA et al (2013) The influence of fetal ethanol exposure on subsequent development of the cerebral cortex as revealed by magnetic resonance imaging. Alcohol Clin Exp Res 37(6):924–932
Lepiemme F et al (2022) Oligodendrocyte precursors guide interneuron migration by unidirectional contact repulsion. Science 376(6595):eabn6204
Leuner B, Shors TJ (2013) Stress, anxiety, and dendritic spines: what are the connections? Neuroscience 251: 108–119
Li X et al (2021a) Decoding cortical glial cell development. Neurosci Bull 37(4):440–460
Li Y et al (2021b) Prenatal ethanol exposure impairs the formation of radial glial fibers and promotes the transformation of GFAPdelta-positive radial glial cells into astrocytes. Mol Med Rep 23(4)
Li Z et al (2022) Identification of cortical interneuron cell markers in mouse embryos based on machine learning analysis of single-cell transcriptomics. Front Neurosci 16:841145
Liang X et al (2024) Structural brain network organization in children with prenatal alcohol exposure. Neuroimage Clin 44:103690
Licheri V et al (2023) Long-term effects of low prenatal alcohol exposure on GABAergic interneurons of the murine posterior parietal cortex. Alcohol Clin Exp Res (Hoboken) 47(12):2248–2261
Lim L et al (2018) Development and functional diversification of cortical interneurons. Neuron 100(2): 294–313
Limoni G et al (2021) PlexinA4-Semaphorin3A-mediated crosstalk between main cortical interneuron classes is required for superficial interneuron lamination. Cell Rep 34(4):108644
Little G, Reynolds J, Beaulieu C (2018) Altered functional connectivity observed at rest in children and adolescents prenatally exposed to alcohol. Brain Connect 8(8):503–515
Livy DJ, Elberger AJ (2008) Alcohol exposure during the first two trimesters-equivalent alters the development of corpus callosum projection neurons in the rat. Alcohol 42(4):285–293
Llorca A, Deogracias R (2022) Origin, development, and synaptogenesis of cortical interneurons. Front Neurosci 16:929469
Lodato S et al (2011) Excitatory projection neuron subtypes control the distribution of local inhibitory interneurons in the cerebral cortex. Neuron 69(4): 763–779
Long JE et al (2009) Dlx1&2 and Mash1 transcription factors control MGE and CGE patterning and differentiation through parallel and overlapping pathways. Cereb Cortex 19(Suppl 1):196
Long X et al (2018) Sensorimotor network alterations in children and youth with prenatal alcohol exposure. Hum Brain Mapp 39(5):2258–2268
Long M et al (2024) Sex and age effects on gray matter volume trajectories in young children with prenatal alcohol exposure. Front Hum Neurosci 18:1379959
Louth EL et al (2018) Developmental ethanol exposure alters the morphology of mouse prefrontal neurons in a layer-specific manner. Brain Res 1678:94–105

Lu L et al (2023) Ethanol exposure disrupted the formation of radial glial processes and impaired the generation and migration of outer radial glial cells in forebrain organoids derived from human embryonic stem cells. Exp Neurol 362:114325

Ma L, Tymanskyj SR (2020) Axon growth and branching. In: Cellular migration and formation of axons and dendrites, pp 57–85

Maier SE, West JR (2001) Drinking patterns and alcohol-related birth defects. Alcohol Res Health 25(3): 168–174

Marguet F et al (2020) Prenatal alcohol exposure is a leading cause of interneuronopathy in humans. Acta Neuropathol Commun 8(1):208

Marguet F et al (2022) Oligodendrocyte lineage is severely affected in human alcohol-exposed foetuses. Acta Neuropathol Commun 10(1):74

Marín O, Rubenstein JL (2001) A long, remarkable journey: tangential migration in the telencephalon. Nat Rev Neurosci 2(11):780–790

Marín O et al (2001) Sorting of striatal and cortical interneurons regulated by semaphorin-neuropilin interactions. Science 293(5531):872–875

Marques-Smith A et al (2016) A transient translaminar GABAergic interneuron circuit connects thalamocortical recipient layers in neonatal somatosensory cortex. Neuron 89(3):536–549

Marshall SA et al (2013) Microglial activation is not equivalent to neuroinflammation in alcohol-induced neurodegeneration: the importance of microglia phenotype. Neurobiol Dis 54:239–251

Mattson SN, Crocker N, Nguyen TT (2011) Fetal alcohol spectrum disorders: neuropsychological and behavioral features. Neuropsychol Rev 21(2):81–101

Mattson SN, Bernes GA, Doyle LR (2019) Fetal alcohol spectrum disorders: a review of the neurobehavioral deficits associated with prenatal alcohol exposure. Alcohol Clin Exp Res 43(6):1046–1062

May PA et al (2017) Who is most affected by prenatal alcohol exposure: boys or girls? Drug Alcohol Depend 177:258–267

Mayer C et al (2018) Developmental diversification of cortical inhibitory interneurons. Nature 555(7697): 457–462

McEwen BS, Milner TA (2017) Understanding the broad influence of sex hormones and sex differences in the brain. J Neurosci Res 95(1-2):24–39

McFarlane S (2000) Dendritic morphogenesis: building An Arbor. Mol Neurobiol 22(1-3):1–9

Mi D et al (2018) Early emergence of cortical interneuron diversity in the mouse embryo. Science 360(6384): 81–85

Milbocker KA et al (2022) Reduced and delayed myelination and volume of corpus callosum in an animal model of Fetal Alcohol Spectrum Disorders partially benefit from voluntary exercise. Sci Rep 12(1):10653

Mildner A et al (2007) Microglia in the adult brain arise from Ly-6ChiCCR2+ monocytes only under defined host conditions. Nat Neurosci 10(12):1544–1553

Miller MW (1986) Effects of alcohol on the generation and migration of cerebral cortical neurons. Science 233(4770):1308–1311

Miller MW (1987) Effect of prenatal exposure to alcohol on the distribution and time of origin of corticospinal neurons in the rat. J Comp Neurol 257(3):372–382

Miller MW (1993) Migration of cortical neurons is altered by gestational exposure to ethanol. Alcohol Clin Exp Res 17(2):304–314

Miller MW (1996) Limited ethanol exposure selectively alters the proliferation of precursor cells in the cerebral cortex. Alcohol Clin Exp Res 20(1):139–143

Miller MW (1997) Effects of prenatal exposure to ethanol on callosal projection neurons in rat somatosensory cortex. Brain Res 766(1-2):121–128

Miller MW (2017) Effect of prenatal exposure to ethanol on the pyramidal tract in developing rats. Brain Res 1672:122–128

Miller MW, Dow-Edwards DL (1988) Structural and metabolic alterations in rat cerebral cortex induced by prenatal exposure to ethanol. Brain Res 474(2): 316–326

Miller MW, Nowakowski RS (1991) Effect of prenatal exposure to ethanol on the cell cycle kinetics and growth fraction in the proliferative zones of fetal rat cerebral cortex. Alcohol Clin Exp Res 15(2):229–232

Miller MW, Potempa G (1990) Numbers of neurons and glia in mature rat somatosensory cortex: effects of prenatal exposure to ethanol. J Comp Neurol 293(1): 92–102

Mohseni F, Bagheri F, Khaksari M (2020) Hydrogen sulfide attenuates the neurotoxicity in the animal model of fetal alcohol spectrum disorders. Neurotox Res 37(4):977–986

Montoliu C et al (1995) Ethanol increases cytochrome P4502E1 and induces oxidative stress in astrocytes. J Neurochem 65(6):2561–2570

Mooney SM, Siegenthaler JA, Miller MW (2004) Ethanol induces heterotopias in organotypic cultures of rat cerebral cortex. Cereb Cortex 14(10):1071–1080

Moore DB et al (1998) Prenatal ethanol exposure reduces parvalbumin-immunoreactive GABAergic neuronal number in the adult rat cingulate cortex. Neurosci Lett 249(1):25–28

Nadarajah B et al (2001) Two modes of radial migration in early development of the cerebral cortex. Nat Neurosci 4(2):143–150

Nash R et al (2012) Human embryonic stem cell model of ethanol-mediated early developmental toxicity. Exp Neurol 234(1):127–135

Newville J et al (2017) Acute oligodendrocyte loss with persistent white matter injury in a third trimester equivalent mouse model of fetal alcohol spectrum disorder. Glia 65(8):1317–1332

Noctor SC et al (2004) Cortical neurons arise in symmetric and asymmetric division zones and migrate through specific phases. Nat Neurosci 7(2):136–144
Norton S et al (1988) Early motor development and cerebral cortical morphology in rats exposed perinatally to alcohol. Alcohol Clin Exp Res 12(1):130–136
O'Leary-Moore SK et al (2010) Magnetic resonance microscopy-based analyses of the brains of normal and ethanol-exposed fetal mice. Birth Defects Res A Clin Mol Teratol 88(11):953–964
Padilla-Valdez MM et al (2024) Neuroinflammation in fetal alcohol spectrum disorders and related novel therapeutic approaches. Biochim Biophys Acta Mol Basis Dis 1870(1):166854
Pal S, Lim JWC, Richards LJ (2024) Diverse axonal morphologies of individual callosal projection neurons reveal new insights into brain connectivity. Curr Opin Neurobiol 84:102837
Parnell SE et al (2009) Magnetic resonance microscopy defines ethanol-induced brain abnormalities in prenatal mice: effects of acute insult on gestational day 8. Alcohol Clin Exp Res 33(6):1001–1011
Parnell SE et al (2013) Magnetic resonance microscopy-based analyses of the neuroanatomical effects of gestational day 9 ethanol exposure in mice. Neurotoxicol Teratol 39:77–83
Pascual M, Guerri C (2007) The peptide NAP promotes neuronal growth and differentiation through extracellular signal-regulated protein kinase and Akt pathways, and protects neurons co-cultured with astrocytes damaged by ethanol. J Neurochem 103(2):557–568
Patten AR, Fontaine CJ, Christie BR (2014) A comparison of the different animal models of fetal alcohol spectrum disorders and their use in studying complex behaviors. Front Pediatr 2:93
Paul AP, Medina AE (2012) Overexpression of serum response factor in astrocytes improves neuronal plasticity in a model of early alcohol exposure. Neuroscience 221:193–202
Paul A et al (2017) Transcriptional architecture of synaptic communication delineates GABAergic neuron identity. Cell 171(3):522–539.e20
Popova EN (2004) Structure of the sensorimotor area of the cerebral cortex in the offspring of alcoholized rats. Neurosci Behav Physiol 34(7):663–669
Popova S, Dozet D (2023) Epidemiology of prenatal alcohol exposure. Springer, pp 1–16
Popova S et al (2017) Estimation of national, regional, and global prevalence of alcohol use during pregnancy and fetal alcohol syndrome: a systematic review and meta-analysis. Lancet Glob Health 5(3):e290–e299
Priya R et al (2018) Activity regulates cell death within cortical interneurons through a calcineurin-dependent mechanism. Cell Rep 22(7):1695–1709
Qiang M, Wang MW, Elberger AJ (2002) Second trimester prenatal alcohol exposure alters development of rat corpus callosum. Neurotoxicol Teratol 24(6):719–732
Quattrocolo G, Fishell G, Petros TJ (2017) Heterotopic transplantations reveal environmental influences on interneuron diversity and maturation. Cell Rep 21(3): 721–731
Radley JJ et al (2008) Repeated stress alters dendritic spine morphology in the rat medial prefrontal cortex. J Comp Neurol 507(1):1141–1150
Rajaprakash M et al (2014) Cortical morphology in children with alcohol-related neurodevelopmental disorder. Brain Behav 4(1):41–50
Rakic P (1972) Mode of cell migration to the superficial layers of fetal monkey neocortex. J Comp Neurol 145(1):61–83
Riar AK et al (2016) Ethanol induces cytostasis of cortical basal progenitors. J Biomed Sci 23:6
Riley EP, Infante MA, Warren KR (2011) Fetal alcohol spectrum disorders: an overview. Neuropsychol Rev 21(2):73–80
Robertson FC et al (2016) Prenatal alcohol exposure is associated with regionally thinner cortex during the preadolescent period. Cereb Cortex 26(7):3083–3095
Rodriguez CI et al (2016) Moderate prenatal alcohol exposure alters functional connectivity in the adult rat brain. Alcohol Clin Exp Res 40(10):2134–2146
Rubert G et al (2006) Ethanol exposure during embryogenesis decreases the radial glial progenitorpool and affects the generation of neurons and astrocytes. J Neurosci Res 84(3):483–496
Rudolph J et al (2010) Ephrins guide migrating cortical interneurons in the basal telencephalon. Cell Adh Migr 4(3):400–408
Saito K et al (2019) Dorsal-to-ventral cortical expansion is physically primed by ventral streaming of early embryonic preplate neurons. Cell Rep 29(6):1555–1567.e5
Sambo D et al (2022) Cell type-specific changes in Wnt signaling and neuronal differentiation in the developing mouse cortex after prenatal alcohol exposure during neurogenesis. Front Cell Dev Biol 10:1011974
Santillano DR et al (2005) Ethanol induces cell-cycle activity and reduces stem cell diversity to alter both regenerative capacity and differentiation potential of cerebral cortical neuroepithelial precursors. BMC Neurosci 6:59
Sarieva K, Mayer S (2021) The effects of environmental adversities on human neocortical neurogenesis modeled in brain organoids. Front Mol Biosci 8: 686410
Schneider ML, Moore CF, Adkins MM (2011) The effects of prenatal alcohol exposure on behavior: rodent and primate studies. Neuropsychol Rev 21(2):186–203
Scott HM, Mason JI, Sharpe RM (2009) Steroidogenesis in the fetal testis and its susceptibility to disruption by exogenous compounds. Endocr Rev 30(7):883–925
Sepulveda B et al (2011) L1 cell adhesion molecule promotes resistance to alcohol-induced silencing of growth cone responses to guidance cues. Neuroscience 180:30–40
Silva CG et al (2018) Cell-intrinsic control of interneuron migration drives cortical morphogenesis. Cell 172(5): 1063–1078.e19

Simons M, Nave KA (2015) Oligodendrocytes: myelination and axonal support. Cold Spring Harb Perspect Biol 8(1):a020479
Skorput AG, Yeh HH (2016) Chronic gestational exposure to ethanol leads to enduring aberrances in cortical form and function in the medial prefrontal cortex. Alcohol Clin Exp Res 40(7):1479–1488
Skorput AG et al (2015) Persistent interneuronopathy in the prefrontal cortex of young adult offspring exposed to ethanol in utero. J Neurosci 35(31):10977–10988
Skorput AG et al (2019) The NKCC1 antagonist bumetanide mitigates interneuronopathy associated with ethanol exposure in utero. Elife:8
Smiley JF et al (2015) Selective reduction of cerebral cortex GABA neurons in a late gestation model of fetal alcohol spectrum disorder. Alcohol 49(6): 571–580
Smith IF, Gursky ZH, Klintsova AY (2022) Representation of prefrontal axonal efferents in the thalamic nucleus reuniens in a rodent model of fetal alcohol exposure during third trimester. Front Behav Neurosci 16:993601
Southwell DG et al (2012) Intrinsically determined cell death of developing cortical interneurons. Nature 491(7422):109–113
Sowell ER et al (2008) Abnormal cortical thickness and brain-behavior correlation patterns in individuals with heavy prenatal alcohol exposure. Cereb Cortex 18(1): 136–144
Stoufflet J, Tielens S, Nguyen L (2023) Shaping the cerebral cortex by cellular crosstalk. Cell 186(13): 2733–2747
Stuempflen M et al (2023) Fetal MRI based brain atlas analysis detects initial in utero effects of prenatal alcohol exposure. Cereb Cortex 33(11):6852–6861
Sundermann B et al (2023) Functional connectivity of cognition-related brain networks in adults with fetal alcohol syndrome. BMC Med 21(1):496
Tabata H, Nakajima K (2003) Multipolar migration: the third mode of radial neuronal migration in the developing cerebral cortex. J Neurosci 23(31):9996–10001
Takahashi T, Nowakowski RS, Caviness VS Jr (1993) Cell cycle parameters and patterns of nuclear movement in the neocortical proliferative zone of the fetal mouse. J Neurosci 13(2):820–833
Takahashi T et al (1999) Sequence of neuron origin and neocortical laminar fate: relation to cell cycle of origin in the developing murine cerebral wall. J Neurosci 19(23):10357–10371
Taléns-Visconti R et al (2011) Neural differentiation from human embryonic stem cells as a tool to study early brain development and the neuroteratogenic effects of ethanol. Stem Cells Dev 20(2):327–339
Tang S et al (2019) Functional connectivity and metabolic alterations in medial prefrontal cortex in a rat model of fetal alcohol spectrum disorder: a resting-state functional magnetic resonance imaging and in vivo proton magnetic resonance spectroscopy study. Dev Neurosci 41(1-2):67–78
Tasic B et al (2018) Shared and distinct transcriptomic cell types across neocortical areas. Nature 563(7729): 72–78
Taverna E, Huttner WB (2010) Neural progenitor nuclei IN motion. Neuron 67(6):906–914
Thanh NX et al (2014) Incidence and prevalence of fetal alcohol spectrum disorder by sex and age group in Alberta. Canada. J Popul Ther Clin Pharmacol 21(3): e395–e404
Tielens S et al (2016) Elongator controls cortical interneuron migration by regulating actomyosin dynamics. Cell Res 26(10):1131–1148
Tobet S et al (2009) Brain sex differences and hormone influences: a moving experience? J Neuroendocrinol 21(4):387–392
Tomás M et al (2005) Ethanol perturbs the secretory pathway in astrocytes. Neurobiol Dis 20(3):773–784
Toudji I et al (2023) Interneuron odyssey: molecular mechanisms of tangential migration. Front Neural Circ 17:1256455
Treit S et al (2013) Longitudinal MRI reveals altered trajectory of brain development during childhood and adolescence in fetal alcohol spectrum disorders. J Neurosci 33(24):10098–10109
Treit S et al (2017) Sexual dimorphism of volume reduction but not cognitive deficit in fetal alcohol spectrum disorders: a combined diffusion tensor imaging, cortical thickness and brain volume study. Neuroimage Clin 15:284–297
Tsai PC et al (2014) MiR-153 targets the nuclear factor-1 family and protects against teratogenic effects of ethanol exposure in fetal neural stem cells. Biol Open 3(8): 741–758
van Tilborg E et al (2018) Origin and dynamics of oligodendrocytes in the developing brain: Implications for perinatal white matter injury. Glia 66(2):221–238
Vemuri MC, Chetty CS (2005) Alcohol impairs astrogliogenesis by stem cells in rodent neurospheres. Neurochem Int 47(1-2):129–135
Villalba A, Gotz M, Borrell V (2021) The regulation of cortical neurogenesis. Curr Top Dev Biol 142:1–66
Wang B et al (2013) Loss of Gsx1 and Gsx2 function rescues distinct phenotypes in Dlx1/2 mutants. J Comp Neurol 521(7):1561–1584
Ware AL, Long X, Lebel C (2021) Functional connectivity of the attention networks is altered and relates to neuropsychological outcomes in children with prenatal alcohol exposure. Dev Cogn Neurosci 48:100951
Whitcher LT, Klintsova AY (2008) Postnatal binge-like alcohol exposure reduces spine density without affecting dendritic morphology in rat mPFC. Synapse 62(8): 566–573
Williams JF, Smith VC (2015) Fetal alcohol spectrum disorders. Pediatrics 136(5):e1395–e1406

Wong FK et al (2018) Pyramidal cell regulation of interneuron survival sculpts cortical networks. Nature 557(7707):668–673

Wozniak JR et al (2013) Global functional connectivity abnormalities in children with fetal alcohol spectrum disorders. Alcohol Clin Exp Res 37(5):748–756

Xu W et al (2019) Genome-wide transcriptome landscape of embryonic brain-derived neural stem cells exposed to alcohol with strain-specific cross-examination in BL6 and CD1 mice. Sci Rep 9(1):206

Yang Y et al (2012) Abnormal cortical thickness alterations in fetal alcohol spectrum disorders and their relationships with facial dysmorphology. Cereb Cortex 22(5):1170–1179

Yanni PA et al (2002) Astrocyte-derived factors modulate the inhibitory effect of ethanol on dendritic development. Glia 38(4):292–302

Yu Y et al (2021) Interneuron origin and molecular diversity in the human fetal brain. Nat Neurosci 24(12): 1745–1756

Zavalin K et al (2022) Loss of KCC2 in GABAergic neurons causes seizures and an imbalance of cortical interneurons. Front Mol Neurosci 15:826427

Zelner I, Koren G (2013) Pharmacokinetics of ethanol in the maternal-fetal unit. J Popul Ther Clin Pharmacol 20(3):e259–e265

Zhang J, Liu Q (2015) Cholesterol metabolism and homeostasis in the brain. Protein Cell 6(4):254–264

Zhang CR et al (2019) Early gestational ethanol exposure in mice: effects on brain structure, energy metabolism and adiposity in adult offspring. Alcohol 75:1–10

Zhou D et al (2011) Developmental cortical thinning in fetal alcohol spectrum disorders. Neuroimage 58(1): 16–25

Zhou C et al (2014) Prenatal ethanol exposure up-regulates the cholesterol transporters ATP-binding Cassette A1 and G1 and reduces cholesterol levels in the developing rat brain. Alcohol Alcohol 49(6):626–634

Zhu Y et al (1999) Cellular and molecular guidance of GABAergic neuronal migration from an extracortical origin to the neocortex. Neuron 23(3):473–485

Prenatal Alcohol Exposure: Impact on Neuroimmune Function in the Stress Response and Pain

7

Justine R. Zimmerly, Shahani Noor, and Erin D. Milligan

Abstract

Fetal alcohol spectrum disorder (FASD) encompasses a broad range of central nervous system (CNS)-related disabilities representing a mild-to-severe continuum of neurodevelopmental disorders that include mood and sensory function. The prevalence of FASD is estimated at ~5% in school-aged children who are prone to develop inappropriate responses to stressful stimuli leading to higher rates of anxiety and low touch tolerance. Low touch tolerance has been self-reported in 33.6% of FASD-affected individuals. The FASD manifestations of sensory abnormalities like pathological light-touch hypersensitivity, a hallmark of chronic pain may be a result of abnormal neurological relays the spinal cord, and from spinal cord to brain. Animal modeling of FASD that utilize prenatal alcohol exposure (PAE) demonstrate mood disorders such as anxiety-like behavior and low touch tolerance, which support these clinical observations of mood and tactile dysregulation.

In an effort to contextualize central nervous system (CNS) processing of stress and resultant mood disorders that are exacerbated by PAE, this review outlines the fundamentals of the neurocircuitry of stress from the perspective of the central autonomic network (CAN), differentiating physiological vs. psychological stressors with a focus on elements of the limbic system, including the medial prefrontal cortex (mPFC), amygdala (AMG), hippocampus (HIPP), hypothalamus, cingulate cortex, and brainstem periaqueductal gray (PAG), locus coeruleus (LC), and the nucleus of the solitary tract (NTS) of the medulla. The review addresses stress-sensitized CNS circuits and the underlying immune signaling molecules that may be responsible for heightened stress responses. Adolescence will be discussed as a critical corticolimbic developmental period that is itself highly susceptible to stressors, which is further impacted by PAE leading to stress-related anxiety with lifelong consequences.

Linking the heightened neuroimmune response of offspring with PAE, a discussion is included of rodent models demonstrating PAE as a risk factor for developing painful tactile neuropathies following sciatic nerve injury mediated by sensitized and over-active spinal glial cytokine actions. Included in this

J. R. Zimmerly · S. Noor · E. D. Milligan (✉)
Department of Neurosciences, University of New Mexico School of Medicine, UNM Health Sciences Center, Albuquerque, NM, USA
e-mail: EMilligan@salud.unm.edu

A. N. Bukiya, D. W. Ali (eds.), *Molecular Mechanisms and Lifelong Consequences of Prenatal Exposure to Psychoactive Substances*, Advances in Experimental Medicine and Biology 1500,
https://doi.org/10.1007/978-3-032-12741-9_7

discussion is the role of limbic forebrain, subcortical and even brainstem circuits that process and regulate mood and stress also engage the emotional and sensory-discriminative aspects of pain processing. Lastly, the impact of PAE on sensitized neuroimmune factors that link stress to touch allodynia in the absence of nerve injury is briefly discussed. These topics aim to help the reader gauge the profound impact of PAE on the CAN, and immune signaling molecules in limbic areas and spinal cord that drive sensitized stress sequelae, which should now include exaggerated pain states as well as anxiety disorders.

Keywords

Fetal Alcohol Spectrum Disorder (FASD) · Anxiety · Limbic forebrain · Immune · Allodynia

7.1 Introduction

Fetal alcohol spectrum disorder (FASD) encompasses a broad range of central nervous system (CNS)-related disabilities representing a mild-to-severe continuum of neurodevelopmental disorders that are related, but not limited to, cognitive, emotional, mood, and sensory function (Coles et al. 2022; May et al. 2018; Reid et al. 2015). Case studies in several communities in the United States suggest that the prevalence of FASD is estimated at about 5% in school-aged children (May et al. 2018; Lebel et al. 2021) who are prone to develop inappropriate responses to stressful stimuli leading to higher rates of psychiatric symptoms and mood disorders such as depression and anxiety (Garrison et al. 2019; Hagan et al. 2016; Khoury et al. 2018; Lynch et al. 2017). Significant individual differences of neurocognitive behaviors result from varying degrees of prenatal alcohol exposure (PAE) in terms of gestational timing, magnitude, and duration, yet all can lead to an FASD (Khoury et al. 2018). Children, adolescents and adults experience anxiety and depression often co-morbid with FASD despite broad PAE patterns (Coles et al. 2022; Khoury et al. 2018; Flannigan et al. 2023). In efforts to gain a better understanding of the underlying factors that lead to depression and anxiety resulting from PAE, animal modeling of FASD supports observations seen clinically, including mood dysregulation. Preclinical literature reports that chronic unpredictable mild stress in animals with PAE induces adverse behavioral consequences such as the emergence of anxiety- and depressive-like behaviors (Bodnar et al. 2018; Hellemans et al. 2010; Schneiderman et al. 2005). Further, work that examines the impact of PAE on stress responses in adolescent offspring demonstrates altered expression of stress-associated factors (e.g., stress peptides) in corticolimbic areas that integrate and regulate mood (Schneiderman et al. 2005; Bangasser et al. 2019). Additionally, co-morbid with FASD-associated neurodevelopmental disorders are sensory processing disorders (Breuer et al. 2024; Franklin et al. 2008). Clinically, sensory processing disorders are identified as inappropriate behavioral reactions to environmental stimuli manifested as (a) sensory-based motor disorder, (b) sensory discrimination disorder, and/or (c) sensory modulation disorder (Miller et al. 2009).

Low touch tolerance, otherwise referred to as tactile hypersensitivity, is identified as a sensory discrimination disorder (Breuer et al. 2024), which has been self-reported in 33.6% of FASD-affected individuals (Himmelrich et al. 2020). In support of these clinical observations, preclinical longitudinal experiments modeling FASD in adult rhesus monkeys exposed prenatally to low/moderate levels of alcohol reveal touch abnormalities such as tactile hypersensitivity (Schneider et al. 2007, 2008). The FASD manifestations of sensory abnormalities like pathological light-touch hypersensitivity that is a hallmark in many chronic pain patients is known as tactile allodynia and could be the result of abnormal neurological relays to spinal cord-to-brain and vice versa. In support, rodent models demonstrate that PAE is a risk factor for developing tactile neuropathies and that the underlying tactile hypersensitivity following sciatic nerve injury appears to occur as a consequence of sensitized, or over-active, spinal glial responses and spinal cytokine actions (Noor et al. 2017; Sanchez et al. 2017). These initial studies laid the groundwork for subsequent reports that revealed PAE potentiated allodynia with corresponding spinal glial and proinflammatory cytokine signaling as drivers of pathological light touch sensitivity (Noor et al. 2018, 2019, 2020, 2023a; Sanchez et al. 2019). The sensitized glial-cytokine responses to secondary challenges observed in offspring with PAE extend to the adverse actions of opioids in the CNS to treat pain in those with PAE (Noor et al. 2023a)· Interestingly, limbic forebrain, subcortical and even brainstem circuits that process and regulate mood and stress responses also engage the emotional and sensory-discriminative aspects of pain processing (De Ridder et al. 2021; Johnstone et al. 2012; Seminowicz and Moayedi 2017; Xiao and Zhang 2018). The culmination of research suggests that PAE, acting through heightened CNS proinflammatory signaling, significantly sensitizes stress responses leading to anxiety, among other mood disorders, and is also a risk factor for chronic neuropathy after minor injury (Carloni et al. 2021; Noor and Milligan 2018; Ruffaner-Hanson et al. 2022). However, with ever-increasing information, more contemporary views of the clinical stress sequelae of individuals with FASD may now include allodynia pain (Madison et al. 2023) in the absence of overt injury.

This review outlines the fundamentals of the neurocircuitry of stress from the perspective of the central autonomic network (CAN), with a focus on elements of the limbic system, including the medial prefrontal cortex (mPFC), amygdala (AMG), hippocampus (HIPP), hypothalamus, cingulate cortex, and brainstem periaqueductal gray (PAG), locus coeruleus (LC) and the nucleus of the solitary tract (NTS) of the medulla. The review then discusses how stress sensitizes CNS circuits responsible for generating a stress response and the underlying neural and immune signaling molecules that manifest the behavioral responses to such stress, as well as the impact of PAE on the stress response. Additionally discussed is adolescence as a critical corticolimbic developmental period that is highly susceptible to stressors, and the further risk that PAE imposes on the developing adolescent brain leading to stress-related anxiety. Additionally reviewed is the sensitization of spinal immune signaling is caused by PAE, generating sensory abnormalities such as allodynia following minor peripheral injury and the potential molecular mechanisms that drive immune dysregulation leading to allodynia. We end with a discussion about the impact of PAE on sensitized neuroimmune factors that link stress to touch allodynia in the absence of nerve injury; a sensory disorder often co-morbid in individuals with FASD. These topics aim to help the reader gauge the profound impact of PAE on immune signaling molecules in the brain and spinal cord that drive sensitized stress sequelae and the potential of controlling neuroimmune signaling for the treatment of stress-related mood and sensory pathologies.

7.2 The Neurocircuitry of Stress

Stress is defined as the response of the body to a real or perceived threat (Garrison et al. 2019). The stress response network consists of several distinct, yet linked, systems such as the autonomic nervous system (ANS), the immune system (for review, see Boahen, and colleagues (Boahen et al. 2023)), and the neuroendocrine hypothalamic pituitary adrenal (HPA) axis (Mueller et al. 2022). The function of the ANS is for continuous monitoring of the body's various organ systems such as cardiovascular, pulmonary, blood chemistry detection, core body temperature, etc., which, when altered, elicits reflexive adjustments to maintain physiological homeostasis (Benarroch 2020). However, the ANS also performs simultaneous monitoring of external environmental cues such as fearful situations or threatening environments, and coordinates responses derived from internal and environmental cues requiring the activation of the entire peripheral and central ANS neuroaxis (both within the CNS and in the peripheral nervous system) (Wehrwein et al. 2016). The stress response of the central aspect of the ANS, often referred to as the central autonomic network (CAN), requires coordination of a number of cortical and subcortical brain and brainstem regions (Wehrwein et al. 2016; Benarroch 1993). These CAN circuits include mPFC, AMG, HIPP, specific sub-nuclei of the hypothalamus (noted further below) and the insular cortex that communicates to the cingulate cortex, HIPP and AMG (Uddin et al. 2017) (Fig. 7.1), as well as brainstem regions including the PAG of the midbrain and the NTS of the medulla (Mueller et al. 2022; Thome et al. 2017; Zhang et al. 2024) (Fig. 7.2). At the level of the brainstem, both the NTS and PAG receive information from the body, either directly (NTS) or indirectly (PAG) through visceral afferent fibers, that relay this information to not only other brainstem pontine and medullary areas, but also rostrally to supra-brainstem areas such as hypothalamic subnuclei to induce efferent (e.g., sympathetic) physiological adjustments to maintain bodily homeostasis (Benarroch 2020). Additionally important are projections from PAG and NTS that directly project caudally to various spinal cord regions (Holt 2022; Linnman et al. 2012). Thus, the anatomical brainstem site of the PAG and NTS allows for direct, and even reciprocal communication to ascending forebrain regions via the HYP and descending spinal regions (Fig. 7.3).

It is important to further emphasize the critical role of the HYP because it functions to integrate and produce patterned autonomic (via parasympathetic and sympathetic projections) and endocrine responses (hormones) to achieve the maintenance of bodily homeostasis and allostasis in response to stress. Several hypothalamic

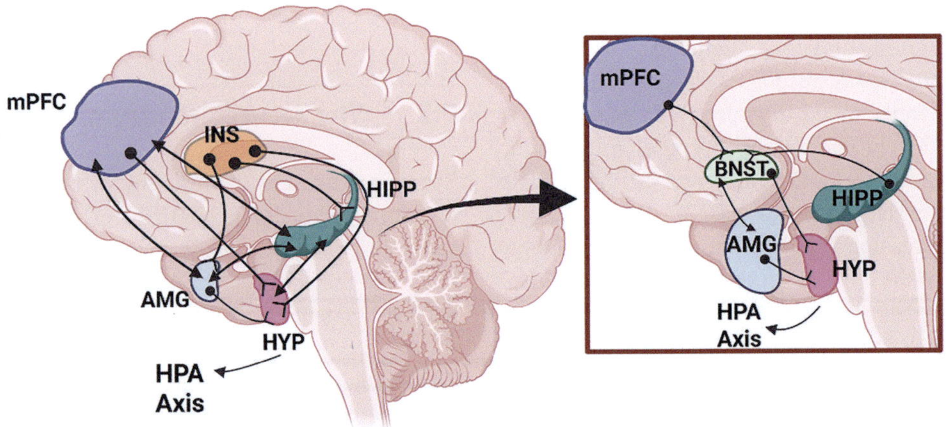

Fig. 7.1 *Central autonomic network circuits*: Reciprocal projections between the amygdala and the medial prefrontal cortex, as well as reciprocal projections between the amygdala and the hippocampus, facilitate the emotional response to psychological stress. The medial prefrontal cortex projects to the hypothalamus to generate the endocrine response to a perceived stressor. Reciprocal projections between the medial prefrontal cortex and the hippocampus further facilitate the cognitive response to stress. The insular cortex (anatomically lateral to its depiction in the figure) communicates to the amygdala, the hippocampus, and to the periventricular nucleus of the hypothalamus, ultimately resulting in HPA axis activation. Projections from the hippocampus to the hypothalamus are crucial for initial activation of the HPA, as well as the negative feedback inhibition of the HPA stress response, while reciprocal projections from the hypothalamus to the hippocampus allow for integration of stress context and stress processing. Projections from the BNST to the amygdala and the hypothalamus also result in the endocrine response to stress. The BNST receives reciprocal projections from the amygdala as well as projections from the medial prefrontal cortex and the hippocampus to facilitate the emotional response to psychological stress. All reciprocal projections between regions are represented by bidirectional arrows. mPFC medial prefrontal cortex, INS insular cortex, AMG amygdala, HIPP hippocampus, HYP hypothalamus, BNST bed nucleus of the stria terminalis, HPA hypothalamic pituitary adrenal axis

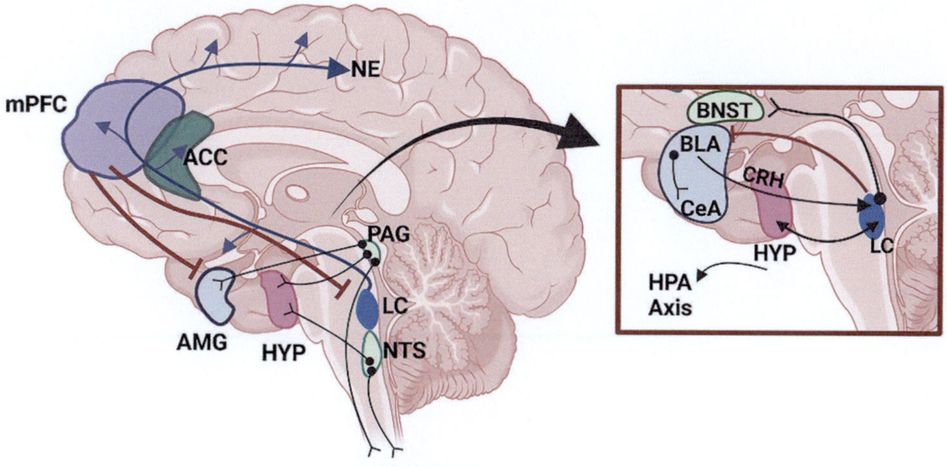

Fig. 7.2 *Projections of the LC, the PAG, and the NTS to corticolimbic structures*: The circuitry between the LC and the amygdala is critical for the development of stress-induced anxiety. The LC has efferent projections to the BLA, which also plays a key role in the regulation of stress and anxiety-like behaviors. The behavioral consequences of stress may be mediated by release of NE to the BLA and the BNST, as well as by reciprocal projections from the BLA to the LC and to the CeA. Additionally, the amygdala releases the stress peptide CRH to the LC, further implicating the role of the amygdala in the central autonomic response to stress and development of anxiety-like behaviors. The LC also projects to the hypothalamus and acts in an excitatory manner to facilitate activation of the HPA axis, but the hypothalamus also has glutamatergic afferent projections to the LC. Projections from the LC to the prefrontal cortex are crucial for the initial response to stress as well as for the regulation of the emotional and autonomic responses to stress. Reciprocal, inhibitory projections from the frontal cortex to the amygdala and LC mitigate the emotional response to the stress and serves to prevent development of anxiety-like behaviors following stress. At the level of the brainstem, the PAG and the NTS send monosynaptic projections to the amygdala and the anterior hypothalamus, as well as caudal projections to the spinal cord. NE norepinephrine, mPFC medial prefrontal cortex, ACC anterior cingulate cortex, PAG periaqueductal gray, AMG amygdala, LC locus coeruleus, NTS nucleus of the solitary tract, HYP hypothalamus, BNST bed nucleus of the stria terminalis, BLA basolateral amygdala, CeA central nucleus of the amygdala, CRH corticotropin releasing hormone, HPA hypothalamic-pituitary-adrenal axis

subnuclei engage the CAN to respond to stress, and key among them are the periventricular nucleus (PVN) of the HYP and the dorsomedial nucleus (DMH) of the HYP (Lamotte et al. 2021). Direct monosynaptic NTS projections to the PVN/DMH of the HYP occur, as well projections to subcortical limbic regions including several subnuclei of the AMG, allowing for the coordination of information of body physiology to brain CAN areas (Holt 2022). Similarly, the PAG sends monosynaptic projections to the AMG and the anterior HYP where PVN neurons are located (Linnman et al. 2012; Brandao and Lovick 2019; Iremonger and Power 2025). However, while neither the NTS nor PAG directly project the HIPP (Castle et al. 2005), these brainstem areas can influence hippocampal output through indirect projections via the PVN of the HYP, which in turn projects to the HIPP (Castle et al. 2005; Reis et al. 2023). The HIPP in turn is capable of engaging the CAN through communication to the prefrontal cortex, HYP and the AMG, thereby generating and regulating aspects of sympathetic outflow (Castle et al. 2005; Henderson et al. 2002; Valenza et al. 2024) (Fig. 7.2).

Given the broad functions of the ANS, both physiological stressors initiated by internal changes in homeostatic physiology, or psychological stressors triggered by environmental threats that impact behavioral responses to a challenge (fight, flight, or inaction) require

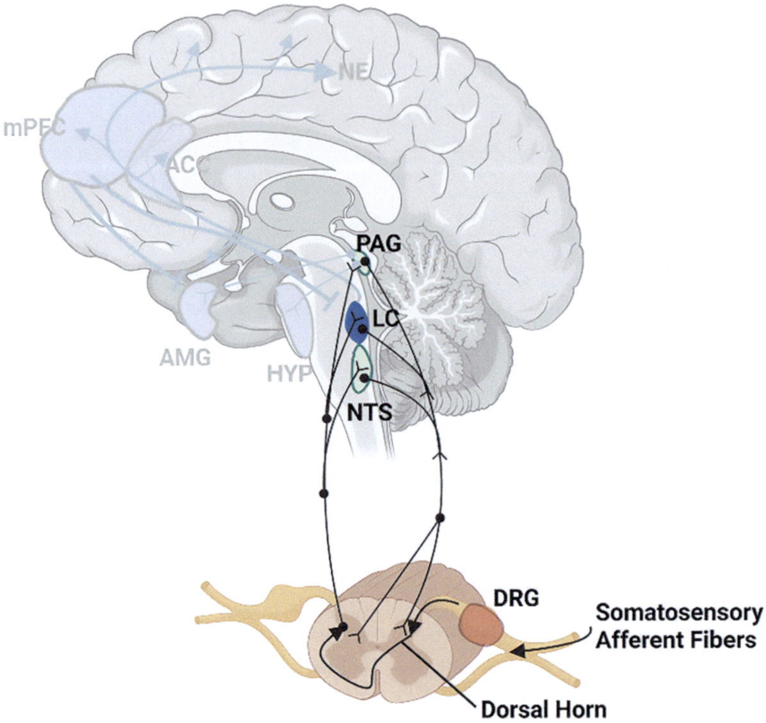

Fig. 7.3 *Projections of the PAG, LC, and NTS to the dorsal horn of the spinal cord.* The brainstem and its communication with the spinal cord facilitates the response to pain and allows for communication to ascending forebrain regions. At the level of the spinal cord, somatosensory afferents synapse onto neurons whose bodies are located in the DRG. Axons from the DRG project to areas of the brainstem, which include the LC, the NTS, and the PAG. These regions project reciprocally to the spinal cord, allowing for bidirectional communication between the brain and spinal cord. PAG periaqueductal gray, LC locus coeruleus, NTS nucleus of the solitary tract, DRG dorsal root ganglion

CAN-HPA circuit actions (Mueller et al. 2022), which make up the basic elements of what is referred to as the limbic system (Morgane and Mokler 2006; Rajmohan and Mohandas 2007). As noted, the HYP is critical for the stress response triggered by coordinated input from the CAN brain and/or brainstem areas to the PVN/DHN of the HYP, and in doing so, engages the neuroendocrine HPA axis with consequent release of circulating glucocorticoids to prepare multiple bodily systems for adequate responses upon a stress challenge (Mueller et al. 2022). For example, systemic stress signals include hypoglycemia, circulating immune signaling molecules such as cytokines, and nociceptive/noxious stimuli (i.e., acute pain) to name a few, all of which are conveyed via afferent nerve fibers of mostly the parasympathetic axons and some sympathetic, which along with efferent sympathetic and parasympathetic fibers, make up the peripheral elements of the ANS (Wehrwein et al. 2016; Vandewalle and Libert 2020). Nociceptive/noxious stimuli are conveyed via afferent axons belonging to the somatosensory system. Consequently, rapid NTS and PAG responses allow for adjustments needed to maintain physiological homeostasis. Thus, the coordination of the ANS-HPA physiological stress response occurs through synaptic inputs from brainstem nuclei (e.g., NTS, PAG) and also through forebrain structures that are involved in higher-order autonomic control to process sensory input (nociceptive/noxious); forebrain areas such as the primary visceromotor (in medial prefrontal cortex) and sensory cortex (in insular cortex). In turn, these cortical areas directly communicate to (1) the HIPP that projects the PVN, (2) amygdala (Benarroch 1993) that also projects to the PVN, and (3) the PVN, generating and integrating HPA axis activation (Mueller et al. 2022; Lamotte et al. 2021; Herman and Cullinan 1997) (Fig. 7.2).

However, it is notable that the physiological ANS-HPA stress responses involving limbic brainstem regions (e.g., PAG and NTS) does not require limbic forebrain CAN activation (Morgane and Mokler 2006), thus certain homeostatic stressors are limbic forebrain insensitive. Yet, it is the limbic system that links emotions to the ANS, with the CAN becoming engaged upon perceived stressors, ultimately resulting in activation of the HPA axis and hormonal release of glucocorticoids (cortisol in humans and corticosterone in rodents). For example, noxious stimuli relayed by somatosensory afferent fibers conveying nociceptive signals to key areas within the brainstem, HYP, and thalamus, are ultimately processed as pain in the limbic insular cortex (Lamotte et al. 2021), and thus are limbic forebrain sensitive. Thus, specific acute stressors can act as limbic insensitive or sensitive depending on the attributes of the triggering stimulus (Herman and Cullinan 1997). Importantly, these limbic areas are also implicated in the development of anxiety and other mood disorders (Schneider et al. 2007).

7.3 Central Autonomic Response and Psychological Stress

Most behaviors and emotions are generated and processed not by a particular limbic structure but rather by circuits that are part of the CAN. The prefrontal cortex plays a key role in the top-down modulation of emotional processes in response to psychological stressors and this region of the cortex has direct impacts on the regulation of CAN-HPA activity (Benarroch 1993; Lamotte et al. 2021). Top-down and bottom-up circuitry provide inputs along their trajectory; that is, limbic mPFC-to-HYP -to-brainstem and vice versa, which are activated by perceived or emotional stress (Morgane and Mokler 2006; Shin and Liberzon 2010), that drives the activity of the HPA axis and autonomic responses (Mueller et al. 2022). Thus, the emotional autonomic network engages emotion regulation and coordinates stress output, which is processed by limbic CAN regions including the prefrontal cortex, HIPP, AMG, the bed nucleus of the stria terminalis (BNST) (discussed further, below), and PAG, as identified through both animal tracing and human imaging studies (Thome et al. 2017; Westerhaus and Loewy 2001; Mantyh 1982, 1983; Rizvi et al. 1991; Lebow and Chen 2016).

Strong reciprocal communication between the amygdaloid complex and the mPFC (dorsal and ventral) facilitates the emotional link to stressors (Lamotte et al. 2021; Morgane and Mokler 2006). Notably, while the AMG is characterized to prompt cardiovascular responses to stress, it also sends projections to the mPFC (Marek et al. 2013). As an additional integrative region, the mPFC receives processed sensory afferents (e.g., noxious input coded as pain) and provides cortical influence over visceral functions while also exerting key roles in cognitive and emotional processes. Its major cortical output region relative to the CAN response to stress includes the PVN of the HYP, and as noted, generates the endocrine response to a perceived stressor. Following perceived stress signals, the AMG projects to additional limbic areas including the HIPP, with reciprocal projections from the HIPP. For example, increased expression of c-fos in the HIPP following acute restraint stress in rats (Chowdhury et al. 2000) has strongly implicated the hippocampal role in impacting the AMG in stress regulation. Hippocampal input to the PVN of the HYP is critical for the subsequent negative feedback inhibition of the HPA stress response (Benarroch 2020). In addition to hippocampal projections to key nuclei of the AMG, the HIPP also projects to the BNST, which in turn directly facilitates the HPA axis response to psychological stress (Choi et al. 2008a).

The BNST, which is considered a part of the extended amygdala, plays a significant role in anxiety disorders such as posttraumatic stress disorder, panic disorder, social phobia, specific phobia and generalized anxiety disorder, based on preclinical animal and clinical studies, and is becoming a recognized region in stress circuitry (Shin and Liberzon 2010). This critical limbic forebrain structure is also part of the CAN and functions to link regions such as the AMG and HIPP with the output of hypothalamic PVN and brainstem regions in controlling vital homeostatic functions (Lamotte et al. 2021; Herman and Cullinan 1997). The communication of the BNST with the AMG and the HIPP acts to generate anxiety-like behaviors (Davis et al. 2010; Lee and Davis 1997). The BNST is located anterior to the HYP and, as implicated, has diverse connectivity with other limbic structures. For example, reports from rodent studies demonstrate the BNST is comprised of up to 18 subregions (Bota et al. 2012), and integrates information about mood and negative emotion via the stress peptide, corticotrophin releasing hormone (CRH, also known as corticotrophin releasing factor), in addition to several other neuropeptides, and excitatory and inhibitory neurotransmitters such a GABA and glutamate, to promote anxiety-related disorders (Lebow and Chen 2016). Through the actions of neuropeptides and neurotransmitters, the BNST processes stress information and readiness for threatening responses by receiving direct connections from not only the AMG but also mPFC (Radley and Sawchenko 2011). Additionally, it is well-characterized from a number of rodent studies that CRH critically facilitating BNST's function as a center for integration of stress information with negative emotion and anxiety-like states. That is, BNST neurons synthesizing CRH project directly to the central AMG and directly to the HYP. In turn, central amygdaloid projections that contain CRH also activate the PVN of the HYP. Together, both the BNST and AMG are capable of activating the HPA axis in response to perceived stressors (Lebow and Chen 2016), with these stressors expressed as either acute, fear-like behavior or more chronic anxiety-like behavior. Thus, Lebow and Chen (2016) have proposed a unified role of the BNST for collecting, monitoring and parsing information to then distill such information into meaningful action, with the aid of the HPA axis to tune the physiological response. Moreover, BNST connections with pain systems may adjust information on mood and sensory systems.

Stressors and anxiety As noted, a distinction exists between physiological stressors along with its related ANS-HPA circuitry, and the perception of an environmental challenge, a perceived (i.e., psychological) stress along with its related limbic forebrain circuitry. For the remainder of this review, the CNS processing of a psychological stressor will be discussed, and it is defined as "a particular relationship between the subject and the environment that is appraised by the subject as taxing or exceeding resources and endangering well-being" (Peterson 2000). Individuals experiencing repeated and chronic stress report long-term anxiety disorders such as generalized anxiety disorder (GAD), PTSD, and social anxiety (Bekhbat and Neigh 2018; Iwata et al. 2013; Serrats et al. 2017). Often, individuals become sensitized to stressors due to their prior stress experience, and this vulnerability is marked by heightened stress responses resulting in disorders of anxiety (Penninx et al. 2021). It is important to emphasize that anxiety disorders are the most common type of affective illness (social anxiety and GAD) capable of emerging at any developmental stage throughout life, including adulthood, with a lifetime prevalence in the US at ~32% (Kessler et al. 2005). Stress-associated anxiety disorders are a considerable burden to the quality of life worldwide, with GAD and other anxiety disorders ranked by WHO as the ninth most health-related cause of disability globally (Disease et al. 2017), with a lifetime prevalence of ~32% just within the US (Kessler et al. 2005; Copeland et al. 2014; Ormel et al. 2015). Several studies suggest that ~20–30% of children and adolescents have an anxiety disorder at some point (Copeland et al. 2014; Ormel et al. 2015).

7.4 FASD, Stress, and Anxiety

Often, symptoms associated with FASD include heightened stress reactivity with an increased risk for developing anxiety disorders (Coles et al. 2022; Khoury et al. 2018; Clark et al. 2024). Reports using adult animal models of PAE show the development of anxiety-like behavior following chronic stress (Hellemans et al. 2008; Lam et al. 2018; Raineki et al. 2016). In populations with FASD, adolescents, and adults report greater rates of anxiety compared to non-FASD individuals (Wolff et al. 2023), with females experiencing higher rates of anxiety disorders that are more apparent in adolescents and adults (Flannigan et al. 2023). Notably, clinical research shows that typical stressors precipitate anxiety disorders that do not become apparent in early childhood, but rather, often manifest in adolescence or later (Baker et al. 2014; Coles et al. 2010; Cook et al. 2016), with observed sex differences in mood dysregulation (Raineki et al. 2016). The data further support that PAE-induced vulnerability to anxiety may be driven by dysfunctional corticolimbic circuit function that also involves immune-like glial cells and their signaling molecules (Bodnar et al. 2018, 2020; Drew and Kane 2014; Ruyak et al. 2022; Wilhelm and Guizzetti 2015) (discussed further below).

Adolescent vulnerability to stress and its impact on corticolimbic dysfunction Nervous system development continues postnatally, with substantial structural remodeling, reorganization, and synaptic functional connectivity within cortical and limbic areas involved in affective processing (Vijayakumar et al. 2018), cognitive and impulse control (Giedd and Rapoport 2010). Notably, neural connections between the mPFC and the subcortical limbic regions, the AMG, and HIPP extensively change during adolescence (Steinberg 2005; Tamnes et al. 2010; Zhang et al. 2016)., The communication between the mPFC and various limbic structures such as the AMG and HIPP support elemental aspects of emotional and cognitive function and stress regulation (Cardinal et al. 2002; Gee 2016; Tottenham and Galvan 2016). The transition between youth and adulthood in both humans and rodents is concurrent with development of an engaged mPFC communicating to limbic pathways necessary for emotion and cognition. These changes occur predominantly during adolescence, a critical period of brain development until young adulthood (Dennis et al. 2013; Shaw et al. 2006), with social interaction facilitating the maturation of corticolimbic circuits. The developmental features occurring at key postnatal periods strongly suggests that the period of adolescence is more susceptible and vulnerable than adulthood to stress challenges (Furuyashiki and Kitaoka 2019), due to this aforementioned substantial structural remodeling, reorganization, and functional connectivity of corticolimbic regions involved in cognitive and mood function (Vijayakumar et al. 2018; Giedd and Rapoport 2010; Dennis et al. 2013; Shaw et al. 2006; Eiland and Romeo 2013; Holder and Blaustein 2014).

A number of early studies support the need for social interaction to optimize corticolimbic circuit development. Neural and behavioral development of rodents is thought to mirror stages of human development (Andersen 2003). In rodent studies, adolescence is imposed on postnatal day (PND) 21, and comparative studies indicate that rodent PND34–P46 corresponds to mid-adolescence in human life and >PND70 corresponds to young adulthood in humans (Braun-Lewensohn et al. 2022; Chulani and Gordon 2014). Similar to human adolescent development when social interactions serve to promote adaptive behavioral patterns for later life challenges, rodent adolescents exhibit a greater preference for social stimuli (Douglas et al. 2004); this period of adolescence is marked by increased social play and emerging cognitive strategies that lead to effective coping with later-life unpredictable challenges in adulthood (Spear 2000; Vanderschuren et al. 2016). Juvenile play is one of the essential mechanisms for healthy maturation of the social brain, as studies have illustrated the negative consequences from altered play exposure (Bell et al. 2010; Burke et al. 2017; Ham et al. 2024; Pellis and Pasztor 1999; Pellis et al. 2023; Stark et al. 2023). Thus, the notion that disruption of adolescent social play reprograms the adult limbic stress response has been gaining attention and support.

Reports have investigated how adolescent stress may exert enduring changes that impact later-life stress responses. For example, juvenile play disruption by repeated 1 h isolation stress for as little as ~2wks during mid-adolescence in rodent models results in stress-sensitized corticosterone release in the presence of unfamiliar conspecifics, while adults lacking a history of adolescent stress showed no such sensitization (Hodges and McCormick 2015). Additionally, while acute stress during adolescence (PND 29–31) exerts minimal impact on adult HPA activity from a 1 h acute restraint stress (Lovelock and Deak 2020), adult stress (30 min forced swim test) in rodents with a history of adolescent acute stress results in increased anxiety and depressive-like behavior as well as increases in gene activation as reflected by semi-quantitative analysis of cFos immunoreactivity in the AMG (Lovelock and Deak 2019). In other studies, adolescents reared in social isolation reveal reduced axonal dendritic pruning and reduced complex arborization in the mPFC (Bell et al. 2010), thus supporting the notion that adolescent stress alters limbic programing that persists into adulthood. In further support, female rodents that experienced pre-to-mid-adolescence social isolation, or more acute isolation schedules from PND30–35 or PND40–45 demonstrated anxiety-like behavior in the open field test or following in the elevated plus maze when tested either during adolescence or later. These behavioral changes co-occur with decreases in synaptic-associated protein expression in the prefrontal cortex (Arakawa 2007; Hermes et al. 2011; Leussis and Andersen 2008). Several reports have shown that the impact of adolescent stress from altered social experiences also results in altered stress limbic circuits (Burke et al. 2017). For example, mice exposed to repeated social defeat stress beginning in late adolescence demonstrated adult anxiety-like behavior (Weber et al. 2019). Thus, part of the stress sequelae observed from repeated psychosocial stress can include adult anxiety, and together, these studies support a greater vulnerability to adolescent psychosocial stressors.

Adult stress disruptions in corticolimbic circuit maturation Studies in adult rodent models show that either acute or chronic stress alters corticolimbic function with resultant behavioral consequences. Acute stress in adults, such as 30 min restraint stress, impacts the excitation of the mPFC via the action of the endocannabinoid receptors by mediating inhibition of the mPFC resulting in the termination of stress-induced HPA axis activation (Hill et al. 2011). To further support the impact of stress-induced mPFC neuronal action in modulating fear/anxiety, optogenetic manipulation increased inhibitory interneuron density (via PV+ expression), which surround glutamatergic neurons projecting to the mPFC and the BNST, which resulted in fear inhibition. This experiment utilized cue-dependent fear conditioning, where mice were exposed to a series of five tones paired with footshock. Mice were then tested for fear extinction, retention, and re-instatement, during which they were presented with tones, but no shock. For the fear acquisition and extinction procedures, optogenetic stimulation coterminated with the stressful stimuli. Mice were then placed into the open field chamber and allowed to explore for 5 min without optogenetic stimulation, and then for 5 min with optogenetic stimulation. This study showed decreased inhibitory interneuron density, which surround glutamatergic neurons projecting to the AMG, generated fear (Jasnow et al. 2013). Within the mPFC circuits, the effect of acute stress on interneuron activity is currently not well-characterized, yet overall, a number of reports demonstrate increased inhibitory activity immediately following acute stressor exposure, with interneurons comprising diverse connectivity and firing patterns suggesting their critical role in balancing both excitatory and inhibitory activity not only in the mPFC, but also to the HIPP, AMG, and BNST. Ultimately, adult chronic or prolonged stress exposure can lead to an imbalance of inhibitory interneuron activity and disrupted corticolimbic function that result in adult behavioral alterations such as impaired spatial memory, elevations in anxiety-like behavior and impaired reward-seeking (Perez-Rando et al. 2022), deficits in learning and memory or dysregulated mood such as depression and anxiety (Popoli et al. 2011; Sousa and Almeida 2012). In addition, chronic stress can lead to structural changes and damage in and between the HIPP and mPFC resulting in impaired plasticity and reduced neural coherence as a consequence of chronic stress (Cerqueira et al. 2007a, b; Liston et al. 2009; Sousa et al. 2000).

PAE enhances the stress impact on corticolimbic function PAE exacerbates the negative consequences of stress, either acute or chronic, and either during adolescence or adulthood, inducing alterations in brain corticolimbic circuits. A number of studies have reported that PAE alters cognitive development, creates deficits in performance after stress during adolescence and/or adulthood (Breton et al. 2021), and creates a vulnerability to stress responses leading to anxiety-like disorders (Hellemans et al. 2008). Preclinical literature reports that chronic unpredictable mild stress in animals with PAE induces adverse behavioral consequences such as the emergence of anxiety- and depressive-like behaviors (Hagan et al. 2016; Schneiderman et al. 2005; Bangasser et al. 2019). One of the limbic regions highly associated with anxiety in children and adolescents with generalized anxiety disorder is the anterior cingulate cortex (ACC), which directly communicates to the AMG. Interestingly, in a study examining mice with PAE (4.0 g/kg of 25% via intraperitoneal injection at E16 and E17), a strong association of the activation states between the ACC and the basolateral AMG was observed, as assessed by immunohistochemical analysis of the immediate early gene cFos that is a marker of neuronal activity. Specifically, activity of ACC neurons was reduced while activity of AMG neurons was increased, with this pattern of activation strongly correlated with anxiety-like behavior as measured by the elevated plus maze. These data support that the PAE-induced increases in anxiety in mice that may be driven dysregulated connectivity between the ACC and the basolateral AMG (Hwang and Hashimoto-Torii 2022). The observed anxiety-like behavior after chronic mild stress is more pronounced by PAE (Lam et al. 2019), and such a stressor increases mRNA levels of the stress peptide, CRH, in the PVN of the hypothalamus in offspring with PAE. And, regardless of stress manipulations, mRNA for CRH is elevated in the central nucleus of the AMG (Lan et al. 2015). As previously suggested, the impact of PAE on glucocorticoid receptor HPA axis function begins during gestation (Lan et al. 2017), and several studies have demonstrated that PAE worsens stress-induced HPA axis functional changes via changes in glucocorticoid receptor expression in cortical and limbic areas (Raineki et al. 2018, 2019). Early studies demonstrated that offspring with PAE showed deficits in HPA feedback inhibition; that is female offspring showed increased levels of stress-induced circulating glucocorticoids when the stressor was applied at the trough circadian cycle, and after stress at their peak circadian cycle, while both males and females with PAE showed increased circulating glucocorticoids compared to controls. These data suggest a potential sex-specific difference in sensitivity of the glucocorticoid response implicating a stress-induced HPA chronic hyperresponsiveness (Osborn et al. 1996). Moreover, PAE creates a vulnerability to developing adverse stress responses that endures when chronic mild stress exposure is initiated during adolescence that leads to anxiety-like behavior in adulthood, along with an increase in mRNA expression for the CRH receptor, CRHR1 in the AMG (Raineki et al. 2016), and in the HIPP (Raineki et al. 2018)· Notably, PAE effects were more pronounced during adolescence, with changes in CRHR1 mRNA expression profiles observed in adult females but not males. Taken together, corticolimbic changes appear to be sensitized in offspring with PAE from adolescent stressors that extend to adulthood.

7.5 The Impact of PAE on the Locus Coeruleus

The locus coeruleus (LC) is a heterogenous cell cluster of noradrenergic neurons located in the brainstem pontine region that serves as the major source of the catecholaminergic neurotransmitter, norepinephrine to most of the limbic forebrain (Poe et al. 2020; Robertson et al. 2013). For example, LC projections to forebrain structures include the mPFC, cingulate cortex, AMG, HIPP, and the BNST, which were identified based on retrograde tracing using rabies virus targeted at LC-norepinephrine neurons in mice (Breton-Provencher et al. 2021). While projections to and from the LC vary across brain areas, crucial stress-responsive regions that are densely innervated by the LC include the limbic-related CAN areas of the prefrontal cortex, the anterior cingulate cortex (Arnsten 2009; Hirschberg et al. 2017), the hypothalamus, and several subnuclei of the AMG (McCall et al. 2015, 2017), and to a lesser extent, the BNST (Hammack et al. 2021) (Fig. 7.2). The LC plays a key role in the CAN response to stress as levels of NE are increased following various psychological stress manipulations, including restraint, foot shock (Smith et al. 1991), and auditory stressors (Britton et al. 1992). There is a growing body of research in recent years indicating that the LC plays a key role in mediating anxiety disorders through its role in the stress response (McCall et al. 2015; Valentino and Van Bockstaele 2008). Stressors engage the LC-noradrenaline system through the actions of limbic-derived CRH, which, via reciprocal communication, increases LC activity (Koob 1999). While LC axons project to regions of the CAN in response to stress that support anxiety/mood integration, the LC also sends descending projections to the spinal cord dorsal horn where the first synaptic relays of incoming noxious signals from peripheral nociceptors communicate to spinal cord pain projection neurons. These descending LC-spinal communication can promote analgesia (Seibt and Schlichter 2015; Li et al. 2022; Millan 2002) or heightened pain (e.g., hyperalgesia and allodynia) (Gao et al. 2025; Kawanabe-Kobayashi et al. 2024).

PAE alters stress-induced activation of LC neurons An interesting observation as a consequence of PAE revealed reduced neuron numbers in the LC, an effect that was also present in a separate cohort of offspring that were derived from dams that were nutritional matches to alcohol-consuming dams; the dam's blood alcohol concentrations were 303 ± 38 mg/dl (Maier and West 2003). In this study, dam rats were given a daily single gavage of alcohol at 6.0–6.5 g/kg, as a 22.5% (weight/volume) solution mixed with sterile water and received ad libitum access to laboratory chow and tap water. A separate study showed that despite no changes within the LC in the number of immunoreactive neurons expressing tyrosine hydroxylase, the enzyme required to catalyze the initial step in catecholamine biosynthesis, rat offspring with PAE (dams blood alcohol concentrations 180–200 mg/dl via vapor chamber) exposed to an acute stressor of a short schedule of footshocks revealed stress-induced increases in the activity of C1 adrenergic neurons in the brain stem (Choi et al. 2008b). In this report, dam's blood ethanol levels averaged 188.6 ± 10 mg/dl, with experiments performed on 2–3-month offspring. Notably, C1 adrenergic neurons are located in the rostral medulla and activate sympathetic output as well as stimulate the HPA axis. Evidence from optogenetic stimulation in a separate study showed that in anaesthetized rats, C1 neurons form direct excitatory synapses with LC neurons, and selective stimulation of C1 neurons activates LC through the release of glutamate (Abbott et al. 2012). Importantly studies aiming to generate moderate PAE, pregnant dams achieve blood alcohol concentrations within the range of 0.08–0.17 g/dl (80–170 mg/dl). For reference, 0.08 g/dl is considered the US legal intoxication limit. Additionally, those studies that model binge drinking, dams' blood alcohol concentrations achieve levels ranging 120–200 mg/dl, and high levels of alcohol consumption achieve blood alcohol concentrations of 400 mg/dl or higher

(Nogales et al. 2025 #2630). In considering the effects of alcohol exposure during development, these studies suggest that a range of prenatal alcohol exposures enhances stress-induced excitation of LC neurons that may act in concert with limbic areas of the CAN to increase the magnitude of a perceived stress along with the response.

The cocaine- and amphetamine-regulated transcript peptide (CART) is a neuropeptide abundantly expressed in several stress-related limbic processing areas that are part of the CAN; such areas include BNST, HIPP, HYP, LC and spinal cord (Koylu et al. 1998; Seress et al. 2004; Dandekar et al. 2008). In response to stress at PND 25 and PND 85, CRH and glucocorticoids increase the transcriptional activity of CART gene expression in the HYP and AMG (Koylu et al. 2006). Direct administration of CART into the lateral ventricle or into the CeA of adult rats led to a decrease in social interaction, indicating a direct link between expression of CART in stress-related brain regions and anxiety-like behavior (Dandekar et al. 2008 #2565). In a more recent study, PAE induced a down-regulation of immunoreactive CART fibers in the HIPP, HYP, BNST, the nucleus accumbens shell and the LC of offspring compared to age-matched controls. These changes in CART expression occurred in the same rat offspring that demonstrated increased anxiety-like behavior as assessed by the elevated plus maze and the forced swim test (Dandekar et al. 2019). While primarily correlational, these studies indicate a relationship between expression of CART in offspring with PAE and development of anxiety-like behaviors. The persistent changes in CART suggest that the CART and LC-noradrenergic stress system can be reprogramed by PAE, creating a vulnerability to stress that leads to mood disorders such as anxiety.

7.6 The Role of Neuroimmune Factors Underlying Sensitized Stress Responses from PAE

Neuroimmune factors and anxiety A growing body of literature suggests that the underlying mechanisms of adverse psychological stress responses in adolescents and adult individuals with FASD involve glial-derived cytokines. While neuroimmune factors can play beneficial roles, the most widely characterized role for glial cytokines in the CNS reflect their detrimental impact. Data are accumulating that adverse glial-cytokine actions in the limbic CAN are strongly linked to the development of mood and cognitive disorders in individuals with FASD. Below, a discussion of the beneficial roles of cytokines is followed by their harmful impact on the CNS.

Beneficial roles of cytokines on CNS synaptic development and plasticity In the CNS, microglia and astrocytes function as mediators of the central immune response to pathogens and stressors. The release of cytokines from these parenchymal glial cells, as well as from infiltrating leukocytes, mediates the innate and adaptive immune response to infection or stress challenges. Cytokines function in a pleiotropic manner and can consequently influence a wide range of signals and processes. There is growing evidence in the literature that cytokines also serve to modulate neuronal activity and viability. This can occur directly, by activation of their receptors on neurons (Marin and Kipnis 2013; Vezzani 2008; Viviani et al. 2007), or indirectly, by promoting the release of molecules from glial cells (Montgomery and Bowers 2012) (Table 7.1). Under certain conditions, cytokines, for example, interleukin-1β (IL-1β) and tumor necrosis factor-α (TNFα), facilitate healthy neuronal function including synaptic pruning, synaptic transmission and neuroplasticity and/or communication (Lima 2023; Pan et al. 1997).

Homeostatic synaptic scaling is a form of synaptic plasticity that adjusts the strength of a cell's synapses in response to prolonged alterations in the electrical activity of the cell, which can occur when a reduction in presynaptic activity leads to a reduction in postsynaptic excitability (Turrigiano 2008). The cytokine TNFα has been found to play a critical and beneficial role in this process, and has been shown to impact the membrane expression, phosphorylation, and subunit composition of AMPAR and GABA-A-receptors on the

Table 7.1 Impact of PAE on sensitizing corticolimbic and spinal immune actions

Region	PAE-induced cytokine alterations	PAE- and cytokine-induced behavioral alterations	References
Hypothalamus	↓IL-2, ↑CCL2, ↑CCR2, ↑TNFa, ↑IL-6		Bodnar et al. (2016), Chang et al. (2018), and Kim et al. (1999)
Amygdala	↑CXCL2; ↑IL-10, ↑IL-1β	Increased anxiety-like behaviors following early life stress	Raineki et al. (2018) and Ruffaner-Hanson et al. (2022)
Hippocampus	↑IFN-y, ↑IL-1β, ↑IL-4, ↑TNF-a, ↑IL-5, ↑IL-2		Bodnar et al. (2016) and Ruffaner-Hanson et al. (2022)
Medial prefrontal cortex	↑IL-6, ↑IL-5, ↓TNFa, ↓IL-1β		Bodnar et al. (2016) and Shamakina et al. (2024)
Locus Coeruleus			
Nucleus of the solitary tract			
Periaqueductal gray			
Dorsal root ganglion	↓IL10, ↑CX3CL1, ↑CXCL1	Allodynia following chronic constriction injury (CCI)	Noor et al. (2017) and Sanchez et al. (2019)
Spinal cord	↓IL10, ↑CCL2, ↑TNFa,	Allodynia following chronic constriction injury (CCI)	Noor et al. (2017) and Sanchez et al. (2019)

postsynaptic membrane, which in turn impact the excitability of the post-synaptic cell (Beattie et al. 2002; Stellwagen et al. 2005; Stellwagen and Malenka 2006). The necessity of TNFα signaling for synaptic scaling in hippocampal neurons was shown in an experiment during which TNFα signaling was blocked by applying a TNF-receptor antagonist during prolonged tetrodotoxin treatment, which blocks voltage-gated sodium channels to propagate action potentials along the axons to reach the axon terminal, thus preventing presynaptic release of neurotransmitters. In this experiment, neurons were unable to communicate to the post-synaptic membrane, and blocking TNFα binding to its receptor expressed on the post-synaptic neurons in turn, prevented the ability of the pre- and post-synaptic neurons to scale up excitatory synapses (Stellwagen et al. 2005). However, in neurons derived from the striatum, TNFα downregulated AMPAR membrane expression, indicating the potential for an adaptive role of TNFα to limit the strength of cortical synaptic drive (Lewitus et al. 2014). Another experiment, which utilized a cell-specific transgenic Cre line, demonstrated that TNFα drives the internalization of synaptic AMPA receptors, decreases synaptic strength, and suppresses behavioral sensitization following repeated administration of cocaine (Lewitus et al. 2016).

Given the crucial role of TNFα in the synaptic tuning of neurons, it is reasonable to speculate that dysregulation in levels of TNFα, or the receptors by which it activates cell signaling (TNF-R1 and TNF-R2) would lead to dysregulated neuronal firing rates with consequent underdeveloped synaptic connectivity in corticolimbic regions. One study which sought to examine the impact of microglia-derived cytokine signaling on expression of glutamatergic receptors demonstrated that increases in TNFα concentration resulted in a twofold increase expression of AMPARs in cultured hippocampal neurons (Beattie et al. 2002). In mice with a genetic deletion of either TNF-R1 or TNF-R2, modifications in the level of hippocampal NMDAR, AMPAR, and KA receptor subunits were observed and associated with alterations in the basal firing rate of hippocampal neurons (Balosso et al. 2009). It is therefore possible that PAE induced CNS pathological conditions that impact TNFα levels (either blunted or heightened) would impact synaptic tuning and synaptic connectivity in different regions of the brain involved in the stress response. There are currently no published reports that explore the impact of PAE on the function of TNFα synaptic scaling in corticolimbic circuits.

Stress-induced cytokine expression in corticolimbic areas Despite evidence for homeostatic functions of cytokines, decades of research demonstrate a detrimental impact of cytokines, transcription factors and chemokines in stress-induced anxiety. Microglia and astrocytes are well characterized to significantly influence the CNS response to psychological stressors (Biltz et al. 2022; Murphy-Royal et al. 2019; Sugama and Kakinuma 2021). This process is driven by activation of toll-like receptors (specifically TLR2 and TLR4), which become activated from their binding to endogenous damage-associated molecular patterns (DAMPs), such as heat shock proteins and high-mobility group box 1 (HMGB1) (Colleselli et al. 2023; Fleshner et al. 2017). Notably, DAMPs are released from all cell types including neurons when the neurons are undergoing a state of cellular stress or challenge. A number of factors that are released by cells in distress include reactive oxygen species, heat-shock proteins, and the nuclear protein, HMGB1 (Fleshner 2013). This process is known as stress-evoked sterile inflammation, which ultimately results in the production of cytokines such as IL-1β and TNFα (Fleshner et al. 2017). Studies have indicated increases in hypothalamic IL-1β mRNA (Shintani et al. 1995; Suzuki et al. 1997), IL-1β protein (Turnbull and Rivier 1999), and IL1RA mRNA (Suzuki et al. 1997) levels following acute restraint stress in experimental mice and rats. The activation of the endocrine HPA axis occurs as a direct consequence of these cytokine-driven responses to stress (Lan et al. 2015). However, while the stress-peptide, CRH, is critical for HPA axis activation, the function of CRH extends beyond its actions to simply engage the HPA axis and is now well-characterized to impact prefrontal cortical and other limbic regions that are part of the CAN. Interestingly, elevated CRH in the AMG has been shown to drive anxiety (Raineki et al. 2016; Ishikawa and Furuyashiki 2022), and anxiety-like behaviors in animal models of stress are additionally linked to overactive glial cells and the production of proinflammatory cytokines that include IL-1β and TNFα in the PFC, hypothalamus, HIPP, and AMG (Bekhbat and Neigh 2018; Hudson et al. 2014; Vecchiarelli et al. 2016; Zerbi et al. 2019). Work to date strongly support that stress leads to increases in IL-1β, TNF-α, and other cytokines within the hypothalamus, HIPP, and PFC after either acute or chronic stress exposure. Thus, taken together, the role of glial cells (astrocytes and microglia) and their signaling cytokines in the development of anxiety disorders as a maladaptive consequence of exposure to stressors, even mild stressors, throughout the lifetime has been well-established.

The impact of PAE exacerbates the vulnerability to developing anxiety due to a sensitization to stressors, and this vulnerability is thought to be driven by heightened actions of cytokines, chemokines, and their related factors. For example, male offspring prenatally exposed to a moderate dose of ethanol (dam's blood alcohol concentrations 50–90 mg/dl) are associated with an elevation in the C-C chemokine motif (*CCL2*), and its receptor, CCR2, in the brain following a secondary insult of adult alcohol exposure (Chang et al. 2015; He and Crews 2008), which builds on evidence that insults in adult individuals with PAE increase neuroinflammatory brain responses. Other work in animal models of PAE showed that glia in adults are highly activated in the HIPP and cortex, along with elevations in the proinflammatory cytokines IL-1β, and TNFα), and the chemokine CCL2 (Drew and Kane 2014; Chang et al. 2015; Bodnar et al. 2016; Boschen et al. 2016; Drew et al. 2015; Kane et al. 2011; Terasaki and Schwarz 2016; Tiwari and Chopra 2011).

In the adolescent, blunted cytokines in the hypothalamus occur in parallel with elevated IL-1β in the cortex of PAE stress-exposed offspring (Bodnar et al. 2016). Other studies examining hypothalamic regulation of stress in adolescent and adult PAE offspring demonstrate increased CCL2, CCR2, TNFα, and the cytokine,

IL-6, that is identified as mostly proinflammatory (Chang et al. 2018; Kim et al. 1999). Neuroimmune dysregulation within the AMG from PAE has been shown in studies of postnatal day 12 PAE offspring revealing elevations in the C-X-C motif chemokine ligand 1 (*CXCL1*) (Raineki et al. 2017), and offspring with a later-life adult alcohol challenge revealed a trend toward potentiated IL6 and the cytokine transcription factor, NfkB, in the AMG (Doremus-Fitzwater et al. 2020). These cytokines/chemokines are not just simply increased in parallel with neuronal changes, but are functionally important because blocking the actions of proinflammatory factors released from glia with an agonist that binds to the peroxisome proliferator-activator receptor-γ (e.g., pioglitazone), prevented microglial and neuronal cell loss and also prevented elevations in IL-1β, TNFα and CCL2 gene expression. Pioglitazone is a drug developed to facilitate insulin sensitivity, but also acts to inhibit proinflammatory gene expression of TNFα and IL-6 (Drew et al. 2015; Cippitelli et al. 2017). Additionally, PAE can prime the immune system in adolescence and adulthood, as evidenced by greater disease severity of adjuvant-induced arthritis and increased joint inflammation, and greater brain glial activation and cytokine expression in neonates, adolescents, and adults (Deak et al. 2022). A better understanding of the underlying mechanisms which contribute to development of adverse stress responses, that is, anxiety disorders in adolescence and adulthood can pave the way for developing potential treatments for individuals experiencing anxiety disorders as a result of PAE.

7.7 Neuroimmune Communication in the Spinal Cord: Neuropathy from PAE

PAE is a risk factor for developing sensory neuropathy Sensory neuropathy resulting from peripheral nerve damage is a common pain condition. A significant number of Americans (25%) experience persistent pain (>6 mo) caused by neuropathy (Cohen et al. 2021). Neuropathies can occur within the CNS or in the peripheral nervous system, often occurring after an injury that leads to a dysfunction of neurons responsible for relaying pain. The cellular components of the pain pathway consists of axons of nociceptors with their cell bodies located in the dorsal root ganglia (DRG), and axon projections from the DRG into the superficial laminae of the dorsal horn of the spinal cord where resident neurons are exquisitely responsive to incoming nociceptive information (Costigan et al. 2009). Work in animal models of neuropathy has overwhelmingly demonstrated that idiopathic sensory signals develop from hyperactive nociceptive neurons as well as neurons within the dorsal horn of the spinal cord that receive such signals as a consequence of nerve damage. In addition, other cells are now recognized to be key players in the overactive nociceptor and spinal relay, and these cells include activated peripheral immune (e.g., monocytes, macrophages and T cells) and CNS glial cell (astrocytes and microglia) in responses to nerve injury (Grace et al. 2014, 2021). Within the spinal cord, feed-forward bi-directional neuron-to-glial responses facilitate chronic pain. For example, activation markers for satellite glial cells located within the DRG are profoundly elevated following sciatic nerve injury in a rat model, along with immune cell accumulation around the injured peripheral nerve (Stoll et al. 1993), sensory ganglia (i.e., DRG) (Dubovy et al. 2007; Hu et al. 2007; Hu and McLachlan 2002; Lu and Richardson 1993; Morin et al. 2007; Shaw et al. 2008; Vega-Avelaira et al. 2009), and the dorsal horn of the spinal cord (Hu et al. 2007; Morin et al. 2007; Shaw et al. 2008; Kim and Moalem-Taylor 2011; Kleinschnitz et al. 2006). Under these pathological conditions, non-nociceptors that convey light touch information to the brain become dysregulated and inappropriately activate pain projection neurons within the spinal cord. Consequently, light mechanical touch is miscoded as pathologically painful, referred to as allodynia (Sandkuhler 2009), and is observed in pain patients where touch from clothes is intolerable (Basbaum et al. 2009; Woolf 2011). In animal models of neuropathy, allodynia is assessed by hindpaw responses to light mechanical touch stimulation (Barrot 2012).

These nociceptive-responsive neurons (also referred to as pain projection neurons) within the dorsal horn of the spinal cord possess ascending axons to various brainstem and corticolimbic areas (Costigan et al. 2009), and enroute, send collaterals to the PAG (Mantyh 1983; Ghilardi et al. 2012), LC (Gao et al. 2025) and the NTS (Holt 2022). Thus, spinal nociceptive projections occur via multiple pathways (Grace et al. 2014; Ossipov et al. 2010). Pain signals from the spinal cord are substantially modulated at key brainstem and brain areas (Mantyh 1983; Costigan et al. 2009; Neugebauer et al. 2023) that also serve other functions including stress responses and mood regulation (Vachon-Presseau 2018). Critical pain modulatory sites that overlap with stress and mood regulation include, but are not limited to, the hypothalamus, central AMG, and anterior cingulate cortex (Vachon-Presseau 2018). The most widely studied pain-pathway structures have focused on the nociceptive input to the dorsal horn of the spinal cord; that is, at the first synapse in the spinal cord where very powerful pain modulation occurs, where incoming pain signals can be suppressed or amplified (Grace et al. 2014; Basbaum et al. 2009; Milligan and Watkins 2009; Woolf and Salter 2000; Calvo and Bennett 2012). Thus, understanding cellular adaptations at the level of the dorsal horn of the spinal cord where the first CNS synaptic nociceptive relay occurs before ascending signals reach other CNS areas, provides an excellent opportunity to understand pain regulation, particularly in the context of individuals with PAE.

7.7.1 Pain in PAE Offspring

A number of published reports demonstrate that PAE amplifies nociceptive processing at the level of the injured nerve (sciatic nerve), the sensory ganglia (e.g., DRG) and the dorsal horn of the spinal cord (Noor et al. 2017, 2018; Sanchez et al. 2017). These published reports revealed an insidious immune cell sensitization caused by moderate PAE in rats that was unmasked by a discrete and well-characterized model of sciatica, that is, a localized sciatic nerve injury that generates tactile allodynia of the hindpaw. For example, these reports showed increased spinal macrophage infiltration and heightened astrocyte and microglial activation in a spinal region targeted by the central projections of damaged sciatic nerves, observed in young adult and middle-aged PAE offspring (Noor et al. 2017; Sanchez et al. 2017), suggests that an immune sensitization may be driving lifelong risk for neuropathy. In addition, increases in peri-sciatic nerve IL-1β, TNFα, IL-6, and the chemokine, CXCL1, as well as a blunted expression of the powerful anti-inflammatory cytokine, interleukin-10 were observed. Peripheral immune organs are also sensitized, as increases in IL-1β and TNFα protein production and release from peripheral immune cells arising from the spleen of middle-aged PAE offspring are observed (Noor et al. 2017; Sanchez et al. 2017), suggesting a lifelong sensitized peripheral immune-cell cytokine response from PAE.

Interestingly, a 75% reduction in the sciatic nerve injury paradigm, which is a minor injury, generated a robust hindpaw allodynia observed in offspring with PAE, while non-PAE rats failed to develop allodynia. Applying the minor injury model in mice further established that PAE is a risk factor for developing allodynia (Noor et al. 2019). The sensory changes leading to allodynia appeared to be mediated, again, by immune cell sensitization, which was unmasked by minor injury. Utilizing a low to moderate PAE paradigm in rats, with peak serum ethanol levels in dams of about 60–80 mg/dl followed by a minimal nerve injury in adulthood, we observed development of chronic allodynia only in PAE offspring, with virtually no changes in normal sensory thresholds in control rats (Noor et al. 2019, 2020; Sanchez et al. 2019). More recently, these observations were reproduced in adult (2–7 month-old) PAE mice using two different PAE paradigms. While both paradigms involved exposure to alcohol throughout gestation, one paradigm involved daily 2-h access to 20% unsweetened alcohol with dams' BEC levels reaching about 116 mg/dl, whereas another PAE paradigm involved daily 4-h access to 10% saccharin-sweetened alcohol solution in dams with BEC levels reported 68 mg/dl after 2 h of drinking (Brady et al. 2012 #2214; Myrick et al. 2024 #2574). Studies utilizing these paradigms have reported PAE-induced susceptibility in allodynia development following minor nerve injury during adulthood, regardless of sex (Myrick et al. 2024 #2574; Noor et al. 2023a #2422; Pasmay et al. 2025 #2631).

Following peripheral nerve injury, the release of endogenous factors (DAMPs) initiates the innate immune activation via TLR4, which is expressed on peripheral immune cells and spinal glia. While proinflammatory activation of innate immune cells such as spinal glia promotes the development and maintenance of allodynia, adaptive immune cells also play a critical role in nociceptive sensitization. Following nerve injury, T cells undergo activation and differentiation. Activated T cells are recruited at the nerve injury site as well as in the spinal cord. Proinflammatory Th1 and Th17 cells can further interact with activated astrocytes, microglia, and pain projection neurons, propagating neuroinflammation and maintaining chronic allodynia. While PAE-induced susceptibility to develop neuropathy did not display sex differences, pain literature from non-PAE studies suggests that the underlying neuroimmune factors or mediators of peripheral nerve injury-induced allodynia may involve sex-specific dimorphic mechanisms. Interestingly, studies utilizing the peripheral nerve injury model (spared nerve injury) in non-PAE rodents suggest that females depend on adaptive immune cells (likely T cells), while males predominantly use microglia-mediated immune actions during allodynia (Sorge et al. 2015 #1677). Interestingly, in the absence of an intact adaptive immune system, females also utilize innate immune cells (microglia)-mediated mechanisms, and the involvement of astrocytes appears to be sex-independent (Chen et al. 2017 #1837).

We speculate that while allodynia in PAE may involve sensitization of the microglia, astrocytes, and T cell-specific immune reactivity differently based on sex, the underlying immune mediators may stem from activation of common immune signaling pathways. Prior studies in PAE confirmed enhanced activation of both microglia and astrocytes in both males and females (Noor et al. 2020 #1879; Noor et al. 2017 #1817; Sanchez et al. 2023 #2410; Sanchez et al. 2017 #1986). These studies reported augmented levels of proinflammatory and pain signaling cytokines like IL-1b and TNF that are often consequent of TLR4 and NFKb activation, which is linked to aberrant activation of Nod-like receptor protein 3 (NLRP3, discussed below). These proinflammatory cytokines were concurrent with increased DRG and spinal glial activation phenotypes, as well as increased peripheral immune cell activity of PAE macrophages from activation with TLR4 agonist (e.g., lipopolysaccharide). These studies support that enhanced TLR4 activity on innate immune cells due to PAE.

While a side-by-side comparison of the adaptive immune profile of PAE offspring following minor injury is yet to be explored, a prior study demonstrated dysregulated adaptive immune responses in PAE female rat offspring following minor nerve injury (Noor et al. 2020 #1879). An increased accumulation of proinflammatory perisciatic and dorsal root ganglia Th1 and Th17 cells from nerve-injured offspring with PAE along with elevated levels of proinflammatory T cell cytokines such as IL-17A, IL-21 (Noor et al. 2020). Gene expression mRNA levels of several key T cell cytokines are increased including T-bet, ROR-γt and IFN-γ in the dorsal horn of the spinal cord from PAE female offspring with allodynia, supporting the involvement of Th1- and Th17-differentiated proinflammatory T cell subpopulations in neuroinflammation during neuropathy in PAE rats, all of which were absent in non-allodynic rats. Moreover, a lack of anti-inflammatory T regulatory cells was present in PAE, indicating an augmented proinflammatory cytokine phenotype creates an imbalance in the activated T cell profile that contributes to chronic allodynia in PAE offspring (Noor et al. 2020).

Even with a reduction in injury, blunted dorsal spinal cord IL-10 protein (produced by both T cells and innate immune cells) expression is observed in PAE offspring (Sanchez et al. 2019).

Lastly, a consistent observation of these studies is that light touch sensory responses appeared to be similar between PAE and non-PAE offspring; that is, a complete lack of pathological light touch is present under basal conditions. Only after the secondary challenge of an injury, did a profound allodynia develop. One possibility for this observation is that the underlying glia are sensitized, but remain quiescent. Thus, examining markers indicative of an immune sensitization in offspring under basal conditions could lead to potential mechanisms that drive heightened immune-like responses in the CNS after an injury has occurred. For example, under *basal* conditions, prior to sciatic nerve injury, lymphocyte function-associated antigen-1 (LFA-1), which is a transmembrane β_2-adhesion receptor αLβ2; CD11a/CD18β2 expressed on leukocytes (e.g., T cell and myeloid cells) and possibly microglia are significantly elevated in the spinal cord dorsal horn in PAE offspring. LFA-1 is further upregulated following minor nerve injury in PAE offspring, and blocking its actions in the spinal cord reversed PAE allodynia (Sanchez et al. 2019). Interestingly, LFA-1 interacts with the intercellular adhesion molecule (ICAM-1) expressed on blood vessel walls (Azcutia et al. 2013; Evans et al. 2009; Walzog et al. 1999), and while speculative, PAE may predispose peripheral immune cell infiltration upon even subtle CNS injuries.

7.8 PAE Impact on the Molecular Tuning of Spinal Neuroimmune Factors and Pain

A possible mechanism that leads to CNS proinflammatory cytokine production from PAE may be through the actions of the NLRP3 inflammasomes. When the complete intracellular complex is formed, it allows for the production and secretion of mature IL-1β from glial-immune cells. Thus, NLRP3 is a critical step for mature IL-1β release, and a recent report demonstrated that in offspring with PAE, spinal IL-1RA (an IL-1β receptor antagonist) transiently reversed sciatic nerve injury-induced allodynia (Sanchez et al. 2019). A separate study showed that peripheral administration of an NLRP3 inhibitor (MCC950) profoundly reversed allodynia in offspring with PAE with sciatic injury (Noor et al. 2023a). Together, these reports support that PAE promotes the action of NLRP3 in facilitating the development of nerve injury-induced allodynia that more readily develops from minor injury. This aberrant activation of NLRP3 is likely generated by the enhanced transcription of signaling components of the NLRP3 protein complex, which are products of the TLR4-NF-κB pathway. Additionally, PAE-induced enhanced production and/or persistent release of DAMPs from damaged neurons and activated glia, in combination with the dysregulation of anti-inflammatory molecule production (e.g., IL-10) may play regulatory roles.

Emerging literature suggests that the involvement of epigenetic modification and altered non-coding RNA molecules, such as microRNA is associated with adverse outcomes of FASD (Balaraman et al. 2016; Bestry et al. 2022; Popova et al. 2023). Interestingly, the pain-inducing spinal neuroimmune factors (mRNA and protein) remain largely unaltered in adult PAE offspring at basal levels. A recent exploration of whether alterations in epigenetic factors may be key in driving dysregulation of the neuroimmune response in PAE. For example, non-coding circular RNAs may act as a novel molecular priming mechanism of PAE, modulating PAE-induced neuroimmune activity. Circular RNAs (circRNAs) are a novel category of long non-coding RNAs that are derived from the circularization and covalent joining of back-spliced exons and/or introns, compared to linear mRNA transcripts generated from canonical splicing (Barrett and Salzman 2016; Hansen et al. 2013; Memczak et al. 2013). To date, several circular RNAs have been reported to regulate CNS glial-immune function, via binding and sequestering microRNAs, regulating immune gene expression (Curry-Hyde et al. 2020). In a recent study, under basal levels, PAE leads to long-term alterations in the circRNA profile of the spinal cord. Moreover, under neuropathic conditions from minor nerve injury that causes allodynia, PAE further dysregulates and creates a unique spinal circRNA profile (Noor et al. 2023b). Strikingly, these circRNAs were preferentially derived from NFkB-related genes, which is a critical transcription factor that mediates transcription of TLR4-related proinflammatory factors, and acts as a critical upstream regulator of NLRP3 inflammasome activation (Chen and Jiang 2013). A number of circRNAs, previously characterized to play immune modulatory roles (such as circ*Itch*, circ*Stag1*, circ*Tttc3* and circ*Vopp1*) were dysregulated in PAE offspring (Noor et al. 2023b). These studies suggest that spinal circRNA alterations may influence the TLR4-NLRP3-IL-1β axis in glial cells (reviewed in (Pritha et al. 2025)), thereby contributing to PAE-induced spinal neuroimmune activation during chronic pain.

7.9 Stress-Induced Allodynia: Nociplastic Pain

Nociplastic pain is a prominent clinical manifestation commonly co-occurring with anxiety disorders, including generalized anxiety disorder (Bandelow 2015; Meng et al. 2024; Romera et al. 2010). Nociplastic pain originates from within the CNS and does not emanate from any known/overt tissue damage (Romera et al. 2010; Kosek et al. 2016; Fitzcharles et al. 2021), and this ambiguity renders this condition a very difficult-to-treat clinical pain problem (Madison et al. 2023; Bandelow 2015; Meng et al. 2024; Kosek et al. 2016) that often manifests as tactile allodynia (Kaplan et al. 2024). Indeed, while therapeutics to treat anxiety disorders are typically minimally effective (~50%) to achieve only partial alleviation (Garakani et al. 2020), correspondingly, there are no available therapeutics that effectively control nociplastic pain from anxiety. The ambiguous features of anxiety-induced nociplastic pain underscore that neuronal function within corticolimbic, brainstem, and spinal circuits has become pathological. But how? Decades of accumulating evidence show stress, leading to anxiety and depression impacts CNS inflammatory states (as discussed above) (Ishikawa and Furuyashiki 2022), and this co-occurrence offers potential opportunities to explore novel therapeutic targets.

Supraspinal pain regions integrate with stress limbic areas Some aspects of pain-related supraspinal regions have been elucidated in terms of the functional anatomy of corticolimbic areas that process sensory information about incoming pain as well as some emotional features of the pain stimulus. Notably, information about tissue trauma occurring in the body, along the peripheral nervous system or in the CNS, is relayed to brainstem areas such as the LC, NTS and PAG, and other limbic areas such as the hypothalamus and AMG, as well as cortical areas such as the prefrontal cortex, anterior cingulate cortex and the BNST, which assign emotional value to the pain signal. Tissue damage-induced pain triggers spinal-to-brainstem and to brain relays, and the assignment and emotional processing occurs from brain-to-brainstem, and even back to spinal cord (Johnstone et al. 2012; Seminowicz and Moayedi 2017; Xiao and Zhang 2018; Hammack et al. 2021; Millan 2002; Ossipov et al. 2010).

It is now becoming increasingly recognized that pain can arise without an overt pathological condition such as from tissue trauma. How might this happen? One possibility is through overactive immune glial cells (e.g., astrocytes and microglia) and the actions of proinflammatory cytokines that these glia release within limbic areas including the mPFC, AMG, HIPP, BNST, PAG, and LC. Psychosocial stress in rodent models show increased CNS immune signaling; referred to as stress-evoked sterile CNS inflammation including microglial activation in the PFC and HIPP (Mondelli et al. 2017; Reus et al. 2015), which also results in anxiety-like behavior. Thus, stress-evoked sterile inflammation of limbic areas has been proposed to underlie mood disorders including prolonged anxiety (Biltz et al. 2022; Ishikawa and Furuyashiki 2022; McKim et al. 2018; Wohleb et al. 2011; Zhang et al. 2019). In clinical studies, populations with psychosocial stress also experience anxiety disorders (Penninx et al. 2021; Kessler et al. 2005; Copeland et al. 2014; Ormel et al. 2015; Clark et al. 2024). Pain is a prominent clinical manifestation commonly co-occurring with anxiety disorders such as GAD (Bandelow 2015 #2443). A recent clinical study of people with GAD that were also experiencing pain underwent functional and structural magnetic resonance imaging, examining the corticolimbic areas of the insula (region of the cortex that receives somatosensory cortical information about pain), thalamus, PAG, PFC, anterior cingulate cortex, AMG, and HIPP. Exclusion criteria included severe physical illness and CNS disease. Compared to healthy controls, structural and functional abnormalities in these corticolimbic areas were present and correlated with pain symptoms (Meng et al. 2024), suggesting that anxiety and pain are served by common corticolimbic substrates. The stress sequelae observed clinically (Madison et al. 2023) and from repeated psychosocial stress in mice include anxiety and pain (Rodriguez-Palma et al. 2023). Observing pain like allodynia in the absence of an overt injury in not expected, as pain is typically understood to be a symptom due to overt tissue or nerve damage. Therefore, experiencing pain as a consequence of stress and in the absence of overt injury is surprising because the underlying neurological mechanism is not well understood. These preclinical studies identified pain in the form of allodynia, as assessed by pathological light touch sensitivity of hindpaws (i.e., tactile allodynia). In the field of pain research, animal models employed to understand allodynia typically induce direct nerve and/or tissue trauma to identify factors and cell types responsible for conveying pain signals to the brain. A large body of evidence has accumulated showing that allodynia produced from a variety of animal models occurs in parallel with glial activation and proinflammatory cytokine signaling in the spinal cord (Costigan et al. 2009 #1007; Grace et al. 2014 #1799). Thus, observing microglial activation from stress in the absence of tissue trauma offered a new approach to understanding the development of pain (Biltz et al. 2022). Notably, stress-induced allodynia requires pathological spinal sensory processing (Sawicki et al. 2018, 2021). Corticolimbic and spinal cord TNFα (Rodriguez-Palma et al. 2023) and IL-1β expression was elevated in these mice (Sawicki et al. 2018) despite the absence of tissue or nerve damage. This stress-evoked allodynia is referred to as nociplastic pain, that as previously noted, is observed clinically (Madison et al. 2023; Bandelow 2015; Meng et al. 2024; Kosek et al. 2016; Kaplan et al. 2024) and further supported in a mouse model of repeated psychosocial stress resulting in anxiety-like behavior and tactile allodynia (Rodriguez-Palma et al. 2023).

In populations with FASD, adolescent and adults report greater rates of anxiety compared to non-FASD individuals (Wolff et al. 2023), with females experiencing higher rates of anxiety disorders that were more apparent in adolescents and adults (Flannigan et al. 2023). Additionally, sensory abnormalities like pathological light-touch sensitivity is a prominent co-morbidity (Himmelrich et al. 2020). While speculative, tactile hypersensitivity reported in individuals with FASD may be driven by enduring stress-evoked corticolimbic, brainstem *and* spinal heightened neuroinflammatory actions. The impact of PAE impact on stress-induced anxiety and allodynia needs further research and exploration.

7.10 Conclusions

Fetal Alcohol Spectrum Disorder (FASD) encompasses disorders that are related to emotional, mood, and sensory function. The US prevalence is ~5% in school-aged children who are particularly vulnerable to experiencing typical, daily stressors, but respond with heightened reactivity leading to higher rates of depression and anxiety, which are frequent co-morbidities with FASD. Low touch tolerance is also frequently associated with FASD. The sensory abnormalities like pathological light-touch hypersensitivity (i.e., allodynia) are a hallmark of pathological pain, and both stress-induced anxiety and sensory disorders are processed by similar corticolimbic and brainstem circuits. The central autonomic network (CAN) is a key aspect of perceived stress responses, and represents circuits that also process pain; these engaged overlapping limbic areas include the medial prefrontal cortex, anterior cingulate cortex, amygdala, hippocampus, bed nucleus of the stria terminalis, and the hypothalamus, as well as brainstem regions such as the periaqueductal gray, the nucleus of the solitary tract and the locus coeruleus. Preclinical literature shows that chronic unpredictable mild stress in animals with PAE induces adverse behavioral consequences such as the emergence of anxiety- and depressive-like behaviors as well as pathological light-touch hypersensitivity. While speculative, some works suggests that an engaged stress-induced CAN communicates with spinal sensory processing areas via several critical brainstem nuclei such as the periaqueductal gray, the nucleus of the solitary tract and the locus coeruleus.

Rodent models demonstrate that PAE is a risk factor for developing anxiety disorders and tactile neuropathies and that the underlying mechanism may be due to sensitized, or over-active corticolimbic, brainstem, and spinal glial activation with consequent neuroimmune actions such as the exaggerated release of the proinflammatory cytokines, interleukin-1β (IL-1β) and tumor necrosis factor-α (TNFα), among others. Work examining the risk of PAE in driving allodynia shows that overt neuroimmune gene and protein increases are not observed under basal conditions, but rather, are triggered following a secondary challenge such as minor peripheral nerve damage. The culmination of research suggests that PAE, acting through heightened CNS proinflammatory signaling significantly sensitizes stress responses leading to anxiety, and is also a risk factor for chronic neuropathy after minor injury.

The clinical stress sequelae of individuals with FASD may now include allodynia pain in the absence of overt injury. Stress sensitizes CNS circuits responsible for generating immune signaling molecules that may underlie nociplastic allodynia.

Lastly, adolescence, as a critical corticolimbic developmental period, is highly susceptible to stressors, and PAE worsens these effects. PAE may reprogram future stress responses leading to stress-related anxiety through the actions of sensitized immune signaling. Understanding the CNS circuits and the neuroimmune factors that play an important role in dysregulating circuit function will provide insight into potential therapeutic targets to mitigate stress-related anxiety and sensory pathologies.

Bibliography

Abbott SB et al (2012) C1 neurons excite locus coeruleus and A5 noradrenergic neurons along with sympathetic outflow in rats. J Physiol 590(12):2897–2915

Andersen SL (2003) Trajectories of brain development: point of vulnerability or window of opportunity? Neurosci Biobehav Rev 27(1–2):3–18

Arakawa H (2007) Ontogeny of sex differences in defensive burying behavior in rats: effect of social isolation. Aggress Behav 33(1):38–47

Arnsten AF (2009) Stress signalling pathways that impair prefrontal cortex structure and function. Nat Rev Neurosci 10(6):410–422

Azcutia V et al (2013) CD47 plays a critical role in T-cell recruitment by regulation of LFA-1 and VLA-4 integrin adhesive functions. Mol Biol Cell 24(21): 3358–3368

Baker AL et al (2014) Randomized controlled trial of MICBT for co-existing alcohol misuse and depression: outcomes to 36-months. J Subst Abus Treat 46(3): 281–290

Balaraman S et al (2016) Plasma miRNA profiles in pregnant women predict infant outcomes following prenatal alcohol exposure. PLoS One 11(11):e0165081

Balosso S et al (2009) Molecular and functional interactions between tumor necrosis factor-alpha receptors and the glutamatergic system in the mouse hippocampus: implications for seizure susceptibility. Neuroscience 161(1):293–300

Bandelow B (2015) Generalized anxiety disorder and pain. Mod Trends Pharmacopsychiatry 30:153–165

Bangasser DA, Eck SR, Ordones Sanchez E (2019) Sex differences in stress reactivity in arousal and attention systems. Neuropsychopharmacology 44(1):129–139

Barrett SP, Salzman J (2016) Circular RNAs: analysis, expression and potential functions. Development 143(11):1838–1847

Barrot M (2012) Tests and models of nociception and pain in rodents. Neuroscience 211:39–50

Basbaum AI et al (2009) Cellular and molecular mechanisms of pain. Cell 139(2):267–284

Beattie EC et al (2002) Control of synaptic strength by glial TNFalpha. Science 295(5563):2282–2285

Bekhbat M, Neigh GN (2018) Sex differences in the neuro-immune consequences of stress: focus on depression and anxiety. Brain Behav Immun 67:1–12

Bell HC, Pellis SM, Kolb B (2010) Juvenile peer play experience and the development of the orbitofrontal and medial prefrontal cortices. Behav Brain Res 207(1):7–13

Benarroch EE (1993) The central autonomic network: functional organization, dysfunction, and perspective. Mayo Clin Proc 68(10):988–1001

Benarroch EE (2020) Physiology and pathophysiology of the autonomic nervous system. Continuum (Minneap Minn) 26(1):12–24

Bestry M et al (2022) Association of prenatal alcohol exposure with offspring DNA methylation in mammals: a systematic review of the evidence. Clin Epigenetics 14(1):12

Biltz RG et al (2022) The neuroimmunology of social-stress-induced sensitization. Nat Immunol 23(11): 1527–1535

Boahen A et al (2023) Bidirectional crosstalk between the peripheral nervous system and lymphoid tissues/ organs. Front Immunol 14:1254054

Bodnar TS, Hill LA, Weinberg J (2016) Evidence for an immune signature of prenatal alcohol exposure in female rats. Brain Behav Immun 58:130

Bodnar TS et al (2018) Altered maternal immune networks are associated with adverse child neurodevelopment: impact of alcohol consumption during pregnancy. Brain Behav Immun 73:205–215

Bodnar TS et al (2020) Immune network dysregulation associated with child neurodevelopmental delay: modulatory role of prenatal alcohol exposure. J Neuroinflammation 17(1):39

Boschen KE, Ruggiero MJ, Klintsova AY (2016) Neonatal binge alcohol exposure increases microglial activation in the developing rat hippocampus. Neuroscience 324:355–366

Bota M, Sporns O, Swanson LW (2012) Neuroinformatics analysis of molecular expression patterns and neuron populations in gray matter regions: the rat BST as a rich exemplar. Brain Res 1450:174–193

Brady ML, Allan AM, Caldwell KK (2012) A limited access mouse model of prenatal alcohol exposure that produces long-lasting deficits in hippocampal-dependent learning and memory. Alcohol Clin Exp Res 36 (3):457–466

Brandao ML, Lovick TA (2019) Role of the dorsal periaqueductal gray in posttraumatic stress disorder: mediation by dopamine and neurokinin. Transl Psychiatry 9(1):232

Braun-Lewensohn O et al (2022) Salutogenesis and the sense of coherence during the adolescent years. In: Mittelmark MB et al (eds) The handbook of salutogenesis. Springer, Cham, pp 139–150

Breton JM et al (2021) Juvenile exposure to acute traumatic stress leads to long-lasting alterations in grey matter myelination in adult female but not male rats. Neurobiol Stress 14:100319

Breton-Provencher V, Drummond GT, Sur M (2021) Locus coeruleus norepinephrine in learned behavior: anatomical modularity and spatiotemporal integration in targets. Front Neural Circuits 15:638007

Breuer L, Greenmyer JR, Wilson T (2024) Clinical diagnosis and management of fetal alcohol spectrum disorder and sensory processing disorder in children. Children (Basel) 11(1):108

Britton KT et al (1992) Dissociation between in vivo hippocampal norepinephrine response and behavioral/ neuroendocrine responses to noise stress in rats. Brain Res 574(1–2):125–130

Burke AR et al (2017) Impact of adolescent social experiences on behavior and neural circuits implicated in mental illnesses. Neurosci Biobehav Rev 76 (Pt B):280–300

Calvo M, Bennett DL (2012) The mechanisms of microgliosis and pain following peripheral nerve injury. Exp Neurol 234(2):271–282

Cardinal RN et al (2002) Emotion and motivation: the role of the amygdala, ventral striatum, and prefrontal cortex. Neurosci Biobehav Rev 26(3):321–352

Carloni E, Ramos A, Hayes LN (2021) Developmental stressors induce innate immune memory in microglia and contribute to disease risk. Int J Mol Sci 22(23): 13035

Castle M, Comoli E, Loewy AD (2005) Autonomic brainstem nuclei are linked to the hippocampus. Neuroscience 134(2):657–669

Cerqueira JJ et al (2007a) The prefrontal cortex as a key target of the maladaptive response to stress. J Neurosci 27(11):2781–2787

Cerqueira JJ et al (2007b) Specific configuration of dendritic degeneration in pyramidal neurons of the medial prefrontal cortex induced by differing corticosteroid regimens. Cereb Cortex 17(9):1998–2006

Chang GQ, Karatayev O, Leibowitz SF (2015) Prenatal exposure to ethanol stimulates hypothalamic CCR2 chemokine receptor system: possible relation to increased density of orexigenic peptide neurons and ethanol drinking in adolescent offspring. Neuroscience 310:163–175

Chang GQ et al (2018) Hypothalamic CCL2/CCR2 chemokine system: role in sexually dimorphic effects of maternal ethanol exposure on melanin-concentrating hormone and behavior in adolescent offspring. J Neurosci 38(42):9072–9090

Chen H, Jiang Z (2013) The essential adaptors of innate immune signaling. Protein Cell 4(1):27–39

Chen G et al (2017) Sex-dependent glial signaling in pathological pain: distinct roles of spinal microglia and astrocytes. Neurosci Bull

Choi DC et al (2008a) The anteroventral bed nucleus of the stria terminalis differentially regulates hypothalamic-pituitary-adrenocortical axis responses to acute and chronic stress. Endocrinology 149(2):818–826

Choi IY, Lee S, Rivier C (2008b) Novel role of adrenergic neurons in the brain stem in mediating the hypothalamic-pituitary axis hyperactivity caused by prenatal alcohol exposure. Neuroscience 155(3): 888–901

Chowdhury GM, Fujioka T, Nakamura S (2000) Induction and adaptation of Fos expression in the rat brain by two types of acute restraint stress. Brain Res Bull 52(3): 171–182

Chulani VL, Gordon LP (2014) Adolescent growth and development. Prim Care 41(3):465–487

Cippitelli A et al (2017) Protection against alcohol-induced neuronal and cognitive damage by the PPARgamma receptor agonist pioglitazone. Brain Behav Immun 64:320–329

Clark CA et al (2024) Prevalence of co-occurring diagnoses in people exposed to alcohol prenatally: findings from a meta-analysis. J Affect Disord 358: 163–174

Cohen SP, Vase L, Hooten WM (2021) Chronic pain: an update on burden, best practices, and new advances. Lancet 397(10289):2082–2097

Coles CD et al (2010) Verbal and nonverbal memory in adults prenatally exposed to alcohol. Alcohol Clin Exp Res 34(5):897–906

Coles CD et al (2022) Prenatal alcohol exposure and mental health at midlife: a preliminary report on two longitudinal cohorts. Alcohol Clin Exp Res 46(2): 232–242

Colleselli K, Stierschneider A, Wiesner C (2023) An update on toll-like receptor 2, its function and dimerization in pro- and anti-inflammatory processes. Int J Mol Sci 24(15):12464

Cook JL et al (2016) Fetal alcohol spectrum disorder: a guideline for diagnosis across the lifespan. CMAJ 188(3):191–197

Copeland WE et al (2014) Longitudinal patterns of anxiety from childhood to adulthood: the Great Smoky Mountains Study. J Am Acad Child Adolesc Psychiatry 53(1):21–33

Costigan M, Scholz J, Woolf CJ (2009) Neuropathic pain: a maladaptive response of the nervous system to damage. Annu Rev Neurosci 32:1–32

Curry-Hyde A et al (2020) Cell type-specific circular RNA expression in human glial cells. Genomics 112(6): 5265–5274

Dandekar MP et al (2008) Importance of cocaine- and amphetamine-regulated transcript peptide in the central nucleus of amygdala in anxiogenic responses induced by ethanol withdrawal. Neuropsychopharmacology 33(5):1127–1136

Dandekar MP et al (2019) Maternal ethanol exposure reshapes CART system in the rat brain: correlation with development of anxiety, depression and memory deficits. Neuroscience 406:126–139

Davis M et al (2010) Phasic vs sustained fear in rats and humans: role of the extended amygdala in fear vs anxiety. Neuropsychopharmacology 35(1):105–135

De Ridder D, Adhia D, Vanneste S (2021) The anatomy of pain and suffering in the brain and its clinical implications. Neurosci Biobehav Rev 130:125–146

Deak T et al (2022) Prenatal and adolescent alcohol exposure programs immunity across the lifespan: CNS-mediated regulation. Pharmacol Biochem Behav 216:173390

Dennis EL et al (2013) Development of brain structural connectivity between ages 12 and 30: a 4-Tesla diffusion imaging study in 439 adolescents and adults. NeuroImage 64:671–684

Disease GBD, Injury I, Prevalence C (2017) Global, regional, and national incidence, prevalence, and years lived with disability for 328 diseases and injuries for 195 countries, 1990–2016: a systematic analysis for the Global Burden of Disease Study 2016. Lancet 390(10100):1211–1259

Doremus-Fitzwater TL et al (2020) Lingering effects of prenatal alcohol exposure on basal and ethanol-evoked expression of inflammatory-related genes in the CNS of adolescent and adult rats. Front Behav Neurosci 14: 82

Douglas LA, Varlinskaya EI, Spear LP (2004) Rewarding properties of social interactions in adolescent and adult male and female rats: impact of social versus isolate housing of subjects and partners. Dev Psychobiol 45(3):153–162

Drew PD, Kane CJ (2014) Fetal alcohol spectrum disorders and neuroimmune changes. Int Rev Neurobiol 118:41–80

Drew PD et al (2015) Pioglitazone blocks ethanol induction of microglial activation and immune responses in the hippocampus, cerebellum, and cerebral cortex in a mouse model of fetal alcohol spectrum disorders. Alcohol Clin Exp Res 39(3):445–454

Dubovy P et al (2007) Increased invasion of ED-1 positive macrophages in both ipsi- and contralateral dorsal root ganglia following unilateral nerve injuries. Neurosci Lett 427(2):88–93

Eiland L, Romeo RD (2013) Stress and the developing adolescent brain. Neuroscience 249:162–171

Evans R et al (2009) Integrins in immunity. J Cell Sci 122 (Pt 2):215–225

Fitzcharles MA et al (2021) Nociplastic pain: towards an understanding of prevalent pain conditions. Lancet 397(10289):2098–2110

Flannigan K et al (2023) Sex-related differences among individuals assessed for fetal alcohol spectrum disorder in Canada. Alcohol Clin Exp Res 47:613

Fleshner M (2013) Stress-evoked sterile inflammation, danger associated molecular patterns (DAMPs), microbial associated molecular patterns (MAMPs) and the inflammasome. Brain Behav Immun 27(1):1–7

Fleshner M, Frank M, Maier SF (2017) Danger signals and inflammasomes: stress-evoked sterile inflammation in mood disorders. Neuropsychopharmacology 42(1): 36–45

Franklin L et al (2008) Children with fetal alcohol spectrum disorders: problem behaviors and sensory processing. Am J Occup Ther 62(3):265–273
Furuyashiki T, Kitaoka S (2019) Neural mechanisms underlying adaptive and maladaptive consequences of stress: roles of dopaminergic and inflammatory responses. Psychiatry Clin Neurosci 73(11):669–675
Gao Y et al (2025) The locus coeruleus-periaqueductal gray GABAergic projection regulates comorbid pain and depression. Adv Sci (Weinh) 12:e2503739
Garakani A et al (2020) Pharmacotherapy of anxiety disorders: current and emerging treatment options. Front Psych 11:595584
Garrison L et al (2019) Forty years of assessing neurodevelopmental and behavioral effects of prenatal alcohol exposure in infants: what have we learned? Alcohol Clin Exp Res 43(8):1632–1642
Gee DG (2016) Sensitive periods of emotion regulation: influences of parental care on frontoamygdala circuitry and plasticity. New Dir Child Adolesc Dev 2016(153): 87–110
Ghilardi JR et al (2012) Neuroplasticity of sensory and sympathetic nerve fibers in a mouse model of a painful arthritic joint. Arthritis Rheum 64(7):2223–2232
Giedd JN, Rapoport JL (2010) Structural MRI of pediatric brain development: what have we learned and where are we going? Neuron 67(5):728–734
Grace PM et al (2014) Pathological pain and the neuroimmune interface. Nat Rev Immunol 14(4): 217–231
Grace PM et al (2021) The Neuroimmunology of chronic pain: from rodents to humans. J Neurosci 41(5):855–865
Hagan JF et al (2016) Neurobehavioral disorder associated with prenatal alcohol exposure. Pediatrics 138(4): e20151553
Ham JR et al (2024) Quality not quantity: deficient juvenile play experiences lead to altered medial prefrontal cortex neurons and sociocognitive skill deficits. Dev Psychobiol 66(2):e22456
Hammack SE, Braas KM, May V (2021) Chemoarchitecture of the bed nucleus of the stria terminalis: neurophenotypic diversity and function. Handb Clin Neurol 179:385–402
Hansen TB et al (2013) Natural RNA circles function as efficient microRNA sponges. Nature 495(7441): 384–388
He J, Crews FT (2008) Increased MCP-1 and microglia in various regions of the human alcoholic brain. Exp Neurol 210(2):349–358
Hellemans KG et al (2008) Prenatal alcohol exposure increases vulnerability to stress and anxiety-like disorders in adulthood. Ann N Y Acad Sci 1144:154–175
Hellemans KGC et al (2010) Prenatal alcohol exposure: fetal programming and later life vulnerability to stress, depression and anxiety disorders. Neurosci Biobehav Rev 34(6):791–807
Henderson LA et al (2002) Brain responses associated with the Valsalva maneuver revealed by functional magnetic resonance imaging. J Neurophysiol 88(6): 3477–3486
Herman JP, Cullinan WE (1997) Neurocircuitry of stress: central control of the hypothalamo-pituitary-adrenocortical axis. Trends Neurosci 20(2):78–84
Hermes G et al (2011) Post-weaning chronic social isolation produces profound behavioral dysregulation with decreases in prefrontal cortex synaptic-associated protein expression in female rats. Physiol Behav 104(2): 354–359
Hill MN et al (2011) Recruitment of prefrontal cortical endocannabinoid signaling by glucocorticoids contributes to termination of the stress response. J Neurosci 31(29):10506–10515
Himmelrich M, Lutke CJ, Hargrove ET (2020) The lay of the land: fetal alcohol spectrum disorder (FASD) as a whole body diagnosis. In: Begun AL, Murray MM (eds) The Routledge handbook of social work and addictive behaviors. Routledge, London
Hirschberg S et al (2017) Functional dichotomy in spinal- vs prefrontal-projecting locus coeruleus modules splits descending noradrenergic analgesia from ascending aversion and anxiety in rats. elife 6:e29808
Hodges TE, McCormick CM (2015) Adolescent and adult male rats habituate to repeated isolation, but only adolescents sensitize to partner unfamiliarity. Horm Behav 69:16–30
Holder MK, Blaustein JD (2014) Puberty and adolescence as a time of vulnerability to stressors that alter neurobehavioral processes. Front Neuroendocrinol 35(1):89–110
Holt MK (2022) The ins and outs of the caudal nucleus of the solitary tract: an overview of cellular populations and anatomical connections. J Neuroendocrinol 34(6): e13132
Hu P, McLachlan EM (2002) Macrophage and lymphocyte invasion of dorsal root ganglia after peripheral nerve lesions in the rat. Neuroscience 112(1):23–38
Hu P et al (2007) Immune cell involvement in dorsal root ganglia and spinal cord after chronic constriction or transection of the rat sciatic nerve. Brain Behav Immun 21(5):599–616
Hudson SP, Jacobson-Pick S, Anisman H (2014) Sex differences in behavior and pro-inflammatory cytokine mRNA expression following stressor exposure and re-exposure. Neuroscience 277:239–249
Hwang HM, Hashimoto-Torii K (2022) Activation of the anterior cingulate cortex ameliorates anxiety in a preclinical model of fetal alcohol spectrum disorders. Transl Psychiatry 12(1):24
Iremonger KJ, Power EM (2025) The paraventricular nucleus of the hypothalamus: a key node in the control of behavioural states. J Physiol 603(8):2231–2243
Ishikawa Y, Furuyashiki T (2022) The impact of stress on immune systems and its relevance to mental illness. Neurosci Res 175:16–24

Iwata M, Ota KT, Duman RS (2013) The inflammasome: pathways linking psychological stress, depression, and systemic illnesses. Brain Behav Immun 31:105–114

Jasnow AM et al (2013) Thy1-expressing neurons in the basolateral amygdala may mediate fear inhibition. J Neurosci 33(25):10396–10404

Johnstone T et al (2012) Turning on the alarm: the neural mechanisms of the transition from innocuous to painful sensation. NeuroImage 59(2):1594–1601

Kane CJ et al (2011) Protection of neurons and microglia against ethanol in a mouse model of fetal alcohol spectrum disorders by peroxisome proliferator-activated receptor-gamma agonists. Brain Behav Immun 25(Suppl 1):S137–S145

Kaplan CM et al (2024) Deciphering nociplastic pain: clinical features, risk factors and potential mechanisms. Nat Rev Neurol 20(6):347–363

Kawanabe-Kobayashi R et al (2024) Descending locus coeruleus noradrenergic signaling to spinal astrocyte subset is required for stress-induced pain facilitation. bioRxiv. https://doi.org/10.1101/2024.11.14.623627

Kessler RC et al (2005) Prevalence, severity, and comorbidity of 12-month DSM-IV disorders in the National Comorbidity Survey Replication. Arch Gen Psychiatry 62(6):617–627

Khoury JE, Jamieson B, Milligan K (2018) Risk for childhood internalizing and externalizing behavior problems in the context of prenatal alcohol exposure: a meta-analysis and comprehensive examination of moderators. Alcohol Clin Exp Res 42:1358

Kim CF, Moalem-Taylor G (2011) Detailed characterization of neuro-immune responses following neuropathic injury in mice. Brain Res 1405:95–108

Kim CK et al (1999) Effects of prenatal exposure to alcohol on the release of adenocorticotropic hormone, corticosterone, and proinflammatory cytokines. Alcohol Clin Exp Res 23(1):52–59

Kleinschnitz C et al (2006) T cell infiltration after chronic constriction injury of mouse sciatic nerve is associated with interleukin-17 expression. Exp Neurol 200(2): 480–485

Koob GF (1999) Corticotropin-releasing factor, norepinephrine, and stress. Biol Psychiatry 46(9):1167–1180

Kosek E et al (2016) Do we need a third mechanistic descriptor for chronic pain states? Pain 157(7): 1382–1386

Koylu EO et al (1998) Cocaine- and amphetamine-regulated transcript peptide immunohistochemical localization in the rat brain. J Comp Neurol 391(1): 115–132

Koylu EO et al (2006) Cocaine and amphetamine regulated transcript (CART) and the stress response. Peptides 27(8):1956–1969

Lam VYY et al (2018) Interactive effects of prenatal alcohol exposure and chronic stress in adulthood on anxiety-like behavior and central stress-related receptor mRNA expression: sex- and time-dependent effects. Psychoneuroendocrinology 97:8–19

Lam VYY et al (2019) Role of corticosterone in anxiety- and depressive-like behavior and HPA regulation following prenatal alcohol exposure. Prog Neuro-Psychopharmacol Biol Psychiatry 90:1–15

Lamotte G, Shouman K, Benarroch EE (2021) Stress and central autonomic network. Auton Neurosci 235: 102870

Lan N et al (2015) Exposure to chronic mild stress differentially alters Corticotropin-releasing hormone and arginine vasopressin mRNA expression in the stress-responsive Neurocircuitry of male and female rats prenatally exposed to alcohol. Alcohol Clin Exp Res 39(12):2414–2421

Lan N et al (2017) Prenatal alcohol exposure and prenatal stress differentially alter glucocorticoid signaling in the placenta and fetal brain. Neuroscience 342:167–179

Lebel CA et al (2021) Prenatal exposure and child brain and mental health (PEACH) study: protocol for a cohort study of children and youth with prenatal alcohol exposure. BMJ Open 11(5):e051660

Lebow MA, Chen A (2016) Overshadowed by the amygdala: the bed nucleus of the stria terminalis emerges as key to psychiatric disorders. Mol Psychiatry 21(4): 450–463

Lee Y, Davis M (1997) Role of the hippocampus, the bed nucleus of the stria terminalis, and the amygdala in the excitatory effect of corticotropin-releasing hormone on the acoustic startle reflex. J Neurosci 17(16): 6434–6446

Leussis MP, Andersen SL (2008) Is adolescence a sensitive period for depression? Behavioral and neuroanatomical findings from a social stress model. Synapse 62(1):22–30

Lewitus GM et al (2014) An adaptive role of TNFalpha in the regulation of striatal synapses. J Neurosci 34(18): 6146–6155

Lewitus GM et al (2016) Microglial TNF-alpha suppresses cocaine-induced plasticity and behavioral sensitization. Neuron 90(3):483–491

Li J et al (2022) Activation of locus coeruleus-spinal cord noradrenergic neurons alleviates neuropathic pain in mice via reducing neuroinflammation from astrocytes and microglia in spinal dorsal horn. J Neuroinflammation 19(1):123

Lima TS (2023) Beyond an inflammatory mediator: interleukin-1 in neurophysiology. Exp Physiol 108(7):917–924

Linnman C et al (2012) Neuroimaging of the periaqueductal gray: state of the field. NeuroImage 60(1):505–522

Liston C, McEwen BS, Casey BJ (2009) Psychosocial stress reversibly disrupts prefrontal processing and attentional control. Proc Natl Acad Sci USA 106(3): 912–917

Lovelock DF, Deak T (2019) Acute stress imposed during adolescence yields heightened anxiety in Sprague Dawley rats that persists into adulthood: sex differences and potential involvement of the medial amygdala. Brain Res 1723:146392

Lovelock DF, Deak T (2020) Acute stress imposed during adolescence has minimal effects on hypothalamic-pituitary-adrenal (HPA) axis sensitivity in adulthood in female Sprague Dawley rats. Physiol Behav 213: 112707

Lu X, Richardson PM (1993) Responses of macrophages in rat dorsal root ganglia following peripheral nerve injury. J Neurocytol 22(5):334–341

Lynch ME, Kable JA, Coles CD (2017) Effects of prenatal alcohol exposure in a prospective sample of young adults: mental health, substance use, and difficulties with the legal system. Neurotoxicol Teratol 64:50–62

Madison AA et al (2023) Conflicts hurt: social stress predicts elevated pain and sadness after mild inflammatory increases. Pain 164(9):1985–1994

Maier SE, West JR (2003) Alcohol and nutritional control treatments during neurogenesis in rat brain reduce total neuron number in locus coeruleus, but not in cerebellum or inferior olive. Alcohol 30(1):67–74

Mantyh PW (1982) Forebrain projections to the periaqueductal gray in the monkey, with observations in the cat and rat. J Comp Neurol 206(2):146–158

Mantyh PW (1983) Connections of midbrain periaqueductal gray in the monkey. I Ascending efferent projections. J Neurophysiol 49(3):567–581

Marek R et al (2013) The amygdala and medial prefrontal cortex: partners in the fear circuit. J Physiol 591(10): 2381–2391

Marin I, Kipnis J (2013) Learning and memory ... and the immune system. Learn Mem 20(10):601–606

May PA et al (2018) Prevalence of fetal alcohol Spectrum disorders in 4 US communities. JAMA 319(5): 474–482

McCall JG et al (2015) CRH engagement of the locus coeruleus noradrenergic system mediates stress-induced anxiety. Neuron 87(3):605–620

McCall JG et al (2017) Locus coeruleus to basolateral amygdala noradrenergic projections promote anxiety-like behavior. elife 6:e18247

McKim DB et al (2018) Microglial recruitment of IL-1beta-producing monocytes to brain endothelium causes stress-induced anxiety. Mol Psychiatry 23(6): 1421–1431

Memczak S et al (2013) Circular RNAs are a large class of animal RNAs with regulatory potency. Nature 495(7441):333–338

Meng J et al (2024) Functional and structural abnormalities in the pain network of generalized anxiety disorder patients with pain symptoms. Neuroscience 543:28–36

Millan MJ (2002) Descending control of pain. Prog Neurobiol 66(6):355–474

Miller LJ et al (2009) Perspectives on sensory processing disorder: a call for translational research. Front Integr Neurosci 3:22

Milligan ED, Watkins LR (2009) Pathological and protective roles of glia in chronic pain. Nat Rev Neurosci 10(1):23–36

Mondelli V et al (2017) Brain microglia in psychiatric disorders. Lancet Psychiatry 4(7):563–572

Montgomery SL, Bowers WJ (2012) Tumor necrosis factor-alpha and the roles it plays in homeostatic and degenerative processes within the central nervous system. J Neuroimmune Pharmacol 7(1):42–59

Morgane PJ, Mokler DJ (2006) The limbic brain: continuing resolution. Neurosci Biobehav Rev 30(2): 119–125

Morin N et al (2007) Neutrophils invade lumbar dorsal root ganglia after chronic constriction injury of the sciatic nerve. J Neuroimmunol 184(1–2):164–171

Mueller B, Figueroa A, Robinson-Papp J (2022) Structural and functional connections between the autonomic nervous system, hypothalamic-pituitary-adrenal axis, and the immune system: a context and time dependent stress response network. Neurol Sci 43(2):951–960

Murphy-Royal C, Gordon GR, Bains JS (2019) Stress-induced structural and functional modifications of astrocytes-further implicating glia in the central response to stress. Glia 67(10):1806–1820

Myrick A et al (2024) Maternal alcohol drinking patterns predict offspring neurobehavioral outcomes. Neuropharmacology 257:110044

Neugebauer V et al (2023) Pain-related cortico-limbic plasticity and opioid signaling. Neuropharmacology 231:109510

Nogales F et al (2025) Rat models of fetal alcohol spectrum disorders for studying the critical role of cerebellar damage: A scoping review. Alcohol Clin Exp Res (Hoboken) 49(9):1855–1876

Noor S, Milligan ED (2018) Lifelong impacts of moderate prenatal alcohol exposure on neuroimmune function. Front Immunol 9:1107

Noor S et al (2017) Prenatal alcohol exposure potentiates chronic neuropathic pain, spinal glial and immune cell activation and alters sciatic nerve and DRG cytokine levels. Brain Behav Immun 61:80–95

Noor S, Sanchez JJ, Pervin Z, Sanchez JE, Sun MS, Epler L, Davies S, Savage DD, Mellios N, Jantzie LL, Milligan ED (2018) Neuropathic pain susceptibility in prenatal alcohol exposed (PAE) females is mediated by the proinflammatory actions of lymphocyte function-associated antigen (LFA)-1 on immune and glial cells neuroscience meeting planner. Society for Neuroscience, San Diego. Peripheral mechanisms of neuropathic pain (Poster #: 666.18/EE2 Topic: D.03. Somatosensation: Pain)

Noor S et al (2019) LFA-1 antagonist (BIRT377) similarly reverses peripheral neuropathic pain in male and female mice with underlying sex divergent peripheral immune proinflammatory phenotypes. Neuroimmunol Neuroinflamm 6(10):1–32

Noor S et al (2020) The LFA-1 antagonist BIRT377 reverses neuropathic pain in prenatal alcohol-exposed female rats via actions on peripheral and central neuroimmune function in discrete pain-relevant tissue regions. Brain Behav Immun 87:339–358

Noor S et al (2023a) Prenatal alcohol exposure promotes NLRP3 inflammasome-dependent immune actions following morphine treatment and paradoxically prolongs nerve injury-induced pathological pain in female mice. Alcohol Clin Exp Res 47(12):2262–2277

Noor S et al (2023b) Prenatal alcohol exposure dysregulates spinal and circulating immune cell circular RNA expression in adult female rats with chronic sciatic neuropathy. Front Neurosci 17:1180308

Ormel J et al (2015) Mental health in Dutch adolescents: a TRAILS report on prevalence, severity, age of onset, continuity and co-morbidity of DSM disorders. Psychol Med 45(2):345–360

Osborn JA et al (1996) Fetal ethanol exposure alters pituitary-adrenal sensitivity to dexamethasone suppression. Psychoneuroendocrinology 21(2):127–143

Ossipov MH, Dussor GO, Porreca F (2010) Central modulation of pain. J Clin Invest 120(11):3779–3787

Pan W et al (1997) Tumor necrosis factor-alpha: a neuromodulator in the CNS. Neurosci Biobehav Rev 21(5):603–613

Pellis SM, Pasztor TJ (1999) The developmental onset of a rudimentary form of play fighting in C57 mice. Dev Psychobiol 34(3):175–182

Pellis SM et al (2023) Play fighting and the development of the social brain: the rat's tale. Neurosci Biobehav Rev 145:105037

Penninx BW et al (2021) Anxiety disorders. Lancet 397(10277):914–927

Perez-Rando M et al (2022) Impact of stress on inhibitory neuronal circuits, our tribute to Bruce McEwen. Neurobiol Stress 19:100460

Pasmay AA et al (2025) Prenatal alcohol exposure promotes nerve injury-induced pathological pain following morphine treatment via NLRP3-mediated peripheral and central proinflammatory immune actions. bioRxiv

Peterson RA (2000) Handbook of stress, medicine and health. J Health Psychol 5(2):255–256

Poe GR et al (2020) Locus coeruleus: a new look at the blue spot. Nat Rev Neurosci 21(11):644–659

Popoli M et al (2011) The stressed synapse: the impact of stress and glucocorticoids on glutamate transmission. Nat Rev Neurosci 13(1):22–37

Popova S et al (2023) Fetal alcohol spectrum disorders. Nat Rev Dis Primers 9(1):11

Pritha AN, Pasmay AA, Noor S (2025) Recent advances in the role of non-coding RNAs in fetal alcohol spectrum disorders. In: Valenzuela CF, Linsenbardt DN, Weiner JL (eds) Effects of alcohol on the brain across the lifespan. Springer, Cham

Radley JJ, Sawchenko PE (2011) A common substrate for prefrontal and hippocampal inhibition of the neuroendocrine stress response. J Neurosci 31(26):9683–9695

Raineki C et al (2016) Short- and long-term effects of stress during adolescence on emotionality and HPA function of animals exposed to alcohol prenatally. Psychoneuroendocrinology 74:13–23

Raineki C et al (2017) Effects of early-life adversity on immune function are mediated by prenatal environment: role of prenatal alcohol exposure. Brain Behav Immun 66:210–220

Raineki C, Ellis L, Weinberg J (2018) Impact of adolescent stress on the expression of stress-related receptors in the hippocampus of animals exposed to alcohol prenatally. Hippocampus 28(3):201–216

Raineki C et al (2019) Glucocorticoid receptor expression in the stress-limbic circuitry is differentially affected by prenatal alcohol exposure and adolescent stress. Brain Res 1718:242–251

Rajmohan V, Mohandas E (2007) The limbic system. Indian J Psychiatry 49(2):132–139

Reid N et al (2015) Systematic review of fetal alcohol spectrum disorder interventions across the life span. Alcohol Clin Exp Res 39(12):2283–2295

Reis F et al (2023) Orchestration of innate and conditioned defensive actions by the periaqueductal gray. Neuropharmacology 228:109458

Reus GZ et al (2015) The role of inflammation and microglial activation in the pathophysiology of psychiatric disorders. Neuroscience 300:141–154

Rizvi TA et al (1991) Connections between the central nucleus of the amygdala and the midbrain periaqueductal gray: topography and reciprocity. J Comp Neurol 303(1):121–131

Robertson SD et al (2013) Developmental origins of central norepinephrine neuron diversity. Nat Neurosci 16(8):1016–1023

Rodriguez-Palma EJ et al (2023) Spinal alarmin HMGB1 and the activation of TLR4 lead to chronic stress-induced nociceptive hypersensitivity in rodents. Eur J Pharmacol 952:175804

Romera I et al (2010) Generalized anxiety disorder, with or without co-morbid major depressive disorder, in primary care: prevalence of painful somatic symptoms, functioning and health status. J Affect Disord 127(1–3):160–168

Ruffaner-Hanson C et al (2022) The maternal-placental-fetal interface: adaptations of the HPA axis and immune mediators following maternal stress and prenatal alcohol exposure. Exp Neurol 355:114121

Ruyak SL et al (2022) Effects of prenatal opioid and alcohol exposures on immune and serotonin factors in human placenta. Exp Neurol 353:114057

Sanchez JJ et al (2017) Prenatal alcohol exposure is a risk factor for adult neuropathic pain via aberrant neuroimmune function. J Neuroinflammation 14(1): 254

Sanchez JJ et al (2019) Targeting the beta2-integrin LFA-1, reduces adverse neuroimmune actions in neuropathic susceptibility caused by prenatal alcohol exposure. Acta Neuropathol Commun 7(1):54

Sanchez JE et al (2023) The FDA-approved compound, pramipexole and the clinical-stage investigational drug, dexpramipexole, reverse chronic allodynia from sciatic nerve damage in mice, and alter IL-1beta and IL-10 expression from immune cell culture. Neurosci Lett 814:137419

Sandkuhler J (2009) Models and mechanisms of hyperalgesia and allodynia. Physiol Rev 89(2): 707–758

Sawicki CM et al (2018) Ropivacaine and bupivacaine prevent increased pain sensitivity without altering neuroimmune activation following repeated social defeat stress. Brain Behav Immun 69:113–123

Sawicki CM, Humeidan ML, Sheridan JF (2021) Neuroimmune interactions in pain and stress: an interdisciplinary approach. Neuroscientist 27(2):113–128

Schneider ML et al (2007) Sensory processing disorders in a nonhuman primate model: evidence for occupational therapy practice. Am J Occup Ther 61(2):247–253

Schneider ML et al (2008) Sensory processing disorder in a primate model: evidence from a longitudinal study of prenatal alcohol and prenatal stress effects. Child Dev 79(1):100–113

Schneiderman N, Ironson G, Siegel SD (2005) Stress and health: psychological, behavioral, and biological determinants. Annu Rev Clin Psychol 1:607–628

Seibt F, Schlichter R (2015) Noradrenaline-mediated facilitation of inhibitory synaptic transmission in the dorsal horn of the rat spinal cord involves interlaminar communications. Eur J Neurosci 42(9):2654–2665

Seminowicz DA, Moayedi M (2017) The dorsolateral prefrontal cortex in acute and chronic pain. J Pain 18(9):1027–1035

Seress L et al (2004) Cocaine- and amphetamine-regulated transcript peptide (CART) is a selective marker of rat granule cells and of human mossy cells in the hippocampal dentate gyrus. Neuroscience 125(1):13–24

Serrats J et al (2017) Pro-inflammatory immune-to-brain signaling is involved in neuroendocrine responses to acute emotional stress. Brain Behav Immun 62:53–63

Shamakina IY et al (2024) Neuroimmune characteristics of animals with prenatal alcohol intoxication. Biochem (Mosc) 89(11):1922–1929

Shaw P et al (2006) Intellectual ability and cortical development in children and adolescents. Nature 440(7084): 676–679

Shaw SK et al (2008) Activated polymorphonuclear cells promote injury and excitability of dorsal root ganglia neurons. Exp Neurol 210(2):286–294

Shin LM, Liberzon I (2010) The neurocircuitry of fear, stress, and anxiety disorders. Neuropsychopharmacology 35(1):169–191

Shintani F et al (1995) Involvement of interleukin-1 in immobilization stress-induced increase in plasma adrenocorticotropic hormone and in release of hypothalamic monoamines in the rat. J Neurosci 15(3 Pt 1): 1961–1970

Smith MA et al (1991) Effects of stress and adrenalectomy on tyrosine hydroxylase mRNA levels in the locus ceruleus by in situ hybridization. Brain Res 544(1): 26–32

Sorge RE et al (2015) Different immune cells mediate mechanical pain hypersensitivity in male and female mice. Nat Neurosci 18(8):1081–1083

Sousa N, Almeida OF (2012) Disconnection and reconnection: the morphological basis of (mal)adaptation to stress. Trends Neurosci 35(12):742–751

Sousa N et al (2000) Reorganization of the morphology of hippocampal neurites and synapses after stress-induced damage correlates with behavioral improvement. Neuroscience 97(2):253–266

Spear LP (2000) The adolescent brain and age-related behavioral manifestations. Neurosci Biobehav Rev 24(4):417–463

Stark RA et al (2023) Atypical play experiences in the juvenile period has an impact on the development of the medial prefrontal cortex in both male and female rats. Behav Brain Res 439:114222

Steinberg L (2005) Cognitive and affective development in adolescence. Trends Cogn Sci 9(2):69–74

Stellwagen D, Malenka RC (2006) Synaptic scaling mediated by glial TNF-alpha. Nature 440:1054–1059

Stellwagen D et al (2005) Differential regulation of AMPA receptor and GABA receptor trafficking by tumor necrosis factor-alpha. J Neurosci 25(12):3219–3228

Stoll G et al (1993) Tumor necrosis factor-alpha in immune-mediated demyelination and Wallerian degeneration of the rat peripheral nervous system. J Neuroimmunol 45(1–2):175–182

Sugama S, Kakinuma Y (2021) Noradrenaline as a key neurotransmitter in modulating microglial activation in stress response. Neurochem Int 143:104943

Suzuki E et al (1997) Immobilization stress increases mRNA levels of interleukin-1 receptor antagonist in various rat brain regions. Cell Mol Neurobiol 17(5): 557–562

Tamnes CK et al (2010) Brain maturation in adolescence and young adulthood: regional age-related changes in cortical thickness and white matter volume and microstructure. Cereb Cortex 20(3):534–548

Terasaki LS, Schwarz JM (2016) Effects of moderate prenatal alcohol exposure during early gestation in rats on inflammation across the maternal-fetal-immune Interface and later-life immune function in the offspring. J Neuroimmune Pharmacol 11:680

Thome J et al (2017) Desynchronization of autonomic response and central autonomic network connectivity in posttraumatic stress disorder. Hum Brain Mapp 38(1):27–40

Tiwari V, Chopra K (2011) Resveratrol prevents alcohol-induced cognitive deficits and brain damage by blocking inflammatory signaling and cell death cascade in neonatal rat brain. J Neurochem 117(4): 678–690

Tottenham N, Galvan A (2016) Stress and the adolescent brain: amygdala-prefrontal cortex circuitry and ventral striatum as developmental targets. Neurosci Biobehav Rev 70:217–227

Turnbull AV, Rivier CL (1999) Regulation of the hypothalamic-pituitary-adrenal axis by cytokines: actions and mechanisms of action. Physiol Rev 79(1): 1–71

Turrigiano GG (2008) The self-tuning neuron: synaptic scaling of excitatory synapses. Cell 135(3):422–435

Uddin LQ et al (2017) Structure and function of the human insula. J Clin Neurophysiol 34(4):300–306

Vachon-Presseau E (2018) Effects of stress on the corticolimbic system: implications for chronic pain. Prog Neuro-Psychopharmacol Biol Psychiatry 87 (Pt B):216–223

Valentino RJ, Van Bockstaele E (2008) Convergent regulation of locus coeruleus activity as an adaptive response to stress. Eur J Pharmacol 583(2–3):194–203

Valenza G et al (2024) Sympathetic and parasympathetic central autonomic networks. Imaging Neurosci 2:1–17

Vanderschuren LJ, Achterberg EJ, Trezza V (2016) The neurobiology of social play and its rewarding value in rats. Neurosci Biobehav Rev 70:86–105

Vandewalle J, Libert C (2020) Glucocorticoids in sepsis: to be or not to be. Front Immunol 11:1318

Vecchiarelli HA et al (2016) Divergent responses of inflammatory mediators within the amygdala and medial prefrontal cortex to acute psychological stress. Brain Behav Immun 51:70–91

Vega-Avelaira D, Geranton SM, Fitzgerald M (2009) Differential regulation of immune responses and macrophage/neuron interactions in the dorsal root ganglion in young and adult rats following nerve injury. Mol Pain 5:70

Vezzani A (2008) Innate immunity and inflammation in temporal lobe epilepsy: new emphasis on the role of complement activation. Epilepsy Curr 8(3):75–77

Vijayakumar N et al (2018) Puberty and the human brain: insights into adolescent development. Neurosci Biobehav Rev 92:417–436

Viviani B, Gardoni F, Marinovich M (2007) Cytokines and neuronal ion channels in health and disease. Int Rev Neurobiol 82:247–263

Walzog B et al (1999) A role for beta(2) integrins (CD11/CD18) in the regulation of cytokine gene expression of polymorphonuclear neutrophils during the inflammatory response. FASEB J 13(13):1855–1865

Weber MD et al (2019) The influence of microglial elimination and repopulation on stress sensitization induced by repeated social defeat. Biol Psychiatry 85(8): 667–678

Wehrwein EA, Orer HS, Barman SM (2016) Overview of the anatomy, physiology, and pharmacology of the autonomic nervous system. Compr Physiol 6(3): 1239–1278

Westerhaus MJ, Loewy AD (2001) Central representation of the sympathetic nervous system in the cerebral cortex. Brain Res 903(1–2):117–127

Wilhelm CJ, Guizzetti M (2015) Fetal alcohol Spectrum disorders: an overview from the glia perspective. Front Integr Neurosci 9:65

Wohleb ES et al (2011) β-Adrenergic receptor antagonism prevents anxiety-like behavior and microglial reactivity induced by repeated social defeat. J Neurosci 31(17):6277–6288

Wolff B et al (2023) Neurocognitive and self-reported psychosocial and behavioral functioning in siblings of individuals with neurodevelopmental conditions: a study using remote self-administered testing. J Clin Exp Neuropsychol 45(5):513–536

Woolf CJ (2011) Central sensitization: implications for the diagnosis and treatment of pain. Pain 152(3 Suppl):S2–S15

Woolf G, Salter MW (2000) Neuronal plasticity: increasing the gain in pain. Science 288:1765–1769

Xiao X, Zhang YQ (2018) A new perspective on the anterior cingulate cortex and affective pain. Neurosci Biobehav Rev 90:200–211

Zerbi V et al (2019) Rapid reconfiguration of the functional connectome after chemogenetic locus coeruleus activation. Neuron 103(4):702–718. e5

Zhang F et al (2016) Adolescent social defeat induced alterations in social behavior and cognitive flexibility in adult mice: effects of developmental stage and social condition. Front Behav Neurosci 10:149

Zhang C et al (2019) Minocycline ameliorates depressive behaviors and neuro-immune dysfunction induced by chronic unpredictable mild stress in the rat. Behav Brain Res 356:348–357

Zhang H et al (2024) The contribution of periaqueductal gray in the regulation of physiological and pathological behaviors. Front Neurosci 18:1380171

Prenatal Alcohol Exposure and Mitochondrial Function in the Brain

8

Rika Morales, Shiwani Thapa, and Anna N. Bukiya

Abstract

Prenatal alcohol exposure (PAE) is recognized as a leading preventable cause of birth defects, giving rise to a continuum of cognitive, behavioral, and physical impairments collectively referred to as Fetal Alcohol Spectrum Disorders (FASD). While PAE affects multiple developing organ systems, the fetal brain is particularly vulnerable, exhibiting enduring structural and functional abnormalities in response to alcohol exposure. Recent research highlights mitochondrial dysfunction as an important mechanism in the pathogenesis of alcohol-related neurodevelopmental deficits. Mitochondria are highly susceptible to alcohol-induced damage, and mounting evidence demonstrates mitochondrial impairments across various organ systems following PAE—focusing growing attention on its specific effects within the developing central nervous system. This chapter explores the essential roles of mitochondria throughout key stages of neurodevelopment and evaluates how PAE disrupts mitochondrial function in different organ systems. Special emphasis is placed on the developing brain, with a focus on its three primary cellular populations: neurons, glial cells, and the cerebral vasculature. Current findings indicate that fetal mitochondria are particularly sensitive to alcohol exposure, resulting in altered mitochondrial morphology, increased production of reactive oxygen species (ROS), elevated oxidative stress, and impaired cellular respiration.

Taken together, these data underscore mitochondria as a critical and vulnerable target of PAE—especially in the developing brain—where mitochondrial dysfunction contributes to the neurodevelopmental deficits' characteristic of FASD. Advancing our understanding of these mechanisms opens the door to mitochondria-targeted interventions, offering promising therapeutic avenues to protect mitochondrial function and mitigate the long-term consequences of prenatal alcohol exposure.

Keywords

Prenatal development · Environmental insult · Oxygen consumption · Cerebrovascular development · Fetal alcohol spectrum disorders

R. Morales · S. Thapa · A. N. Bukiya (✉)
Department of Pharmacology, Addiction Science and Toxicology, College of Medicine, The University of Tennessee Health Science Center, Memphis, TN, USA
e-mail: abukiya@uthsc.edu

A. N. Bukiya, D. W. Ali (eds.), *Molecular Mechanisms and Lifelong Consequences of Prenatal Exposure to Psychoactive Substances*, Advances in Experimental Medicine and Biology 1500,
https://doi.org/10.1007/978-3-032-12741-9_8

Abbreviations

4-HNE	4-Hydroxynonenal
AA	Absolute alcohol
AIF	Apoptosis-inducing factor
ARBD	Alcohol-related birth defect
ARND	Alcohol-related neurodevelopmental disorder
CBF	Cerebral blood flow
EC	Endothelial cell
ETC	Electronic transport chain
FAS	Fetal alcohol syndrome
FASD	Fetal alcohol spectrum disorders
GD	Gestational day
GSH	Glutathione
mPTP	Mitochondrial permeability transition pore
ND-PAE	Neurobehavioral disorder associated with PAE
NOX	NADPH oxidase
PAE	Prenatal alcohol exposure
pFAS	Partial fetal alcohol syndrome
PND	Postnatal day
ROS	Reactive oxygen species
VEGF	Vascular endothelial growth factor

8.1 Introduction

Prenatal alcohol exposure (PAE) remains a prominent and preventable cause of neurodevelopmental impairment globally (May et al. 2009; Olivier et al. 2016; Lange et al. 2017; Popova et al. 2019). Despite ongoing public health initiatives and increased awareness of the risks, alcohol use during pregnancy persists at concerning levels across diverse populations (Popova et al. 2019; Gosdin et al. 2022). As a result, many children are affected by a continuum of lifelong physical, cognitive, and behavioral deficits collectively termed Fetal Alcohol Spectrum Disorders (FASD; Basavarajappa 2015; Gosdin et al. 2022). These disorders exert profound emotional, social, and economic burden on individuals, families, and healthcare systems worldwide (Gosdin et al. 2022).

The developing brain is particularly susceptible to environmental insults, and alcohol exposure during pregnancy exerts teratogenic effects through a wide array of molecular and cellular mechanisms (Archibald et al. 2001; Lewis et al. 2016; Caputo et al. 2016; Gao et al. 2019; Wang et al. 2020; Jacobson et al. 2021). Among the critical but frequently underappreciated targets of alcohol-induced toxicity are mitochondria (Fig. 8.1; Hoek et al. 2002; Jung 2014; Bukiya 2019; Thoudam et al. 2024). As the primary energy-producing organelles, mitochondria play indispensable roles in brain development, cellular homeostasis, and synaptic activity (Cooper 2000; Osellame et al. 2012; Chen et al. 2023). Disruption of mitochondrial integrity during key periods of prenatal brain development can result in persistent alternations to brain structure and function. Such disturbances may significantly contribute to the neuropathological features observed in FASD (Clarren et al. 1978; Khacho et al. 2017; Clemente-Suárez et al. 2023; Klemmensen et al. 2023).

An expanding body of research indicates that PAE disrupts mitochondrial bioenergetics, dynamics, and signaling in a manner that is both cell-type-specific and developmentally regulated (Chen et al. 2003; Bukiya 2019). Given the essential roles of mitochondria in neurodevelopment, elucidating how alcohol impairs mitochondrial function is critical for uncovering mechanisms of neural injury and informing the development of targeted therapeutic strategies.

In this chapter, we will first provide an overview of FASD, emphasizing its global prevalence and significance as a public health concern. We will then examine mitochondrial biology, highlighting key structural and functional distinctions between developing and mature mitochondria, and their roles in maintaining cellular health. Finally, we will investigate how alcohol exposure interferes with mitochondrial development and function within the brain's principal cell types and discuss the downstream effects on neurological development and disease susceptibility.

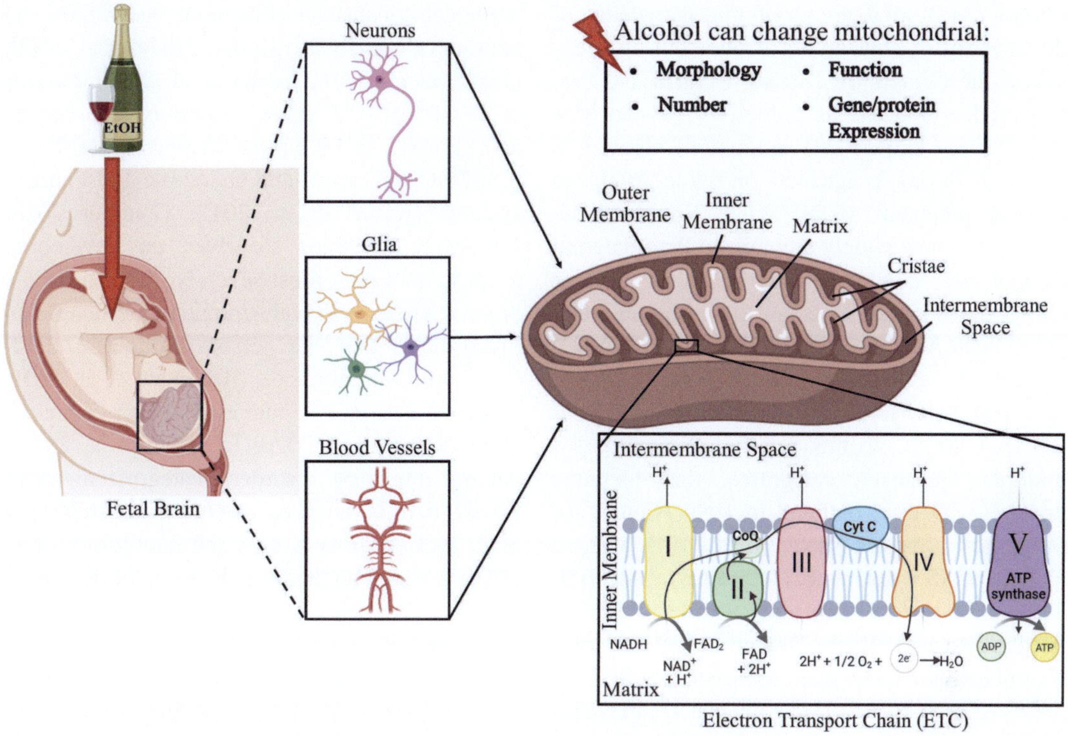

Fig. 8.1 Developing brain mitochondria: a target of prenatal alcohol exposure (PAE). Alcohol consumed during pregnancy crosses the placenta and reaches the fetal brain, where it can impact neurons, glial cells (astrocytes, oligodrocytes, and mircoglai), and cerebral vessels through alcohol-induced mitochondrial dysfunction. As a target of PAE, both mitochondrial formation and function are altered, including specific complexes in the electron transport chain (ETC), which is located within the inner mitochondrial membrane. CoQ, ubiquinone; Cyt C, cytochrome C

8.2 Prenatal Alcohol Exposure

8.2.1 Brief History of Fetal Alcohol Spectrum Disorder

In 1900, Nicloux first discovered that alcohol could cross from the mother to the embryo or fetus through the placenta (Nicloux 1900; Brown et al. 2018). Four years later, in 1904, Ballantyne linked maternal alcohol consumption to an increased risk of adverse birth outcomes, such as structural abnormalities, miscarriage, and premature labor (Ballantyne 1904; Brown et al. 2018). However, it wasn't until the late 1960s that the harmful effects of alcohol as a teratogen and its impact on the cellular development of the embryo and fetus were scientifically established (Lemoine et al. 1968; Brown et al. 2018). Despite these findings, research on the effects of alcohol during pregnancy didn't gain significant attention until 1973, when Jones and Smith documented patterns of malformations in children exposed to maternal alcohol and proposed diagnostic criteria for the condition (Jones and Smith 1973; Brown et al. 2018). They coined the term Fetal Alcohol Syndrome (FAS). Following this, numerous animal and human studies were conducted to validate the existence of FAS. By 1977, the U.S. Food and Drug Administration issued its first public service announcement, warning against alcohol consumption during pregnancy (Brown et al. 2018). Since then, scientific and technological advancements have deepened our understanding of the severe impacts of maternal alcohol use. With a more profound knowledge of the severity of consuming alcohol during pregnancy, the Centers for Disease Control and Prevention has updated its guidelines to state that "there is no known safe amount of alcohol to consume during pregnancy or while trying to become pregnant" (CDC 2024; Brown et al. 2018). It is now widely recognized that maternal alcohol use induces a wide range of adverse effects in offspring. To cover these, the umbrella term "Fetal Alcohol Spectrum Disorder" (FASD) was introduced to encompass the physical, cognitive, and behavioral disorders caused by PAE (NIAAA 2023). As this definition encompasses multiple diagnostic categories, the disorders under FASD were outlined in 1996 (Center for Substance Abuse Prevention 2014). These include FAS, partial FAS (pFAS), Alcohol-Related Neurodevelopmental Disorder (ARND), Alcohol-Related Birth Defects (ARBD), and Neurobehavioral Disorder associated with PAE (ND-PAE; NIAAA 2023). For clarity, the term FASD is explicitly used to refer to the range of diagnoses resulting from PAE (Bertrand et al. 2005).

8.2.2 Developmental Effects of PAE

As previously mentioned, FASD refers to a range of conditions caused by the harmful effects of alcohol consumption during pregnancy (Basavarajappa 2015; Gosdin et al. 2022). In the United States, the rate of alcohol use among pregnant women has increased to 13.5% between 2018 and 2020, which is two percentage points higher than what was reported between 2015 and 2017 (Denny et al. 2019; Gosdin et al. 2022). Globally, FASD occurs in 7.7 cases per 1000 live births, while in specific communities, prevalence rates may be 10–40 times higher (Popova et al. 2019). Unfortunately, there is no cure for the long-term effects of FASD. Despite the known economic and public health challenges associated with FASD, alcohol use by pregnant women, both compulsively and recreationally, remains prevalent (Gosdin et al. 2022). PAE is a primary factor in diagnosing FASD and is a leading preventable cause of congenital disabilities and neurodevelopmental disorders (May et al. 2009; Olivier et al. 2016; Lange et al. 2017; Popova et al. 2019). PAE impacts various fetal organs and systems, including the kidneys, liver, heart, gastrointestinal tract, and endocrine and immune systems (Kenna et al. 2012; Gauthier 2015; Caputo et al. 2016). However, the developing brain is the organ most severely affected. In the brain, PAE leads to both structural and functional impairments that can persist throughout childhood and into adulthood (Archibald et al. 2001; Lewis et al. 2016; Caputo et al. 2016; Gao et al. 2019; Wang et al. 2020; Jacobson et al. 2021). Among the five disorders categorized under FASD, FAS is the most severe form (Streissguth et al. 1980; Manzo-Avalos and Saavedra-Molina 2010) and will be the primary focus of this chapter, but other PAE-associated disorders will be mentioned. In 2002, the U.S. Congress instructed the CDC to revise and improve the diagnostic and referral criteria for FAS, resulting in a report published in 2005 that outlined the updated guidelines (Bertrand et al. 2005). This chapter will apply those criteria to explore the developmental effects of PAE further observed in individuals with FAS. Given the challenges in confirming and documenting PAE, it alone is insufficient to diagnose FAS. An FAS diagnosis requires evidence of three key characteristics: (1) three specific facial abnormalities, (2) growth deficits, and (3) central nervous system (CNS) abnormalities (Bertrand et al. 2005). The following sections will briefly review the effects of PAE on physical growth and cognitive development, as well as the behavioral impacts in individuals diagnosed with FAS.

8.2.3 Growth and Morphological Abnormalities

Based on the CDC guidelines, two of the three criteria that need to be met for an FAS diagnosis in humans include growth delays (i.e., a lower-than-average height) and specific facial anomalies (i.e., smooth philtrum, small palpebral fissures, and a thin vermillion border; Bertrand et al.

2005). PAE is consistently linked to growth deficiencies and morphological abnormalities, with effects observed in both human and animal models. For example, several studies have examined the long-term effects of PAE on growth in humans. A longitudinal study found that heavy PAE is related to prenatal growth restriction that persists through the first 9 years of life (Carter et al. 2012a). Heavy drinking (≥2 drinks/day or ≥4 drinks/occasion) throughout the first trimester of pregnancy was associated with reductions in weight, length/height, and head circumference, corresponding to average decreases of 0.6 and 0.5 standard deviations for weight and length/height, respectively, and 0.9 cm for head circumference, relative to controls (Carter et al. 2012a). Findings from this study are consistent with other prospective studies that examined longitudinal growth deficits in children prenatally exposed to alcohol (Day et al. 2002; Lumeng et al. 2007; Carter et al. 2012b). Notably, another study that defined light-to-moderate alcohol intake as three or more drinks per week found a linear relationship between PAE and growth deficits: the greater the PAE, the more pronounced the delay of postnatal growth was (Larkby and Day 1997). Additionally, numerous studies have compared the physical characteristics of children with and without FAS. The findings from these studies also suggest a potential dose-related association between craniofacial shape development and PAE (Suttie et al. 2013; Muggli et al. 2017; Liu et al. 2023). Facial abnormalities associated with PAE are highly variable. Nonetheless, the classic facial features of FAS include a shortened eye opening, a thin upper lip vermilion border, and a flat area between the nose and the upper lip (Suttie et al. 2013; Jańczewska et al. 2019; Mayo Clinic Staff 2024). One study that examined the association between dose, timing of PAE, frequency, and craniofacial phenotype in children found that at any level of PAE (low, moderate-to-high, or binge-level alcohol exposure), craniofacial development can be influenced (Muggli et al. 2017). Observed differences were concentrated around the eyes, nose, lips, and midface. Still, differences were most pronounced between groups with no exposure and groups with low exposure during the first trimester of pregnancy (Muggli et al. 2017). Low PAE (≤20 g of absolute alcohol [AA] per occasion and ≤70 g of AA/week) resulted in differences in the forehead, while moderate-to-high PAE (21–49 g of AA per occasion and ≤70 g of AA/week; >70 g of AA/week) resulted in differences that were seen in the eyes, chin, midface, and parietal region (Muggli et al. 2017). The binge-level PAE exposure (≥50 g of AA per occasion) led to differences confined to the chin (Muggli et al. 2017). These observed facial phenotype differences exhibited signs of recession and were underdeveloped when compared to children with no exposure. For example, observed differences included the upturning of the nasal tip, midfacial hypoplasia, an elongated or shortened upper lip, and retrognathia (recessed chin; Muggli et al. 2017). Midfacial hypoplasia was evident by the flattening of the nasal bridge and malar regions with reductions in midfacial depth and the overall size of the face (i.e., head circumference and reduced upper facial width) and neurocranium (Muggli et al. 2017).

Due to ethical limitations and numerous confounding variables in human subject research on FASD, animal models have been employed to control for many of these confounds, with rodents being the most frequently used models in FASD research (Patten et al. 2014; Almeida et al. 2020). Although their pregnancies are considerably shorter than those in humans, in rodents, for instance, gestational days (GDs) 1–10/11 roughly correspond to the first trimester of human pregnancy (Patten et al. 2014; Almeida et al. 2020). The second trimester spans GDs 11–21/22, while the third trimester is represented by postnatal days (PNDs) 1–10 (Patten et al. 2014; Almeida et al. 2020). Significant brain development occurs after birth for these animals (Semple et al. 2013). As a result, many studies have focused on the timing and method of alcohol exposure on fetal development and have demonstrated that alcohol disrupts key developmental processes (Sulik et al. 1981; Smith 1997). One study that administered ~143 mM of alcohol to neonatal rats between PNDs 4–10, resulted in blood alcohol levels ranging from 12.3 mM (low) to 90.3 mM (peak; Kelly et al. 1987). To put this in human context, a blood alcohol level of 12.3 mM corresponds to roughly 0.057% blood alcohol concentration, which is just below the legal limit of 0.08% to drive motor vehicle in most U.S. Although this level would not be considered legally intoxicating, it reflects social alcohol consumption and may produce noticeable behavioral effects in humans (SA Health 2022). Despite this relatively low blood alcohol level, the study found notable microencephaly, with a reduction in head size by 20%–25%, and significant growth deficits in the cerebellum, cerebrum, and brain stem of alcohol exposed rats (Kelly et al. 1987). Another study, using baboons, showed that gastric alcohol infusion (~39 mM, with blood alcohol levels of ~17 mM) on three separate occasions during the second trimester equivalent to human pregnancy (GD 90, 100, and 110) led to fetal abdominal and head circumferences being significantly decreased in comparison to alcohol-free controls (Tobiasz et al. 2018). In addition to craniofacial changes (Kotch and Sulik 1992), animal studies have also revealed reduced overall body size and increased postnatal mortality in PAE offspring (Abel 1989). Notably, both human and animal research underline that even moderate levels of PAE can result in subtle but significant developmental disruptions.

8.2.4 Cognitive Impairments

As previously mentioned, PAE directly interferes with the development of the fetal brain, often resulting in impairments across a variety of cognitive domains, which is another requirement for an FAS diagnosis (Bertrand et al. 2005). Cognitive domains that PAE typically influences include overall general intelligence, attention and activity levels, language development, learning and memory, motor function, executive function, and more (Mattson et al. 2019). The severity of these impairments can vary, but they typically lead to long-lasting challenges.

For instance, in humans, deficits in general intelligence can result in below-average IQ scores, making academic achievement and daily tasks more difficult (Streissguth et al. 1996; Mattson and Riley 1998; Mattson et al. 2011). As a reference, an IQ score of <70 typically signifies an intellectual deficit, and the average IQ scores of individuals with FAS range between 68 and 79 (Streissguth et al. 1996). Impairments in learning and memory are also common, with individuals struggling to retain and recall information, which again impacts both academic performance and daily functioning (Mattson and Roebuck 2002; Willoughby et al. 2008; Crocker et al. 2011; O'Leary et al. 2015). This deficiency can be attributed to abnormal hippocampal volumes, where children exposed to alcohol prenatally displayed a smaller hippocampus, a region that plays a key role in learning and memory (Willoughby et al. 2008). One study also assessed spatial working memory performance in children diagnosed with FAS, pFAS, or ARND and found that, regardless of diagnosis, children exhibited clear impairments, with deficits becoming more pronounced as task complexity increased (Green et al. 2009). Executive function deficits, which include impairments in attention, decision-making, problem-solving, and planning, can result in significant challenges in organizing tasks, making decisions, and controlling impulses (Anderson 2002; Mattson et al. 2019). Children with FASD show notable deficits in these domains compared to age-matched controls (Mattson et al. 2019).

Furthermore, multiple studies have demonstrated that children with PAE display impairments in response inhibition—the ability to suppress one response in favor of another (Mattson and Riley 1998; Connor et al. 2000; Mattson et al. 2019). When assessed for response inhibition, children with FASD had significantly slower reaction times (Gerhold et al. 2016). Therefore, due to PAE's disruption of proper brain development, FASD is characterized by distinctive and pervasive cognitive impairments.

These cognitive impairments are paralleled in rodent models of FASD, where controlled alcohol exposure during gestation or early postnatal development produces comparable deficits (Bariselli and Lovinger 2021). For example, a study using a developmental alcohol binge-pattern exposure where mice were exposed to alcohol both prenatally (~43 mM on GDs 10–11 and ~87 mM on GDs 12–18) and postnatally (~33 mM on PNDs 4–5 and ~65 mM on PNDs 6–14), found that adult offspring exhibited impaired performance on the five-choice serial reaction time test (5-CSRTT) for visual attention (Louth et al. 2016). The 5-CSRTT assesses attention by requiring the mouse to respond to brief and unpredictable visual cues presented in one of five locations within the operant chamber (Remmelink et al. 2017). Indicators of impaired attention include reduced response accuracy, longer reaction times, and increased omission rates (no response was made) as conditions became more challenging (Louth et al. 2016). Furthermore, another study using a binge exposure model (141 mM alcohol on PNDs 6–9, with blood alcohol levels reaching ~66 mM) found that rats displayed an impaired ability to relocate the hidden platform during a delayed matching-to-place task in the Morris water maze (Girard et al. 2000). As with human studies, reduced hippocampal volumes can also partially mediate these deficits (Dodge et al. 2020). Overall, the consistency of cognitive impairments across human and animal models highlights the translational relevance of rodent research for understanding FASD.

8.2.5 Behavioral Difficulties

Beyond cognitive deficits, PAE can also significantly contribute to a range of behavioral difficulties in children that impair daily functioning and social development. In humans, individuals with FAS often exhibit problems with self-regulation, neurocognition, and adaptive functioning (Doyle and Mattson 2015; Hagan Jr et al. 2016; Mattson et al. 2019). These deficits often manifest as part of a neurobehavioral disorder called Neurobehavioral Disorder Associated with PAE (ND-PAE), which, as stated above, falls under the FASD umbrella (Doyle and Mattson 2015; Hagan Jr et al. 2016; Mattson et al. 2019). Behaviors associated with ND-PAE often overlap with those seen in Attention-Deficit/Hyperactivity Disorder (Peadon 2010). For example, children with PAE frequently show deficits in reaction time, attention-shifting capacity, and response inhibition (Doyle and Mattson 2015).

Additionally, impulse control is another characteristic challenge, where children with PAE tend to lack the ability to control impulsive responses (Doyle and Mattson 2015). Mood and anxiety disorders are also at higher risk of developing in children with PAE, as they typically have difficulty in mood and behavior regulation (Doyle and Mattson 2015). These impairments may include extreme emotional reactivity, frequent behavioral outbursts, irritability, and overall lack of mood stability (Doyle and Mattson 2015). In addition, children with PAE often display social difficulties, such as understanding social cues, interpreting others' emotions, or maintaining appropriate social interactions (Kelly et al. 2000; Doyle and Mattson 2015).

Animal models of PAE replicate many of these behavioral phenotypes. For example, increased locomotor activity—a commonly used proxy for hyperactivity—has been widely observed in rodents following gestational or early postnatal alcohol exposure (Shah and West 1984; Risbud et al. 2022). For example, one study exposed Sprague-Dawley rats to alcohol during neonatal and adolescent developmental periods: (1) PNDs 4–9 (~54 mM alcohol) and (2) PNDs 28–42 (~87 mM). Findings from this study revealed that neonatal alcohol exposure and adolescent alcohol exposure altered locomotor activity in a sex- and time-dependent manner (Risbud et al. 2022). Neonatal alcohol exposure resulted in increased locomotor activity, while alcohol exposure during adolescence decreased overall locomotor activity in females (Risbud et al. 2022). Impulsivity and poor inhibitory control have also been demonstrated in operant conditioning tasks, such as the go/no-go task, and it was found that chronic PAE of ~87 mM alcohol throughout gestation to guinea pigs resulted in increased no-go but not the go responses (Olmstead et al. 2009). These results are indicative of impulsive control difficulty. Regarding social behavior, rodent studies have shown that PAE impairs social play and social recognition, which are developmentally critical behaviors (Meyer and Riley 1986; Holman et al. 2018; Bariselli et al. 2023). These findings parallel social difficulties seen in humans with FASD. Together, clinical and preclinical studies conclude that PAE leads to persistent behavioral disturbances that span multiple domains.

8.3 Mitochondria

8.3.1 Structure, Function, and Distribution of Mitochondria

The term "mitochondrion" was coined in 1898 by Carl Benda (Helmenstine 2025). Mitochondria, plural of mitochondrion, are multifaceted membrane-bound organelles central to cellular metabolism, cell death regulation, and energy production (Cooper 2000; Osellame et al. 2012; Chen et al. 2023). Because of their essential contribution to many processes of cellular function, mitochondria are often referred to as the "powerhouse of the cell"—a phrase popularized by Philip Siekevitz in 1957 (Nunes 2021).

Their hallmark structure is composed of two membranes: a smooth outer membrane and a highly folded inner membrane that forms cristae, which increases surface area and houses the key protein complexes involved in the electron transport chain (ETC) and ATP synthesis (Cooper 2000; Osellame et al. 2012; Chen et al. 2023). Within the inner compartment, or matrix, reside enzymes for the tricarboxylic acid cycle, mitochondrial DNA (mtDNA), ribosomes, and other necessary components for mitochondrial gene expression (Bornstein et al. 2020; Chen et al. 2023). This architecture enables the mitochondria's primary function: the production of energy, in the form of ATP, through oxidative phosphorylation (Cooper 2000). However, mitochondria are not static entities; they constantly undergo fission, fusion, and transport processes, allowing them to adapt to shifting metabolic demands and spatial needs within the cell (Scott and Youle 2010; Green et al. 2022).

Beyond their structural components, mitochondria are present in nearly all eukaryotic cells and are highly dynamic organelles, forming a dynamic, branched tubular network throughout the cell's cytoplasm (Frederick and Shaw 2007). Their distribution is cell type-specific, aligning closely with areas of high energy demand (Westermann 2012; Safiulina and Kaasik 2013; Son and Han 2018). Cells with high energy demands, like muscle fibers, contain a high concentration of mitochondria (Romanello and Sandri 2023), while others, like red blood cells, lack them entirely (Pretini et al. 2019). Thus, mitochondria morphology and placement are finely tuned by signaling pathways that respond to metabolic cues, developmental state, and external stress (Akbari et al. 2019; Chen et al. 2023). This dynamic adaptability is crucial for meeting energetic demands and regulating cell survival, differentiation, and stress responses (Osellame et al. 2012; Chen et al. 2023).

Given their essential roles, the health of mitochondria is closely linked to cellular function, overall well-being, and even the aging process (San-Millán 2023; Casanova et al. 2023). One critical aspect of mitochondrial function is their dual role in both generating and mitigating reactive oxygen species (ROS; Hoek et al. 2002), which are highly reactive molecules produced as byproducts of oxidative phosphorylation (Nolfi-Donegan et al. 2020). Under physiological conditions, ROS are tightly regulated by mitochondria's protective mechanisms, such as antioxidant enzymes, which neutralize ROS and prevent them from causing cellular damage (Addabbo et al. 2009; He et al. 2017; Napolitano et al. 2021). These defenses comprise enzymatic and non-enzymatic antioxidants (Mailloux 2018; Napolitano et al. 2021). For instance, superoxide dismutase converts the highly reactive superoxide radical into hydrogen peroxide. At the same time, vitamin E quenches singlet oxygen by absorbing its energy, both of which maintain redox balance and protect cells from oxidative damage (Mailloux 2018; Napolitano et al. 2021). However, under stress conditions such as alcohol exposure, ROS production can exceed detoxification capacity, leading to a state known as oxidative stress (Afzal et al. 2023). This imbalance can cause widespread damage to proteins, lipids, and mtDNA, impairing mitochondrial integrity and function (Hoek et al. 2002; Alhowail 2022; Thoudam et al. 2024). As mitochondrial damage accumulates, ATP production becomes increasingly inefficient, further elevating ROS production—amplifying dysfunction in a self-reinforcing cycle (Zhang et al. 2023; Chen et al. 2024a). This vicious cycle of oxidative stress and mitochondrial impairment is implicated in a wide range of diseases, including neurodegenerative conditions such as Alzheimer's and Parkinson's, as well as metabolic disorders like diabetes (San-Millán 2023; Casanova et al. 2023). Without functional mitochondria, cells lose the ability to maintain homeostasis, leading to dysfunction or cell death (Forum on Neuroscience and Nervous System Disorders 2013).

8.3.2 Developing and Mature Mitochondria: What Is the Difference?

The transition from developing to mature mitochondria reflects profound changes in morphology, metabolic activity, and functional specialization, which often mirror the differentiation state of the host cell (Khacho and Slack 2017; Son and Han 2018; Rastogi et al. 2019; Peng et al. 2022). In early-stage or undifferentiated cells, mitochondria are typically small, spherical, and possess sparse or poorly formed cristae, reflecting restricted oxidative capacity and reduced ETC activity (Facucho-Oliveira and St John 2009; Xu et al. 2013; Rastogi et al. 2019). Tissues with immature mitochondria rely predominantly on glycolysis for energy production, which is a metabolic pathway that supports rapid proliferation and biosynthetic activity typical of stem or progenitor cells (Facucho-Oliveira and St John 2009; Xu et al. 2013; Son and Han 2018; Mahmoud 2023). As cells differentiate, mitochondria undergo a maturation process involving increased mitochondrial biogenesis, mtDNA replication, and levels of oxygen consumption and ATP generation through oxidative phosphorylation (Cho et al. 2006; Facucho-Oliveira and St John 2009; Khacho and Slack 2017; Mahmoud 2023). Structurally, mature mitochondria are elongated and exhibit densely packed cristae within a more electron-dense matrix, enabling efficient energy production through oxidative phosphorylation, instead of glycolysis (Facucho-Oliveira and St John 2009; Xu et al. 2013; Mishra and Chan 2014; Khacho and Slack 2017; El-Merhie et al. 2017; Mahmoud 2023).

Functionally, this shift from glycolysis to oxidative phosphorylation results in higher levels of ROS (Facucho-Oliveira and St John 2009; Xu et al. 2013). For undifferentiated cells, low levels of ROS have been shown to have a beneficial role in cell signaling and regulation of proliferation and differentiation (Facucho-Oliveira and St John 2009; Bratic and Larsson 2013; Khacho and Slack 2017; Peng et al. 2022). However, continuous exposure to high ROS levels can have deleterious effects for both undifferentiated and differentiated cells (Facucho-Oliveira and St John 2009; Bratic and Larsson 2013; Xu et al. 2013). In contrast, mature mitochondria are equipped to meet the elevated and localized demands of differentiated cells, such as neurons and cardiomyocytes, and have a larger capacity to neutralize ROS (Addabbo et al. 2009; Xu et al. 2013; He et al. 2017; Napolitano et al. 2021; Peng et al. 2022; Mahmoud 2023). Without proper maturation, mitochondria struggle to maintain cellular homeostasis, often initiating a vicious cycle of impaired energy production and rising oxidative stress (Zhang et al. 2023; Chen et al. 2024a, b). This disruption is implicated in the pathogenesis of several conditions; thus, mitochondrial maturation is not merely a structural transformation, but also a fundamental biological process essential for cellular function and long-term viability (Mishra and Chan 2014; Khacho and Slack 2017; Rastogi et al. 2019; Peng et al. 2022; Mahmoud 2023).

Understanding the distinctions between developing and mature mitochondria is crucial for identifying periods of heightened vulnerability during embryonic and fetal development, particularly in environmental insults, such as PAE. Since developing mitochondria have reduced oxidative capacity, with potential limited ROS defense mechanisms, they are more susceptible to oxidative stress and mitochondrial dysfunction, both of which are hallmark features observed in models of FAS/FASD (Facucho-Oliveira and St John 2009; Xu et al. 2013; Rastogi et al. 2019). Disruption of mitochondrial function due to alcohol-related oxidative damage may compromise the metabolic reprogramming essential for normal cellular differentiation and tissue development. Thus, mitochondrial immaturity not only increases susceptibility to alcohol-induced damage but may also underlie many of the neurodevelopmental and systemic abnormalities characteristic of FASD.

8.3.3 PAE-Induced Mitochondrial Dysfunction in Developing Tissues

Although developing and mature mitochondria differ in structure and dynamics, both remain vulnerable to the harmful effects of alcohol. While it is well established that alcohol disrupts the function of mature mitochondria (Hoek et al. 2002), alcohol exposure also adversely affects the morphology and function of developing mitochondria in various fetal tissues (Henderson et al. 1999). Organs commonly targeted by alcohol-induced mitochondrial damage include the pancreas (Dobson et al. 2012; Srinivasan et al. 2015), skeletal muscles (Olesen and Quintanilla 2023), liver, heart, and the brain. The effects of alcohol on liver and heart mitochondria are briefly discussed here, followed by a more detailed exploration of PAE and its impact on the developing brain in the following section.

Alcohol is primarily metabolized in the liver (Zakhari 2006; Han et al. 2012; NIAAA 2022), where mitochondria play a key role during the breakdown of alcohol due to an increased demand for oxygen and energy (Cunningham et al. 1990; Nassir and Ibdah 2014). Alcohol consumption, however, interferes with this process, reducing the expression of respiratory complexes I, III, IV, and V in the ETC (Han et al. 2016; Sun et al. 2016; Simon and Molina 2022). This disruption in respiratory activity leads to diminished ATP production (Marcinkeviciute et al. 2000), inhibition of ATP synthesis (Cederbaum et al. 1974; Mitchell and Herlong 1986), and, as a result, the overproduction of ROS (Manzo-Avalos and Saavedra-Molina 2010; Siggins et al. 2023), which compromises cell viability (Bailey et al. 1999; Manzo-Avalos and Saavedra-Molina 2010). An in vitro study incubating cultured liver cells from Sprague-Dawley rat fetuses (GD 19) in ~44 mM alcohol solution for up to 24 h revealed three significant mitochondrial dysfunctions: (1) decreased membrane permeability to rhodamine 123, a cationic dye, suggesting a reduction in mitochondrial transmembrane potential due to alcohol, (2) lowered ATP levels, and (3) reduced succinate dehydrogenase activity, as assessed by the MTT (3-(4,5-dimethylthiazol-2-yl)-2,5-diphenyltetrazolium bromide) assay, indicating a loss of mitochondrial membrane integrity (Devi et al. 1993). Higher alcohol concentrations (~54 mM alcohol; 24 h), further reduced mitochondrial complex activity (complex I by 16%, complex IV by 28%), and diminished mitochondrial glutathione (GSH) levels by 20% in cultured rat liver cells (GDs 19–20; Devi et al. 1993). GSH is vital in protecting mitochondrial health by supporting antioxidant defense, detoxification, mtDNA stabilization, and apoptosis regulation (Marí et al. 2009; Chen et al. 2024a, b). Additionally, fetal liver mitochondria exposed to alcohol displayed altered morphology. Liver tissue collected from half-term mini-pig fetuses, whose mothers received daily alcohol feeding (~65 mM alcohol), exhibited abnormal mitochondrial morphology, including changes in shape (ranging from straight rod-shaped to spherical), size/length (spherical mitochondria with a 2 μm diameter or elongated forms up to 7 μm with a normal diameter of 0.5–1 μm), disorientation of cristae, and the appearance of dense material in the matrix (Rømert and Matthiessen 1983).

In the adult heart, mitochondria generate 60%–90% of the energy required to meet cardiac demands (Zuccolotto dos Reis 2024). Therefore, disruptions in mitochondrial function can significantly contribute to cardiac pathology (Nyquist-Battie and Freter 1988; Lemieux and Hoppel 2009; Nguyen et al. 2018; Zuccolotto dos Reis 2024), particularly in conditions like cardiomyopathy (Kim et al. 2001; Vendemiale et al. 2001; Hajnóczky et al. 2005; Piano et al. 2007). Similar to liver mitochondria, alcohol-induced mitochondrial dysfunction in the heart is linked to irregular ETC activity, decreased ATP production, excessive ROS generation, and impaired mitochondrial dynamics (Eisner et al. 2017; Steiner and Lang 2017; Nguyen et al. 2018). Long-term alcohol exposure accelerates mitochondrial dysfunction and apoptosis, leading to compromised cardiac function (Vendemiale et al. 2001; Hajnóczky et al. 2005; Steiner and Lang 2017). In the context of PAE, alcohol-induced mitochondrial impairment can greatly impact both cardiac development and function (Nyquist-Battie and Freter 1988; Su et al. 2024). One study demonstrated that neonatal cardiomyocytes, from 1- to 3-day-old Wistar rats, chronically exposed to 50 mM alcohol for 6 days, exhibited a dose-dependent compromise of mitochondrial function (Laurent et al. 2014). This was evident by a significant decrease in succinate dehydrogenase activity and reduced ATP levels (Laurent et al. 2014). A reduction in succinate dehydrogenase activity indicates the loss of mitochondrial membrane integrity as its proper function is essential for maintaining mitochondrial membrane potential and overall mitochondrial health. Dysfunction of succinate dehydrogenase can compromise the integrity of the inner mitochondrial membrane, leading to leakage of ions and small molecules, impaired ATP production, and the initiation of apoptotic pathways (Tseng et al. 2018; Lee et al. 2022). Furthermore, alcohol exposure significantly increased mitochondrial depolarization: JC1 dye was used to measure changes in mitochondrial membrane potential, with depolarization considered an early indicator of mitochondrial dysfunction (Reers et al. 1995). Alcohol exposure also led to increased mtDNA damage, potentially overwhelming mtDNA repair mechanisms (Laurent et al. 2014). In a recent study, 65 mM alcohol was administered daily to pregnant C57BL/6 mice during GDs 8.5–15.5 (equivalent to the second trimester of human pregnancy), a critical period for cardiac development (Zhang et al. 2022; Su et al. 2024). From this study, primary cultures of cardiomyocytes from neonatal mouse hearts exposed to various alcohol concentrations for 24, 48, and 72 h showed a significant increase in mitochondrial peroxide levels, indicating ROS production, as well as a corresponding rise in ROS levels (Zhang et al. 2022; Su et al. 2024). Moreover, PAE caused a dose-dependent reduction in ATP levels and mitochondrial membrane potential (Zhang et al. 2022; Su et al. 2024). Specifically, PAE induced myocardial mitochondrial damage in offspring, as evidenced by a notable decrease in mitochondrial membrane potential, a significant increase in mitochondrial superoxide (reflecting ROS generation), and sustained opening of the mitochondrial permeability transition pore (mPTP; Zhang et al. 2022; Su et al. 2024). Typically, mPTPs remain closed to preserve membrane integrity (Murphy and Steenbergen 2008; Lam et al. 2015); excessive opening can lead to cell death (Kroemer et al. 2007) through mitochondrial matrix swelling, outer membrane rupture, cytochrome C and apoptosis-inducing factor (AIF) release, and activation of the caspase pathway, ultimately inducing apoptosis (Penna et al. 2013). Additional indicators of mitochondrial dysfunctions included decreased ATP synthesis capacity, reduced ATP content, and a decreased mtDNA copy number (a biomarker of mitochondrial health [Castellani et al. 2020; Su et al. 2024]).

In summary, alcohol-induced mitochondrial dysfunction has been well documented across multiple organ systems, including the liver and heart, as well as other organs not specifically discussed here. These effects on mitochondrial morphology and function are observed in adult and developing tissues, with fetal organ mitochondria exhibiting heightened vulnerability to alcohol-induced mitochondrial damage (Bukiya 2019).

Given the critical role mitochondria play in supporting the energy demands and structural integrity of developing tissues, it is essential to understand how PAE impacts mitochondrial function in the developing brain. The following section will delve into the effects of PAE on mitochondrial health in the fetal brain, highlighting how disruptions in mitochondrial function contribute to the broader neurodevelopmental deficits observed in FASD.

8.4 Effects of PAE on Developing Mitochondria in the Brain

The health of mitochondria is essential for the optimal functioning of the CNS (Arzua et al. 2024), and alcohol, a well-known CNS depressant (Mukherjee 2013), damages mitochondria in the brain. As previously emphasized, the developing brain is particularly vulnerable to PAE, as it is the most profoundly affected organ (Archibald et al. 2001; Lewis et al. 2016; Caputo et al. 2016; Gao et al. 2019; Wang et al. 2020; Jacobson et al. 2021). Alcohol, due to its soluble nature, crosses the blood–brain barrier and placenta (Streissguth et al. 1980; Gupta et al. 2016), rapidly distributing in the fetal circulation system (Paton 2005; Cederbaum 2012; Popova et al. 2021). This exposure significantly disrupts mitochondrial development and function in the growing brain (Chen et al. 2003), with fetal (or developing) mitochondria being more sensitive to alcohol than adult (or mature) mitochondria (Bukiya 2019). Mitochondria in the brain are primary targets of alcohol-induced oxidative stress (Manzo-Avalos and Saavedra-Molina 2010). Several studies, ranging from cell cultures to animal models, report that alcohol-induced mitochondrial dysfunction contributes to alterations in brain structure (Clarren et al. 1978) and function (Khacho et al. 2017; Clemente-Suárez et al. 2023; Klemmensen et al. 2023), ultimately leading to cognitive and behavioral issues (Connor and Streissguth 1996; Marin-Garcia et al. 1996; de la Monte and Wands 2002; Finsterer 2008; Khacho et al. 2017; Sharma et al. 2021; Arzua et al. 2024).

Similar to mitochondria in the liver and heart, brain mitochondria are also significantly affected by PAE; however, some studies indicate tissue-specific responses (Marin-Garcia et al. 1996; Bukiya 2019). Studies have shown that brain mitochondria exhibit reduced respiratory activity in ETC complexes when exposed to alcohol (Bustamante et al. 2012; Simon and Molina 2022). However, one study highlighted the distinct differences in complex activity between the brain and liver tissues in neonates (1-day-old) from alcohol-fed mothers (Sprague-Dawley rats; alcohol providing 36% of the total calories in the liquid diet, though the exact alcohol concentration was not specified; Marin-Garcia et al. 1996). For example, levels of complex V activity were significantly decreased in both the brain (57%) and liver (34%) of alcohol-exposed neonates (Marin-Garcia et al. 1996). In contrast, complex III activity decreased only in the liver (39%) and not in the brain. A notable finding from this study was that complex IV activity in both the brain and liver was not reduced by alcohol exposure in neonates, unlike the reductions typically observed in adults (Marin-Garcia et al. 1996).

Besides affecting the respiratory activity of the ETC, evidence suggests that PAE modifies other markers of mitochondrial dysfunction. Timed pregnant guinea pigs were administered alcohol (~87 mM) daily and chronically (Green et al. 2006). At GD 65 and PD 0, the brains of the offspring were excised, and the hippocampus was dissected. Chronic PAE resulted in decreased brain weight and hippocampal weight, and decreased GSH content in the mitochondrial fraction of hippocampal homogenate at PD 0, with no changes in hippocampal cytosolic GSH concentration (Green et al. 2006). Furthermore, at the same alcohol concentration, fetal rat brains (GDs 17 and 18) exhibited an increase in mitochondrial permeability transition—where the inner mitochondrial membrane becomes more permeable to small molecules (Kwong and Molkentin 2015)—as observed through the increased rate of induced mitochondrial swelling (Ramachandran et al. 2006). This was accompanied by a 62% increase in cytochrome c and a 25% increase in AIF release compared to controls (Ramachandran et al. 2006). These events were linked to a 30% rise in caspase-3 activity and a 25% increase in DNA fragmentation. Levels of 4-HNE (4-hydroxynonenal; a toxic aldehyde generated during lipid peroxidation) were also increased by 23% (Ramachandran et al. 2006). These studies illustrate that PAE can elicit a cascade of fetal brain events that are consistent with mitochondrially mediated apoptotic cell death. A more recent study found that PAE induced mtDNA damage while inhibiting its repair in both fetal brain tissue and fetal brain-derived exosomes (FB-E) from maternal blood (Darbinian et al. 2023). The study also identified a potential correlation between mtDNA damage and reduced eye size, indicating that the level of damaged mtDNA in FB-E might serve as a predictor for identifying fetuses at risk of being born with FAS/FASD (Darbinian et al. 2023).

These findings highlight the widespread impact of PAE on mitochondrial function in the developing brain, further suggesting that alcohol-induced mitochondrial dysfunction could have profound implications for neurodevelopment. Given the central role of mitochondria in energy production and cellular health, these disruptions can significantly affect the functioning of neurons, glial cells, and cerebral vessels. Each of these cellular components is critical for proper brain development and function, and their impairment during key developmental windows may contribute to the neurodevelopmental deficits observed in FASD.

In the following sections, we will explore in greater detail how alcohol-induced mitochondrial dysfunction impacts neurons, glial cells, and cerebral vessels within the developing brain (Table 8.1). Understanding these cellular disruptions is key to comprehending the broader neurobiological consequences of PAE.

8.4.1 Alcohol Modulation of Developing Neuronal Cell Culture Mitochondria

Neurogenesis is a critical process in brain development, resulting in the production of neurons, the fundamental units of the brain (Temple 2001; Ming and Song 2011; Bond et al. 2015; Accogli et al. 2020; Villalba et al. 2021). In humans, neurogenesis begins around the tenth week of gestation (Zecevic 2004; Malik et al. 2013; Gulati 2015). PAE is a major environmental risk factor disrupting neurogenesis with decreased proliferation and differentiation of progenitor neuronal cells that leads to long-term neurodevelopmental impairments (Tyler and Allan 2014; Gil-Mohapel et al. 2014; Hagan et al. 2016; Kable and Mukherjee 2017; Moore and Xia 2022, Muggli et al. 2024). One of the key mechanisms implicated in alcohol-induced disruption of neuronal development is mitochondrial dysfunction. Mitochondria play essential roles in cellular energy production, calcium homeostasis, ROS regulation, and apoptosis, all of which are vital for proper neuronal maturation and survival (Hamanaka and Chandel 2010; Efremov and Sazanov 2011; Martinou and Youle 2011; Nunnari and Suomalainen 2012; Brand et al. 2013; Chen et al. 2023; Casanova et al. 2023). PAE has been shown to alter mitochondrial morphology and function, leading to oxidative stress and membrane damage (Goodlett and Horn 2001; Chen et al. 2023; Alhowail 2022). These changes initiate a cascade culminating in neuronal injury and death (Goodlett and Horn 2001; Chen et al. 2003; Alhowail 2022).

Early studies demonstrated that PAE induced oxidative stress in the fetal brain (Henderson et al. 1995; Marin-Garcia et al. 1996). Sprague Dawley rats exposed to a 2-day binge alcohol treatment (~87 mM) on GDs 17 and 18 (equivalent to the end of the second trimester of pregnancy in humans), with blood alcohol levels of 67 mM, exhibited elevated membrane lipid peroxidation, as indicated by increased levels of malondialdehyde and conjugated dienes, byproducts of ROS-induced lipid damage. This study also revealed depleted GSH levels in fetal brain lysates, underscoring accelerated oxidative stress (Henderson et al. 1995). Following these findings, further research examined alcohol-induced mitochondrial dysfunction and its contribution to apoptotic cell death in the fetal brain. Alcohol exposure was shown to cause mitochondrial swelling, increased inner mitochondrial membrane permeability, and the subsequent leakage of pro-apoptotic proteins such as cytochrome c and AIF. Moreover, accumulation of 4-HNE

Table 8.1 Effects of PAE on mitochondrial structure and function in the developing brain

	Reference	Species	Trimester of exposure	Alcohol exposure	Tissue/cell type	Assay/parameters	Findings
Neurons	Marin-Garcia et al. (1996)	Rat (Sprague Dawley)	Throughout pregnancy	62 mM via liquid diet (23 days)	Brain lysate	Specific enzyme activity assays Northern RNA blots	↓ Complex V activity (57%) No changes in *ATPase6* transcript levels
	Henderson et al. (1995)	Rat (Sprague Dawley)	Second trimester (GD 17–19)	67 mM via intubation (12-h intervals)	Brain lysate	Spectrophotometric scanning method (Tietze 1969; Ohkawa et al. 1979) HPLC	↑ Levels of byproducts of ROS such as MDA (14%) and conjugated dienes (23%) ↓ GSH levels (19%) ↑ Oxidative stress
	Ramachandran et al. (2001)	Rat (Sprague Dawley)	Second trimester (GD 17–19)	67 mM via intubation (12-h intervals)	Brain lysate	Isolated mitochondria HPLC Spectrophotometry Western blots	Mitochondrial swelling ↑ Membrane permeability Leak of pro-apoptotic proteins (cytochrome c & AIF) Accumulation of 4-HNE ↑ Apoptotic signaling
	Ramachandran et al. (2003)	Rat (Sprague Dawley)	Second trimester (GD 17–19)	54 mM in vitro exposure (24 h)	Primary cortical neuron cultures	Trypan blue exclusion HPLC Confocal microscopy Flow cytometry Western blots Annexin V-fluorescein isothiocyanate staining	↑ ROS formation ↑ 4-HNE and MDA levels ↑ Oxidative stress ↑ Cytochrome c release and activation of caspase 3 ↑ Apoptosis
	Chu et al. (2007)	Rat (long Evans)	Throughout pregnancy (GD 6 until delivery)	51 mM via liquid diet	Cerebellum (Purkinje cells)	Real time qPCR Immunohistochemistry MitoTracker fluorescent staining	↓ Mitochondrial complexes II, IV and V coding genes Mitochondrial DNA damage ↑ 8-OHdG and 4-HNE levels ↑ p53 and NADPH oxidase ↑ Oxidative stress
	Ullah et al. (2012)	Rat (Sprague Dawley)	Second trimester (GD 17.5)	100 mM in vitro exposure (12 h)	Primary cortical neuron cultures	MTT assay JC-1 staining Western blots	↓ Cell viability ↓ Mitochondrial membrane potential ↓ Anti-apoptotic protein

						TUNEL and DAPI staining	(Bcl-2) ↑ Pro-apoptotic protein (Bax) Metformin and thymoquinone reversed alcohol effects
	Perez et al. (2020)	Rat (Sprague Dawley)	Second trimester (GD 18)	25 mM 50 mM 75 mM In vitro exposure (24 h)	Hippocampus neuron cultures	Alamar blue assay kit Mito tracker fluorescent staining Bioluminescence assay kit Western blots	↓ Mitochondrial membrane potential ↓ ATP production ↓ Superoxide levels ↓ Mitochondrial Ca^{2+} levels Disrupted Ca^{2+} homeostasis No changes in mitochondria length NOX inhibition restored mitochondrial function
	Lee et al. (2005)	Rat (Wistar)	Second trimester (GD 12)	25–100 mM alcohol 0.1–10 mM acetaldehyde in vitro exposure (48 h)	Midbrain neuron cultures	DCFH-DA assay ELISA assay Cytotoxicity assay Immunohistochemistry	Dose-dependent increase Apoptosis Oxidative stress Calcium dysregulation Acetaldehyde has more toxic effects than alcohol
	Light et al. (2002)	Rat (Sprague Dawley)	Third trimester (PND 4)	46 mM via oral gavage (single dose)	Cerebellum (Purkinje cells)	Immunohistochemistry TUNEL staining Fluorescence microscopy.	Activation of caspase-3 enzyme Mitochondrial release ofCytochrome c ↑ Apoptosis (70%)
	Tong et al. (2011)	Rat (long Evan)	Third trimester (PND 8)	3.5 mM acetaldehyde in vitro exposure (48 h)	Cerebellum neuronal culture	MTT assay ELISA assay Mito tracker staining qPCR	↓ Cell viability ↑ 4-HNE, 8-OHdG, ATP levels and MitoTracker red fluorescence ↑ Oxidative stress ↓ Expression of ADH and ALDH
	Xu et al. (2005)	Mouse (CD-1)	First trimester (GD 6–15)	33 mM 65 mM 130 mM via oral gavage	Cerebral tissue	Isolated mitochondria TUNEL assay Flow cytometry Enzymic activity assays ATP assay kit	↓ Complex I (91.7% and 87.9%) and II (72.4% and 69.7%) activity at 33 and 65 mM

(continued)

Table 8.1 (continued)

	Reference	Species	Trimester of exposure	Alcohol exposure	Tissue/cell type	Assay/parameters	Findings
							↓ ATP synthase activity at 65 mM
	Sari et al. (2010)	Mouse (C57BL/6)	Second trimester (GD 7–13)	12 mM via liquid diet	Brain lysate	LC-MS TUNEL staining	Downregulation of mitochondrial enzymes
	Arzua et al. (2024)	Mouse (C57BL/6)	Third trimester (PND 7)	48 mM via subcutaneous injections	Hippocampus	Bioinformatic analysis (mRNA profiling)	Dysregulated mitochondrial genes Associated with neuronal apoptosis, synaptic dysfunction and behavior deficits
	Green et al. (2006)	Guinea pig (Dunkin Hartley)	First to second trimester (GD 2–64)	87 mM via liquid diet	Hippocampus	Fluorescence assay	↓ Mitochondrial antioxidant (GSH) presence
	de la Monte et al. (2001)	Human		100 mM in vitro exposure (4 days)	PNET2 neuronal cultured cells	TUNEL assay Western blots MitoTracker fluorescence labeling	Damaged mitochondrial DNA ↓ Mitochondrial mass Insulin stimulation rescues mitochondria function
	Darbinian et al. (2023)	Human	First trimester (16 weeks fetal brain)	Reported alcohol drinking	Cortical neurons	qPCR Superoxide activity assay ATP assay	↓ Mitochondrial DNA Damage to mitochondrial DNA as a biomarker
Glia (astrocytes)	Watts et al. (2005)	Rat (Sprague Dawley)	Third trimester (PND 2)	44 mM 88 mM in vitro exposure (24 h)	Cortical astrocyte cultures	Trypan blue exclusion assay MTT assay Flow cytometry DCF-DA assay Fluorometric assays	Resistant to apoptotic death and oxidative stress at 44 mM ↓ Astrocyte (28%) viability at 88 mM Astrocytes co-cultured with cortical neurons Normalize neuronal GSH homeostasis Protect neurons from apoptosis
	Rathinam et al. (2006)	Rat (Sprague Dawley)	Third trimester (PND 2)	44 mM 88 mM in vitro exposure (24 h)	Cortical astrocyte cultures	Fluorometric GSH assays HPLC DCF-DA assay	Astrocytes co-cultured with cortical neurons ↑ GSH efflux from astrocytes

						Enzymic activity assays Western blots	Maintains neuronal GSH homeostasis Protects against ↑ ROS production
	Montoliu et al. (1995)	Rat (Sprague Dawley)	PND 21	25 mM in vitro exposure (14 days)	Cortical astrocyte cultures	Immunofluorescence staining.	↑ Expression of CYP2E1 Acetaldehyde may contribute to oxidative damage
Glia (oligodendrocytes)	Chiappelli and Taylor (1991)	Rat (Sprague Dawley)	Second to third trimester	10 mM via liquid diet (14 days)	Oligodendrocytes cultured	Immunostaining ELISA assay	↓ Expression of myelin basic protein ↓ Mature oligodendrocytes
	Newville et al. (2017)	Mouse (C57Bl/J6)	Third trimester (PND 3–15)	35 mM (BAC) via vapor inhalation chamber	Proliferating and mature oligodendrocytes n corpus callosum	Immunohistochemistry Fluorescent imaging Western blot Magnetic resonance imaging	↓ Mature (58%) and proliferating (75%) oligodendrocytes At PND 50, myelin basic protein damaged Abnormal white matter microstructures
Glia (oligodendrocytes)	Creeley et al. (2013)	Non-human primate (cynomolgus macaque)	Second trimester (GD 120)	65 mM via intravenous injection	Oligodendrocytes	Immunohistochemistry	↑ Oligoapoptosis Disrupts early and late myelination stages
	Darbinian et al. (2021)	Human	Second trimester (20 weeks fetal brain)	Based on PASS study	Cerebral cortex	qPCR Flow cytometry Histological staining	Delayed oligo differentiation ↓ Mature oligodendrocytes ↑ Apoptosis ↓ Myelin basic protein
Glia (microglia)	Boyadjieva and Sarkar (2010)	Rat (Sprague Dawley)	Second trimester (GD 19)	50 mM 100 mM in vitro exposure (24 h)	Hypothalamic microglia cultures	ELISA assay Immunohistochemistry	Activated microglia ↑ Inflammatory cytokines production ↑ Apoptotic death of hypothalamic neurons
	Boyadjieva and Sarkar (2013a)	Rat (Sprague Dawley)	Second trimester (GD 19)	25 mM 50 mM 100 mM in vitro exposure (24 h)	Hypothalamic microglia cultures	ELISA assay DCF-DA assay Nitrite assay GSH assay Calorimetric assay	Dose-dependent effect ↑ Oxidants levels (O2-, ROS, and nitrite) ↓ GSH levels ↑ Oxidative stress ↑ Neuronal cells death
	Boyadjieva and Sarkar (2013b)	Rat (Sprague Dawley)	Second trimester (GD 19)	50 mM in vitro exposure (24 h)	Hypothalamic microglia cultures	ELISA assay DCF-DA assay	Activation of microglial cells ↓ cAMP and BDNF levels in

(continued)

Table 8.1 (continued)

	Reference	Species	Trimester of exposure	Alcohol exposure	Tissue/cell type	Assay/parameters	Findings
						Nitrite assay GSH assay	neurons dbcAMP and BDNF supplementation reversed toxic effects
Cerebrovascular tree	Cananzi and Mayhan (2017)	Rat (Sprague Dawley)	Throughout pregnancy (21–23 days)	13.6 mM via liquid diet	Cerebral arteriole and microvessel tissue	Superoxide level assay Western blots	↑ NOX2 and NOX4 expression levels ↑ Superoxide levels ↑ Oxidative stress
	Jégou et al. (2012)	Mouse	Second trimester (GD 13–19)	22 mM 65 mM via subcutaneous injection	Cortical vascular network	qPCR Western blots Immunohistochemistry Video microscopy	↓ Vascular network density at both 22 and 65 mM Abnormal vascular patterning at 65 mM
	Girault et al. (2017)	Mouse (NMRI)	Second trimester (GD 13–19)	50 mM via subcutaneous injection	Microvascular endothelial cells	Immunolabeling Viability assay qPCR Western blots Real time video microscopy JC-1 staining	↓ Mitochondrial membrane potential ↑ Release of AIF protein Impaired endothelial cell function ↑ Autophagy
	Bisen et al. (2019)	Non-human primate (baboon)	Second trimester (GD 90, 100 and 110)	17 mM (BAC) via gastric infusion	Cerebral arteries	TMT labeling LC-MS	Dysregulation in cerebral artery proteome ↑ Mitochondrial proteome Mitochondrial proteins -critical target

This table summarizes key findings from studies investigating the impact of PAE on mitochondrial parameters in neurons, glia (astrocytes, oligodendrocytes, and microglia), and cerebrovasculature. Studies are grouped by species. Alcohol exposure timing, concentrations, and durations vary across studies. Outcomes include changes in mitochondrial morphology, function (such as membrane potential, ATP production), oxidative stress markers, apoptotic signaling, and gene expression

AIF apoptosis-inducing factor, *DCFH-DA* 2′,7′-dichlorodihydrofluorescein diacetate, *GD* gestational day, *GSH* glutathione, *4-HNE* 4-hydroxynonenal, *MDA* malondialdehyde, *MMP* mitochondrial membrane potential, *MTT* 3-(4,5-dimethylthiazol-2-yl)-2,5-diphenyltetrazolium bromide assay, *NOX* NAPDH oxidase, *8-OHdG* 8-hydroxy-2-′-deoxyguanosine, *PAE* prenatal alcohol exposure, *PND* postnatal day, *ROS* reactive oxygen species further amplified apoptotic signaling (Ramachandran et al. 2001). These effects were validated in fetal rat cortical neurons, where alcohol-induced mitochondrial dysfunction accelerated neuronal apoptosis, evidenced by increased ROS production, elevated 4-HNE levels, and activation of caspase-3 (Ramachandran et al. 2003). Similarly, in another study using CD1 mice, alcohol doses of ~33, 65, and 130 mM administered from GDs 6 to 15 (equivalent to the end of the first trimester throughout mid-pregnancy in humans) caused structural impairments in mitochondria isolated from fetal cerebral tissue on gestation day 18. Electron microscopy revealed an increased mitochondrial matrix volume at 65- and 130-mM doses of alcohol. At the higher dose, functional deficits were observed, including reduced activity in respiratory complexes I and II, ATP synthase impairment, and decreased ATP production (Xu et al. 2005). A study using Sprague Dawley rats demonstrated that a single alcohol dose administered on PND 4 (equivalent to the third trimester of human pregnancy) induced Purkinje cell apoptosis, associated with mitochondrial release of cytochrome c (Light et al. 2002). Further evidence from Long-Evans rats fed liquid diets containing varying alcohol concentrations (0%–9.25%) from GD 6 through delivery showed dose-dependent mitochondrial dysfunction in the cerebellum, with blood alcohol levels reaching up to ~51 mM. Cerebellar tissue collected on PND 1 displayed reduced expression of mitochondrial genes for respiratory complexes II, IV, and V, alongside elevated oxidative stress markers, including the p53 apoptosis gene and NADPH oxidase. Additionally, levels of 8-hydroxydeoxyguanosine (8-OHdG), indicating mitochondrial DNA damage, and 4-HNE, a lipid peroxidation byproduct, were elevated in cerebellar granule and Purkinje cells (Chu et al. 2007). Chronic PAE (~87 mM) in Dunkin-Hartley strain guinea pigs from GDs 2 to 64 (equivalent to first through second trimester in humans), resulting in blood alcohol levels of 61 mM, led to significantly reduced fetal and neonatal brain weights, particularly in the hippocampus. Notably, reduced GSH levels were observed specifically in neonatal hippocampal mitochondria, preceding the loss of CA1 pyramidal neurons (Green et al. 2006; McGoey et al. 2003). These findings highlight the hippocampus as particularly vulnerable to PAE-induced mitochondrial dysfunction. In addition to compromising mitochondrial structure and function, PAE disrupts the expression of mitochondrial genes and proteins essential for energy homeostasis. Binge-like alcohol exposure in C57BL/6 mice (48.4 mM alcohol on postnatal day 7) led to long-term dysregulation of 50 synapse-related and 23 mitochondria-related genes as observed on PND 60 in the hippocampus. These gene networks were implicated in neuronal apoptosis, synaptic dysfunction, and behavioral deficits such as memory impairment and anxiety (Arzua et al. 2024). Proteomic analysis of C57BL/6 mice exposed to a 25% alcohol liquid diet from GD 7 to 13 (blood alcohol levels ~11.9 mM) revealed decreased expression of mitochondrial enzymes, including ubiquinol-cytochrome c reductase complex core proteins I and II, ADP/ATP translocase, and ATP synthase subunit α. These enzymes are critical for maintaining mitochondrial membrane potential and energy homeostasis (Sari et al. 2010). Translational studies involving human fetal brain tissue from mothers reporting alcohol consumption have revealed similar mitochondrial vulnerability. They found reduced mitochondrial DNA levels in both human cortical neurons and rat pup cortical neurons, highlighting mitochondrial DNA damage as a potential biomarker for FASD (Darbinian et al. 2023). Importantly, these findings underscore that PAE affects multiple brain regions, including the cortex, cerebellum, and hippocampus, with each exhibiting distinctive alterations in mitochondrial function and oxidative damage that contribute to region-specific neurodevelopmental impairments.

As the primary metabolite of alcohol, acetaldehyde has also been widely studied for its impact on neuron health. Both in vivo rat models and in vitro mouse embryonic cortical cultures demonstrated that alcohol and acetaldehyde exposures induced dose-dependent neurotoxicity during embryonic development. In mouse embryonic cortical cultures, 24-h-long exposure to alcohol (25–100 mM) or acetaldehyde (0.1–10 mM) led to oxidative stress, calcium dysregulation, and apoptosis, with acetaldehyde showing greater toxicity than alcohol (Lee et al. 2005). Furthermore, acetaldehyde exposure in primary neuronal cultures derived from PND 8 rat pups resulted in dose-dependent reductions in cell viability and mitochondrial function, with decreased ATP content observed at 3.5 mM acetaldehyde concentration. PAE downregulated the expression of alcohol- and acetaldehyde-metabolizing enzymes in the cerebellum, exacerbating mitochondrial vulnerability (Tong et al. 2011). Given the accumulating evidence of alcohol-induced mitochondrial dysfunction leading to neuronal injury, several studies have focused on identifying potential neuroprotective strategies. In vitro models using immature human PNET2 neuronal cells showed that prolonged alcohol exposure reduced mitochondrial mass and function, effects mitigated by inhibitors of multiple caspase isoforms and fully reversed by nerve growth factor treatment (de la Monte and Wands 2001). Similarly, cortical neurons from GD 17.5 Sprague Dawley rats exposed to 100 mM alcohol for 12 h exhibited increased mitochondrial membrane depolarization, upregulation of the pro-apoptotic protein Bax, and downregulation of the anti-apoptotic protein Bcl-2. Treatment with metformin and thymoquinone reversed these detrimental changes, suggesting potential pharmacological protection against alcohol-induced mitochondrial dysfunction (Ullah et al. 2012). More recently, an in vitro study using hippocampal neurons from GD 18 Sprague Dawley rats exposed to alcohol concentrations of 25, 50, and 75 mM for 24 h showed elevated ROS levels and, at higher alcohol concentrations, reduced mitochondrial membrane potential, ATP production, superoxide generation, and mitochondrial calcium levels. Mitochondrial length remained unchanged, implying that alcohol disrupts mitochondrial function and calcium homeostasis without altering mitochondrial morphology. Inhibition of NADPH oxidase (NOX) restored mitochondrial function, reinforcing the role of ROS in alcohol-induced mitochondrial dysfunction (Perez et al. 2020).

These studies demonstrate that PAE disrupts mitochondrial morphology and function, impairs respiratory chain activity, increases oxidative stress, triggers apoptotic signaling, and contributes to mitochondrial DNA damage in developing neurons. Together, these mechanisms play a central role in the neurodevelopmental deficits associated with FASD. Future studies are required to elucidate the precise molecular pathways connecting alcohol exposure to impaired mitochondrial biogenesis and dynamics. Moreover, translational studies are warranted to evaluate whether mitochondria-targeted antioxidants or biogenesis enhancers offer therapeutic potential in mitigating FASD outcomes.

8.4.2 Alcohol Modulation of Developing Glial Cell Mitochondria

During brain development, glial cell generation occurs after neurogenesis (Götz and Huttner 2005) and generally starts in the later stages of gestation, around 18–20 weeks in humans (Sasaki et al. 1988; de Azevedo et al. 2003; Zecevic 2004; Howard et al. 2008; Jakovcevski et al. 2009; Zhang et al. 2016). Glial cells, including astrocytes, oligodendrocytes, and microglia, play crucial roles in the development and maturation of the brain. These cells act as nursing cells providing support, protection, and myelination to neurons (Fields and Stevens-Graham 2002; Hanisch and Kettenmann 2007; Feinberg et al. 2010; Allen and Lyons 2018). Given their significant role in regulating neuronal metabolism and managing oxidative stress, glial cell mitochondria are essential for proper glial cell functioning and subsequent neuronal maintenance (Dienel 2017; Barros et al. 2018; Jha and Morrison 2018; McAvoy and Kawamata 2019). PAE can severely affect the mitochondrial function in these glial cells, thus affecting energy production and enhancing oxidative stress (Wilhelm and Guizzetti 2016; Kane and Drew 2021). These mitochondrial alterations may compromise glial cell viability and function, ultimately hindering the proper development of neurons, affecting overall brain growth.

Astrocytes Astrocytes are supporting cells that provide a structural framework for neurons and respond to neuronal injury (Dringen et al. 1999; Wang and Cynader 2000; Sidoryk-Wegrzynowicz et al. 2011; Verkhratsky et al. 2023; Gradisnik and Velnar 2023). PAE has been shown to cause morphological changes, impaired proliferation, and increased oxidative stress in astrocytes (Miller and Potempa 1990; Montoliu et al. 1995; Guizzetti and Costa 2000, 2002; Guizzetti et al. 2003, 2004, 2014; Tsuji et al. 2003; Blanco et al. 2004). Specifically, cortical astrocyte cultures from 2-day-old Sprague Dawley rats (equivalent to the third trimester of human pregnancy; Oberheim et al. 2012) were intermittently treated with 44 and 88 mM alcohol and showed resistance to alcohol-induced oxidative stress and subsequent apoptosis. However, treatment with the higher alcohol concentration (88 mM) for a longer duration (24 h) resulted in a significant decrease in astrocyte cell viability, as revealed by trypan blue exclusion assay and MTT assay (based on mitochondrial succinate dehydrogenase activity; Watts et al. 2005). This study further demonstrated that coculture of fetal cortical neurons with astrocytes in the presence of alcohol (44 and 88 mM) protected the neurons against increased reactive oxygen species (ROS) production and accelerated cell death. This protective effect was attributed to the efflux of GSH from astrocytes, followed by the increased neuronal GSH synthesis.

Furthermore, chronic alcohol exposure (both 44 and 88 mM) for up to 6 days did not significantly alter the GSH content in astrocytes (Rathinam et al. 2006). GSH plays a key role in mitochondrial antioxidant defense and thus is crucial for protecting against oxidative damage. These findings reveal an essential aspect of glial-neuronal interaction, where the astrocytes provide the structural framework for neurons and contribute to sustaining a cellular redox balance and maintaining mitochondrial health. In another study, cortical astrocytes were cultured from 21-day-old rat fetuses and incubated in 25 mM alcohol for 14 days. This treatment enhanced ROS production, increased lipid peroxidation, and reduced GSH content. Notably, this effect was linked to an increased expression of CYP2E1, an alcohol-metabolizing enzyme, as indicated by immunofluorescence staining (Montoliu et al. 1995). This finding suggests that acetaldehyde production in the cultured astrocytes might contribute to the observed oxidative damage. In summary, although astrocytes exhibit protective mechanisms, prolonged or high-level alcohol exposure can overwhelm these defenses and result in mitochondrial dysfunction, which compromises neurodevelopment. The disruption of mitochondrial function and impaired antioxidant systems further exacerbates oxidative damage, which can ultimately impair both glial cell function and neuronal health.

Oligodendrocytes Oligodendrocytes generate myelin, which is crucial for efficient neuronal signal transmission (Barres and Raff 1993; Nave 2010; Gibson et al. 2014; Kuhn et al. 2019). This myelination process begins during gestational week 20 in humans and continues into adulthood (Abraham et al. 2010; Nickel and Gu 2018; Chapman and Hill 2020). PAE leads to disruptions in oligodendrocytes development, increasing apoptotic cell death and impairing myelination (Chiappelli and Taylor 1991; Ozer et al. 2000; Creeley et al. 2013; Newville et al. 2017; Darbinian et al. 2021; Darbinian and Selzer 2022). In an in vitro study, oligodendrocytes cultured from PND 2 Sprague Dawley rats showed that a 10 mM alcohol concentration via liquid diet during the last 2 weeks of gestation decreased the expression of myelin basic protein (MBP), a marker for mature oligodendrocytes (Chiappelli and Taylor 1991). In an FASD mouse model, both acute and long-term impact of alcohol exposure was investigated by administering 35 mM alcohol from postnatal days 3 to 15. This study found a 58% decrease in mature oligodendrocytes and a 75% reduction in proliferating oligodendrocyte in the corpus callosum, as measured by fluorescent staining (Newville et al. 2017). Long-term effects of this alcohol exposure paradigm revealed a recovery in oligodendrocyte numbers by postnatal day 50, though myelin basic protein dysregulation and abnormal white matter microstructures persisted (Newville et al. 2017).

Additionally, a study with non-human primates (Cynomolgus macaques) exposed to a single dose of alcohol (blood alcohol level ~65 mM) during GD 120 (equivalent to the end of second trimester in humans) showed that alcohol exposure triggered oligodendrocytes apoptosis throughout the white matter of the brain (Creeley et al. 2013). In another study, alcohol exposure was found to decrease mature oligodendrocyte numbers, as indicated by increased apoptosis, reduced myelin basic protein expression, and delayed oligodendrocyte differentiation in human fetal brain tissue collected at gestational week 20 (Darbinian et al. 2021). These studies suggest that alcohol exposure likely delays oligodendrocyte maturation and promotes apoptotic signaling, disrupting oligodendrocyte-driven myelination processes. While the mechanisms of these disruptions are still not fully understood, one area that remains particularly underexplored is the role of mitochondria in oligodendrocyte function. Mitochondria play an essential role in cellular health, and their involvement in alcohol-induced damage to oligodendrocyte development and survival could provide valuable insight into the long-term effects of alcohol exposure on myelination.

Microglia Microglia are the primary defense cells that support neurons and help maintain brain homeostasis (Prinz and Mildner 2011; von Bernhardi et al. 2016; Cherry et al. 2016). Both prenatal and postnatal alcohol exposure, studied in vitro (Boyadjieva and Sarkar 2010, 2013a, b) and in vivo (Chastain et al. 2019; Mukherjee et al. 2020) in rat models, has been shown to cause microglial activation in the developing hypothalamus. In one study, cortical microglia cells cultured from GD 19 Sprague Dawley rats were incubated with two different alcohol concentrations (50 and 100 mM) for 24 h. Immunohistochemistry documented that alcohol activated cultured microglia. Alcohol also increased the levels of inflammatory cytokines produced by the microglia. Ultimately, this study showed that alcohol-activated microglia increased apoptotic death in mediobasal hypothalamic neurons (Boyadjieva and Sarkar 2010). In a subsequent study from the same group, the effects of alcohol exposure on cell-cell communication between fetal hypothalamic neurons and microglia were further explored (Boyadjieva and Sarkar 2013a). This study showed that in the presence of microglia, alcohol exposure (25, 50, and 100 mM) for 24 h dose-dependently exacerbated the increase in oxidative stress and promoted increased cell death in neuronal cultures. This effect was attributed to elevated levels of microglial-derived factors, such as oxidants (O_2^-, ROS, and nitrite) and decreased levels of antioxidants (GSH; Boyadjieva and Sarkar 2013b). These studies highlight that microglial activation is closely linked to mitochondrial dysfunction, as alcohol-induced oxidative stress causes an imbalance in mitochondrial dynamics within microglial cells, contributing to the release of harmful ROS, which further exacerbates neuroinflammation.

Furthermore, it was shown that the activation of microglial cells led to decreased production of cyclic adenosine monophosphate (cAMP) and brain-derived neurotrophic factor in neuronal cultures (Boyadjieva and Sarkar 2013b). However, the neuroinflammatory marker was reversed with the supplementation of dibutyryl cyclic adenosine monophosphate (dbcAMP) and brain-derived neurotrophic factor, indicating their protective role against the toxic effects of alcohol-activated microglia (Boyadjieva and Sarkar 2013b). In summary, mitochondrial health in microglia may be crucial in preventing the detrimental outcomes of alcohol-induced damage to both microglia and neurons.

In conclusion, early alcohol exposure significantly impacts glial cell function, particularly mitochondria. Complex interplay among the glial cells and their mitochondrial health maintains neuronal integrity and supports brain maturation. Various studies have shown that prenatal alcohol exposure, both in vitro and in vivo, leads to increased production of oxidants and decreased antioxidant levels. Oxidants or ROS are markers of mitochondrial function, thus suggesting that mitochondria within glial cells are compromised by alcohol exposure. These findings of mitochondrial damage in glial cells highlight a critical pathway through which alcohol may disrupt neuronal maintenance. However, further in vivo and in vitro studies focusing on mitochondrial function, such as oxygen consumption rate assays, are needed to fully elucidate the underlying mechanisms and roles of mitochondria in the pathophysiology of PAE.

8.4.3 Alcohol Modulation of Developing Cerebral Vasculature Mitochondria

The cerebral vasculature, which includes all the arteries, veins, and capillaries responsible for blood circulation within the brain, plays a crucial role in proper neurodevelopment (Agarwal and Carare 2021). These vessels ensure continuous blood flow to various brain regions, supporting progenitor cell migration, oxygen delivery, nutrient supply, and waste removal (Solonskii et al. 2008; Scher 2012; Menshawi et al. 2015)—all of which are essential for brain development (Clarke and Sokoloff 1999). Due to the fundamental role in early brain development, the cerebral vasculature begins to form around 24 days of human gestation. By the beginning of second trimester, the four major arteries comprising the Circle of Willis—the anterior, middle, posterior cerebral arteries, as well as the basilar artery—are formed (Menshawi et al. 2015). Blood flow in these arteries is regulated by myogenic mechanisms, which depend on mitochondrial function (Clarke and Sokoloff 1999). Mitochondria influence numerous cellular processes that are involved in the formation and function of cerebral vasculature (Busija et al. 2016). Some of these include the maintenance of arterial tone (Katakam et al. 2013; Busija et al. 2016), vasoactive responses to physiological and pharmacological stimuli (Xi et al. 2005; Katakam et al. 2014), and apoptosis (Qian et al. 2011; Jiang et al. 2013). Although apoptosis does not directly control moment-to-moment blood flow, it contributes to vascular remodeling, endothelial cell (EC) turnover, and the maintenance of vessel integrity—the essentials for sustaining healthy cerebral circulation over time (Cho et al. 1995, 1997).

While research on PAE and its association with mitochondrial dysfunction in the brain is ongoing (Alhowail 2022), growing evidence suggests that mitochondria within cerebral vasculature may also be a target of PAE (Bukiya 2019). A proteomics study further identified mitochondria-associated proteins as highly sensitive targets for PAE within alcohol-exposed baboon fetal cerebral arteries (Bisen et al. 2019). Despite these findings, there is limited data on mitochondria's physiological role in the developing cerebral vasculature. Even less is known about the pathophysiological consequences of PAE on mitochondrial function within this system. While other studies reported PAE-induced alterations in mitochondrial respiration in brain tissues (previous sections), including specific changes in mitochondrial complex activity, there is virtually no data on such effects in cerebrovascular mitochondria. Given that mitochondria are essential for cellular recovery and neuroprotection following ischemia-reperfusion injury (Lesnefsky et al. 2017; Huang et al. 2023), as well as for regulating blood flow by supplying ECs with the energy required for vascular function (Tang et al. 2014; Wilson et al. 2022), further exploration of mitochondrial dysfunction in the context of PAE is vital for understanding the lasting cerebrovascular effects of FASD.

Studies have demonstrated crosstalk between "NOX and mitochondria," both of which are significant sources of ROS in cerebral vasculature, including endothelial and smooth muscle cells (Paravicini and Touyz 2008; Dikalov 2011; Zorov et al. 2014; Daiber et al. 2016; Schiffer et al. 2020). Under physiological conditions, a delicate balance is maintained to support redox signaling and vascular homeostasis. However, PAE can disrupt this balance by enhancing NOX activation, producing excess ROS (Dong et al. 2009; Drake and Wells 2021). NOX is a family of enzymes that generate ROS by transferring electrons from NADPH to molecular oxygen, primarily producing superoxide and hydrogen peroxide (Ogboo et al. 2022). Emerging evidence highlights a functional link between NOX and mitochondria through redox signaling and oxidative stress (Fukai and Ushio-Fukai 2020). Notably, mitochondria-localized NOX isoforms—particularly NOX2 and NOX4—contribute to a feed-forward loop known as "ROS-induced ROS release," where ROS generated by one source stimulates further ROS production from the other, thereby amplifying oxidative stress (Dong et al. 2009; Dikalov 2011; Fukai and Ushio-Fukai 2020). Acetaldehyde, a toxic metabolite of alcohol, can further stimulate NOX activity, contributing to increased ROS generation and intensifying oxidative damage (Yan and Zhao 2020). As ROS, primarily superoxide, accumulates in response to alcohol-enhanced NOX activity and mitochondrial dysfunction, the cellular antioxidant defenses become overwhelmed (Guo et al. 2013; Bhatti et al. 2017). This excessive ROS content then perpetuates the cycle by further activating NOX, impairing mitochondrial ETC function by inactivating complexes I, II, and III (Ghezzi and Zeviani 2012; Guo et al. 2013). As a result, ATP production is inhibited (Ghezzi and Zeviani 2012), oxidative stress is exacerbated, and both EC and vascular myocyte function are disrupted (Daiber et al. 2016; Bhatti et al. 2017). For example, a study administered Sprague-Dawley dams a liquid diet with or without alcohol (3%) throughout gestation (roughly lasting for 21–23 days; equivalent to the first and second trimester of human pregnancy; Cananzi and Mayhan 2017). Offspring aged 4–6 weeks exhibited impaired cerebral arteriole dilation in response to endothelial agonists, including endothelial nitric oxide synthase (eNOS) and neuronal nitric oxide synthase (nNOS)—both critical in regulating vascular tone and blood flow in the brain. ROS content is known to modulate eNOS and nNOS activity (Tran et al. 2022; Roy et al. 2023), and PAE was found to upregulate NOX2 and NOX4 expression in both parietal cortex tissue and microvessels (Cananzi and Mayhan 2017). Due to the enhanced NOX activity, PAE also increased basal superoxide levels, suggesting that PAE impairs vascular reactivity of eNOS- and nNOS-dependent pathways through increased oxidative stress (Cananzi and Mayhan 2017). Such mitochondrial-NOX crosstalk may represent a key mechanism by which PAE leads to long-term cerebrovascular deficits.

As previously mentioned, cerebral circulation is vital for proper brain function. However, alterations in cerebral blood flow (CBF) and vascular reactivity due to PAE can have profound implications for brain health (Saha and Mayhan 2022; Momin et al. 2023). Mitochondria, which are central to cellular energy production, are particularly sensitive to changes in blood flow and oxygen availability (Schirrmacher 2020). When CBF is compromised, the brain's ability to generate sufficient ATP through oxidative phosphorylation is reduced, potentially resulting in mitochondrial dysfunction (Clemente-Suárez et al. 2023). Studies have shown varied blood flow patterns in response to PAE (Parnell et al. 2007; Bake et al. 2011; Seleverstov et al. 2017; Tobiasz et al. 2018). For example, in a baboon model, repeated PAE (39 mM alcohol) during the second trimester equivalent to human pregnancy—resulting in maternal blood alcohol levels of ~17 mM—led to decreased CBF velocity in the anterior and middle cerebral arteries (Seleverstov et al. 2017; Tobiasz et al. 2018). In a sheep model exposed to a similar alcohol concentration (40 mM), but with higher blood alcohol levels (~40 mM), during the second and third trimester equivalent (GDs 109–132), showed a substantial increase in fetal whole-brain blood perfusion by 37% (Parnell et al. 2007). This increase was region-specific, predominantly occurring in the cerebellum, a region known to be alcohol-sensitive (Parnell et al. 2007). Altered vascular reactivity further contributes to cerebrovascular dysregulation, undermining the brain's ability to maintain adequate CBF (Kunz and Iadecola

2009). Several studies indicate that PAE damages the endothelial lining of blood vessels, impairing their ability to regulate blood flow and contributing to the loss of vascular reactivity (Turcotte et al. 2002). This endothelial dysfunction can promote arterial stiffness (Parkington et al. 2014). In a study examining the susceptibility to brain damage following ischemia/reperfusion injury, offspring prenatally exposed to alcohol (3%) exhibited increased susceptibility due to impaired responses of cerebral arterioles (Cananzi and Mayhan 2019). Similarly, in a mouse FASD model (~52 mM alcohol on GDs 12.5–15.5), normal cerebral artery function was initially observed. Still, adult offspring later demonstrated poorer neurological recovery following transient cerebral ischemia at 3 months of age (Bake et al. 2016). These cerebrovascular alterations suggest that impaired regulation of CBF and oxygen delivery following PAE may be a critical upstream factor contributing to mitochondrial dysfunction and its lasting effects on brain development.

In addition to functional impairments, PAE has also been shown to negatively impact developing cerebral vascular (Momin et al. 2023), which is believed to contribute to alcohol-induced brain abnormalities observed in FAS/FASD cases (Girault et al. 2017). In an in vivo mouse model, subcutaneous injections of either ~22 mM or 65 mM alcohol were administered to pregnant dams from GD 13 throughout GD 19, and brain tissue was harvested from PD2 offspring (Jégou et al. 2012). PAE led to a 30% reduction in vascular network density in the neocortex at the ~22 mM alcohol dose, and a 28% reduction at the 65 mM dose (Jégou et al. 2012). Additionally, the higher alcohol dose significantly altered the orientation of these microvessels (Jégou et al. 2012), suggesting fewer vessels and abnormal vascular patterning. Similarly, in a rat model, oral administration of 143 mM alcohol during PDs 4–10 resulted in enlarged capillary diameters in both the cerebellum and hippocampal—regions especially vulnerable to alcohol-induced injury (Kelly et al. 1990). In cerebral vasculature, ECs contain a higher mitochondrial content than other vascular beds, reflecting the high energetic demands of maintaining the blood-brain barrier (McBride et al. 2006). These cells rely heavily on mitochondrial respiration for energy (Tang et al. 2014; Caja and Enríquez 2017; Wilson et al. 2022). Mitochondrial regulation of vascular tone occurs at the endothelial level, directly influencing vessel diameter and blood flow (Luo et al. 2023; Busija et al. 2016; Reichard and Asosingh 2018). Alcohol's impact on this system is evident in studies showing that PAE alters the activity, plasticity, and survival of ECs (Girault et al. 2017). For instance, incubation of primary mouse brain microvascular endothelial cells (MPMVECs) with 50 mM alcohol for 6 h led to a significant increase in autophagic vacuole concentration in the cortical microvessel endothelium (Girault et al. 2017), indicating mitochondrial stress. Mitochondrial dysfunction within ECs not only impairs vascular tone but also disrupts angiogenesis (Momin et al. 2023), compounding the long-term vascular and metabolic consequences of PAE (Jégou et al. 2012; Girault et al. 2017; Marcu et al. 2017; Saha and Mayhan 2022). These structural abnormalities in the cerebral vasculature may further limit oxygen and nutrient delivery during critical developmental periods, creating an environment of metabolic stress that contributes to mitochondrial dysfunction and impairs long-term neuronal viability.

Beyond its direct effects on cerebral vasculature, PAE has also been shown to suppress autophagy (Girault et al. 2017; Uğuz et al. 2024). The increased frequency of autophagic vacuoles in microvessel endothelium indicates defective or dysregulated autophagy (Girault et al. 2017). Additionally, PD 2 offspring exposed to 65 mM alcohol exhibited decreased expression of vascular endothelial growth factor (VEGF) and its receptors (Jégou et al. 2012). VEGF is a potent regulator of blood vessel formation, and even inactivation of a single VEGF allele has been shown to cause embryonic lethality (Carmeliet et al. 1996). Further evidence suggests that PAE reduces signaling through the VEGF pathway, impairing autophagy by hindering mitochondrial clearance (Momin et al. 2023). Under normal conditions, alcohol activates a protective autophagy response to combat alcohol-mediated neurotoxicity, mainly through the mTOR (mammalian target of rapamycin) pathway (Chen et al. 2012; Pla et al. 2014; Luo 2014; Girault et al. 2017). The mTOR pathway is a central regulator of cell growth, metabolism, and mitochondrial function; when active, it inhibits autophagy, but under stress, its inhibition promotes autophagic clearance of damaged mitochondria (Tang et al. 2014; Li et al. 2022). Disruption of this delicate balance by PAE can impair mitochondrial quality control, accumulation of dysfunctional mitochondria and increased production of ROS (Li et al. 2022). This oxidative stress can induce a paradoxical effect—either suppressing autophagy/mitophagy or triggering excessive mitophagy—which further exacerbate mitochondrial damage and increases apoptosis in developing cerebral arteries (Chen et al. 2012; Bukiya 2019). For instance, PAE in MPMVECs led to a marked decrease in mitochondrial integrity and a significant increase in the release of AIF protein (Girault et al. 2017). This suggests that alcohol-induced EC death is partially mediated by the release of AIF from mitochondria and its subsequent translocation to the nucleus—a hallmark of caspase-independent apoptosis (Girault et al. 2017). These findings indicate that by disrupting key regulators of autophagy and mitochondrial quality control, PAE not only impairs EC function but also initiates a cascade of mitochondrial stress, oxidative damage, and cell death that may underlie persistent cerebrovascular and neural deficits associated with FASD.

In conclusion, mitochondria are integral to the function and health of the cerebrovascular tree, playing a pivotal role in energy production, vascular tone regulation, and EC survival. PAE-induced mitochondrial dysfunction within this system, however, remains understudied. While current evidence indicates significant mitochondrial damage in response to alcohol exposure, particularly in ECs, the precise mechanisms and long-term consequences of this dysfunction in the context of developing cerebrovascular system are not fully understood. Given the critical role of mitochondria in both cerebrovascular and neural health, it is crucial that future research further explores the pathways by which PAE disrupts mitochondrial function within the cerebral vasculature.

8.5 Conclusions

PAE continues to be a major environmental risk factor with lasting consequences for brain development, particularly through its disruption of mitochondrial function (Chen et al. 2003). As central regulators of cellular energy production, oxidative stress balance, and survival pathways, mitochondria are indispensable for supporting healthy neurodevelopment (Cooper 2000; Osellame et al. 2012; Chen et al. 2023). As demonstrated throughout this chapter, PAE can significantly impair mitochondrial function in the developing brain, initiating a cascade of molecular and cellular disturbances that impact both neuronal and vascular integrity.

The deleterious effects of PAE on mitochondria are multifaceted, impairing key functions such as ATP synthesis, mitochondrial dynamics, and the regulation of autophagy and apoptosis. These mitochondrial disruptions compromise the function of neurons and glial cells and extend to the cerebral vasculature, which plays a vital role in brain homeostasis by ensuring adequate blood flow, oxygenation, and metabolic waste clearance. Mitochondria within endothelial and smooth muscle cells of the developing cerebral vasculature appear particularly vulnerable, and their dysfunction may contribute to the structural and functional abnormalities characteristic of FASD.

Despite the advances highlighted here, our understanding of the precise mechanisms by which PAE disrupts mitochondrial function remains incomplete. The complexity of these interactions—spanning diverse brain regions and cell types—underscores the urgent need for continued research. Clarifying the molecular pathways involved in alcohol-induced mitochondrial dysfunction will be crucial for identifying novel therapeutic targets to mitigate or reverse the damage caused by prenatal alcohol exposure.

In conclusion, the evidence presented in this chapter underscores the pivotal role of mitochondria in brain development and illustrates how PAE-induced mitochondrial dysfunction leads to widespread neural and cerebrovascular impairments. Advancing research in this field is essential not only to deepen our understanding of FASD pathophysiology but also to inform the development of effective preventive and therapeutic strategies aimed at improving outcomes for affected individuals.

Acknowledgments Authors deeply thank Dr. Amandeep Bajwa (UT HSC) for critical comments on the manuscript. This work was supported by NIH grant R01 AA028200 (AB).

References

Abel EL (1989) Paternal and maternal alcohol consumption: effects on offspring in two strains of rats. Alcohol Clin Exp Res 13:533–541. https://doi.org/10.1111/j.1530-0277.1989.tb00373.x

Abraham H, Vincze A, Jewgenow I et al (2010) Myelination in the human hippocampal formation from midgestation to adulthood. Int J Dev Neurosci 28:401–410. https://doi.org/10.1016/j.ijdevneu.2010.03.004

Accogli A, Addour-Boudrahem N, Srour M (2020) Neurogenesis, neuronal migration, and axon guidance. Handb Clin Neurol 173:25–42. https://doi.org/10.1016/B978-0-444-64150-2.00004-6

Addabbo F, Montagnani M, Goligorsky MS (2009) Mitochondria and reactive oxygen species. Hypertension 53:885–892. https://doi.org/10.1161/hypertensionaha.109.130054

Afzal S, Abdul Manap AS, Attiq A et al (2023) From imbalance to impairment: the central role of reactive oxygen species in oxidative stress-induced disorders and therapeutic exploration. Front Pharmacol. https://doi.org/10.3389/fphar.2023.1269581

Agarwal N, Carare RO (2021) Cerebral vessels: an overview of anatomy, physiology, and role in the drainage of fluids and solutes. Front Neurol. https://doi.org/10.3389/fneur.2020.611485

Akbari M, Kirkwood TBL, Bohr VA (2019) Mitochondria in the signaling pathways that control longevity and health span. Ageing Res Rev 54:100940. https://doi.org/10.1016/j.arr.2019.100940

Alhowail A (2022) Mechanisms underlying cognitive impairment induced by prenatal alcohol exposure. Brain Sci 12(12):1667. https://doi.org/10.3390/brainsci12121667

Allen NJ, Lyons DA (2018) Glia as architects of central nervous system formation and function. Science 362:181–185

Almeida L, Andreu-Fernández V, Navarro-Tapia E et al (2020) Murine models for the study of fetal alcohol spectrum disorders: an overview. Front Pediatr. https://doi.org/10.3389/fped.2020.00359

Anderson P (2002) Assessment and development of executive function (EF) during childhood. Child Neuropsychol 8:71–82. https://doi.org/10.1076/chin.8.2.71.8724

Archibald S, Fennema-Notestine C, Gamst A et al (2001) Brain dysmorphology in individuals with severe prenatal alcohol exposure. Dev Med Child Neurol 43:148–154. https://pubmed.ncbi.nlm.nih.gov/11263683/. Accessed 14 Apr 2025

Arzua T, Yan Y, Liu X et al (2024) Synaptic and mitochondrial mechanisms behind alcohol-induced imbalance of excitatory/inhibitory synaptic activity and associated cognitive and behavioral abnormalities. Transl Psychiatry 14:51. https://doi.org/10.1038/s41398-024-02748-8

Bailey SM, Pietsch EC, Cunningham CC (1999) Ethanol stimulates the production of reactive oxygen species at mitochondrial complexes I and III. Free Radic Biol Med 27:891–900. https://doi.org/10.1016/s0891-5849(99)00138-0

Bake S, Tingling JD, Miranda RC (2011) Ethanol exposure during pregnancy persistently attenuates cranially directed blood flow in the developing fetus: evidence from ultrasound imaging in a murine second trimester equivalent model. Alcohol Clin Exp Res 36:748–758. https://doi.org/10.1111/j.1530-0277.2011.01676.x

Bake S, Gardner R, Tingling JD et al (2016) Fetal alcohol exposure alters blood flow and neurological responses to transient cerebral ischemia in adult mice. Alcohol Clin Exp Res 41:117–127. https://doi.org/10.1111/acer.13277

Ballantyne JW (1904) Manual of antenatal pathology and hygiene of the embryo. William Green and Sons, Edinburg

Bariselli S, Lovinger DM (2021) Corticostriatal circuit models of cognitive impairments induced by fetal exposure to alcohol. Biol Psychiatry 90:516–528. https://doi.org/10.1016/j.biopsych.2021.05.014

Bariselli S, Reuveni N, Westcott N et al (2023) Postnatal ethanol exposure impairs social behavior and operant extinction in the adult female mouse offspring. Front Neurosci. https://doi.org/10.3389/fnins.2023.1160185

Barres BA, Raff MC (1993) Proliferation of oligodendrocyte precursor cells depends on electrical activity in axons. Nature 361:258–260

Barros LF, Brown A, Swanson RA (2018) Glia in brain energy metabolism: a perspective. Glia 66:1134–1137. https://doi.org/10.1002/glia.23316

Basavarajappa B (2015) Fetal alcohol Spectrum disorder: potential role of endocannabinoids signaling. Brain Sci 5:456–493. https://doi.org/10.3390/brainsci5040456

Bertrand J, Floyd RL, Weber MK (2005) Guidelines for identifying and referring persons with fetal alcohol syndrome. Morb Mortal Wkly Rep Recomm Rep 54:

1-CE. https://www.cdc.gov/mmwr/preview/mmwrhtml/rr5411a1.htm#:~:text=Diagnosis%20of%20FAS%20*%20A%20diagnosis%20ofdocumented%20as%20structural%2C%20neurologic%2C%20or%20functional%20(Box). Accessed 14 Apr 2025

Bhatti JS, Bhatti GK, Reddy PH (2017) Mitochondrial dysfunction and oxidative stress in metabolic disorders—a step towards mitochondria based therapeutic strategies. Biochim Biophys Acta (BBA) - Mol Basis Dis 1863:1066–1077. https://doi.org/10.1016/j.bbadis.2016.11.010

Bisen S, Kakhniashvili D, Johnson DL, Bukiya AN (2019) Proteomic analysis of baboon cerebral artery reveals potential pathways of damage by prenatal alcohol exposure*. Mol Cell Proteomics 18:294–307. https://doi.org/10.1074/mcp.ra118.001047

Blanco AM, Pascual M, Valles SL, Guerri C (2004) Ethanol-induced iNOS and COX-2 expression in cultured astrocytes via NF-κB. Neuroreport 15:681–685. https://doi.org/10.1097/00001756-200403220-00021

Bond AM, Ming GL, Song H (2015) Adult mammalian neural stem cells and neurogenesis: five decades later. Cell Stem Cell 17(4):385–395. https://doi.org/10.1016/j.stem.2015.09.003

Bornstein R, Gonzalez B, Johnson SC (2020) Mitochondrial pathways in human health and aging. Mitochondrion 54:72–84. https://doi.org/10.1016/j.mito.2020.07.007

Boyadjieva NI, Sarkar DK (2010) Role of microglia in ethanol's apoptotic action on hypothalamic neuronal cells in primary cultures. Alcohol Clin Exp Res 34:1835–1842. https://doi.org/10.1111/j.1530-0277.2010.01271.x

Boyadjieva NI, Sarkar DK (2013a) Cyclic adenosine monophosphate and brain-derived neurotrophic factor decreased oxidative stress and apoptosis in developing hypothalamic neuronal cells: role of microglia. Alcohol Clin Exp Res 37:1370–1379. https://doi.org/10.1111/acer.12104

Boyadjieva NI, Sarkar DK (2013b) Microglia play a role in ethanol-induced oxidative stress and apoptosis in developing hypothalamic neurons. Alcohol Clin Exp Res 37:252–262. https://doi.org/10.1111/j.1530-0277.2012.01889.x

Brand MD, Orr AL, Perevoshchikova IV, Quinlan CL (2013) The role of mitochondrial function and cellular bioenergetics in ageing and disease. Br J Dermatol 169 (Suppl 2):1–8. https://doi.org/10.1111/bjd.12208

Bratic A, Larsson N-G (2013) The role of mitochondria in aging. J Clin Invest 123:951–957. https://doi.org/10.1172/jci64125

Brown JM, Bland R, Jonsson E, Greenshaw AJ (2018) A brief history of awareness of the link between alcohol and fetal alcohol spectrum disorder. Can J Psychiatry 64:164–168. https://doi.org/10.1177/0706743718777403

Bukiya AN (2019) Fetal cerebral artery mitochondrion as target of prenatal alcohol exposure. Int J Environ Res Public Health 16:1586. https://doi.org/10.3390/ijerph16091586

Busija DW, Rutkai I, Dutta S, Katakam PV (2016) Role of mitochondria in cerebral vascular function: energy production, cellular protection, and regulation of vascular tone. Compr Physiol:1529–1548. https://doi.org/10.1002/cphy.c150051

Bustamante J, Karadayian AG, Lores-Arnaiz S, Cutrera RA (2012) Alterations of motor performance and brain cortex mitochondrial function during ethanol hangover. Alcohol 46:473–479. https://doi.org/10.1016/j.alcohol.2011.09.027

Caja S, Enríquez JA (2017) Mitochondria in endothelial cells: sensors and integrators of environmental cues. Redox Biol 12:821–827. https://doi.org/10.1016/j.redox.2017.04.021

Cananzi SG, Mayhan WG (2017) In utero exposure to alcohol alters reactivity of cerebral arterioles. J Cereb Blood Flow Metab 39:332–341. https://doi.org/10.1177/0271678x17728163

Cananzi SG, Mayhan WG (2019) In utero exposure to alcohol impairs reactivity of cerebral arterioles and increases susceptibility of the brain to damage following ischemia/reperfusion in adulthood. Alcohol Clin Exp Res 43:607–616. https://doi.org/10.1111/acer.13979

Caputo C, Wood E, Jabbour L (2016) Impact of fetal alcohol exposure on body systems: a systematic review. Birth Defects Res C Embryo Today 108:174–180. https://doi.org/10.1002/bdrc.21129

Carmeliet P, Ferreira V, Breier G et al (1996) Abnormal blood vessel development and lethality in embryos lacking a single VEGF allele. Nature 380:435–439. https://doi.org/10.1038/380435a0

Carter RC, Jacobson JL, Molteno CD et al (2012a) Effects of heavy prenatal alcohol exposure and iron deficiency anemia on child growth and body composition through age 9 years. Alcohol Clin Exp Res 36:1973–1982. https://doi.org/10.1111/j.1530-0277.2012.01810.x

Carter RC, Jacobson JL, Sokol RJ et al (2012b) Fetal alcohol-related growth restriction from birth through young adulthood and moderating effects of maternal prepregnancy weight. Alcohol Clin Exp Res 37:452–462. https://doi.org/10.1111/j.1530-0277.2012.01940.x

Casanova A, Wevers A, Navarro-Ledesma S, Pruimboom L (2023) Mitochondria: it is all about energy. Front Physiol 14:1114231. https://doi.org/10.3389/fphys.2023.1114231

Castellani CA, Longchamps RJ, Sun J et al (2020) Thinking outside the nucleus: mitochondrial DNA copy number in health and disease. Mitochondrion 53:214–223. https://doi.org/10.1016/j.mito.2020.06.004

Cederbaum AI (2012) Alcohol metabolism. Clin Liver Dis 16:667–685. https://doi.org/10.1016/j.cld.2012.08.002

Cederbaum AI, Lieber CS, Rubin E (1974) Effects of chronic ethanol treatment on mitochondrial functions damage to coupling site I. Arch Biochem Biophys 165:560–569. https://doi.org/10.1016/0003-9861(74)90283-5

Center for Substance Abuse Prevention (US) (2014) Literature review. In: Addressing fetal alcohol spectrum disorders (FASD). https://www.ncbi.nlm.nih.gov/books/NBK344235/. Accessed 14 Apr 2025

Centers for Disease Control and Prevention (CDC) (2024) About alcohol use during pregnancy. Clin Obstet Gynecol 62:142–155. https://www.cdc.gov/alcohol-pregnancy/about/index.html#:~:text=Alcohol%20use%20during%20pregnancy%20mightare%20trying%20to%20get%20pregnant. Accessed 1 May 2025

Chapman TW, Hill RA (2020) Myelin plasticity in adulthood and aging. Neurosci Lett 715:134645. https://doi.org/10.1016/j.neulet.2019.134645

Chastain LG, Franklin T, Gangisetty O et al (2019) Early life alcohol exposure primes hypothalamic microglia to later-life hypersensitivity to immune stress: possible epigenetic mechanism. Neuropsychopharmacology 44:1579–1588

Chen WJ, Maier SE, Parnell SE et al (2003) Alcohol and the developing brain: neuroanatomical studies. Alcohol Res Health 27(2):174–180

Chen G, Ke Z, Xu M et al (2012) Autophagy is a protective response to ethanol neurotoxicity. Autophagy 8: 1577–1589. https://doi.org/10.4161/auto.21376

Chen W, Zhao H, Li Y (2023) Mitochondrial dynamics in health and disease: mechanisms and potential targets. Signal Transduct Target Ther 8(1):333. https://doi.org/10.1038/s41392-023-01547-9

Chen T-H, Wang H-C, Chang C-J, Lee S-Y (2024a) Mitochondrial glutathione in cellular redox homeostasis and disease manifestation. Int J Mol Sci 25:1314. https://doi.org/10.3390/ijms25021314

Chen X, Luo Y, Zhu Q et al (2024b) Small extracellular vesicles from young plasma reverse age-related functional declines by improving mitochondrial energy metabolism. Nat Aging 4:814–838. https://doi.org/10.1038/s43587-024-00612-4

Cherry JD, Tripodis Y, Alvarez VE et al (2016) Microglial neuroinflammation contributes to tau accumulation in chronic traumatic encephalopathy. Acta Neuropathol Commun 4:112

Chiappelli F, Taylor AN, de los Monteros AE, de Vellis J (1991) Fetal alcohol delays the developmental expression of myelin basic protein and transferrin in rat primary oligodendrocyte cultures. Int J Dev Neurosci 9:67–75. https://doi.org/10.1016/0736-5748(91)90074-v

Cho A, Courtman DW, Langille BL (1995) Apoptosis (programmed cell death) in arteries of the neonatal lamb. Circ Res 76:168–175

Cho A, Mitchell L, Koopmans D, Langille BL (1997) Effects of changes in blood flow rate on cell death and cell proliferation in carotid arteries of immature rabbits. Circ Res 81:328–337

Cho YM, Kwon S, Pak YK et al (2006) Dynamic changes in mitochondrial biogenesis and antioxidant enzymes during the spontaneous differentiation of human embryonic stem cells. Biochem Biophys Res Commun 348:1472–1478. https://doi.org/10.1016/j.bbrc.2006.08.020

Chu J, Tong M, de la Monte SM (2007) Chronic ethanol exposure causes mitochondrial dysfunction and oxidative stress in immature central nervous system neurons. Acta Neuropathol 1174:142–151. https://doi.org/10.1007/s00401-007-0199-4

Clarke DD, Sokoloff L (1999) Circulation and energy metabolism of the brain. In: Basic neurochemistry: molecular, cellular and medical aspects, 6th edn https://www.ncbi.nlm.nih.gov/books/NBK20413/. Accessed 1 May 2025

Clarren SK, Alvord EC, Sumi SM et al (1978) Brain malformations related to prenatal exposure to ethanol. J Pediatr 92:64–67. https://doi.org/10.1016/s0022-3476(78)80072-9

Clemente-Suárez V, Redondo-Flórez L, Beltrán-Velasco A et al (2023) Mitochondria and brain disease: a comprehensive review of pathological mechanisms and therapeutic opportunities. Biomedicine 11:2488. https://doi.org/10.3390/biomedicines11092488

Connor PD, Streissguth AP (1996) Effects of prenatal exposure to alcohol across the life span. Alcohol Health Res World 20:170–174

Connor PD, Sampson PD, Bookstein FL et al (2000) Direct and indirect effects of prenatal alcohol damage on executive function. Dev Neuropsychol 18:331–354. https://pubmed.ncbi.nlm.nih.gov/11385829/. Accessed 14 Apr 2025

Cooper GM (2000) Mitochondria. In: The cell: a molecular approach, 2nd edn https://www.ncbi.nlm.nih.gov/books/NBK9896/#:~:text=Mitochondria%20are%20surrounded%20by%20amajor%20working%20compartments%20of%20mitochondria. Accessed 14 Apr 2025

Creeley CE, Dikranian KT, Johnson SA et al (2013) Alcohol-induced apoptosis of oligodendrocytes in the fetal macaque brain. Acta Neuropathol Commun 1:23. https://doi.org/10.1186/2051-5960-1-23

Crocker N, Vaurio L, Riley EP, Mattson SN (2011) Comparison of verbal learning and memory in children with heavy prenatal alcohol exposure or attention-deficit/hyperactivity disorder. Alcohol Clin Exp Res 35: 1114–1121. https://doi.org/10.1111/j.1530-0277.2011.01444.x

Cunningham CC, Coleman WB, Spach PI (1990) The effects of chronic ethanol consumption on hepatic mitochondrial energy metabolism. Alcohol Alcohol 25:127–136. https://doi.org/10.1093/oxfordjournals.alcalc.a044987

Daiber A, Di Lisa F, Oelze M et al (2016) Crosstalk of mitochondria with NADPH oxidase via reactive oxygen and nitrogen species signalling and its role for vascular function. Br J Pharmacol 174:1670–1689. https://doi.org/10.1111/bph.13403

Darbinian N, Selzer ME (2022) Oligodendrocyte pathology in fetal alcohol spectrum disorders. Neural Regen Res 17:497–502. https://doi.org/10.4103/1673-5374.314294

Darbinian N, Darbinyan A, Merabova N et al (2021) Ethanol-mediated alterations in oligodendrocyte differentiation in the developing brain. Neurobiol Dis 148:105181. https://doi.org/10.1016/j.nbd.2020.105181

Darbinian N, Darbinyan A, Merabova N et al (2023) In utero ethanol exposure induces mitochondrial DNA damage and inhibits mtDNA repair in developing brain. Front Neurosci. https://doi.org/10.3389/fnins.2023.1214958

Day NL, Leech SL, Richardson GA et al (2002) Prenatal alcohol exposure predicts continued deficits in offspring size at 14 years of age. Alcohol Clin Exp Res 26:1584–1591. https://pubmed.ncbi.nlm.nih.gov/12394293/. Accessed 14 Apr 2025

de Azevedo LC, Fallet C, Moura-Neto V et al (2003) Cortical radial glial cells in human fetuses: depth-correlated transformation into astrocytes. J Neurobiol 55:288–298. https://doi.org/10.1002/neu.10205

de la Monte SM, Wands JR (2001) Mitochondrial DNA damage and impaired mitochondrial function contribute to apoptosis of insulin-stimulated ethanol-exposed neuronal cells. Alcohol Clin Exp Res 25(6):898–906

de la Monte SM, Wands JR (2002) Chronic gestational exposure to ethanol impairs insulin-stimulated survival and mitochondrial function in cerebellar neurons. Cell Mol Life Sci 59:882–893. https://doi.org/10.1007/s00018-002-8475-x

Denny CH, Acero CS, Naimi TS, Kim SY (2019) Consumption of alcohol beverages and binge drinking among pregnant women aged 18–44 years—United States, 2015–2017. MMWR Morb Mortal Wkly Rep 68:365–368. https://doi.org/10.15585/mmwr.mm6816a1

Devi BG, Henderson GI, Frosto TA, Schenker S (1993) Effect of ethanol on rat fetal hepatocytes: studies on cell replication, lipid peroxidation and glutathione. Hepatology 18:648–659. https://doi.org/10.1002/hep.1840180325

Dienel GA (2017) The metabolic trinity, glucose-glycogen-lactate, links astrocytes and neurons in brain energetics, signaling, memory, and gene expression. Neurosci Lett 637:18–25

Dikalov S (2011) Cross talk between mitochondria and NADPH oxidases. Free Radic Biol Med 51:1289–1301. https://doi.org/10.1016/j.freeradbiomed.2011.06.033

Dobson CC, Mongillo DL, Brien DC et al (2012) Chronic prenatal ethanol exposure increases adiposity and disrupts pancreatic morphology in adult guinea pig offspring. Nutr Diabetes. https://doi.org/10.1038/nutd.2012.31

Dodge NC, Thomas KG, Meintjes EM et al (2020) Reduced hippocampal volumes partially mediate effects of prenatal alcohol exposure on spatial navigation on a virtual water maze task in children. Alcohol Clin Exp Res 44:844–855. https://doi.org/10.1111/acer.14310

Dong J, Sulik KK, Chen S (2009) The role of NOx enzymes in ethanol-induced oxidative stress and apoptosis in mouse embryos. Toxicol Lett 193:94–100. https://doi.org/10.1016/j.toxlet.2009.12.012

Doyle LR, Mattson SN (2015) Neurobehavioral disorder associated with prenatal alcohol exposure (ND-pae): review of evidence and guidelines for assessment. Curr Dev Disord Rep 2:175–186. https://doi.org/10.1007/s40474-015-0054-6

Drake DM, Wells PG (2021) Novel mechanisms in alcohol neurodevelopmental disorders via BRCA1 depletion and BRCA1-dependent NADPH oxidase regulation. Redox Biol 48:102148. https://doi.org/10.1016/j.redox.2021.102148

Dringen R, Pfeiffer B, Hamprecht B (1999) Synthesis of the antioxidant glutathione in neurons: supply by astrocytes of CysGly as precursor for neuronal glutathione. J Neurosci 19:562–569. https://doi.org/10.1523/JNEUROSCI.19-02-00562.1999

Efremov RG, Sazanov LA (2011) Respiratory complex I: 'steam engine' of the cell? Curr Opin Struct Biol 21(4):532–540. https://doi.org/10.1016/j.sbi.2011.07.002

Eisner V, Cupo RR, Gao E et al (2017) Mitochondrial fusion dynamics is robust in the heart and depends on calcium oscillations and contractile activity. Proc Natl Acad Sci. https://doi.org/10.1073/pnas.1617288114

El-Merhie N, Baumgart-Vogt E, Pilatz A et al (2017) Differential alterations of the mitochondrial morphology and respiratory chain complexes during postnatal development of the mouse lung. Oxid Med Cell Longev. https://doi.org/10.1155/2017/9169146

Facucho-Oliveira JM, St John JC (2009) The relationship between pluripotency and mitochondrial DNA proliferation during early embryo development and embryonic stem cell differentiation. Stem Cell Rev Rep 5:140–158. https://pubmed.ncbi.nlm.nih.gov/19521804/. Accessed 14 Apr 2025

Feinberg K, Eshed-Eisenbach Y, Frechter S et al (2010) A glial signal consisting of gliomedin and NrCAM clusters axonal Na+ channels during the formation of nodes of Ranvier. Neuron 65:490–502. https://doi.org/10.1016/j.neuron.2010.02.004

Fields RD, Stevens-Graham B (2002) New insights into neuron–glia communication. Science 298:556–562

Finsterer J (2008) Cognitive decline as a manifestation of mitochondrial disorders (mitochondrial dementia). J Neurol Sci 272:20–33. https://doi.org/10.1016/j.jns.2008.05.011

Forum on Neuroscience and Nervous System Disorders (2013) Mitochondrial pathology. In: Neurodegeneration: exploring commonalities across diseases: workshop summary. https://www.ncbi.nlm.nih.gov/books/NBK208519/#:~:text=Mitochondria%20are%20cellular%20organelles%20responsibleconsumes%2020%20percent%20of%20oxygen. Accessed 14 Apr 2025

Frederick RL, Shaw JM (2007) Moving mitochondria: establishing distribution of an essential organelle. Traffic 8:1668–1675. https://doi.org/10.1111/j.1600-0854.2007.00644.x

Fukai T, Ushio-Fukai M (2020) Cross-talk between NADPH oxidase and mitochondria: role in ROS Signaling and angiogenesis. Cells 9(8):1849. https://doi.org/10.3390/cells9081849

Gao L, Grebogi C, Lai Y-C et al (2019) Quantitative assessment of cerebral connectivity deficiency and cognitive impairment in children with prenatal alcohol exposure. Chaos. https://doi.org/10.1063/1.5089527

Gauthier TW (2015) Prenatal alcohol exposure and the developing immune system. Alcohol Res Curr Rev 37:279. https://pmc.ncbi.nlm.nih.gov/articles/PMC4590623/. Accessed 14 Apr 2025

Gerhold MM, Jacobson SW, Jacobson JL et al (2016) An ERP study of response inhibition in the auditory domain in children with fetal alcohol spectrum disorders. Alcohol Clin Exp Res 41:96–106. https://doi.org/10.1111/acer.13263

Ghezzi D, Zeviani M (2012) Assembly factors of human mitochondrial respiratory chain complexes: physiology and pathophysiology. Adv Exp Med Biol:65–106. https://doi.org/10.1007/978-1-4614-3573-0_4

Gibson EM, Purger D, Mount CW et al (2014) Neuronal activity promotes oligodendrogenesis and adaptive myelination in the mammalian brain. Science 344: 1252304

Gil-Mohapel J, Titterness AK, Patten AR, Taylor S, Ratzlaff A, Ratzlaff T, Helfer J, Christie BR (2014) Prenatal ethanol exposure differentially affects hippocampal neurogenesis in the adolescent and aged brain. Neuroscience 273:174–188. https://doi.org/10.1016/j.neuroscience.2014.05.012

Girard TA, Xing HC, Ward GR, Wainwright PE (2000) Early postnatal ethanol exposure has long-term effects on the performance of male rats in a delayed matching-to-place task in the Morris water maze. Alcohol Clin Exp Res 24:300–306. https://pubmed.ncbi.nlm.nih.gov/10776666/. Accessed 14 Apr 2025

Girault V, Gilard V, Marguet F et al (2017) Prenatal alcohol exposure impairs autophagy in neonatal brain cortical microvessels. Cell Death Dis. https://doi.org/10.1038/cddis.2017.29

Goodlett CR, Horn KH (2001) Mechanisms of alcohol-induced damage to the developing nervous system. Alcohol Res Health 25(3):175–184

Gosdin LK, Deputy NP, Kim SY et al (2022) Alcohol consumption and binge drinking during pregnancy among adults aged 18–49 years—United States, 2018–2020. MMWR Morb Mortal Wkly Rep 71:10–13. https://doi.org/10.15585/mmwr.mm7101a2

Götz M, Huttner WB (2005) The cell biology of neurogenesis. Nat Rev Mol Cell Biol 6:777–788

Gradisnik L, Velnar T (2023) Astrocytes in the central nervous system and their functions in health and disease: a review. World J Clin Cases 11:3385–3394. https://doi.org/10.12998/wjcc.v11.i15.3385

Green CR, Watts LT, Kobus SM et al (2006) Effects of chronic prenatal ethanol exposure on mitochondrial glutathione and 8-iso-prostaglandin F2alpha concentrations in the hippocampus of the perinatal guinea pig. Reprod Fertil Dev 18(5):517–524. https://doi.org/10.1071/rd05128

Green CR, Mihic AM, Nikkel SM et al (2009) Executive function deficits in children with fetal alcohol spectrum disorders (FASD) measured using the Cambridge neuropsychological tests automated battery (CANTAB). J Child Psychol Psychiatry Allied Discip 50:688–697. https://pubmed.ncbi.nlm.nih.gov/19175817/. Accessed 14 Apr 2025

Green A, Hossain T, Eckmann DM (2022) Mitochondrial dynamics involves molecular and mechanical events in motility, fusion and fission. Front Cell Dev Biol. https://doi.org/10.3389/fcell.2022.1010232

Guizzetti M, Costa LG (2000) Possible role of protein kinase C zeta in muscarinic receptor-induced proliferation of astrocytoma cells. Biochem Pharmacol 60: 1457–1466. https://doi.org/10.1016/s0006-2952(00)00468-8

Guizzetti M, Costa LG (2002) Effect of ethanol on protein kinase Czeta and p70S6 kinase activation by carbachol: a possible mechanism for ethanol-induced inhibition of glial cell proliferation. J Neurochem 82:38–46. https://doi.org/10.1046/j.1471-4159.2002.00942.x

Guizzetti M, Bordi F, Dieguez-Acuña FJ et al (2003) Nuclear factor kappaB activation by muscarinic receptors in astroglial cells: effect of ethanol. Neuroscience 120:941–950. https://doi.org/10.1016/s0306-4522(03)00401-9

Guizzetti M, Thompson BD, Kim Y et al (2004) Role of phospholipase D signaling in ethanol-induced inhibition of carbachol-stimulated DNA synthesis of 1321N1 astrocytoma cells. J Neurochem 90:646–653. https://doi.org/10.1111/j.1471-4159.2004.02541.x

Guizzetti M, Zhang X, Goeke C, Gavin DP (2014) Glia and neurodevelopment: focus on fetal alcohol spectrum disorders. Front Pediatr 2:123. https://doi.org/10.3389/fped.2014.00123

Gulati A (2015) Understanding neurogenesis in the adult human brain. Indian J Pharmacol 47(6):583–584. https://doi.org/10.4103/0253-7613.169598

Guo C, Sun L, Chen X, Zhang D (2013) Oxidative stress, mitochondrial damage and neurodegenerative diseases. Neural Regen Res 8:2003–2014

Gupta KK, Gupta VK, Shirasaka T (2016) An update on fetal alcohol syndrome—pathogenesis, risks, and treatment. Alcohol Clin Exp Res 40:1594–1602. https://doi.org/10.1111/acer.13135

Hagan JF Jr, Balachova T, Bertrand J et al (2016) Neurobehavioral disorder associated with prenatal alcohol exposure. Pediatrics 138(4):e20151553. https://doi.org/10.1542/peds.2015-1553

Hajnóczky G, Buzas CJ, Pacher P et al (2005) Alcohol and mitochondria in cardiac apoptosis: mechanisms and visualization. Alcohol Clin Exp Res 29:693–701. https://doi.org/10.1097/01.alc.0000163493.45344.7a

Hamanaka RB, Chandel NS (2010) Mitochondrial reactive oxygen species regulate cellular signaling and dictate biological outcomes. Trends Biochem Sci 35(9): 505–513. https://doi.org/10.1016/j.tibs.2010.04.002

Han D, Ybanez MD, Johnson HS et al (2012) Dynamic adaptation of liver mitochondria to chronic alcohol feeding in mice. J Biol Chem 287:42165–42179. https://doi.org/10.1074/jbc.m112.377374

Han D, Johnson HS, Rao MP et al (2016) Mitochondrial remodeling in the liver following chronic alcohol feeding to rats. Free Radic Biol Med 102:100–110. https://doi.org/10.1016/j.freeradbiomed.2016.11.020

Hanisch UK, Kettenmann H (2007) Microglia: active sensor and versatile effector cells in the normal and pathologic brain. Nat Neurosci 10:1387–1394. https://doi.org/10.1038/nn1997

He L, He T, Farrar S et al (2017) Antioxidants maintain cellular redox homeostasis by elimination of reactive oxygen species. Cell Physiol Biochem 44:532–553. https://doi.org/10.1159/000485089

Helmenstine A (2025) Mitochondria—definition, structure, function. Sci Notes Proj. https://sciencenotes.org/mitochondria-definition-structure-function/. Accessed 14 Apr 2025

Henderson GI, Chen JJ, Schenker S (1995) In utero ethanol elicits oxidative stress in the rat fetus. Alcohol Clin Exp Res 19(3):714–720. https://doi.org/10.1111/j.1530-0277.1995.tb01572.x

Henderson GI, Chen JJ, Schenker S (1999) Ethanol, oxidative stress, reactive aldehydes, and the fetus. Front Biosci 4:541–550. https://pubmed.ncbi.nlm.nih.gov/10369807/. Accessed 14 Apr 2025

Hoek JB, Cahill A, Pastorino JG (2002) Alcohol and mitochondria: a dysfunctional relationship. Gastroenterology 122:2049–2063. https://doi.org/10.1053/gast.2002.33613

Holman PJ, Ellis L, Morgan E, Weinberg J (2018) Prenatal alcohol exposure disrupts male adolescent social behavior and oxytocin receptor binding in rodents. Horm Behav 105:115–127. https://doi.org/10.1016/j.yhbeh.2018.08.004

Howard BM, Mo Z, Filipovic R et al (2008) Radial glia cells in the developing human brain. Neuroscientist 14: 459–473. https://doi.org/10.1177/1073858407313512

Huang J, Chen L, Yao Z et al (2023) The role of mitochondrial dynamics in cerebral ischemia-reperfusion injury. Biomed Pharmacother 162:114671. https://doi.org/10.1016/j.biopha.2023.114671

Jacobson JL, Akkaya-Hocagil T, Ryan LM et al (2021) Effects of prenatal alcohol exposure on cognitive and behavioral development: findings from a hierarchical meta-analysis of data from six prospective longitudinal U.S. cohorts. Alcohol Clin Exp Res 45:2040–2058. https://doi.org/10.1111/acer.14686

Jakovcevski I, Filipovic R, Mo Z et al (2009) Oligodendrocyte development and the onset of myelination in the human fetal brain. Front Neuroanat 3:5. https://doi.org/10.3389/neuro.05.005.2009

Jańczewska I, Wierzba J, Cichoń-Kotek M, Jańczewska A (2019) Fetal alcohol spectrum disorders—diagnostic difficulties in the neonatal period and new diagnostic approaches. Dev Period Med 23:60. https://doi.org/10.34763/devperiodmed.20192301.6066. Accessed 14 Apr 2025

Jégou S, El Ghazi F, de Lendeu PK et al (2012) Prenatal alcohol exposure affects vasculature development in the neonatal brain. Ann Neurol 72:952–960. https://doi.org/10.1002/ana.23699

Jha MK, Morrison BM (2018) Glia-neuron energy metabolism in health and diseases: new insights into the role of nervous system metabolic transporters. Exp Neurol 309:23–31. https://doi.org/10.1016/j.expneurol.2018.07.009

Jiang L, Liu Y, Ma M-M et al (2013) Mitochondria dependent pathway is involved in the protective effect of bestrophin-3 on hydrogen peroxide-induced apoptosis in basilar artery smooth muscle cells. Apoptosis 18: 556–565. https://doi.org/10.1007/s10495-013-0828-4

Jones KL, Smith DW (1973) Recognition of the fetal alcohol syndrome in early infancy. Lancet 302:999–1001. https://doi.org/10.1016/s0140-6736(73)91092-1

Jung ME (2014) Alcohol withdrawal and cerebellar mitochondria. Cerebellum 14:421–437. https://doi.org/10.1007/s12311-014-0598-8

Kable JA, Mukherjee RA (2017) Neurodevelopmental disorder associated with prenatal exposure to alcohol (ND-PAE): a proposed diagnostic method of capturing the neurocognitive phenotype of FASD. Eur J Med Genet 60(1):49–54. https://doi.org/10.1016/j.ejmg.2016.09.013

Kane CJM, Drew PD (2021) Neuroinflammatory contribution of microglia and astrocytes in fetal alcohol spectrum disorders. J Neurosci Res 99:1973–1985. https://doi.org/10.1002/jnr.24735

Katakam PVG, Wappler EA, Katz PS et al (2013) Depolarization of mitochondria in endothelial cells promotes cerebral artery vasodilation by activation of nitric oxide synthase. Arterioscler Thromb Vasc Biol 33: 752–759. https://doi.org/10.1161/atvbaha.112.300560

Katakam PV, Gordon AO, Sure VN et al (2014) Diversity of mitochondria-dependent dilator mechanisms in vascular smooth muscle of cerebral arteries from normal and insulin-resistant rats. Am J Phys Heart Circ Phys. https://doi.org/10.1152/ajpheart.00091.2014

Kelly SJ, Pierce DR, West JR (1987) Microencephaly and hyperactivity in adult rats can be induced by neonatal exposure to high blood alcohol concentrations. Exp Neurol 96:580–593. https://doi.org/10.1016/0014-4886(87)90220-2

Kelly SJ, Mahoney JC, West JR (1990) Changes in brain microvasculature resulting from early postnatal alcohol exposure. Alcohol 7:43–47. https://doi.org/10.1016/0741-8329(90)90059-1

Kelly SJ, Day N, Streissguth AP (2000) Effects of prenatal alcohol exposure on social behavior in humans and

other species. Neurotoxicol Teratol 22:143–149. https://doi.org/10.1016/s0892-0362(99)00073-2
Kenna K, Sozo F, De Matteo R et al (2012) Alcohol exposure during late gestation: multiple developmental outcomes in sheep. J Dev Orig Health Dis 3:224–236. https://doi.org/10.1017/s2040174412000244
Khacho M, Slack RS (2017) Mitochondrial dynamics in the regulation of neurogenesis: from development to the adult brain. Dev Dyn 247:47–53. https://doi.org/10.1002/dvdy.24538
Khacho M, Clark A, Svoboda DS et al (2017) Mitochondrial dysfunction underlies cognitive defects as a result of neural stem cell depletion and impaired neurogenesis. Hum Mol Genet 26:3327–3341. https://doi.org/10.1093/hmg/ddx217
Kim S, Beck J, Bieniarz T et al (2001) A rodent model of alcoholic heart muscle disease and its evaluation by echocardiography. Alcohol Clin Exp Res 25:457–463
Klemmensen MM, Borrowman SH, Pearce C et al (2023) Mitochondrial dysfunction in neurodegenerative disorders. Neurotherapeutics. https://doi.org/10.1016/j.neurot.2023.10.002
Kotch LE, Sulik KK (1992) Experimental fetal alcohol syndrome: proposed pathogenic basis for a variety of associated facial and brain anomalies. Am J Med Genet 44:168–176. https://doi.org/10.1002/ajmg.1320440210
Kroemer G, Galluzzi L, Brenner C (2007) Mitochondrial membrane permeabilization in cell death. Physiol Rev 87:99–163. https://doi.org/10.1152/physrev.00013.2006
Kuhn S, Gritti L, Crooks D, Dombrowski Y (2019) Oligodendrocytes in development, myelin generation and beyond. Cells 8:1424. https://doi.org/10.3390/cells8111424
Kunz A, Iadecola C (2009) Chapter 14 cerebral vascular dysregulation in the ischemic brain. Handb Clin Neurol:283–305. https://doi.org/10.1016/s0072-9752(08)01914-3
Kwong JQ, Molkentin JD (2015) Physiological and pathological roles of the mitochondrial permeability transition pore in the heart. Cell Metab 21:206–214. https://doi.org/10.1016/j.cmet.2014.12.001
Lam CK, Zhao W, Liu G-S et al (2015) Hax-1 regulates cyclophilin-D levels and mitochondria permeability transition pore in the heart. Proc Natl Acad Sci. https://doi.org/10.1073/pnas.1508760112
Lange S, Probst C, Gmel G et al (2017) Global prevalence of fetal alcohol spectrum disorder among children and youth. JAMA Pediatr 171:948. https://doi.org/10.1001/jamapediatrics.2017.1919
Larkby C, Day N (1997) The effects of prenatal alcohol exposure. Alcohol Health Res World 21:192. https://pmc.ncbi.nlm.nih.gov/articles/PMC6826810/. Accessed 14 Apr 2025
Laurent D, Mathew JE, Mitry M et al (2014) Chronic ethanol consumption increases myocardial mitochondrial DNA mutations: a potential contribution by mitochondrial topoisomerases. Alcohol Alcohol 49: 381–389. https://doi.org/10.1093/alcalc/agu029
Lee RD, An SM, Kim SS et al (2005) Neurotoxic effects of alcohol and acetaldehyde during embryonic development. J Toxicol Environ Health A 68(23–24): 2147–2162. https://doi.org/10.1080/15287390500177255
Lee S, Xu H, Van Vleck A et al (2022) B-cell succinate dehydrogenase deficiency triggers metabolic dysfunction and insulinopenic diabetes. Diabetes 71:1439–1453. https://doi.org/10.2337/db21-0834
Lemieux H, Hoppel CL (2009) Mitochondria in the human heart. J Bioenerg Biomembr 41:99–106. https://doi.org/10.1007/s10863-009-9211-0
Lemoine P, Harousseau H, Borteyru JP et al (1968) Les enfants de parents alcooliques: anomalies observes a propos de 127 cases (children of alcohol parents: abnormalities observed in 127 cases). Ouest Med 25: 476–482
Lesnefsky EJ, Chen Q, Tandler B, Hoppel CL (2017) Mitochondrial dysfunction and myocardial ischemia-reperfusion: implications for novel therapies. Annu Rev Pharmacol Toxicol 57:535–565. https://doi.org/10.1146/annurev-pharmtox-010715-103335
Lewis CE, Thomas KG, Molteno CD et al (2016) Prospective memory impairment in children with prenatal alcohol exposure. Alcohol Clin Exp Res 40:969–978. https://doi.org/10.1111/acer.13045
Li A, Gao M, Liu B et al (2022) Mitochondrial autophagy: molecular mechanisms and implications for cardiovascular disease. Cell Death Dis. https://doi.org/10.1038/s41419-022-04906-6
Light KE, Belcher SM, Pierce DR (2002) Time course and manner of Purkinje neuron death following ethanol exposure on postnatal day 4 in the rat. Neuroscience 114(2):327–337. https://doi.org/10.1016/s0306-4522(02)00344-5
Liu X, Kayser M, Kushner SA et al (2023) Association between prenatal alcohol exposure and children's facial shape: a prospective population-based cohort study. Hum Reprod 38:961–972. https://doi.org/10.1093/humrep/dead006
Louth EL, Bignell W, Taylor CL, Bailey CDC (2016) Developmental ethanol exposure leads to long-term deficits in attention and its underlying prefrontal circuitry. eNeuro. https://doi.org/10.1523/eneuro.0267-16.2016
Lumeng JC, Cabral HJ, Gannon K et al (2007) Pre-natal exposures to cocaine and alcohol and physical growth patterns to age 8 years. Neurotoxicol Teratol 29:446–457. https://doi.org/10.1016/j.ntt.2007.02.004
Luo J (2014) Autophagy and ethanol neurotoxicity. Autophagy 10:2099–2108. https://doi.org/10.4161/15548627.2014.981916
Luo Z, Yao J, Wang Z, Xu J (2023) Mitochondria in endothelial cells angiogenesis and function: current understanding and future perspectives. J Transl Med. https://doi.org/10.1186/s12967-023-04286-1

Mahmoud AI (2023) Metabolic switches during development and regeneration. Development. https://doi.org/10.1242/dev.202008

Mailloux RJ (2018) Mitochondrial antioxidants and the maintenance of cellular hydrogen peroxide levels. Oxid Med Cell Longev. https://doi.org/10.1155/2018/7857251

Malik S, Vinukonda G, Vose LR et al (2013) Neurogenesis continues in the third trimester of pregnancy and is suppressed by premature birth. J Neurosci 33(2):411–423. https://doi.org/10.1523/JNEUROSCI.4445-12.2013

Manzo-Avalos S, Saavedra-Molina A (2010) Cellular and mitochondrial effects of alcohol consumption. Int J Environ Res Public Health 7:4281–4304. https://doi.org/10.3390/ijerph7124281

Marcinkeviciute A, Mildaziene V, Crumm S et al (2000) Kinetics and control of oxidative phosphorylation in rat liver mitochondria after chronic ethanol feeding. Biochem J 349:519–526. https://doi.org/10.1042/bj3490519

Marcu R, Zheng Y, Hawkins BJ (2017) Mitochondria and angiogenesis. Adv Exp Med Biol:371–406. https://doi.org/10.1007/978-3-319-55330-6_21

Marí M, Morales A, Colell A et al (2009) Mitochondrial glutathione, a key survival antioxidant. Antioxid Redox Signal 11:2685–2700. https://doi.org/10.1089/ars.2009.2695

Marin-Garcia J, Ananthakrishnan R, Goldenthal MJ (1996) Mitochondrial dysfunction after fetal alcohol exposure. Alcohol Clin Exp Res 20(6):1029–1032. https://doi.org/10.1111/j.1530-0277.1996.tb01942.x

Martinou JC, Youle RJ (2011) Mitochondria in apoptosis: Bcl-2 family members and mitochondrial dynamics. Dev Cell 21(1):92–101. https://doi.org/10.1016/j.devcel.2011.06.017

Mattson SN, Riley EP (1998) A review of the neurobehavioral deficits in children with fetal alcohol syndrome or prenatal exposure to alcohol. Alcohol Clin Exp Res 22:279–294. https://doi.org/10.1111/j.1530-0277.1998.tb03651.x

Mattson SN, Roebuck TM (2002) Acquisition and retention of verbal and nonverbal information in children with heavy prenatal alcohol exposure. Alcohol Clin Exp Res 26:875–882. https://pubmed.ncbi.nlm.nih.gov/12068257/. Accessed 14 Apr 2025

Mattson SN, Crocker N, Nguyen TT (2011) Fetal alcohol spectrum disorders: neuropsychological and behavioral features. Neuropsychol Rev 21:81–101. https://doi.org/10.1007/s11065-011-9167-9

Mattson SN, Bernes GA, Doyle LR (2019) Fetal alcohol spectrum disorders: a review of the neurobehavioral deficits associated with prenatal alcohol exposure. Alcohol Clin Exp Res 43:1046–1062. https://doi.org/10.1111/acer.14040

May PA, Gossage JP, Kalberg WO et al (2009) Prevalence and epidemiologic characteristics of FASD from various research methods with an emphasis on recent in-school studies. Dev Disabil Res Rev 15:176–192. https://doi.org/10.1002/ddrr.68

Mayo Clinic Staff (2024) Fetal alcohol syndrome. Mayo Clinic. https://www.mayoclinic.org/diseases-conditions/fetal-alcohol-syndrome/symptoms-causes/syc-20352901. Accessed 14 Apr 2025

McAvoy K, Kawamata H (2019) Glial mitochondrial function and dysfunction in health and neurodegeneration. Mol Cell Neurosci 101:103417. https://doi.org/10.1016/j.mcn.2019.103417

McBride HM, Neuspiel M, Wasiak S (2006) Mitochondria: more than just a powerhouse. Curr Biol. https://doi.org/10.1016/j.cub.2006.06.054

McGoey TN, Reynolds JN, Brien JF (2003) Chronic prenatal ethanol exposure-induced decrease of guinea pig hippocampal CA1 pyramidal cell and cerebellar Purkinje cell density. Can J Physiol Pharmacol 81(5):476–484. https://doi.org/10.1139/y03-048

Menshawi K, Mohr JP, Gutierrez J (2015) A functional perspective on the embryology and anatomy of the cerebral blood supply. J Stroke 17:144. https://doi.org/10.5853/jos.2015.17.2.144

Meyer LS, Riley EP (1986) Social play in juvenile rats prenatally exposed to alcohol. Teratology 34:1–7. https://pubmed.ncbi.nlm.nih.gov/3764769/. Accessed 14 Apr 2025

Miller MW, Potempa G (1990) Numbers of neurons and glia in mature rat somatosensory cortex: effects of prenatal exposure to ethanol. J Comp Neurol 293:92–102. https://doi.org/10.1002/cne.902930108

Ming GL, Song H (2011) Adult neurogenesis in the mammalian brain: significant answers and significant questions. Neuron 70(4):687–702. https://doi.org/10.1016/j.neuron.2011.05.001

Mishra P, Chan DC (2014) Mitochondrial dynamics and inheritance during cell division, development and disease. Nat Rev Mol Cell Biol 15:634–646. https://doi.org/10.1038/nrm3877

Mitchell MC, Herlong HF (1986) Alcohol and nutrition: caloric value, bioenergetics, and relationship to liver damage. Annu Rev Nutr 6:457–474. https://doi.org/10.1146/annurev.nu.06.070186.002325

Momin SZ, Le JT, Miranda RC (2023) Vascular contributions to the neurobiological effects of prenatal alcohol exposure. Adv Drug Alcohol Res. https://doi.org/10.3389/adar.2023.10924

Montoliu C, Sancho-Tello M, Azorin I et al (1995) Ethanol increases cytochrome P4502E1 and induces oxidative stress in astrocytes. J Neurochem 65:2561–2570. https://doi.org/10.1046/j.1471-4159.1995.65062561.x

Moore EM, Xia Y (2022) Neurodevelopmental trajectories following prenatal alcohol exposure. Front Hum Neurosci 15:695855. https://doi.org/10.3389/fnhum.2021.695855

Muggli E, Matthews H, Penington A et al (2017) Association between prenatal alcohol exposure and craniofacial shape of children at 12 months of age. JAMA Pediatr 171:771. https://doi.org/10.1001/jamapediatrics.2017.0778

Muggli E, Halliday J, Hearps S et al (2024) Low to moderate prenatal alcohol exposure and neurodevelopment in a prospective cohort of early school aged children. Sci Rep 14(1):7302. https://doi.org/10.1038/s41598-024-57938-7

Mukherjee S (2013) Alcoholism and its effects on the central nervous system. Curr Neurovasc Res 10:256–262. https://doi.org/10.2174/15672026113109990004

Mukherjee S, Cabrera MA, Boyadjieva NI et al (2020) Alcohol increases exosome release from microglia to promote complement C1q-induced cellular death of proopiomelanocortin neurons in the hypothalamus in a rat model of fetal alcohol spectrum disorders. J Neurosci 40:7965–7979

Murphy E, Steenbergen C (2008) Mechanisms underlying acute protection from cardiac ischemia-reperfusion injury. Physiol Rev 88:581–609. https://doi.org/10.1152/physrev.00024.2007

Napolitano G, Fasciolo G, Venditti P (2021) Mitochondrial management of reactive oxygen species. Antioxidants 10:1824. https://doi.org/10.3390/antiox10111824

Nassir F, Ibdah JA (2014) Role of mitochondria in alcoholic liver disease. World J Gastroenterol 20:2136. https://doi.org/10.3748/wjg.v20.i9.2136

Nave KA (2010) Myelination and support of axonal integrity by glia. Nature 468:244–248. https://doi.org/10.1038/nature09614

Newville J, Valenzuela CF, Li L et al (2017) Acute oligodendrocyte loss with persistent white matter injury in a third trimester equivalent mouse model of fetal alcohol spectrum disorder. Glia 65:1317–1332. https://doi.org/10.1002/glia.23164

Nguyen BY, Ruiz-Velasco A, Bui T et al (2018) Mitochondrial function in the heart: the insight into mechanisms and therapeutic potentials. Br J Pharmacol 176:4302–4318. https://doi.org/10.1111/bph.14431

NIAAA (2022) Alcohol metabolism. National Institute on Alcohol Abuse and Alcoholism. https://www.niaaa.nih.gov/publications/alcohol-metabolism#:~:text=Most%20of%20the%20ethanol%20inCH3CHO)%2C%20a%20known%20carcinogen. Accessed 14 Apr 2025

NIAAA (2023) Understanding fetal alcohol spectrum disorders. National Institute on Alcohol Abuse and Alcoholism. https://www.niaaa.nih.gov/publications/brochures-and-fact-sheets/understanding-fetal-alcohol-spectrum-disorders#:~:text=The%20term%20fetal%20alcohol%20spectrumof%20Fetal%20Alcohol%20Spectrum%20Disorders? Accessed 13 Apr 2025

Nickel M, Gu C (2018) Regulation of central nervous system myelination in higher brain functions. Neural Plast 2018:6436453. https://doi.org/10.1155/2018/6436453

Nicloux M (1900) Passage de l'alcool ingéré de la mere au foetus et passage de l'alcool ingere dans le lait, en paticulier chez la femme. Bull Mus Natl Hist Nat Obstet 5:97–132

Nolfi-Donegan D, Braganza A, Shiva S (2020) Mitochondrial electron transport chain: oxidative phosphorylation, oxidant production, and methods of measurement. Redox Biol 37:101674. https://doi.org/10.1016/j.redox.2020.101674

Nunes L (2021) Mighty mitochondria. Association for Psychological Science - APS. https://www.psychologicalscience.org/observer/mighty-mitochondria#:~:text=1948%E2%80%931951:%20American%20biochemist%20Albert%20Lehninger%20and%20studentsenzymes%20to%20oxidize%20nutrients%20and%20produce%20energy.&text=1957:%20American%20cell%20biologist%20Philip%20Siekevitz%20wrote,coining%20a%20term%20still%20in%20use%20today. Accessed 14 Apr 2025

Nunnari J, Suomalainen A (2012) Mitochondria: in sickness and in health. Cell 148(6):1145–1159. https://doi.org/10.1016/j.cell.2012.02.035

Nyquist-Battie C, Freter M (1988) Cardiac mitochondrial abnormalities in a mouse model of the fetal alcohol syndrome. Alcohol Clin Exp Res. https://doi.org/10.1111/j.1530-0277.1988.tb00192.x

O'Leary CE, Thomas KG, Dodge NC et al (2015) Verbal learning and memory impairment in children with fetal alcohol spectrum disorders. Alcohol Clin Exp Res 39:724–732. https://doi.org/10.1111/acer.12671

Oberheim NA, Goldman SA, Nedergaard M (2012) Heterogeneity of astrocytic form and function. Methods Mol Biol 814:23–45

Ogboo BC, Grabovyy UV, Maini A et al (2022) Architecture of the NADPH oxidase family of enzymes. Redox Biol 52:102298. https://doi.org/10.1016/j.redox.2022.102298

Ohkawa H, Ohishi N, Yagi K (1979) Assay for lipid peroxides in animal tissues by thiobarbituric acid reaction. Anal Biochem 95(2):351–358. https://doi.org/10.1016/0003-2697(79)90738-3

Olesen MA, Quintanilla RA (2023) The effects of alcohol abuse against the mitochondria: functional consequences for liver, muscle, and the brain. In: Mitochondrial intoxication, pp 181–204. https://doi.org/10.1016/b978-0-323-88462-4.00003-1

Olivier L, Curfs LM, Viljoen DL (2016) Fetal alcohol spectrum disorders: prevalence rates in South Africa. S Afr Med J 106:103. https://doi.org/10.7196/samj.2016.v106i6.11009

Olmstead MC, Martin A, Brien JF, Reynolds JN (2009) Chronic prenatal ethanol exposure increases disinhibition and perseverative responding in the adult guinea pig. Behav Pharmacol 20:554–557. https://doi.org/10.1097/fbp.0b013e3283305e27

Osellame LD, Blacker TS, Duchen MR (2012) Cellular and molecular mechanisms of mitochondrial function. Best Pract Res Clin Endocrinol Metab 26:711–723. https://doi.org/10.1016/j.beem.2012.05.003

Ozer E, Sarioglu S, Gure A (2000) Effects of prenatal ethanol exposure on neuronal migration, neurogenesis and brain myelination in the mouse brain. Clin Neuropathol 19:21–26

Paravicini TM, Touyz RM (2008) NADPH oxidases, reactive oxygen species, and hypertension. Diabetes Care. https://doi.org/10.2337/dc08-s247

Parkington HC, Kenna KR, Sozo F et al (2014) Maternal alcohol consumption in pregnancy enhances arterial stiffness and alters vasodilator function that varies between vascular beds in fetal sheep. J Physiol 592: 2591–2603. https://doi.org/10.1113/jphysiol.2013.262873

Parnell SE, Ramadoss J, Delp MD et al (2007) Chronic ethanol increases fetal cerebral blood flow specific to the ethanol-sensitive cerebellum under normoxaemic, hypercapnic and acidaemic conditions: ovine model. Exp Physiol 92:933–943. https://doi.org/10.1113/expphysiol.2007.038091

Paton A (2005) Alcohol in the body. BMJ 330:85–87. https://doi.org/10.1136/bmj.330.7482.85

Patten AR, Fontaine CJ, Christie BR (2014) A comparison of the different animal models of fetal alcohol spectrum disorders and their use in studying complex behaviors. Front Pediatr. https://doi.org/10.3389/fped.2014.00093

Peadon E (2010) Distinguishing between attention-deficit hyperactivity and fetal alcohol spectrum disorders in children: clinical guidelines. Neuropsychiatr Dis Treat:509. https://doi.org/10.2147/ndt.s7256

Peng J, Ramatchandirin B, Pearah A et al (2022) Development and functions of mitochondria in early life. Newborn 1:131–141. https://doi.org/10.5005/jp-journals-11002-0013

Penna C, Perrelli M-G, Pagliaro P (2013) Mitochondrial pathways, permeability transition pore, and redox signaling in cardioprotection: therapeutic implications. Antioxid Redox Signal 18:556–599. https://doi.org/10.1089/ars.2011.4459

Perez MJ, Loyola R, Canelo F et al (2020) NADPH oxidase contributes to oxidative damage and mitochondrial impairment induced by acute ethanol treatment in rat hippocampal neurons. Neuropharmacology 171: 108100. https://doi.org/10.1016/j.neuropharm.2020.108100

Piano MR, Geenen DL, Schwertz DW et al (2007) Long-term effects of alcohol consumption in male and female rats. Cardiovasc Toxicol 7:247–254. https://doi.org/10.1007/s12012-007-9002-y

Pla A, Pascual M, Renau-Piqueras J, Guerri C (2014) TLR4 mediates the impairment of ubiquitin-proteasome and autophagy-lysosome pathways induced by ethanol treatment in brain. Cell Death Dis. https://doi.org/10.1038/cddis.2014.46

Popova S, Lange S, Shield K et al (2019) Prevalence of fetal alcohol spectrum disorder among special subpopulations: a systematic review and meta-analysis. Addiction 114:1150–1172. https://doi.org/10.1111/add.14598

Popova S, Dozet D, Shield K et al (2021) Alcohol's impact on the fetus. Nutrients 13:3452. https://doi.org/10.3390/nu13103452

Pretini V, Koenen MH, Kaestner L et al (2019) Red blood cells: chasing interactions. Front Physiol. https://doi.org/10.3389/fphys.2019.00945

Prinz M, Mildner A (2011) Microglia in the CNS: immigrants from another world. Glia 59:177–187

Qian Y, Du Y-H, Tang Y-B et al (2011) CLC-3 chloride channel prevents apoptosis induced by hydrogen peroxide in basilar artery smooth muscle cells through mitochondria dependent pathway. Apoptosis 16:468–477. https://doi.org/10.1007/s10495-011-0584-2

Ramachandran V, Perez A, Chen J et al (2001) In utero ethanol exposure causes mitochondrial dysfunction, which can result in apoptotic cell death in fetal brain: a potential role for 4-hydroxynonenal. Alcohol Clin Exp Res 25(6):862–871

Ramachandran V, Watts LT, Maffi SK et al (2003) Ethanol-induced oxidative stress precedes mitochondrially mediated apoptotic death of cultured fetal cortical neurons. J Neurosci Res 64(4):456–469. https://doi.org/10.1002/jnr.1081

Ramachandran V, Perez A, Chen J et al (2006) In utero ethanol exposure causes mitochondrial dysfunction, which can result in apoptotic cell death in Fetal brain: a potential role for 4-hydroxynonenal. Alcohol Clin Exp Res 25:862–871. https://doi.org/10.1111/j.1530-0277.2001.tb02292.x

Rastogi A, Joshi P, Contreras E, Gama V (2019) Remodeling of mitochondrial morphology and function: an emerging hallmark of cellular reprogramming. Cell Stress 3:181–194. https://doi.org/10.15698/cst2019.06.189

Rathinam ML, Watts LT, Stark AA et al (2006) Astrocyte control of fetal cortical neuron glutathione homeostasis: up-regulation by ethanol. J Neurochem 96:1289–1300. https://doi.org/10.1111/j.1471-4159.2006.03674.x

Reers M, Smiley ST, Mottola-Hartshorn C et al (1995) [29] mitochondrial membrane potential monitored by JC-1 dye. In: Methods in enzymology. Academic Press, pp 406–417. https://doi.org/10.1016/0076-6879(95)60154-6

Reichard A, Asosingh K (2018) The role of mitochondria in angiogenesis. Mol Biol Rep 46:1393–1400. https://doi.org/10.1007/s11033-018-4488-x

Remmelink E, Chau U, Smit A et al (2017) A one-week 5-choice serial reaction time task to measure impulsivity and attention in adult and adolescent mice. Sci Rep 7:42519. https://doi.org/10.1038/srep42519

Risbud RD, Breit KR, Thomas JD (2022) Early developmental alcohol exposure alters behavioral outcomes following adolescent re-exposure in a rat model. Alcohol Clin Exp Res 46:1993–2009. https://doi.org/10.1111/acer.14950

Romanello V, Sandri M (2023) Implications of mitochondrial fusion and fission in skeletal muscle mass and

health. Semin Cell Dev Biol 143:46–53. https://doi.org/10.1016/j.semcdb.2022.02.011
Rømert P, Matthiessen ME (1983) Alcohol-induced injury of mitochondria in hepatocytes of mini-pig fetuses. Virchows Arch A Pathol Anat Histopathol 399:299–305. https://doi.org/10.1007/bf00612947
Roy R, Wilcox J, Webb AJ, O'Gallagher K (2023) Dysfunctional and dysregulated nitric oxide synthases in cardiovascular disease: mechanisms and therapeutic potential. Int J Mol Sci 24:15200. https://doi.org/10.3390/ijms242015200
SA Health (2022) Blood alcohol concentration (BAC) and the effects of alcohol. Government of South Australia. https://www.sahealth.sa.gov.au/wps/wcm/connect/public+content/sa+health+internet/conditions/alcohol/blood+alcohol+concentration+bac+and+the+effects+of+alcohol. Accessed 7 Jul 2025
Safiulina D, Kaasik A (2013) Energetic and dynamic: how mitochondria meet neuronal energy demands. PLoS Biol. https://doi.org/10.1371/journal.pbio.1001755
Saha PS, Mayhan WG (2022) Prenatal exposure to alcohol: mechanisms of cerebral vascular damage and lifelong consequences. Adv Drug Alcohol Res. https://doi.org/10.3389/adar.2022.10818
San-Millán I (2023) The key role of mitochondrial function in health and disease. Antioxidants 12:782. https://doi.org/10.3390/antiox12040782
Sari Y, Zhang M, Mechref Y (2010) Differential expression of proteins in fetal brains of alcohol-treated prenatally C57BL/6 mice: a proteomic investigation. Electrophoresis 31:483–496. https://doi.org/10.1002/elps.200900385
Sasaki A, Hirato J, Nakazato Y, Ishida Y (1988) Immunohistochemical study of the early human fetal brain. Acta Neuropathol 76:128–134. https://doi.org/10.1007/BF00688096
Scher MS (2012) Developmental origins of cerebrovascular disease I: prenatal cerebrovascular development--classic findings in the context of advances in genetic and fetal surveillance evaluations. J Child Neurol (1): 121–131: https://doi.org/10.1177/0883073811417714
Schiffer TA, Lundberg JO, Weitzberg E, Carlström M (2020) Modulation of mitochondria and NADPH oxidase function by the nitrate-nitrite-no pathway in metabolic disease with focus on type 2 diabetes. Biochim Biophys Acta (BBA) - Mol Basis Dis 1866:165811. https://doi.org/10.1016/j.bbadis.2020.165811
Schirrmacher V (2020) Mitochondria at work: new insights into regulation and dysregulation of cellular energy supply and metabolism. Biomedicine 8:526. https://doi.org/10.3390/biomedicines8110526
Scott I, Youle RJ (2010) Mitochondrial fission and fusion. Essays Biochem 47:85–98. https://doi.org/10.1042/bse0470085
Seleverstov O, Tobiasz A, Jackson JS et al (2017) Maternal alcohol exposure during mid-pregnancy dilates fetal cerebral arteries via endocannabinoid receptors. Alcohol 61:51–61. https://doi.org/10.1016/j.alcohol.2017.01.014
Semple BD, Blomgren K, Gimlin K et al (2013) Brain development in rodents and humans: identifying benchmarks of maturation and vulnerability to injury across species. Prog Neurobiol 106–107:1–16. https://doi.org/10.1016/j.pneurobio.2013.04.001
Shah KR, West M (1984) Behavioral changes in rat following perinatal exposure to ethanol. Neurosci Lett 47: 145–148. https://doi.org/10.1016/0304-3940(84)90420-8
Sharma C, Kim S, Nam Y et al (2021) Mitochondrial dysfunction as a driver of cognitive impairment in Alzheimer's disease. Int J Mol Sci 22:4850. https://doi.org/10.3390/ijms22094850
Sidoryk-Wegrzynowicz M, Wegrzynowicz M, Lee E et al (2011) Role of astrocytes in brain function and disease. Toxicol Pathol 39:115–123. https://doi.org/10.1177/0192623310385254
Siggins RW, McTernan PM, Simon L et al (2023) Mitochondrial dysfunction: at the nexus between alcohol-associated immunometabolic dysregulation and tissue injury. Int J Mol Sci 24:8650. https://doi.org/10.3390/ijms24108650
Simon L, Molina PE (2022) Cellular bioenergetics: experimental evidence for alcohol-induced adaptations. Function. https://doi.org/10.1093/function/zqac039
Smith SM (1997) Alcohol-induced cell death in the embryo. Alcohol Health Res World 21:287. https://pmc.ncbi.nlm.nih.gov/articles/PMC6827686/#:~:text=Studies%20using%20mice%20and%20chicks%20show%20thatfacial%20structures%20(i.e.%2C%20cranial%20neural%20crest%20cells). Accessed 14 Apr 2025
Solonskii AV, Logvinov SV, Kutepova NA (2008) Development of brain vessels in human embryos and fetuses in conditions of prenatal exposure to alcohol. Neurosci Behav Physiol 38:373–376. https://doi.org/10.1007/s11055-008-0053-8
Son G, Han J (2018) Roles of mitochondria in neuronal development. BMB Rep 51:549–556. https://doi.org/10.5483/bmbrep.2018.51.11.226
Srinivasan P, Nabokina S, Said HM (2015) Chronic alcohol exposure affects pancreatic acinar mitochondrial thiamin pyrophosphate uptake: studies with mouse 266-6 cell line and primary cells. Am J Physiol Gastrointest Liver Physiol. https://doi.org/10.1152/ajpgi.00226.2015
Steiner JL, Lang CH (2017) Etiology of alcoholic cardiomyopathy: mitochondria, oxidative stress and apoptosis. Int J Biochem Cell Biol 89:125–135. https://doi.org/10.1016/j.biocel.2017.06.009
Streissguth AP, Landesman-Dwyer S, Martin JC, Smith DW (1980) Teratogenic effects of alcohol in humans and laboratory animals. Science 209:353–361. https://doi.org/10.1126/science.6992275
Streissguth AP, Barr HM, Kogan J, Bookstein FL (1996) Final report: Understanding the occurrence of secondary disabilities in clients with fetal alcohol syndrome (FAS) and fetal alcohol effects (FAE)

Su Y, Yu Y, Quan J et al (2024) Alcohol exposure during pregnancy induces cardiac mitochondrial damage in offspring mice. Birth Defects Res. https://doi.org/10.1002/bdr2.2369

Sulik KK, Johnston MC, Webb MA (1981) Fetal alcohol syndrome: embryogenesis in a mouse model. Science 214:936–938. https://doi.org/10.1126/science.6795717

Sun Q, Zhong W, Zhang W, Zhou Z (2016) Defect of mitochondrial respiratory chain is a mechanism of ROS overproduction in a rat model of alcoholic liver disease: role of zinc deficiency. Am J Physiol Gastrointest Liver Physiol. https://doi.org/10.1152/ajpgi.00270.2015

Suttie M, Foroud T, Wetherill L et al (2013) Facial dysmorphism across the fetal alcohol spectrum. Pediatrics. https://doi.org/10.1542/peds.2012-1371

Tang X, Luo Y-X, Chen H-Z, Liu D-P (2014) Mitochondria, endothelial cell function, and vascular diseases. Front Physiol. https://doi.org/10.3389/fphys.2014.00175

Temple S (2001) The development of neural stem cells. Nature 414:112–117. https://doi.org/10.1038/35102174

Thoudam T, Gao H, Jiang Y et al (2024) Mitochondrial quality control in alcohol-associated liver disease. Hepatol Commun. https://doi.org/10.1097/hc9.0000000000000534

Tietze F (1969) Enzymic method for quantitative determination of nanogram amounts of total and oxidized glutathione: applications to mammalian blood and other tissues. Anal Biochem 27(3):502–522. https://doi.org/10.1016/0003-2697(69)90064-5

Tobiasz AM, Duncan JR, Bursac Z et al (2018) The effect of prenatal alcohol exposure on fetal growth and cardiovascular parameters in a baboon model of pregnancy. Reprod Sci 25:1116–1123. https://doi.org/10.1177/1933719117734317

Tong M, Longato L, Nguyen QG et al (2011) Acetaldehyde-mediated neurotoxicity: relevance to fetal alcohol spectrum disorders. Oxid Med Cell Longev 2011:213286. https://doi.org/10.1155/2011/213286

Tran N, Garcia T, Aniga M et al (2022) Endothelial nitric oxide synthase (eNOS) and the cardiovascular system: in physiology and in disease states. Am J Biomed Sci Res 15:153–177

Tseng P-L, Wu W-H, Hu T-H et al (2018) Decreased succinate dehydrogenase B in human hepatocellular carcinoma accelerates tumor malignancy by inducing the Warburg effect. Sci Rep. https://doi.org/10.1038/s41598-018-21361-6

Tsuji R, Guizzetti M, Costa LG (2003) In vivo ethanol decreases phosphorylated MAPK and p70S6 kinase in the developing rat brain. Neuroreport 14:1395–1399. https://doi.org/10.1097/00001756-200307180-00023

Turcotte L-A, Aberle NS, Norby FL et al (2002) Influence of prenatal ethanol exposure on vascular contractile response in rat thoracic aorta. Alcohol 26:75–81. https://doi.org/10.1016/s0741-8329(01)00198-7

Tyler CR, Allan AM (2014) Prenatal alcohol exposure alters expression of neurogenesis-related genes in an ex vivo cell culture model. Alcohol 48(5):483–492. https://doi.org/10.1016/j.alcohol.2014.06.001

Uğuz AC, Okan A, Doğanyiğit Z et al (2024) Evaluation of TRPM2 channel-mediated autophagic signaling pathway in hippocampus and cortex tissues of rat offspring following prenatal exposure to elevated alcohol levels. Environ Toxicol 40:222–244. https://doi.org/10.1002/tox.24427

Ullah I, Ullah N, Naseer MI et al (2012) Neuroprotection with metformin and thymoquinone against ethanol-induced apoptotic neurodegeneration in prenatal rat cortical neurons. BMC Neurosci 19(13):11. https://doi.org/10.1186/1471-2202-13-11

Vendemiale G, Grattagliano I, Altomare E et al (2001) Mitochondrial oxidative damage and myocardial fibrosis in rats chronically intoxicated with moderate doses of ethanol. Toxicol Lett 123:209–216. https://doi.org/10.1016/s0378-4274(01)00401-5

Verkhratsky A, Butt A, Li B et al (2023) Astrocytes in human central nervous system diseases: a frontier for new therapies. Signal Transduct Target Ther 8:396. https://doi.org/10.1038/s41392-023-01628-9

Villalba A, Götz M, Borrell V (2021) The regulation of cortical neurogenesis. Curr Top Dev Biol 142:1–66. https://doi.org/10.1016/bs.ctdb.2020.10.003

von Bernhardi R, Heredia F, Salgado N, Muñoz P (2016) Microglia function in the normal brain. In: von Bernhardi R (ed) Glial cells in health and disease of the CNS. Springer, Cham, pp 67–92

Wang XF, Cynader MS (2000) Astrocytes provide cysteine to neurons by releasing glutathione. J Neurochem 74:1434–1442. https://doi.org/10.1046/j.1471-4159.2000.0741434.x

Wang R, Martin CD, Lei AL et al (2020) Prenatal ethanol exposure leads to attention deficits in both male and female rats. Front Neurosci. https://doi.org/10.3389/fnins.2020.00012

Watts LT, Rathinam ML, Schenker S, Henderson GI (2005) Astrocytes protect neurons from ethanol-induced oxidative stress and apoptotic death. J Neurosci Res 80:655–662. https://doi.org/10.1002/jnr.20502

Westermann B (2012) Bioenergetic role of mitochondrial fusion and fission. Biochim Biophys Acta (BBA) - Bioenergetics 1817:1833–1838. https://doi.org/10.1016/j.bbabio.2012.02.033

Wilhelm CJ, Guizzetti M (2016) Fetal alcohol spectrum disorders: an overview from the glia perspective. Front Integr Neurosci 9:65. https://doi.org/10.3389/fnint.2015.00065

Willoughby KA, Sheard ED, Nash K, Rovet J (2008) Effects of prenatal alcohol exposure on hippocampal volume, verbal learning, and verbal and spatial recall in late childhood. J Int Neuropsychol Soc 14:1022–1033. https://doi.org/10.1017/s1355617708081368

Wilson C, Lee MD, Buckley C et al (2022) Mitochondrial ATP production is required for endothelial cell control of vascular tone. Function. https://doi.org/10.1093/function/zqac063

Xi Q, Cheranov SY, Jaggar JH (2005) Mitochondria-derived reactive oxygen species dilate cerebral arteries by activating Ca2+ sparks. Circ Res 97:354–362. https://doi.org/10.1161/01.res.0000177669.29525.78

Xu Y, Sladek NE, Shen J et al (2005) Impaired development of mitochondria plays a role in the central nervous system defects of fetal alcohol syndrome. Birth Defects Res A Clin Mol Teratol 73(2):83–91. https://doi.org/10.1002/bdra.20110

Xu X, Duan S, Yi F, Ocampo A, Liu GH, Belmonte J (2013) Mitochondrial regulation in pluripotent stem cells. Cell Metab 18:325–332. https://www.cell.com/cell-metabolism/fulltext/S1550-4131(13)00249-0. Accessed 14 Apr 2025

Yan T, Zhao Y (2020) Acetaldehyde induces phosphorylation of dynamin-related protein 1 and mitochondrial dysfunction via elevating intracellular ROS and ca2+ levels. Redox Biol 28:101381. https://doi.org/10.1016/j.redox.2019.101381

Zakhari S (2006) Overview: How is alcohol metabolized by the body? Alcohol Res Health 29:245. https://pmc.ncbi.nlm.nih.gov/articles/PMC6527027/#:~:text=After%20alcohol%20is%20swallowed%2C%20it exposed%20to%20enzymes%20and%20metabolized. Accessed 14 Apr 2025

Zecevic N (2004) Specific characteristics of radial glia in the human fetal telencephalon. Glia 47(1):37–43. https://doi.org/10.1002/glia.20044

Zhang Y, Sloan SA, Clarke LE et al (2016) Purification and characterization of progenitor and mature human astrocytes reveals transcriptional and functional differences with mouse. Neuron 89:37–53. https://doi.org/10.1016/j.neuron.2015.11.013

Zhang L, Liu B, Li H et al (2022) Epidemiology of congenital heart disease in Jinan, China from 2005 to 2020: a time trend analysis. Front Cardiovasc Med. https://doi.org/10.3389/fcvm.2022.815137

Zhang H, Yu X, Ye J et al (2023) Systematic investigation of mitochondrial transfer between cancer cells and T cells at single-cell resolution. Cancer Cell. https://doi.org/10.1016/j.ccell.2023.09.003

Zorov DB, Juhaszova M, Sollott SJ (2014) Mitochondrial reactive oxygen species (ROS) and ROS-induced ROS release. Physiol Rev 94:909–950. https://doi.org/10.1152/physrev.00026.2013

Zuccolotto dos Reis FH (2024) Mitochondria and the heart. Eur Heart J 45:1963–1964. https://doi.org/10.1093/eurheartj/ehae031

Prenatal Cannabis and Tobacco: Studies in Animal Models 9

R. Clayton Edenfield, Rahul D'Mello, Lyndsey E. Shorey-Kendrick, B. Adam Crosland, Olivia L. Hagen, Cindy T. McEvoy, Eliot R. Spindel, Susan K. Murphy, Jamie O. Lo, and Margeaux W. Marbrey

Abstract

Prenatal exposure to cannabis and tobacco can significantly disrupt critical stages of fetal development, resulting in long-lasting consequences for offspring's health. Prenatal THC exposure has been shown to impair offspring neurodevelopment, alter metabolic and cardiovascular function, and disrupt reproductive health, with sex-specific effects that persist into adulthood. Similarly, nicotine exposure during pregnancy is associated with structural and functional deficits in the offspring's pulmonary, neurological, behavioral, cardiac, and renal systems. Epigenetic modifications are a key mechanism through which both THC and nicotine exert their developmental effects, including widespread changes in DNA methylation that influence gene expression and may mediate long-term health outcomes. The rapidly changing landscape of prenatal cannabis and nicotine use, including rising rates of co-use and novel product formulations, highlights the need for ongoing, mechanistic research. Further studies are required to define how these substances impact fetal development and identify shared and distinct molecular pathways, particularly in the context of polysubstance exposure and

Rahul D'Mello, Jamie O. Lo, and Margeaux W. Marbrey have equally contributed to this chapter.

R. C. Edenfield (✉) · O. L. Hagen
Division of Reproductive and Developmental Science, Oregon National Primate Research Center, Oregon Health & Science University, Beaverton, OR, USA
e-mail: edenfiel@ohsu.edu; hageno@ohsu.edu

R. D'Mello · B. A. Crosland · J. O. Lo
Division of Reproductive and Developmental Science, Oregon National Primate Research Center, Oregon Health & Science University, Beaverton, OR, USA

Division of Maternal Fetal Medicine, Department of Obstetrics and Gynecology, Oregon Health & Science University, Portland, OR, USA
e-mail: dmello@ohsu.edu; crosland@ohsu.edu; loj@ohsu.edu

L. E. Shorey-Kendrick · E. R. Spindel
Division of Neuroscience, Oregon National Primate Research Center, Oregon Health & Science University, Beaverton, OR, USA
e-mail: shorey@ohsu.edu; spindele@ohsu.edu

C. T. McEvoy
Division of Neonatology, Department of Pediatrics, Oregon Health & Science University, Portland, OR, USA
e-mail: mcevoyc@ohsu.edu

S. K. Murphy · M. W. Marbrey
Division of Reproductive Sciences, Department of Obstetrics and Gynecology, Duke University School of Medicine, Durham, NC, USA
e-mail: susan.murphy@duke.edu; Margeaux.marbrey@duke.edu

A. N. Bukiya, D. W. Ali (eds.), *Molecular Mechanisms and Lifelong Consequences of Prenatal Exposure to Psychoactive Substances*, Advances in Experimental Medicine and Biology 1500,
https://doi.org/10.1007/978-3-032-12741-9_9

contemporary delivery methods. Animal models are pivotal in dissecting these pathways and evaluating the direct effects of exposure, free from confounding variables common in human studies. Importantly, they provide a platform to examine both the individual and synergistic effects of THC and nicotine, as well as to uncover underlying mechanisms that may inform intervention strategies and guide public health policy.

Keywords

Prenatal exposure · Cannabis · Tobacco · Animal models · Developmental toxicology

9.1 Introduction

Pregnancy is a dynamic process consisting of tightly regulated periods of fetal and placental development, during which the intrauterine environment directly affects fetal development and plays a critical role in shaping long-term health outcomes (Olyaei et al. 2022; Duko et al. 2024; Ainiti et al. 2023). This period marks a critical window of vulnerability, as organogenesis, neuronal differentiation, and placental morphogenesis proceed in tightly regulated sequences that are especially susceptible to disruption by environmental exposures that can also impact maternal physiology, which can indirectly impact intrauterine development. The Barker Hypothesis, also known as the Fetal Origins of Adult Disease (FOAD) or Developmental Origins of Health and Disease (DOHaD), suggests that adverse conditions in utero, including exposure to toxicants and nutrient deficiency, can result in fetal adaptations which predispose individuals to chronic diseases in later life (Calkins and Devaskar 2011), highlighting the importance of maternal behavior and lifestyle factors during this time.

Cannabis and tobacco are the most commonly used illicit (based on jurisdiction) and licit substances, respectively, in pregnancy (SAMHSA 2023). Used independently, both can have adverse short and long-term developmental effects on offspring (Olyaei et al. 2022; Duko et al. 2024; Ainiti et al. 2023). There are also increasing rates of co-use, which is associated with a higher risk of neonatal complications than just cannabis or nicotine alone (Crosland et al. 2024). These substances, through various biological mechanisms, can disrupt normal fetal growth and increase susceptibility to chronic diseases in adulthood. However, underreporting, especially of illicit substances, can make it difficult to accurately determine the prevalence of cannabis and nicotine use in pregnancy (Olyaei et al. 2022).

Studying the impact of substance use in pregnancy is challenging due to the limitations of retrospective and observational study designs, which are often limited by self-reported data, a lack of data regarding timing of use and dose, and inadequate adjustment for confounding variables, including polysubstance use. To overcome these limitations and gain a deeper understanding of the effects of maternal substance use, animal models are necessary (Fig. 9.1). Animal models offer controlled conditions that allow for standardized methodology, reduction of confounders, and the ability to collect longitudinal samples in order to elucidate underlying biological mechanisms (Olyaei et al. 2022). In summary, prenatal cannabis and tobacco use are both prevalent and harmful, yet human studies are limited in the data they can provide; consequently, animal models are essential for generating insights that inform clinical guidance and advance scientific research.

9.2 Cannabis

Cannabis is the most used illicit drug among reproductive-aged and pregnant individuals in the United States (Abuse 2019) and is associated with an increased risk of adverse fetal and neonatal outcomes, including preterm birth and decreased birthweight (Gunn et al. 2016). Cannabis use has varying rates by geographic region. In the United States, a 2017 study of 14,400 pregnant women found that 3.8% used cannabis during pregnancy, with usage rates varying by trimester: 6.5% in the first, 3.3% in the second,

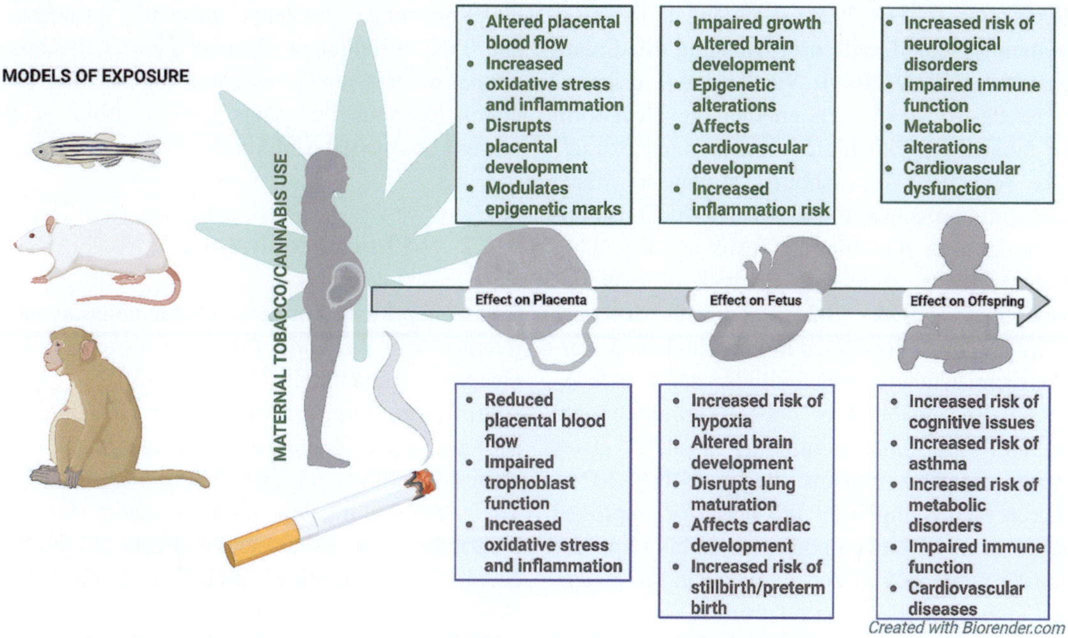

Fig. 9.1 *Models of exposure for maternal cannabis/tobacco use*. Zebrafish, rodents, and rhesus macaques are commonly used to model maternal exposure of cannabis and tobacco and their effects on the mother, placenta, fetus, and offspring

and 1.8% in the third (Volkow et al. 2017). A California-based study showed that cannabis use increased more than two-fold from 3.4% to 7.0% between 2002 and 2017(Young-Wolff et al. 2021). A recent California-based study from 2024 reported that 20,053 individuals (6.3%) screened positive for prenatal cannabis use, with 2.9% identified through self-report, 5.3% through toxicology testing, and 1.8% by both methods (Young-Wolff et al. 2024). The reported frequency of use was 0.6% (1930) daily, 0.7% (2345) weekly, 1.5% (4892) monthly or less, and 3.4% (10,886) unknown (Young-Wolff et al. 2024). However, the true prevalence of prenatal cannabis use is likely higher because patient underreporting of cannabis use can be as high as 60–70% (National Academies of Sciences, Engineering, and Medicine, Health and Medicine Division, Board on Population Health and Public Health Practice 2017; Metz and Stickrath 2015). Furthermore, self-report does not accurately capture the frequency and potency of the cannabis products used, which vary with different strains and delivery mechanisms and inconsistent in formulation and labeling (Olyaei et al. 2022).

9.2.1 Route of Exposure

Assessing cannabis dosage is challenging, as studies often rely on frequency of use rather than precise measurements of delta-9-tetrahydrocannabinol (THC, the main psychoactive component of cannabis) exposure. Researchers often categorize the degree of use based on cannabis cigarette consumption without including potency, which has significantly increased in cannabis products over time (Cupo et al. 2024). THC content has increased drastically over the past two decades from approximately 4% in 1995 to 14% in 2019 (ElSohly et al. 2016, 2021). The method of cannabis use further complicates exposure assessment, as THC absorption varies by route of administration. Common methods of cannabis use include inhalation, ingestion, and topical application (NIDA 2024). Smoking is the most common method, with users inhaling dried plant material (NIDA 2024). Vaporization, using e-cigarette-like devices, is another prevalent form of inhalation, with highly concentrated extracts like wax used for dabbing, a way to inhale concentrated cannabis (NIDA 2024). Consumption/ingestion of edibles can result in delayed but potent effects, increasing the risk of overconsumption (NIDA 2024). Topical exposure includes cannabis-infused lotions and balms. Furthermore, synthetic cannabinoids, such as delta-8-tetrahydrocannabinol or delta-10-tetrahydrocannabinol, are more commonly used in states where cannabis remains illegal (NIDA 2024). These factors highlight the need for improved assessment of contemporary cannabis exposure during pregnancy to better understand its potential long-term effects on offspring.

Animal models, including zebrafish, chickens, rodents, and nonhuman primates (NHPs), offered valuable insights into the developmental and behavioral outcomes associated with prenatal cannabinoid exposure (Olyaei et al. 2022). However, there are several limitations to the available preclinical literature; the route of THC administration has varied in existing studies, ranging from injected cannabinoids, commonly used in rodent studies, to vaporizing and ingestion, which more closely recapitulate typical human use. The administration route also influences the compounds studied; vaporization allows for naturalistic cannabis preparations, while injected or oral methods typically use isolated THC, avoiding potential entourage effects. Additionally, synthetic cannabinoids used in research differ functionally from plant-derived cannabinoids. Dosing poses another limitation, as available research studies frequently use higher THC concentrations than typical human exposure. Finally, differences in gestational timelines between species complicate direct comparisons, as rodents have a shorter gestational length than humans and give birth at a developmental stage equivalent to the late second trimester. Among animal models, NHPs provide the strongest translational strength due to their similarities to humans in reproductive physiology, developmental ontogeny, placental structure, and THC metabolism. Despite these challenges, animal models remain essential for isolating the effects of prenatal cannabis exposure from social and environmental confounders in human studies.

9.2.2 Pharmacokinetics

Cannabis primarily consists of cannabinoids that interact with the body's main endocannabinoid receptors, cannabinoid 1 (CB1) and CB2. THC is the most abundant and active cannabinoid, acting as a partial agonist at both receptors, with a stronger affinity for CB1 (Monfort et al. 2022). This interaction with CB1 receptors largely contributes to its psychoactive effects, leading to changes in cognition, mood, and emotions (Mannekote Thippaiah et al. 2021).

THC can also cross the placental and blood–brain barrier and activate endogenous cannabinoid receptors located on the placenta and major fetal organs, including the brain, heart, and lung (Monfort et al. 2022). THC is lipophilic and distributes in adipose tissues (Monfort et al. 2022). THC is metabolized in the liver by cytochrome P450 enzymes, CYP2C9, CYP2C19, and CYP3A4, to the active 11-hydroxy-delta-9-tetrahydrocannabinol (11-OH-THC), then oxidized to the inactive 11-nor-9-carboxy-delta-9-tetrahydrocannabinol (THC-COOH). THC-COOH undergoes glucuronidation by glucuronosyltransferases (UGT1A1, 1A3, 1A9, and 1A10) becoming the inactive 11-nor-9-carboxy-delta-9-tetrahydrocannabinol glucuronide (Dinis-Oliveira 2016). THC is also metabolized by UDP-glucosyltransferase (UGT) to inactive delta-9-tetrahydrocannabinol glucuronide. Active metabolites of THC can be used as biomarkers of cannabis exposure, such as 8-hydroxy-THC and 8β,11-dihydroxy-THC, as can inactive compounds such as THC-COOH (Dinis-Oliveira 2016). During pregnancy, THC metabolism is altered as CYP2C19, CYP3A4, and UGT activity is increased, and CYP2C9 activity is decreased (Ward and Varner 2019).

Preclinical models, including rats, mice, dogs, rhesus macaques, sheep, guinea pigs, rabbits, and pigs, have been used to assess the pharmacokinetics of cannabinoids (Monfort et al. 2022). THC, cannabidiol (CBD), 11-OH-THC, and THC-COOH were detected in plasma for at least 24 h in all animal models, except for guinea pigs (Monfort et al. 2022). Cannabinoid pharmacokinetics in animals, especially NHPs, closely mirror those in humans, making them relevant models for predicting fetal and neonatal cannabinoid transfer (Moore et al. 2022). Physiologically based pharmacokinetic models have been developed in mice, rats, and pigs (Methaneethorn et al. 2020).

Pharmacokinetics of THC, 11-OH-THC, and THC-COOH can differ with age and other co-exposures (Torrens et al. 2020; Breit et al. 2020). Cannabinoid pharmacokinetics must be evaluated in fetuses and newborns, as their metabolic and elimination pathways differ markedly. Controlling for fed versus fasting state is essential to minimize variability (Fernández-Trapero et al. 2020). Given the close resemblance of THC pharmacokinetics in rhesus macaques to humans (Ginsburg et al. 2014; Perlin et al. 1985), data from this model, particularly in pregnant and lactating subjects, should be prioritized for predicting human cannabinoid exposure (Monfort et al. 2022).

In rat models, fetal THC concentrations are approximately 10% of maternal levels 60 min after THC is administered via gastric gavage (Hutchings et al. 1989). A study using rhesus macaques measuring THC and THC-COOH levels in maternal and fetal plasma following intravenous administration of 0.3 mg/kg THC (Bailey et al. 1987) reported that THC concentration peaked at 3 min in maternal plasma and at 15 min in fetal plasma, indicating rapid transfer across the placenta. Three hours post-administration, THC levels in maternal and fetal plasma were equal, and THC-COOH was not detected at significant levels in fetal plasma (Bailey et al. 1987). In sheep exposed to inhaled cannabis smoke containing 3.19% THC, THC appeared in maternal plasma at 3 min, peaking at 10 min, while it was first detected in fetal plasma at 10 min, reaching its peak at 90 min (Abrams et al. 1985). Throughout the 24 h, THC concentrations remained lower in fetal plasma than in maternal plasma. Multiple animal models show that THC consistently crosses the placenta with a 10–15 min lag period and clears slowly from the fetal compartment for up to 3 h after peaking (Monfort et al. 2022). Furthermore, the route of exposure in pregnant rats produces markedly different physiological effects (Black et al. 2023). All of these animal models provide invaluable insight into metabolism, but it is important to note that rhesus macaques are most similar to humans.

THC and metabolites can cross the placenta and accumulate in the fetal brain, though their distribution and effects differ. Inhalation and injection models show significant transfer of THC and its active metabolite, 11-OH-THC, into the fetal brain without altering endocannabinoid (e.g., anandamide) concentrations or feedback regulation. Anandamide levels in the fetal brain positively correlate with THC, while 2-arachidonoylglycerol levels show a negative correlation (Baglot et al. 2022).

9.3 Maternal and Gestational Outcomes

9.3.1 Pregnancy Hormones

Key hormones essential for pregnancy include estradiol, follicle-stimulating hormone, luteinizing hormone, progesterone, prolactin, and chorionic gonadotropin, which regulate fetal development and maternal physiology. These hormones interact with enzymes involved in the clearance of THC and its metabolites (Authement and Isoherranen 2024). Prenatal THC exposure can influence pregnancy hormone levels, with evidence suggesting increases in estradiol, while prolactin, chorionic gonadotropin, and progesterone remain largely unaffected. Pregnant rhesus macaques receiving daily intramuscular injections of THC (2.5 mg/kg/day) exhibited elevated estradiol levels compared to vehicle-treated controls (Asch and Smith 1986). However, no significant changes were observed in prolactin, macaque chorionic gonadotropin (mCG), or progesterone levels (Asch and Smith 1986). In non-pregnant rhesus macaques, exposure to THC increased menstrual cycle length and basal follicle-stimulating hormone, but plateaued basal estradiol and luteinizing hormone concentrations, suggesting ovulatory dysfunction (Ryan et al. 2021).

9.3.2 Maternal Weight

Cannabis is an appetite stimulant and may contribute to maternal weight gain during pregnancy. However, few studies have evaluated maternal weight following cannabis use during pregnancy (Olyaei et al. 2022). Pregnant mice exposed to daily low-dose cannabis smoke (5 min of 0.2 grams of cannabis) from gestational day 5.5 to 17.5 showed a significant reduction in net body weight ($p = 0.03$), despite a slight increase in daily food intake compared to controls (Benevenuto et al. 2017). This association was not observed in pregnant rats receiving daily intraperitoneal injections of 3 mg/kg THC from embryonic day 6.5 to 22(Natale et al. 2020) or those exposed to moderate THC doses (100 mg/mL) via e-cigarette vapors from gestational day 5 to 20 (Breit et al. 2020). Rats exposed to vaporized THC (100 mg/mL) did not have altered maternal weight or food consumption (Hume et al. 2024). The effect of the route of THC administration on these differing outcomes remains unclear. In rhesus macaques exposed to edible THC (0.36 mg/kg), there were no significant changes to maternal, fetal, or placental weight observed (Roberts et al. 2022). However significant increase in the male-to-female ratio was noted in the THC vapor-exposed litters and a decrease in maternal body temperature (Sandini et al. 2023).

9.3.3 Gestational Length

There is evidence that cannabis use may be linked to preterm birth in humans (National Academies of Sciences, Engineering, and Medicine, Health and Medicine Division, Board on Population Health and Public Health Practice 2017; Marchand et al. 2022; Conner et al. 2016; Lo et al. 2024), but this has not been demonstrated in animal studies. Although there is limited preclinical literature examining this, several studies have reported that cannabis use does not affect gestational length (Breit et al. 2020; Natale et al. 2020). Gestational length remained unchanged in pregnant rats receiving daily intraperitoneal injections of 3 mg/kg THC from embryonic day 6.5 to 22(Natale et al. 2020) or those exposed to moderate THC doses (100 mg/mL) via e-cigarette vapors from gestational day 5 to 20 (Breit et al. 2020). In rhesus macaques, THC may cause ovulatory dysfunction characterized by altered hormones resulting in reduced fecundity (Ryan et al. 2021).

9.3.4 Pregnancy Loss

The association between cannabis use and pregnancy loss is inconsistent (Table 9.1). In humans, the relationship between cannabis use and pregnancy loss remains unclear. These mixed findings across species underscore the complexity of assessing cannabis-related pregnancy outcomes. While some rodent studies suggest a potential association, the findings are not statistically significant. A prior study showed that pregnant mice exposed to daily low-dose cannabis smoke (5 min of 0.2 grams of cannabis) exhibited a post-implantation loss index nearly twice that of controls (Benevenuto et al. 2017), but the difference was not statistically significant (Benevenuto et al. 2017). Similarly, in a different study where mice were given daily intraperitoneal injections of 3 mg/kg THC from E6.5–22, there was no significant difference in the number of reabsorptions compared to the control (Natale et al. 2020). In contrast, pregnant rats exposed to 10 g/kg of cannabis smoke showed an increase in spontaneous abortions (Akingbade et al. 2021). There was also no difference in the rates of miscarriage, dystocia, or cannibalization between pregnant rats exposed to THC vapor and the control (Breit et al. 2020). In another study of pregnant rats, exposure to 18% THC smoke also showed fewer offspring and increased reabsorption events (Black et al. 2023).

Table 9.1 Impact of THC exposure on maternal and pregnancy outcomes in animal studies

Study	Year	Primary measures	Species	Conditions	Results
Black et al. (2023)	2023	Litter size, reabsorption, histology, cytokine levels, plasma levels	Rat ($n = 76$)	0.7–18% THC smoke via inhalation or 3 mg/kg THC via intraperitoneal injection	Decreased offspring, increased reabsorption events
Natale et al. (2020)	2020	Immunohistochemistry, Iso-lectin B4 staining, placental composition, cell culture, RNA isolation, and real-time PCR	Rat ($n = 8$)	3 mg/kg THC via injection	Symmetrical intrauterine growth restriction, labyrinth-specific changes, reduced GLUT1, increased pericytes and collagen
Hutchings et al. (1989)	1989	Litter outcomes, plasma concentration	Rat ($n = 8$–10)	15–50 mg/kg THC via intraperitoneal injection	Dose-related increase in the sex-ratio offspring, inhibition of brain growth protein synthesis
Akingbade et al. (2021)	2021	Litter outcomes	Rat ($n = 5$)	10 g/kg cannabis via inhalation	Spontaneous abortion
Breit et al. (2020)	2020	Core body temperature, birth and litter monitoring, plasma concentration	Rat ($n = 10$–13)	100 mg/mL THC via inhalation	THC levels accumulate in dams
Hume et al. (2024)	2024	Litter outcomes	Rat ($n = 24$)	100 mg/mL THC via inhalation	Transient decreased pup weight
Sandini et al. (2023)	2023	Behavior testing, RNA extraction, differential gene expression, litter outcomes, body temperature	Rat ($n = 49$)	200 mg cannabis via inhalation	Decreased body temperature in dams, increase in male to female ratio
Roberts et al. (2022)	2022	Gross fetal measurements, MRI	Rhesus ($n = 5$)	0.36 mg/kg THC via ingestion	No change to maternal, fetal, or placental weight
Asch and Smith (1986)	1986	Litter outcomes, plasma concentration	Rhesus ($n = 5$)	2.5 mg/kg THC via injection	Increased estradiol, abortion, stillbirth

One study examined pregnant rhesus macaques receiving daily intramuscular injections of THC (2.5 mg/kg/day) at different gestational stages: from pregnancy confirmation to cesarean section, from gestational day (GD) 55–109 (full term is ~168 days), or from GD 110 until delivery (Asch and Smith 1986). Among those exposed throughout pregnancy, four out of five experienced pregnancy loss, including three spontaneous abortions shortly after THC administration began, one stillbirth at GD 140, and one live birth of a healthy infant. The authors suggest that the spontaneous abortions may have resulted from a rapid decline in macaque chorionic gonadotropin (mCG) levels due to THC exposure (Asch and Smith 1986). In macaques administered THC later in gestation, one stillbirth and two preterm deliveries with neonatal demise were observed, while the remaining infants were born healthy.

9.4 Placental Outcomes

The placenta is a critical organ at the maternal-fetal interface that serves as a barrier between the two compartments. Key functions include selective transfer of growth factors, hormones, cytokines, gases, water, nutrients, and waste products for normal fetal growth and development, biosynthesis of growth factors, hormones, and cytokines, and immune protection of the fetal allograft from pathogens and the maternal immune system.

The vertebrate placenta is a product of convergent evolution on the macro- and microscale, resulting in interspecies heterogeneity (Roberts et al. 2016). As a result, animal models investigating placental biology have different limitations in translatability of results to human disease compared to other organ systems. In this section, we will review the different animal models used to investigate the effects of cannabis exposure during pregnancy on the placenta. The first study suggesting transplacental passage of cannabis was performed in mice in 1967 (Persaud and Ellington 1967). Shortly after, several studies in rats, hamsters, and rabbits reported teratogenic effects from cannabis extracts (Persaud and Ellington 1968; Geber and Schramm 1969). This was followed by a study using hamsters that demonstrated placental transfer of tritiated-1-delta-9-tetrahydrocannabinol (THC) in 1969 (Idänpään-Heikkilä et al. 1969). Of note, placental accumulation of THC, identified by gas chromatography and quantified by thin-layer chromatography, was shown to be more than twice as much THC in the placenta compared to the fetus. This was the first study to suggest that cannabis exposure may have an impact on placental function.

Early investigations using rodent models (hamster, mouse) demonstrated placental accumulation of THC following exposure. The first study used pregnant Syrian golden hamsters injected intraperitoneally ($n = 16$) with THC-H^3 (THC radiolabeled with tritium-hydrogen) on gestational day (GD) 6 ($n = 8$) and on GD 15 ($n = 8$) (Idänpään-Heikkilä et al. 1969). A second group of hamsters were injected subcutaneously with THC-^{3}H on GD 6 ($n = 4$) and on GD 15 ($n = 4$). The animals were necropsied at 15, 30, 120 min and 24 h, and specific tissues (fetus, placenta, maternal brain, maternal blood) were homogenized and radioactivity assayed. Across all groups, a 2- to three-fold higher concentration of THC in the placenta compared to the fetus was observed. A second study using pregnant mice administered either intravenous ($n = 4$) or oral ($n = 4$) THC-^{14}C (THC radiolabeled with carbon-14) on GD 15 (Freudenthal et al. 1972). The animals were euthanized with control animals at 30 min ($n = 2$) and 120 min ($n = 2$). Whole body autoradiography was used to identify tissue distribution of THC-^{14}C, which demonstrated high concentrations in the yolk sac placenta.

The expression of the cannabinoid receptors CB1 and CB2 were first demonstrated in rat placentas as receptors for the endocannabinoid anandamide (Cella et al. 2008). These receptors were previously reported to be expressed in human placentas from the first- and third-trimesters (Kenney et al. 1999; Park et al. 2003; Habayeb et al. 2008). Characterization of the endocannabinoid system in the placenta was performed in pregnant rats and demonstrated the system was active in the placenta throughout development with CB1 and CB2 expressed in giant trophoblast (CB1 > CB2), spongiotrophoblasts (CB1 = CB2), and in syncytiotrophoblasts (CB1 > CB2) (Fonseca et al. 2012). Pregnant mice deficient in either of the cannabinoid receptors (CB1 or *Cnr1−/−* and CB2 or *Cnr2−/−*) had abnormal placentation (Sun et al. 2010). CB1-deficient mice had placentas with lower weight, decreased differentiated spongiotrophoblast cells, and decreased proliferation of trophoblast progenitor cells in the ecoplacental cone. Mouse trophoblast stem cells cultured in vitro that were deficient in CB1 and CB2 had slower proliferation, preferentially differentiated into trophoblast giant cells, and were less invasive. In addition, CB1 directly interacts with VANGL2, a core planar cell polarity component that regulates trophoblast migration (Kim et al. 2021). Loss of either of these proteins resulted in decreased trophoblast migration. Cannabinoid signaling is also important for decidual development. Mice deficient in both CB1 and CB2 demonstrated compromised primary decidual zone with dysregulated angiogenic factors (Li et al. 2020). In vitro culture of CB1-deficient stromal cells induced to a decidual reaction showed decreased expression of markers of decidualization. Expression of CB1 is increased in control stromal cells induced to a decidual reaction in vitro, and treatment of control cells with CB1 antagonists compromised decidualization, suggesting CB1 is important for endometrial decidualization.

Pregnant mice exposed to inhaled cannabis smoke had a sex-specific increase in placental weight in male fetuses, with female fetuses having increased weight that was not statistically significant (Benevenuto et al. 2017). THC administered during pregnancy to pregnant rats from GD 6.5 to GD 22 had placentas with increased labyrinth area, reduced labyrinth trophoblast progenitors, increased maternal blood space, decreased fetal capillary area, and increased recruitment of pericytes with greater collagen deposition, when compared to controls (Natale et al. 2020). In addition, labyrinth trophoblasts had lower expression of glucose transporter 1 (GLUT1) and glucocorticoid receptor (GR).

The rhesus macaque placenta is the most similar in structure and function to humans, sharing a hemochorial villous structure that is bi-discoid. The first study that evaluated placenta effects of THC in rhesus macaques reported no difference in placental morphology on gross and histologic examination, and no difference in placental weights (Table 9.2) (Asch and Smith 1986). More recently, pregnant rhesus macaques chronically exposed to edible THC throughout gestation demonstrated placental insufficiency with decreased amniotic fluid volume, placental perfusion, and fetal oxygen availability when compared to control animals (Roberts et al. 2022). Ultrasound and magnetic resonance imaging (MRI) evaluation during pregnancy showed decreasing levels of amniotic fluid from GD 85 to GD 155 in THC-exposed animals, compared to increasing levels of amniotic fluid in control animals as observed normally in pregnancy. Dynamic contrast-enhanced (DCE) MRI analysis of placental blood flow showed decreased placental blood flow at GD 135 and 155 and blood oxygen level-dependent (BOLD) MRI analysis of placental oxygenation showed decreased oxygen availability from GD 85 to GD 155. Histological examination of placentas revealed evidence of THC-induced ischemic injury with both acute and remote microinfarctions and increased syncytial knotting in placentas. Gene expression analysis showed a unique signature in the placentas from THC-exposed animals, with gene ontology analysis demonstrating changes in vascular development and angiogenesis pathways. Further association between DNA methylation and differentially expressed genes identified significant epigenetic regulation of gene expression (eQTM), with the top differentially expressed gene *DNAJA4* correlated with methylation of 12 CpGs (Shorey-Kendrick et al. 2023a).

9.5 Fetal, Newborn, and Infant Outcomes

9.5.1 Fetal Growth and Birthweight

Prenatal cannabis exposure has been shown to result in fetal growth restriction and low birth weight in humans (Marchand et al. 2022; Conner et al. 2016; Lo et al. 2024), but it is unclear whether this is secondary to THC or the toxins from smoked cannabis, the most common mode of cannabis use in pregnancy. In animal models, however, the impact of cannabis use in pregnancy on fetal growth and birth weight remains unclear (Olyaei et al. 2022). Several rodent studies have reported growth restriction following exposure during pregnancy (Table 9.3) (Benevenuto et al. 2017; Natale et al. 2020; Lee et al. 2021; Gillies et al. 2020). Pregnant mice exposed to daily low-dose cannabis smoke (5 min of 0.2 grams of cannabis) from GD 5.5 to 17.5 had litters with 9.9% lower fetal weight compared to controls (Benevenuto et al. 2017). Fetal organs, including the lungs ($p = 0.001$), brain ($p = 0.002$), thymus ($p = 0.003$), and liver ($p = 0.008$), also showed a significant weight reduction. Daily intraperitoneal injections of 3 mg/kg THC from GD 6 to 22 have also been shown to cause fetal growth restriction in pregnant rats (Lee et al. 2021). Symmetrical fetal growth restriction post E19.5 is demonstrated in rats and may be caused by placental defects (Natale et al. 2020). Rats prenatally exposed to THC display altered expression of nutrient

Table 9.2 Effects of THC exposure on placental outcomes in animal studies

Study	Year	Primary measures	Species	Conditions	Results
Freudenthal et al. (1972)	1972	Whole body autoradiography	Mouse ($n = 4$)	~ 20 mg/kg THC via oral gavage or injection	High placental concentrations
Benevenuto et al. (2017)	2017	Body weight	Mouse ($n = 8$)	1 cannabis cigarette via smoke inhalation	Sex specific weight increase
Idänpään-Heikkilä et al. (1969)	1969	Gas chromatography, thin-layer chromatography	Syrian Golden hamster ($n = 8$)	2 mg/kg THC via injection	THC crosses the placenta and gathers in the fetus
Natale et al. (2020)	2020	Immunohistochemistry, Iso-lectin B4 staining, placental composition, cell culture, RNA isolation, and real-time PCR	Rat ($n = 8$)	3 mg/kg THC via injection	Symmetrical intrauterine growth restriction, labyrinth-specific changes, reduced GLUT1, increased pericytes, and collagen
Roberts et al. (2022)	2022	Ultrasound, histology, MRI, RNA-seq	Rhesus ($n = 5$)	0.36 mg/kg THC via ingestion	Placental insufficiency with decreased amniotic fluid volume, decreased placental perfusion, altered placental transcriptome, and decreased fetal oxygen availability
Shorey-Kendrick et al. (2023a)	2023	DNA extraction and DNA methylation array acquisition and preprocessing, gene ontology, enrichment analysis, expression quantitative trait methylation, enrichment analysis of candidate autism disorder genes	Rhesus ($n = 5$)	0.36 mg/kg THC via ingestion	Differential methylation in all tissues, placental MEGF10 hypermethylation, and autism spectrum disorder gene enrichment
Asch and Smith (1986)	1986	Litter outcomes, plasma concentration	Rhesus ($n = 5$)	2.5 mg/kg THC via injection	Increased estradiol, abortion, stillbirth

transporters and changes to the placental fetal vasculature, which may underlie the reduced fetal growth (Allen et al. 2024).

Conversely, NHP and rodent studies have found no association between prenatal cannabis exposure and fetal growth or birthweight (Breit et al. 2020; Asch and Smith 1986; Weimar et al. 2020). Fetal growth measurements showed no significant differences among infants born to rhesus macaques receiving intramuscular THC injections (2.5 mg/kg/day) throughout pregnancy, during the latter two-thirds, or near term (Asch and Smith 1986). Similarly, birth weights did not differ between THC-exposed and control groups, though infants from THC-treated mothers exhibited reduced postnatal weight gain (Asch and Smith 1986). Pregnant rats exposed to THC vapors (100 mg/2 mL at 2 L/min airflow) showed no difference in birthweight compared to the control (Breit et al. 2020). Twice-daily exposure to cannabis vapors (400 mg/mL) in pregnant rats led to reduced postnatal weight gain in offspring compared to those from untreated mothers; however, this may have been from stress related to vapor delivery (Weimar et al. 2020). Another study in rats also showed a decrease in birth weight while not affecting maternal weight (Gillies et al. 2020).

9.5.2 Neurodevelopmental Effects

Prenatal THC exposure has been shown to adversely affect fetal brain development. In

Table 9.3 Impact of THC exposure on fetal and newborn outcomes in animal studies

Study	Year	Primary measures	Species	Conditions	Results
Roeder et al. (2024)	2024	Gross measurements	Mouse ($n = 32$)	40 mg THC via inhalation	Maternal weight gain and birth weight
Rouzer et al. (2024)	2024	Ultrasonography	Mouse ($n = 7$ dams)	750 μg/kg CP-55940 via IP	Decreased cranial blood flow, reduced cerebroplacental ratios
Robinson et al. (2024)	2024	Histology, immunohistochemistry, AMIRA 3 dimensional reconstructions	Mouse ($n = 67$)	5–10 mg/kg THC via oral gavage	Ventricular septal defect, enlarged semilunar valves, increased wall thickness and cell proliferation, reduced cardiac transcription factor expression
Weimar et al. (2020)	2020	Gross measurements, behavioral testing	Rat ($n = 21$–36)	400 mg/mL cannabis via inhalation	Reduced weight
Akingbade et al. (2021)	2021	Histology, biochemical assays	Rat ($n = 5$)	10 g/kg cannabis via inhalation	Altered neuronal morphology in SC and LGN, changed enzyme activity levels
Frau et al. (2019)	2019	Behavioral testing, electrophysiology, immunostaining, correlated confocal and STORM imaging	Rat ($n = 8$–18)	2 mg/kg THC via subcutaneous injection	Sex-specific ventral tegmental area changes, altered excitation-inhibition balance, reversed synaptic plasticity polarity
Gillies et al. (2020)	2020	Intraportal insulin challenge, protein extraction, and western blot, immunohistochemistry, endocrine pancreas morphometry, gross weights	Rat ($n = 5$–7)	3 mg/kg THC via injection	Reduced birthweight
Natale et al. (2020)	2020	Histology, immunohistochemistry, cell culture, RNA isolation and real-time PCR	Rat ($n = 8$)	3 mg/kg THC via injection	Symmetrical intrauterine fetal growth restriction, labyrinth-specific changes, reduced GLUT1, increased pericytes and collagen
Oke et al. (2021)	2021	Morphometry, gross weights	Rat ($n = 14$)	3 mg/kg THC via intraperitoneal injection	Reduced liver-to-body weight ratio
Lee et al. (2021)	2021	Echocardiography, RNA extraction and real-time RT-qPCR, protein extraction and western blot	Rat ($n = 8$)	3 mg/kg THC via injection	Fetal growth restriction, lower heart-to-body weight, thicker left ventricular wall, reduced cardiac output, increased collagen, and cardiac remodeling
Beggiato et al. (2017)	2017	[3H]-GABA outflow and uptake experiments, binding experiments	Rat ($n = 7$–10)	5 mg/kg THC via oral gavage	Disrupted hippocampal GABA function, reduced [3H]-GABA outflow and uptake, and lower CB1 receptor density
Moellmer et al. (2024)	2024	RNA isolation, NanoString neuroinflammatory panel, histology	Rhesus ($n = 3$–6)	0.36 mg/kg THC via ingestion	Differential gene expression in skeletal muscle, altered PI3K-Akt signaling, IL-24 upregulated in fetal, IL-4/IL-13/IL-10 upregulated in infants
Roberts et al. (2022)	2022	Gross fetal measurements, MRI	Rhesus ($n = 5$)	0.36 mg/kg THC via ingestion	Nonsignificant reduction in whole brain growth rate

(continued)

Table 9.3 (continued)

Study	Year	Primary measures	Species	Conditions	Results
Shorey-Kendrick et al. (2023a, b)	2023	DNA extraction and DNA methylation (DNAm) array acquisition and pre-processing, gene ontology, expression quantitative trait methylation, enrichment analysis of candidate autism disorder genes	Rhesus ($n = 5$)	0.36 mg/kg THC via ingestion	Differential methylation with 98% in the placenta, enriched at autism spectrum disorder genes
Le et al. (2024)	2024	Tissue histology, western blot, RNA isolation, bulk RNA-sequencing	Rhesus ($n = 5$)	0.36 mg/kg THC via ingestion	Decreased heart weight-to-body weight ratio, altered fetal vascular transcriptome, upregulated metabolism and inflammation genes
Ryan et al. (2024)	2024	Fetal pathology, fetal brain histology, multiplex immunohistochemistry	Rhesus ($n = 5$)	0.36 mg/kg THC via ingestion	Increased Iba-1/GFAP staining, sex/age-dependent brain changes
Shorey-Kendrick et al. (2025)	2025	MRI, pulmonary function test, bronchial alveolar lavage, whole genome bisulfite sequencing, RNA sequencing	Rhesus ($n = 5$)	0.36 mg/kg THC via ingestion	Reduced forced residual capacity, decreased lung capacity, diffusion capacity, and fetal lung perfusion, lower oxygen availability and lung volume, decreased pulmonary growth factors, altered methylation in lung development, ECM organization, and immune signaling
Carty et al. (2017)	2017	Lethality and morphology, behavior, RT-qPCR	Zebrafish	1–16; 0.25–4 μM THC via media	Malformation, differential C-FOS, DAZL, and VASA expression
Ahmed et al. (2018)	2018	Electrophysiology, gross morphology, motor neuron immunolabelling, nAChR labeling	Zebrafish ($n = 61$)	2–10; 1–4 mg/L THC via media	Reduced body length, survival, hatch rates, heart rate, mEPC frequency, motor neuron branching, C-start response

rodent models, offspring of pregnant rats exposed to daily moderate doses of THC (5 mg/kg) exhibited long-term alterations in the hippocampal GABAergic system, including decreased [3H]-GABA uptake and significantly reduced CB1 receptor binding in the hippocampus at 90 days of age (Beggiato et al. 2017). Exposure to cannabis smoke during gestation also impaired the visual pathway, leading to histological and biochemical changes in the superior colliculus and lateral geniculate nucleus, likely due to oxidative damage (Akingbade et al. 2021).

Sex-specific neurodevelopmental effects have also been observed, with male offspring more affected. Daily subcutaneous administration of low-dose THC (2 mg/kg) throughout gestation in mice induced a hyperdopaminergic state in male offspring, characterized by enhanced dopamine release and heightened excitability of the ventral tegmental area dopamine neurons (Frau et al. 2019). These male offspring also exhibited increased behavioral sensitivity to acute THC exposure during pre-adolescence. Notably, postnatal administration of pregnenolone reversed these THC-induced effects. Female offspring, however, did not develop a hyperdopaminergic state or increased THC sensitivity (Table 9.3) (Traccis et al. 2021). Additional studies have reported spatial memory impairment, brain hyperexcitability, and altered hippocampal oscillations, particularly in male offspring (Beggiato et al. 2017, 2020).

In rhesus macaques, THC-exposed fetuses showed a slight but nonsignificant reduction in whole-brain growth rate, with the most pronounced effects in the cortical plate, white matter, brainstem, and cerebellum. These findings suggest that THC exposure alters fetal brain growth trajectories, with significant age-by-sex interactions. Molecular analyses further revealed that THC exposure disrupts extracellular vesicle-associated (Roberts et al. 2022) miRNAs in fetal cerebrospinal fluid, particularly in pathways related to axonal guidance and netrin signaling (de Salas-Quiroga et al. 2020). Furthermore, THC exposure alters fetal DNA methylation in multiple tissue types, including placenta, lung, heart, and brain, at genes involved in neurobehavioral development (Shorey-Kendrick et al. 2023b).

9.5.3 Cardiovascular, Cerebrovascular, and Pulmonary Effects

Prenatal THC exposure has been linked to cardiac abnormalities and impaired cerebrovascular function. In rodent models, maternal THC exposure resulted in ventricular septal defects, semilunar valve thickening, and myocardial hyperplasia in 44–55% of E17.5 fetuses (Robinson et al. 2024). Additionally, THC exposure at E12.5 increased ventricular myocardium proliferation and downregulated key cardiac transcription factors, suggesting an increased risk of postnatal cardiac dysfunction.

THC exposure also impacts fetal cerebral blood flow. In a study evaluating prenatal alcohol and cannabinoid co-exposure, THC decreased cerebroplacental ratios, which correlated with an increased risk of perinatal mortality (Rouzer et al. 2024). These vascular alterations highlight the potential impact of THC on fetal cerebrovascular health and long-term cardiovascular function. In rhesus macaques, in utero THC exposure causes decreased heart weight-to-body weight ratio (Le et al. 2024).

Pulmonary effects have also been observed in in utero THC exposure. In rhesus macaques, infants exposed to THC in utero display significantly reduced forced residual capacity ($p = 0.015$), correlated with nonsignificant decreases in total lung capacity, lung diffusion capacity and lower fetal lung perfusion, oxygen availability, and lung volume measured by MRI (Shorey-Kendrick et al. 2025). Pulmonary growth factor levels in bronchial alveolar lavage were diminished at 6 months. Infant lungs exhibited altered epigenetic regulation of gene expression, particularly in genes associated with extracellular matrix organization, lung development, and immune signaling activation (Shorey-Kendrick et al. 2025).

9.5.4 Hepatic and Metabolic Effects

Prenatal THC exposure has been associated with liver abnormalities and metabolic alterations. In rodent models, THC exposure at 3 mg/kg during pregnancy resulted in a decreased liver-to-body weight ratio at birth, followed by catch-up growth postnatally (Oke et al. 2021). Changes in fetal liver composition suggest disruptions in metabolic programming, which may have long-term consequences for offspring health.

9.5.5 Epigenetic Effects

THC exposure during pregnancy alters epigenetic regulation of gene expression. Analysis of placental and fetal tissue (lung, brain, and heart) from rhesus macaques revealed significant DNA methylation changes at genes involved in neurobehavioral development (Shorey-Kendrick et al. 2023a). Notably, 98% of differentially methylated CpGs were found in the placenta, with many genes overlapping with those associated with autism spectrum disorder (Shorey-Kendrick et al. 2023b). In the same model, infant lungs have shown altered epigenetic regulation of gene expression, including at genes involved in the extracellular matrix organization and lung development, and activation of immune signaling (Shorey-Kendrick et al. 2025).

These findings indicate that THC exposure may have lasting epigenetic consequences beyond immediate fetal development.

9.5.6 Inflammatory Effects

Although prenatal THC exposure has minimal effects on overall muscle development, it alters inflammation-related pathways, particularly cytokine signaling. In rhesus macaques, differential gene expression was more pronounced in infants than fetuses, with upregulation of *IL-24*, *IL-4*, *IL-13*, and *IL-10* signaling genes (Moellmer et al. 2024). Despite PI3K-Akt pathway involvement, the absence of *IGF-1* upregulation suggests that prenatal THC exposure does not significantly impact skeletal muscle mass.

In the same model, THC-exposed offspring exhibited a decreased heart-to-body weight ratio, altered fetal vascular transcriptome, and upregulation of metabolism and inflammation-related genes (Le et al. 2024). These findings suggest that THC exposure may contribute to inflammatory dysregulation in multiple organ systems, warranting further investigation into potential long-term health implications. Pregnant rats exposed to 18% THC smoke had an increase in proinflammatory cytokines in the placenta and fetal brain (Black et al. 2023).

9.5.7 Comparative Model Insights

Zebrafish models provide additional insights into prenatal cannabinoid exposure, though their relevance to mammalian systems remains debated. THC exposure during key developmental stages, such as gastrulation, led to adverse outcomes in zebrafish embryos, including reduced body length, altered motor neuron development, and decreased survival rates (Ahmed et al. 2018). Additional defects, such as jaw malformations, axis curvature, and trunk degradation were also observed (Carty et al. 2017). However, no primate or rodent studies have reported similar fetal malformations, which may suggest translational limitations of zebrafish models for predicting human developmental outcomes.

9.6 Pre-pubertal

9.6.1 Neurodevelopmental Effects

Prenatal THC exposure alters brain function and behavior in a sex-specific manner in pre-pubertal offspring, with male offspring most affected. In rodent models, daily subcutaneous injections of 2 mg/kg THC throughout gestation induced a hyperdopaminergic state in male offspring but not in females (Table 9.4) (Frau et al. 2019). Male offspring exhibited increased dopamine release, heightened excitability of ventral tegmental area dopamine neurons, and greater sensitivity to acute THC exposure in pre-adolescence. In contrast, female offspring did not develop this heightened THC sensitivity (Traccis et al. 2021).

THC exposure also impacts cognitive function and spatial learning. In female rats, prenatal THC exposure impaired spatial memory and learning (Lei et al. 2021). Co-exposure to ethanol did not exacerbate these deficits but did reduce thigmotaxis, potentially indicating increased risk-taking behavior (Lei et al. 2021). At the molecular level, prenatal THC exposure led to significant downregulation of docosahexaenoic acid and arachidonic acid signaling pathways in the prefrontal cortex and ventral hippocampus at postnatal day 21, particularly in females (Sarikahya et al. 2023). This was linked to decreased expression of PPARα, potentially due to initial overactivation by both THC and estrogen (Sarikahya et al. 2023).

Further, THC exposure disrupted neuronal composition and gene expression in the hippocampus, particularly in pathways associated with neurogenesis and neural differentiation (Peng et al. 2023). THC impaired neural stem cell differentiation by downregulating MEF2C, a transcription factor critical for neurodevelopment (Peng et al. 2023). This effect was reversed by CB1 receptor inhibition, suggesting that THC disrupts hippocampal development through CB1

Table 9.4 Effect of prenatal THC exposure on pre-pubertal outcomes in animal studies

Study	Year	Primary measures	Species	Conditions	Results
Roeder et al. (2024)	2024	Circadian activity, open field locomotor activity, exercise, wheel running	Mouse ($n = 32$)	40 mg THC via inhalation	Affects dark-cycle activity, locomotion, exploratory behavior
Peng et al. (2023)	2023	Immunofluorescence staining of GFAP and NEUN, whole transcriptome analysis of the fetal hippocampus, qPCR	Mouse ($n = 4$)	5 mg/kg THC via intraperitoneal injection	Altered hippocampal development, neurogenesis, and differentiation, via mef2c
Robinson et al. (2024)	2024	Morphologic abnormalities via histology, echocardiography	Mouse ($n = 67$)	5–10 mg/kg THC via oral gavage	Compromised heart function
Lei et al. (2023)	2023	Behavior testing	Rat ($n = 26$)	100 mg/mL THC via inhalation	Sex-specific impaired spatial learning and memory
Weimar et al. (2020)	2020	Behavioral testing	Rat ($n = 21$–36)	400 mg/mL cannabis via inhalation	Decreased play behavior, sex-specific decreased social investigation
Frau et al. (2019)	2019	Cerebral microdialysis, behavioral analysis, electrophysiological recordings, and immunostaining	Rat ($n = 8$–18)	2 mg/kg THC via subcutaneous injection	Sex-specific hypodopaminergic state
Traccis et al. (2021)	2021	Behavioral testing, cerebral microdialysis, and electrophysiological recordings	Rat ($n = 6$–12)	2 mg/kg THC via subcutaneous injection	Delayed risk-taking, increased locomotion in females
Murru et al. (2024)	2024	HPLC, GC, DNA isolation from rat caecal samples, and sequencing	Rat ($n = 5$)	2 mg/kg THC via subcutaneous injection	Alterations in liver fatty acid profile, altered liver gene expression, and reduction in fasting glycemia
Sarikahya et al. (2022)	2022	Behavior testing, extracellular recording of the ventral tegmental area, mass spectrometry, protein extraction, and western blotting	Rat ($n = 13$ dams, 63 pups)	3 mg/kg THC via intraperitoneal injection	Sex-specific dysregulation of fatty acid pathways in the brain lipidome
Sarikahya et al. (2023)	2023	Behavior testing, extracellular recordings of the prefrontal cortex and vHIPP, MALDI IMS, protein expression analyses	Rat ($n = 13$ dams, 37 pups)	3 mg/kg THC via intraperitoneal injection	Sex-specific PPARα expression

receptor-mediated MEF2C regulation (Peng et al. 2023).

9.6.2 Metabolic, Endocrine, and Cardiovascular Effects

Prenatal THC exposure has broad metabolic consequences, with sex-specific alterations in lipid metabolism and gut microbiota composition. In pre-adolescent rats, prenatal THC exposure (2 mg/kg, GD 5–20) increased liver de novo lipogenesis and altered fatty acid profiles in both sexes (Murru et al. 2024). However, the metabolic effects were distinct between males and females. In females, THC exposure affected *PPAR-α* and *Fgf21* gene expression, while in males, it resulted in reduced fasting glycemia and altered midbrain N-acylethanolamine levels (Murru et al. 2024). Male offspring also showed increased Ileibacterium abundance, a microbiota shift linked to metabolic dysfunction and a potential contributor to their heightened susceptibility to psychopathology (Murru et al. 2024).

Additionally, prenatal THC exposure influenced pre-pubertal offspring activity patterns. THC reduced dark-cycle activity and increased locomotion in open-field tests, with male offspring exhibiting greater exploratory behavior (Table 9.4) (Roeder et al. 2024). These behavioral shifts suggest a potential link between THC exposure and altered activity or obesity risk later in life, particularly in males.

Prenatal THC exposure also adversely affects early cardiac function. In pups of both sexes at postnatal day 21, THC exposure led to compromised heart function, characterized by reduced left ventricular ejection fraction, fractional shortening, and cardiac output (Robinson et al. 2024).

9.7 Post-pubertal/Adulthood

After puberty, sex becomes an increasingly important biological factor in the effects of THC exposure. The hormonal and physiological changes that occur during this stage heighten the potential for sex-specific responses, influencing the way males and females process and are affected by THC. These post-pubertal differences emphasize the need for a detailed understanding of THC's impact on both sexes as they mature.

9.7.1 Neurodevelopmental and Behavioral Effects

Prenatal THC exposure leads to long-lasting effects on brain function and behavior, with sex-specific alterations in neuronal activity, neurotransmitter signaling, and cognitive function. Electrophysiological recordings in rodents showed hyperactivity in the prefrontal cortex of both sexes but divergent activity in the ventral hippocampus, with males exhibiting hypoactivity and females showing hyperactivity (Sarikahya et al. 2023). Protein expression analysis revealed disturbances in dopamine and N-methyl-D-aspartate (NMDA) receptors, including increased D1R and decreased D2R and NMDAR2B expression in the prefrontal cortex and ventral hippocampus of adult males, with more selective downregulation of these markers in the ventral hippocampus of females, particularly at postnatal day 120(Sarikahya et al. 2023).

MALDI-IMS imaging identified sex- and region-specific deficiencies in docosahexaenoic acid and arachidonic acid in the prefrontal cortex and hippocampus, highlighting THC-induced prefrontal cortex-hippocampal dysfunction and polyunsaturated fatty acid signaling abnormalities (Sarikahya et al. 2023). THC-exposed rats exhibited higher basal kynurenic acid (KYNA) levels and lower basal glutamate levels, along with impaired short-term memory in adulthood. Following an acute kynurenine challenge in adulthood, the increase in KYNA levels in the medial prefrontal cortex was more pronounced in THC-exposed rats, suggesting a potential link between KYNA dysregulation and cognitive dysfunction (Table 9.5) (Beggiato et al. 2020).

Beyond cognitive and neural alterations, prenatal THC exposure may increase susceptibility to addiction-like behaviors. THC-exposed rats developed a supra-motivational phenotype independent of value-based processing, which was linked to an enhanced reinforcing efficiency of opioid rewards. This phenotype was associated with increased cue-evoked dopamine responses and altered striatal encoding patterns, with males showing greater vulnerability to relapse (Luján et al. 2024). However, while prenatal cannabis exposure disinhibited ventral tegmental area dopamine neuron activity, it did not influence cocaine preference in offspring (Peterson et al. 2024). In humans, increased drug-seeking behavior is associated with methylation changes in the brain (Kozlenkov et al. 2017).

9.7.2 Metabolic, Endocrine, and Cardiovascular Effects

Prenatal THC exposure disrupts metabolic function in a sex-dependent manner in post-pubertal offspring. In male and female rats, THC exposure led to reduced body weight during adolescence (Breit et al. 2020). Females exhibited elevated blood glucose levels following a glucose challenge, along with increased serum insulin concentrations (Gillies et al. 2020). Additionally, females showed a significantly reduced ratio of phosphorylated Akt [Ser 473] to total Akt2

Table 9.5 Effect of THC exposure on post-pubertal outcomes in animal studies

Study	Year	Primary measures	Species	Conditions	Results
Peterson et al. (2024)	2024	LC–MS/MS analysis, electrophysiology	Mouse ($n = 18$)	5 mg/kg cannabis oil via ingestion	Sex-specific decreased GABAergic input and increased
Navarro et al. (2024)	2024	Emotional, cognitive evaluations, and oral ethanol self-administration	Mouse ($n = 131$)	10 mg/kg dronabinol via oral gavage	Sex-specific increased anxiety, depression, cognitive impairment, neurodevelopmental changes, and alcohol motivation
Breit et al. (2020)	2020	Adolescent body weights	Rat ($n = 10$–13)	100 mg/mL THC via inhalation	Decreased body weight in THC-exposed adolescents
Hume et al. (2024)	2024	Adiposity, glucose metabolism, and feeding behavior tests	Rat ($n = 24$)	100 mg/mL THC via inhalation	Reduced body weight gain on HFD/LFD, sex- and diet-dependent glucose metabolism and feeding effects
Sandini et al. (2023)	2023	Behavioral testing, differential gene expression, and gene ontology analysis	Rat ($n = 49$)	200 mg of cannabis via inhalation	Sex-specific increased exploration behavior, gene changes in development, cellular function, and nervous system disease
Weimar et al. (2020)	2020	Emotional reactivity, social and novel environment-induced anxiety-like behavior, and behavioral flexibility at neonatal, juvenile, and adult timepoints	Rat ($n = 21$–36)	400 mg/mL cannabis via inhalation	Increased anxiety, impaired behavioral flexibility
Luján et al. (2024)	2024	Fiber photometry, electrophysiological recordings, tensor component analysis	Rat ($n = 22$)	2 mg/kg THC via intraperitoneal injection	Increased cue-evoked dopamine responses, susceptibility to addiction-like disorders
Gillies et al. (2020)	2020	Fasting blood glucose, insulin, and sex steroid levels; immunohistochemistry and endocrine pancreas morphometry	Rat ($n = 5$–7)	3 mg/kg THC via injection	Sex-specific glucose intolerance, insulin sensitivity, and decreased total islet cell number.
Oke et al. (2021)	2021	Circulating, hepatic triglyceride, cholesterol, RNA isolation, quantitative real-time PCR analysis, protein extraction, and western immunoblot	Rat ($n = 14$)	3 mg/kg THC via intraperitoneal injection	Sex-specific increased adipose/body weight ratio, elevated hepatic lipogenic enzymes, oxidative stress, mitochondrial dysfunction, and altered miRNA expression
Martínez-Peña et al. (2021)	2021	Hormone levels, follicle quantitation, immunohistochemistry, and immunofluorescence	Rat ($n = 5$–6)	3 mg/kg THC via intraperitoneal injection	Accelerated folliculogenesis, reduced ovarian blood vessel density, altered VEGF/TSP-1 expression, and increased transitioning follicles
Sarikahya et al. (2022)	2022	Behavioral testing, electrophysiology, imaging mass spectrometry, protein extraction and Western blotting	Rat ($n = 13$ dams, 63 pups)	3 mg/kg THC via intraperitoneal injection	Sex-specific behavioral, neuronal, and molecular alterations in the mesolimbic system, dysregulation of fatty acid pathways in brain lipidome
Martínez-Peña et al. (2022)	2022	Nanostring analysis, miRNA real-time quantitative PCR, and immunohistochemistry	Rat ($n = 5$)	3 mg/kg THC via intraperitoneal injection	Differential miRNA expression, specifically miR-122-5p

(continued)

Table 9.5 (continued)

Study	Year	Primary measures	Species	Conditions	Results
Sarikahya et al. (2023)	2023	Cognitive/memory task, in vivo electrophysiology, imaging mass spectrometry, protein expression analyses	Rat ($n = 13$ dams, 37 pups)	3 mg/kg THC via intraperitoneal injection	Sex-specific cognitive deficits, hyperactive prefrontal cortex, disturbances in dopamine receptors and other proteins, differences in neural polyunsaturated fatty acids
Oke et al. (2021)	2020	In vivo microdialysis, dialysate, glutamate was measured by high-performance liquid chromatography, behavior testing	Rat ($n = 3$–5)	5 mg/kg THC via oral gavage	Prenatal THC increased basal KYNA, reduced glutamate in mPFC, increased adult KAT I, and impaired short-term memory

protein expression after an insulin challenge, as well as a decrease in the total number of islet cells, indicating impaired insulin signaling (Gillies et al. 2020).

At 6 months of age, THC-exposed male offspring showed increased visceral adiposity, higher hepatic triglyceride levels, and elevated expression of enzymes involved in triglyceride synthesis. These metabolic changes were accompanied by mitochondrial dysfunction and oxidative stress (Oke et al. 2021). Further molecular analysis revealed decreases in miR-203a-3p and miR-29a/b/c, microRNAs linked to dyslipidemia, suggesting a possible mechanism underlying THC-induced metabolic dysfunction (Oke et al. 2021).

In addition, prenatal THC exposure has been shown to have lasting effects on post-pubertal cardiovascular health. Offspring exposed to THC in utero exhibited lower left ventricular ejection fraction, fractional shortening, and cardiac output at postnatal day 21 (Robinson et al. 2024). These structural and functional deficits suggest that THC exposure during gestation may predispose offspring to long-term cardiovascular dysfunction.

9.7.3 Reproductive Effects

Prenatal THC exposure may have long-term consequences for reproductive health. Female C57BL/6 J mice exposed to dronabinol (a synthetic THC) (10 mg/kg/12 h, p.o.) from gestational day 5 to postnatal day 21 exhibited increased anxiogenic and depressive-like behaviors, cognitive impairments, and increased alcohol consumption by postnatal day 60 (Navarro et al. 2024). These behavioral alterations were linked to changes in neurodevelopment-related gene and protein expression and disruptions in the reward system, emphasizing the long-lasting neurobehavioral effects of prenatal and lactational cannabinoid exposure.

At 6 months of age, THC-exposed rat offspring exhibited accelerated folliculogenesis and follicular development arrest, despite no changes in circulating steroid levels (Martínez-Peña et al. 2021). Ovaries from THC-exposed offspring showed reduced blood vessel density, decreased VEGF and VEGFR-2 expression, and increased thrombospondin 1 (TSP-1), indicating disrupted follicular dynamics that could impact long-term fertility (Martínez-Peña et al. 2021).

Epigenetic changes were also observed in THC-exposed rat offspring, with altered expression of 12 out of 420 evaluated miRNAs. Among these, miR-122-5p was the only upregulated target and showed the greatest fold change (Martínez-Peña et al. 2022). RT-qPCR confirmed the upregulation of miR-122-5p and the downregulation of its target, insulin-like growth factor 1 receptor (Igf1r). Ovarian tissue exhibited decreased IGF-1R-positive follicular cells, increased follicular apoptosis, and reduced Igf1r expression in ovarian explants and granulosa cells. These molecular disruptions, linked to diminished ovarian health and fertility, suggest that prenatal THC exposure may lead to subfertility or premature reproductive senescence (Martínez-Peña et al. 2022).

9.8 Harm Reduction of Gestational THC Exposure

Prenatal THC exposure is associated with oxidative stress, mitochondrial dysfunction, and deficiencies in DHA and ARA in the prefrontal cortex and hippocampus (Sarikahya et al. 2023). Given the adverse effects of prenatal THC exposure, interventions are required. Nutritional and pharmacological interventions targeting oxidative stress, metabolic dysfunction, and neurodevelopmental disruptions have been explored. Antioxidants such as N-acetylcysteine and α-lipoic acid have shown potential in reducing THC-induced neuroinflammation, synaptic deficits, and oxidative damage (Beggiato et al. 2020; Sarikahya et al. 2023). THC also disrupts glucose homeostasis and increases hepatic triglyceride accumulation in male offspring (Gillies et al. 2020; Oke et al. 2021). PPARα and PPARγ agonists, including rosiglitazone, have been proposed to restore insulin sensitivity and lipid metabolism (Oke et al. 2021). Additionally, omega-3 fatty acids may counteract excessive CB1 receptor activation, mitigating THC-induced neurodevelopmental deficits (Sarikahya et al. 2023; Peng et al. 2023). THC exposure impairs ovarian folliculogenesis, VEGF expression, and follicular survival, potentially affecting long-term fertility (Martínez-Peña et al. 2021, 2022). Postnatal IGF-1 administration has been investigated to restore ovarian function, while maternal choline supplementation may normalize THC-induced DNA methylation changes (Martínez-Peña et al. 2022). These findings suggest that antioxidant, metabolic, and endocrine-targeted interventions may mitigate the effects of prenatal THC exposure, though further research is needed to confirm their efficacy and safety.

9.9 Nicotine

Despite shifting public perception, traditional combusted cigarettes are still used by up to 12% of pregnant individuals in the United States with similar rates in Canada, though as high as 60% in native populations in Canada (Tong et al. 2013; Cui et al. 2014). A recent NCHS report showed an overall decrease in cigarette smoking during pregnancy in the US from 2016–2021 from 7.2% to 4.6%, however, it did not account for vaping (Martin et al. 2023). Use of these products in pregnancy is exceedingly dangerous as nicotine levels can often concentrate in fetal tissues, representing a higher percentage in fetal circulation compared to maternal (Maritz and Harding 2011).

E-cigarettes are one of the most popular forms of nicotine (Cherian et al. 2020). Originally considered less harmful than cigarettes (Goniewicz et al. 2014), e-cigarettes now deliver higher levels of nicotine than combustible cigarettes while still containing toxic compounds (Margham et al. 2016), that can be harmful (Cherian et al. 2020). In addition to e-cigarette use, smokeless tobacco and nicotine pouches are gaining popularity among adolescents (Nemeth et al. 2024; Giovenco et al. 2025). Smokeless tobacco allows for diffusion of nicotine across the oral tissue membranes and into the bloodstream (Nemeth et al. 2024). Other waning tobacco products include hookah or water pipe, cigars, and pipe tobacco (O'Connor 2012). These nicotine products, however, are less commonly used by pregnant women in the US, though are popular in other countries (Brinchmann et al. 2023). In contrast, nicotine replacement products (e.g., patch, gum) are frequently used by pregnant women as a cigarette smoking cessation aid (O'Connor 2012; Lassen et al. 2010) Secondary or tertiary nicotine exposure, involving secondhand inhalation of cigarette or e-cigarette vapors or tertiary surface touch of e-cigarette liquid or cigarette residues on household surfaces is also of concern (Bush and Goniewicz 2015).

Disentangling the effects of nicotine from cigarette smoke is challenging as cigarette-associated combustion produces over 5000 chemical constituents and smoke exposure has considerable effects on maternal and fetal health (Talhout et al. 2011; Siddiqui et al. 2008). Cigarette smoke or side-stream secondhand smoke is unique in that it contains nicotine with a smoke vehicle, representing a dual exposure to nicotine with combustion. Similarly, e-cigarettes require a base liquid of propylene glycol and vegetable glycerin aerosolized as a delivery mechanism for nicotine. Aerosolization of just the base liquid is known to elicit detrimental health effects in the absence of nicotine (Wieslander et al. 2001). Thus, for the below-reported studies, the type of nicotine exposure might vary significantly from injection to cigarette or side-stream exposure and from nicotine formulations such as free base vs salt.

Nicotine levels can vary by the product and frequency of use. Individual cigarettes typically contain 8–12 mg of nicotine, smokeless nicotine products contain 2–48 mg (Mallock et al. 2024), nicotine gum or lozenges have 2–4 mg, patches have 12–21 mg, and e-cigarettes can contain 0 to 50 mg/mL with dosage determined by self-administration (Benowitz et al. 2009). The addiction threshold, the point at which a person's behavior becomes addictive, is typically 5 mg of nicotine per day, plasma cotinine (the primary metabolite of nicotine) at 50 ng/ml/day (Sofuoglu and LeSage 2012). Serum cotinine levels across tobacco products have been reviewed and compared (Whittington et al. 2018). Measured serum cotinine levels of e-cigarette users indicate 373 ng/mL, cigarette smokers at 310 ng/mL, and nicotine patch users at 167 ng/mL (Whittington et al. 2018). Current measurements of nicotine in pregnancy have determined 0.7 mg/kg of free nicotine in serum in pregnant smokers (Lo et al. 2015). Typical doses of administered nicotine salt in pregnant animals have centered on 1–2 mg/kg per day, as that is consistent with blood nicotine concentrations of a pregnant smoker consuming 20 cigarettes per day (Roy et al. 2002). This is important to consider for comparison with animal studies. Newer generations of e-cigarettes and pouches that use nicotine salts can have even higher concentrations of nicotine than combustible cigarettes.

Human studies have demonstrated that nicotine exhibits significant implications on the future health of in utero exposed children and grandchildren, affecting the pulmonary, neurological, metabolic, and behavioral systems and the epigenome (Li et al. 2005; Neuman et al. 2012; Joubert et al. 2016; Xepapadaki et al. 2009; England et al. 2015; Chan et al. 2020; Li et al. 2018; Suter et al. 2011; McEvoy and Spindel 2017). Although these findings clarify the implications of nicotine exposure in pregnancy, they are often limited in scope with reduced sample size, confounding variables such as use of multiple substances, variability in patient demographics, and limitations in sample collection.

To circumvent these limitations, the field has employed extensive use of animal models to understand the implications of nicotine exposure on early fetal development and future health. This section describes the current state of research using rodents and NHPs with some embryonic models. The described studies employ daily subcutaneous, intravenous, or intraperitoneal administration of nicotine through gestation or an implanted osmotic mini-pump to sustain drug delivery. Furthermore, some experiments have expanded exposure time beyond gestation to a few weeks before the initiation of pregnancy, throughout lactation until weaning of the offspring. By using animal exposure models, the scientific community can accurately evaluate the safety of these nicotine-containing products on the health of the mother and fetus. These findings have been instrumental in informing the public health of the dangers of nicotine on the in utero exposed offspring. Despite these endeavors, further research is still required, especially the examination of novel, emerging nicotine-containing products.

9.10 Pharmacokinetics of Nicotine in Maternal and Fetal Tissue

Nicotine is metabolized by cytochrome P450 enzymes, along with aldehyde oxidase, flavin-containing monooxygenase 3, amine N-methyltransferase, and

UDP-glucuronosyltransferases in the liver to cotinine, its main metabolite (Hukkanen et al. 2005). Other minor metabolites include nornicotine, nicotine *N*'-oxide, 3′-hydroxycotinine, norcotinine, glucuronide, and cotinine glucuronide (Gabrielsson and Gumbleton 1993; Tutka et al. 2005). Cotinine is the major metabolite for most animal species, but rats and guinea pigs metabolize nicotine to roughly equal amounts of nicotine-*N*′-oxide and cotinine and 3′-hydroxycotinine (Matta et al. 2007). Rodents metabolize nicotine faster than humans (Gorrod and Jenner 1975; Seaton and Vesell 1993; Scheline 1978), with a plasma nicotine half-life of 6–7 min in mice, 45 min in the rat, versus 2 h in humans (Matta et al. 2007). Roughly 70% of nicotine in the blood is metabolized as it passes through the liver (Matta et al. 2007). Nicotine metabolism in the liver does not substantially differ between pregnant and nonpregnant animals (Gabrielsson and Gumbleton 1993; Tutka et al. 2008). However, due to increased renal clearance and other physiologic changes, elimination is faster in pregnant than nonpregnant animals (Gabrielsson and Gumbleton 1993; Tutka et al. 2008; Slotkin et al. 2005). This primarily occurs through excretion of the products of liver metabolism into the urine by the kidneys (Gabrielsson and Gumbleton 1993), usually within 24 h (Chellian et al. 2021). Nicotine and metabolites can also be excreted in feces, though less so than in urine (Tutka et al. 2005), in sweat, saliva, during exhalation (Gabrielsson and Gumbleton 1993), and in breast milk. When animals are chronically exposed, nicotine levels are higher in breast milk than in plasma during lactation (roughly three times as high) due to the more acidic nature of milk (Matta et al. 2007).

During pregnancy, nicotine is rapidly distributed throughout the body, including the placenta, which it easily crosses, and the amniotic fluid, exposing the fetus (Matta et al. 2007; Tutka et al. 2008). Nicotine can also cross the blood-brain barrier and bind to receptors in fetal brain tissue (Matta et al. 2007). Of concern is that nicotine levels are often higher in fetal tissues than in the mother (Marzouk et al. 2022). Experiments by Mosier and Jansons (Mosier Jr. and Jansons 1972) in pregnant rats injected intravenously on gestational day 19 with $[^3H](-)$-nicotine (0.019 mg/kg body weight) showed that $[^3H](-)$-nicotine rose rapidly in the maternal decidua and plasma but then declined within 30 min of injection. At this time point, the vast majority of the $[^3H]$ signal was in the form of nicotine in all maternal and fetal tissues measured, except in maternal plasma, which showed equal proportions of nicotine and cotinine. Nicotine and its metabolites were detectable within the fetus 5 min after the injection. The higher levels of nicotine in the fetal plasma and higher proportion of nicotine in the decidua, relative to maternal plasma, were interpreted to suggest that the decidua may serve as a pump, pushing nicotine into the fetal circulation. Amniotic fluid achieved the level of the maternal plasma within 30–60 min. After 30 min and up until 20 h, the fetal plasma had higher levels than the maternal plasma, with the $[^3H]$ signal levels more than doubling in the fetus after 30 min and highest in the gonads. By 60 min, the fetal liver, kidney, adrenals, gonads, placenta, and decidua exceeded that of the whole fetus, while brain, heart, and lung tissues were comparable to the levels in the whole fetus. At 4 h, adrenal and gonads were higher than all other tissues measured, and the authors indicated that these organs had lower levels of nicotine by chromatographic analyses, indicating better metabolizing capacity. The stomach, pancreas, intestine, and spleen were analyzed together as a unit, and levels were comparable over the course of the experiment to the whole fetus. (Mosier Jr. and Jansons 1972).

9.11 Maternal & Gestational Outcomes of Nicotine Exposure

Use of nicotine-containing products during pregnancy invariably results in dual effects on both mother and baby. Nicotine exposure during pregnancy is correlated with fetal growth restriction, fetal developmental abnormalities, and pre-term birth (Tarasi et al. 2022). Neonatally exposed rats exhibit a significant delay to the incidence of pregnancy, a trend toward lower live birth rate, and ovarian dysfunction with a reduced estradiol to progesterone ratio at 6 months of age (Holloway et al. 2006). However, the underlying mechanisms are still poorly understood. Maternal body weight is decreased during gestation with nicotine use in rats (Wang et al. 2009; Mohsenzadeh et al. 2014) as nicotine is known to accelerate metabolic rate. In rats, the impact on fetal weight varies depending on the mode of exposure, with combustion products amplifying growth restriction (Table 9.6) (Wang et al. 2009; Mao et al. 2009). However, e-cigarettes have exhibited variable effects on weight change in both maternal and fetal weights in rodents (Wetendorf et al. 2019; Mills et al. 2025; Orzabal et al. 2019; Li et al. 2012; Walayat et al. 2021). This may be explained by the levels of nicotine in the e-cigarettes, with potentially higher amounts of nicotine correlating with smaller maternal and fetal weights. Additionally, clinical trials are limited and have not been able to successfully correlate differences in birth weight due to the small, reported sample size of e-cigarette users. Nicotine

Table 9.6 Effect of nicotine exposure on maternal and gestational outcomes in animal studies

Study	Year	Primary measures	Species	Conditions	Results
Lee et al. (2018)	2018	Organ weight	Mouse ($n = 10$)	1 cigarette via inhalation	Decreased maternal heart and increased thymus weight
Wetendorf et al. (2019)	2019	Weight, implantation, serum levels, RNA microarray, immunohistochemistry	Mouse ($n = 5$)	E-cigarette via inhalation	Reduced weight gain in offspring
Li et al. (2012)	2012	Body/organ weight, western blot, RT-PCR, EM-seq	Rat ($n = 9$–39)	4 ug/kg/min nicotine via osmotic minipump	Reduced brain and body weights. Sex specific hypoxic ischemic injury
Mao et al. (2009)	2009	Body/organ weight, Western blot	Rat ($n = 10$)	2.1 mg/day nicotine via osmotic minipump	Decreased fetal weight
Mills et al. (2025)	2025	Weight, litter size, and magnetic resonance angiography	Rat ($n = 7$–11)	50 mg/mL nicotine via E-cigarette inhalation	Decreased litter number and pup survival, and altered maternal circulating factors
Orzabal et al. (2019)	2019	Mass spectrometry, body weight/length, heart rate, blood flow	Rat ($n = 5$–15)	100 mg/mL nicotine via E-cigarette inhalation	Reduced fetal weight and length, reduced uterine and umbilical blood flow
Walayat et al. (2021)	2021	Weight, western blot, whole-genome bisulfite sequencing	Rat ($n = 5$–31)	E-cigarette 2.4% nicotine via inhalation	Reduced fetal brain weight, increased brain reactive oxygen species, sex specific increased DNA methylation
Mohsenzadeh et al. (2014)	2014	Cytokine analysis	Rat ($n = 32$)	2–6 mg/kg nicotine tartrate via intraperitoneal injection	Reduced maternal and fetal weight, increased inflammatory markers
Wang et al. (2009)	2009	Enzyme activity, developmental indices, immunohistochemistry	Rat ($n = 4$–16)	1 mg/ per kg 2× per day nicotine via subcutaneous injection	Decreased maternal weight and altered metabolism
Holloway et al. (2006)	2006	Breeding success, hormone analysis	Rat ($n = 5$–6)	1 mg/kg nicotine bitartrate via subcutaneous injection	Ovarian dysfunction; delayed incidence of pregnancy

replacement products, on the other hand, do not result in smaller birth weights (Lassen et al. 2010).

In the context of gestational e-cigarette exposure, e-cigarettes caused significant impacts on maternal health. In addition to decreased body weights, rats exposed to e-cigarettes during gestation exhibited reduced prolactin levels (Mills et al. 2025). Furthermore, cerebrovascular function was blunted and showed marked endothelial vessel dysfunction. Additionally, exposure to e-cigarettes with or without nicotine resulted in distinct patterns of extracellular vesicles, which could be an indicator of abnormal endothelium and vessel shedding. The size and number of vesicles were dependent on nicotine presence, further demonstrating how e-cigarettes can elicit detrimental effects on maternal health (Mills et al. 2025). When considering the health of the fetus, in utero e-cigarette exposure was associated with decreased litter numbers and impaired postnatal survival, ultimately resulting in elevated deaths. These detrimental effects worsened with increased nicotine level and e-cigarette device wattage. This study suggests that e-cigarettes, currently the most popular form of nicotine intake, are not safe to use during pregnancy, regardless of nicotine level.

9.12 Placental Outcomes

Since 2007 and the debut of the Barker hypothesis (Barker 2007), environmental, natural, manufactured, and artificial toxicants were evidenced to dramatically impact mothers and their babies. Nicotine readily crosses the fetal-placental barrier, and the human fetus was identified to be exposed to higher levels of nicotine compared to the smoking mothers (Luck et al. 1985). Nicotine exposure in the fetus has been associated with altered signaling pathways, including inflammatory signaling, oxidative stress response, and endoplasmic reticulum stress (Wong et al. 2015a). Indeed, along with smaller fetal weights, serum inflammatory markers increase in correlation to the increased concentration of nicotine in neonatal rats (Mohsenzadeh et al. 2014). In rats, nicotine treatment throughout gestation demonstrated impaired placental features, including abnormal placental protein expression, decreased labyrinth vascularization, and reduced trophoblast invasion (Holloway et al. 2014). Reduced placental sizes were also observed in mice exposed to nicotine at gestation (Musanejad et al. 2021). Within Rhesus macaques, fetal-side placental blood volume was reduced on MRI across gestation in animals exposed to nicotine, with an increase of syncytiotrophoblast cell sprouting and cytotrophoblast cell island development, historically observed in human placentas exposed to cigarette smoke (Lo et al. 2015; van der Veen and Fox 1982). Rat studies have also shown that neonatal nicotine exposure correlates with increased endoplasmic reticulum stress and impaired disulfide bond formation, which can lead to activation of the unfolded protein response (Table 9.7) (Wong et al. 2015b). These findings suggest nicotine is responsible for the activation of oxidative stress pathways and potential for cytotoxicity.

Human epidemiological studies have suggested that in utero cigarette smoke exposure can cause reduced fecundability in both exposed male and female offspring (Jensen et al. 1998; Weinberg et al. 1989). Experiments in mice demonstrated gestational nicotine exposure impaired successful plug to pregnancy rate and caused a reduction in fetal weights and fetal/placental weight ratios with no reduction in placental weight at midgestation (Greco et al. 2022). Exposure in rats during pregnancy showed a reduction of serum circulating insulin-like growth factor pathway (Gruslin et al. 2009) with decreases in birthweight from nicotine exposure at gestational day 21 and at term. Yet, this weight was recovered at weaning. Additionally, nicotine exposure also activated cytochrome P450 enzymes CYP2E1 and CYP1A1 in the placenta and liver, which might be associated with subsequent increases in oxidative stress and peroxidation of lipids (Wang et al. 2009). Placental P-glycoprotein (ABCB1 glycoprotein), hypothesized to be protective of developmental abnormalities (Lankas et al. 1998) and

Table 9.7 Effect of nicotine exposure on placental outcomes in animal studies

Study	Year	Primary measures	Species	Conditions	Results
Greco et al. (2022)	2022	Organ weight, echocardiograph, immunohistochemistry, histology, heart explants	Mouse ($n = 7$–29)	0.75–1.5 mg/kg/day nicotine via osmotic minipump	Reduction in fetal/placental weight ratio, no change in placental weight at mid-gestation
Musanejad et al. (2021)	2021	Weight, histology, follicle count	Mouse ($n = 8$–35)	1 mg/kg/day nicotine via subcutaneous injection	Smaller placentas
Gruslin et al. (2009)	2009	Weight, western blot	Rat ($n = 10$)	1 mg/kg/day nicotine	Decreased weight at E21; lessened insulin-like growth factor signaling
Wang et al. (2009)	2009	Enzyme activity, developmental indices, IHC	Rat ($n = 4$–16)	1 mg/ per kg twice per day nicotine via subcutaneous injection	Decreased p glycoprotein and increased oxidative stress and lipid peroxidation
Holloway et al. (2014)	2014	Histology, western blot, RT-PCR, in vivo cell migration/invasion	Rat ($n = 5$–6)	1 mg/ per kg nicotine bitartrate via subcutaneous injection	Inhibited trophoblast interstitial invasions; increased placental hypoxia; decreased labyrinth vascularization; impaired placental factors
Wong et al. (2015b)	2015	Western blot, RT-PCR	Rat ($n = 5$–6)	1 mg/kg nicotine bitartrate via subcutaneous injection	Induced ER stress and reduced disulfide bonds leading to oxidative stress
Lo et al. (2015)	2014	Dynamic contrast-enhanced MRI, ultrasound, histology	Rhesus ($n = 27$)	2 mg/kg/day nicotine bitartrate via osmotic pump	Decreased fetal-side placental blood supply; increased cytotrophoblast cell islands; increased syncytiotrophoblast sprouting

upregulated as a defender in response to toxicity (Sun et al. 2006; Abu-Qare et al. 2003), was found to be increased in the nicotine-exposed animals (Wang et al. 2009). Thus, nicotine in the placenta can elicit cytotoxic responses, which can impair fetal and maternal health.

9.13 Fetal and Neonatal Health Outcomes

9.13.1 Pulmonary Health

Although sometimes difficult to link cigarette smoke or secondhand smoke exposure to neonatal lung development deficits in humans (Antonucci et al. 2004; Martinez et al. 2015), animal models have played a pivotal role in defining maternal cigarette exposure risk on offspring health. Furthermore, the use of animal models has successfully identified cigarette- and nicotine-dependent mechanistic effects, a feat near impossible with human tissue due to ethical restrictions. For example, during postnatal lung development, cigarette smoke exposure has been correlated with increased incidence of sudden infant death syndrome (SIDS)(Shea and Steiner 2008) and potential for bronchopulmonary dysplasia (Antonucci et al. 2004), yet the underlying mechanisms have often remained elusive. This has been shown in humans as well, after considering that in utero smoke exposure increased preterm delivery (Morrow et al. 2017). Animal models have successfully shed light on these early correlations and have identified new risks associated with neonatal nicotine exposure on lung development.

In utero exposure studies in rodents have successfully identified nicotine-mediated novel molecular and morphological changes in pulmonary development. Neonatal nicotine exposure in mice was demonstrated to elevate oxidative stress and NF-kB signaling with abnormal alveolar structures in the lungs of exposed offspring (Tsai et al. 2021). Additionally, cigarette smoke exposure increased the risk for wheeze and asthma, impaired airway remodeling, upregulated inflammatory markers, and bronchopulmonary dysplasia with worsened effects on male offspring (Liu et al. 2013). Specifically, nicotine exposure alone was sufficient to elicit an asthma phenotype, including increased airway resistance in rats with changes in acetylation status in pulmonary and gonadal tissues (Table 9.8) (Rehan et al. 2012). This exposure led to the incidence of asthma in the F2 generation. Indeed, these implications on lung health, particularly asthma, are extremely robust and have been observed in subsequent generations, with male offspring more sensitive (Rehan et al. 2012, 2013). Although many of these studies were performed in rats, comparative studies in Rhesus macaque also determined in utero nicotine exposure resulted in decreased lung volume and weight with decreased forced expiratory flows, decreased compliance, and increased pulmonary resistance (Sekhon et al. 2001), confirming the dramatic implications of nicotine on fetal lung

Table 9.8 Effect of nicotine exposure on offspring respiratory health in animal studies

Study	Year	Primary measures	Species	Conditions	Results
Tsai et al. (2021)	2021	Histology, Western blot	Mouse ($n = 10$)	6 mg/kg/day nicotine via osmotic minipump	Upregulated oxidative stress in lung tissue, impaired alveolar structures; elevated NF-KB signaling
Noel et al. (2023)	2023	Gene network analysis	Mouse ($n = 4$–10)	18 mg/mL via e-cigarette inhalation	Abnormal lung gene expression; sex specific asthmatic responses
Singh et al. (2013)	2013	Histology, immunohistochemistry, and western blot	Mouse ($n = 5$)	Secondhand cigarette smoke via inhalation	Molecular and morphological lung impairments
Singh et al. (2015)	2015	Histology, western blot	Mouse ($n = 5$)	Secondhand cigarette smoke via inhalation	Increased lung epithelial cell apoptosis; increased alveolar regions; decreased Hif1a in lung tissues
Singh et al. (2017)	2017	Lung resistance, cytokine analysis, RT-PCR	Mouse ($n = 5$)	Secondhand cigarette smoke via inhalation	Impaired cytokine levels; impaired lung angiogenesis and alveolar development in F1 and F2 generations
Rehan et al. (2012)	2012	Lung resistance/compliance, tracheal constriction, western blot, global DNA methylation	Rat ($n = 10$–12)	1 mg/kg nicotine via subcutaneous injection	Increased airway resistance; sex specific tracheal constriction; abnormal protein accumulates, fibroblasts, acetylation in gonads and lungs
Rehan et al. (2013)	2014	Lung resistance/compliance, tracheal constriction, western blot	Rat ($n = 10$–12)	1 mg/kg nicotine via subcutaneous injection	Increased airway resistance; decreased airway compliance
Liu et al. (2013)	2012	Lung resistance/compliance, tracheal constriction, western blot, immunohistochemistry, histology	Rat ($n = 4$–16)	1 mg/kg nicotine via subcutaneous injection	Increased airway resistance; decreased airway compliance
Sekhon et al. (2001)	2000	Lung function, lung weight/volume, peak tidal expiratory flow, lung resistance/compliance	Rhesus ($n = 7$)	1.5 mg/kg/day nicotine bitartrate via osmotic minipump	Decreased lung weight and volume; increased pulmonary resistance

development. In Rhesus macaques, prenatal nicotine exposure also dramatically upregulated connective tissue in the lung, likely acting through alpha-7 nicotinic receptors (Sekhon et al. 2001, 1999;Arredondo et al. 2003). Showing the importance of animal models to study the effects of prenatal nicotine exposure, studies in NHP also demonstrated that vitamin C supplementation during pregnancy could block some of the effects of nicotine lung exposure (Proskocil et al. 2005), and subsequent clinical trials confirmed this potential therapeutic intervention (Graham and Papandonatos 2008; McEvoy et al. 2023).

Flavored e-cigarette exposure is also related to pulmonary defects in exposed mouse offspring. Gestational exposure to flavored e-cigarettes containing 18 mg/mL nicotine resulted in abnormal lung transcriptome changes at birth related to immune responses and chemokine signaling (Noel et al. 2023). Further, males exposed in utero specifically exhibited asthmatic responses at 7 weeks of age.

Many studies have also examined side stream or secondhand smoke in gestation, matching the exposure to what a pregnant individual would experience sitting in a smoking bar for 3 h per day (1.52 ± 0.41 mg/m^3) (Singh et al. 2009). These studies have determined that secondhand smoke exposure can cause pulmonary deficits in offspring, including morphological and molecular lung impairments (Singh et al. 2009, 2013, 2017). Secondhand smoke exposure in utero has been extensively studied to elicit bronchopulmonary dysplasia, impaired lung angiogenesis and development, and reduced cytokines within exposed offspring and subsequent generations (Singh et al. 2017). Furthermore, secondhand exposure activated apoptotic factors in the lung with concomitant presence of apoptosis in lung epithelial cells with increased alveolar volume (Singh et al. 2015). Interestingly, in addition to effects on in utero exposed offspring, increased incidence of asthma and bronchopulmonary dysplasia was observed in the F2 generation (Singh et al. 2017). Thus, second-hand smoke exposure during gestation is sufficient to impair lung function within in utero exposed offspring and in subsequent generations.

9.13.2 Renal and Cardiovascular Health

In addition to lung development, nicotine exposure at gestation can elicit measurable effects on blood flow, cardiovascular health, and kidney function. At postnatal day 10 and day 21, uterine and umbilical blood flow were decreased with e-cigarette exposure (Orzabal et al. 2019). Nicotine exposure in utero was identified to promote blood pressure in adulthood with subsequent adverse reactions in perivascular adipose tissues (Gao et al. 2008). Within the heart, nicotine exposure during gestation is associated with increased arterial contractions, oxidative stress levels, and decreased superoxide dismutase 1 (SOD1) levels in the aortas of 5-month-old male rats (Xiao et al. 2011). These vascular effects were reversed with an SOD mimetic. In addition to these chronic cardiac effects, female offspring exhibited elevated susceptibility to ischemia/reperfusion injury in adulthood when exposed to nicotine in utero (Lawrence et al. 2008). Mitochondrial damage and oxidative stress have also been observed in cardiac tissue in neonatal nicotine-exposed rats with some antioxidant deficits that persist to adulthood (Barra et al. 2017). Thus, maternal nicotine exposure can cause lifelong cardiac defects.

Embryo culture models using nicotine or smoke exposure mimic gestational effects. Within zebrafish embryo culture, embryos were exposed to media containing e-cigarette vapor, nicotine alone, or a combustible cigarette with matching nicotine content (Palpant et al. 2015). Embryos were exposed for 72 h, and cardiac development was assessed, even 2 days of murine embryo culture at day 8.5 with nicotine can cause abnormal morphology with elevated oxidative stress parameters (Table 9.9) (Lin et al. 2014). In zebrafish embryos, both e-cigarette and traditional cigarette media negatively impaired cardiac development and heart rate, with cigarette media delivering the most severe outcomes, including pericardial edema, unlooped and malformed hearts, and a significant bradycardia (average heart rate reduced to 134 bpm compared to 155 bpm in controls). Corollary studies in

Table 9.9 Effect of nicotine exposure on offspring renal and cardiovascular health in animal studies

Study	Year	Primary measures	Species	Conditions	Results
Lin et al. (2014)	2014	Western blot, lipid peroxidation, embryo morphology	Mouse ($n = 10$)	1 mM nicotine via media	Severe morphological effects; elevated lipid peroxidation; impaired peroxidase enzymes
Greco et al. (2022)	2022	Organ weight, echocardiograph, immunohistochemistry, histology, heart explants	Mouse ($n = 7$–29)	0.75–1.5 mg/kg/day nicotine via osmotic minipump	Reduction in fetal/placental weight ratio, no change in placental weight at mid-gestation
Stangenberg et al. (2019)	2019	EM-seq, IHC, RT-PCR	Mouse ($n = 10$)	4 cigarettes/day via inhalation	Decreased kidney size; increased renal global DNA methylation; reversal with L-carnitine
Xiao et al. (2011)	2011	Vascular oxidative damage, arterial contraction, western blot, histology	Rat ($n = 12$–13)	4 ug/kg/min nicotine via osmotic minipump	Increased oxidative stress; decreased antioxidant expression in adult offspring aortas
Lawrence et al. (2008)	2008	Gestational length, post-ischemic recovery, myocardial infarction size, coronary flow, western blot, NO release	Rat ($n = 4$–6 litters)	6 mg/kg/day nicotine via osmotic minipump	Increased susceptibility to ischemia/reperfusion injury in offspring
Orzabal et al. (2019)	2019	Mass spectrometry, body weight/length, heart rate, blood flow	Rat ($n = 5$–15)	100 mg/mL nicotine via e-cigarette inhalation	Reduced uterine and umbilical artery blood flow
Barra et al. (2017)	2017	Histology, western blot, RT-PCR	Rat ($n = 5$–6)	1 mg/kg/day nicotine bitartrate via subcutaneous injection	Decreased cardiac antioxidant levels in adulthood
Gao et al. (2008)	2008	Histology, arterial contractile response	Rat ($n = 6$)	1 mg/kg/day nicotine via subcutaneous injection	Increased blood pressure with subsequent changes in perivascular adipose tissues
Palpant et al. (2015)	2015	Developmental assessment, embryo larval survival, IHC, RT-PCR	Zebrafish ($n = 48$)	6.8–34 μM nicotine via media	Impaired heart development and function with tobacco exhibiting the most severe effects

mouse models confirmed some of these findings. After gestational nicotine exposure, congenital heart defects were present in offspring with reduced fractional shortening and ejection fraction (Greco et al. 2022). These animals demonstrated coronary artery malformations, impaired cardiac gene expression, and elevated cardiac lipid peroxidation. Thus, nicotine and cigarette exposures can exhibit detrimental consequences on cardiac function and development.

In addition to cardiac development defects, gestational nicotine exposure was sufficient to impair kidney growth and development. Exposure of offspring in utero to nicotine caused reduced kidney weights postnatally with persistence into adulthood (Mao et al. 2009; Li et al. 2019). These studies also determined that angiotensin II receptor mRNA and protein levels were decreased in kidneys throughout life after gestational exposure to nicotine. Cigarette smoke reduced renal methylation, reversible with L-carnitine (Stangenberg et al. 2019). Glomerular density was decreased while renal reactive oxygen species were increased with cigarette or e-cigarette gestational exposure (Li et al. 2019).

Only glomerular density could be recovered by the replacement of gestational cigarette exposure with e-cigarette exposure. Thus, nicotine and cigarette smoke exposure in animal models can impair kidney health with deficits persisting to adulthood.

9.13.3 Neurodevelopmental Health

The developing brain is sensitive to external stimuli, including changes in hormones, the presence of drugs, and/or environmental factors (Castro et al. 2023). In turn, vapors derived from tobacco or nicotine-containing products can dramatically alter brain development and cause measurable changes in developing offspring. Within in utero e-cigarette or nicotine-exposed male and female rodent offspring, total body weights and brain weights were reduced (Li et al. 2012; Walayat et al. 2021), resulting in significantly increased brain-to-body weight ratios compared to controls. Furthermore, hypoxia-ischemic induced brain injury, associated with adverse long-term neurologic problems including cerebral palsy and developmental delays, was elevated in offspring exposed in utero *(*Li et al. 2012*;* Walayat et al. 2021*;* Ferriero 2004*)*. In addition, elevated global DNA methylation was identified specifically in males (Walayat et al. 2021), causing abnormal changes in angiotensin receptor expression levels (Table 9.10) (Li et al. 2012, 2013). Thus, nicotine exposure is associated with sex-specific differences within in utero brain tissues.

Further examination of neuronal function was performed on neonates exposed to nicotine and tobacco products. Gestational cigarette exposure exhibited significant effects on oxidative stress levels in brain regions with elevated glial numbers and concomitant decreases in antioxidants (Lei et al. 2021, 2018). Also, decreased neurons and cell sizes were observed in the hippocampus and somatosensory cortex, suggesting nicotine elicits major deficits in brain function associated with cognition, learning, and memory outputs (Roy et al. 2002). Exposure of animals in utero to nicotine-containing e-cigarette vapors resulted in changes in behavior, including increased activity (Smith et al. 2015). Maternal cigarette smoking in mice also caused an upregulation of brain inflammatory markers and oxidative stress (Chan et al. 2016). Primary neuron cultures from offspring exposed to maternal e-cigarettes showed elevated cytokine and oxidative stress levels and upregulated mitochondrial superoxide (Archie et al. 2023). Furthermore, treatment with nicotine during gestation can impair gliotransmitter release, which is further worsened by lifestyle factors such as diet (Orellana et al. 2014). Thus, neonatal nicotine exposure can elicit changes in neurons associated with behavior, memory, learning, and cognition.

RNA sequencing of mouse frontal cortex from offspring exposed to e-cigarette vapors at gestation showed sex-specific significant changes in genes involved in cancer, organismal injury and abnormalities, neurological disease, psychiatric disorders, and gastrointestinal disorders (Lauterstein et al. 2016). Importantly, e-cigarette vapors without nicotine caused a 1.8–15x increase in the fold change of changed genes in these offspring's exposed brains, suggesting that non-nicotine components of e-cigarette vapor may drive neurodevelopmental disruptions. Interestingly, the inclusion of nicotine appeared to attenuate some of these transcriptomic changes, raising the possibility that nicotine may modulate, rather than exacerbate, certain toxic effects of e-cigarette constituents.

9.13.4 Metabolic Health

Maternal smoking is often correlated with childhood obesity and adult adiposity (Bergmann et al. 2003; Wideroe et al. 2003). To test this using animal models, rats were exposed to nicotine neonatally. At birth, offspring exposed to nicotine were significantly decreased in weight compared to control (saline) exposed offspring (Holloway et al. 2005). However, at the time of weaning, the nicotine-exposed offspring demonstrated no difference in total body weight compared to controls. Offspring were weighed every week until 26 weeks of age (Holloway et al. 2005).

Table 9.10 Effect of nicotine exposure on offspring neurodevelopmental outcomes in animal studies

Study	Year	Primary measures	Species	Conditions	Results
Lauterstein et al. (2016)	2016	Birth weight, real-time PCR, RNA sequencing	Mouse ($n = 2$ litters)	25.6 mg/m^3 e-cigarette aerosol via inhalation	Alterations in cancer gene regulation, psychiatric disorder, and neurological disease, sex-specific
Chan et al. (2016)	2017	Global DNA methylation, body/organ weight	Mouse ($n = 10$)	E-cigarette 18 mg/ml via inhalation	Global lung methylation changes; worsened effects without nicotine; decreased total body weight; increased liver weights
Archie et al. (2023)	2023	Reactive oxygen species, mitochondrial superoxide, western blot, cytokine analysis	Mouse ($n = 3$–10)	E-cigarette 2.4% nicotine via inhalation	Elevated reactive oxygen species and cytokines, and mitochondrial superoxide in neonatal brains
Chan et al. (2016)	2016	Maze, open field test	Mouse ($n = 3$–18)	4 cigarettes/day via inhalation	Upregulated brain inflammatory markers and oxidative stress
Orellana et al. (2014)	2014	Immunohistochemistry, channel uptake, cytokine analysis	Mouse ($n = 5$)	6 mg/kg/day nicotine bitartrate via osmotic minipump	Abnormal gliotransmitter release
Smith et al. (2015)	2015	Weight, serum levels, rotarod test, open field test, maze	Mouse ($n = 7$–31)	E-cigarette 2.4% nicotine via inhalation	Differences in behavior including increased activity
Li et al. (2012)	2012	Body/organ weight, western blot, RT-PCR, enzymatic-methyl-seq	Rat ($n = 9$–39)	4 ug/kg/min nicotine via osmotic minipump	Reduced brain and body weights; increased brain to body weight ratio
Li et al. (2013)	2013	Quantitative methylation-specific PCR, electrophoretic mobility	Rat ($n = 5$)	5 ug/kg/min nicotine via osmotic minipump	Abnormal methylated promoter regions resulting in differential expression of angiotensin receptors in brain
Walayat et al. (2021)	2021	Weight, western blot, whole-genome bisulfite sequencing	Rat ($n = 5$–31)	E-cigarette 2.4% nicotine via inhalation	Increased brain reactive oxygen species; sex specific elevated global DNA methylation
Lei et al. (2021)	2021	Mito sox, western blot	Rat ($n = 4$–6)	20 cigarettes/day via inhalation	Increased oxidative stress and decreased antioxidant in neuronal signaling
Lei et al. (2018)	2018	Oxidative stress, mitochondrial function	Rat ($n = 5$–8)	20 cigarettes/day via inhalation	Increased oxidative stress; abnormal mitochondrial features

Intriguingly, animals exposed to nicotine during gestation exhibited significantly increased body weights and hypertriglyceridemia at adulthood compared to controls. Within the pancreas, neonatal nicotine exposure impaired mitochondria and beta cells (Bruin et al. 2008a, 2012), with one study reporting impaired glucose metabolism (Holloway et al. 2005). Furthermore, regulators of histone methylation were changed in pancreatic tissue after neonatal nicotine exposure, suggesting nicotine can modify the pancreatic epigenome (Raez-Villanueva et al. 2022). Nicotine exposure also promoted glucose intolerance, insulin granule accumulation, and increased oxidative stress in islet cells (Bruin et al. 2008a, b), which likely contribute to dysglycemia. A number of these findings were found to be reversed if nicotine exposure was removed at birth (Bruin et al. 2007) or if dams were co-treated with dietary antioxidants (Bruin et al. 2012). Similar findings were confirmed in another rat study that reported increases in adipose at weaning, with adipocyte hypertrophy that culminated in glucose intolerance and insulin resistance in adulthood (Somm et al. 2008). Finally, in a mouse study, nicotine increased liver size and blood glucose levels that led to increased triglycerides and glucose intolerance by adulthood (Saad et al. 2018). However, these metabolic phenotypes were largely reversed in female offspring if supplemented with L-carnitine. Thus, neonatal nicotine exposure is associated with dysglycemia and metabolic syndrome in exposed offspring that continues to adulthood.

Gestational exposure to nicotine or cigarette vapors can have detrimental consequences on weaning weights of pups and long-term effects on metabolism through adulthood. Exposure in utero and during lactation to e-cigarettes containing 24 mg/mL nicotine resulted in decreased total body weights specifically in adult female exposed offspring (Wetendorf et al. 2019), suggesting long-term implications of nicotine on metabolism. However, these increases were not observed with e-cigarette vapors exhibiting 18 mg/mL nicotine (Chen et al. 2018); in the absence of nicotine, aerosolized e-cigarette vapors alone can elicit larger weights at weaning with increased total fat mass and fat percentage (Table 9.11) (Chen et al. 2018). This suggests that the presence of nicotine within aerosolized e-cigarette vapor is sufficient to elicit reductions in fetal weight, while the e-cigarette vapor alone increases fetal weight. Further studies are required to understand these e-cigarette-specific effects on offspring metabolism.

Nicotine and tobacco exposures at gestation are known to interrupt neurological signals in the brain that control metabolic function. One of these signaling pathways include the pro-opiomelanocortin (POMC) leptin receptor and the melanocortin receptor (MC4R), involved in neurological communications to control metabolic processes (Horvath et al. 2004). Both these receptors were found upregulated in the male offspring (Chen et al. 2018). Upon exposure to cigarette smoke, metabolic regulators of POMC and inducible nitric oxide synthase (iNOS) were increased robustly, yet the changes were reversed if at gestation, the exposure was switched to e-cigarette vapors containing nicotine (Chen et al. 2018). In Rhesus macaque exposed to nicotine at gestation, POMC expression was decreased in the brain with concomitant decreases in normalized fetal weight (Grove et al. 2001). The animals exhibited accelerated metabolism and elevated energy expenditure in the presence of nicotine (Grove et al. 2001). Thus, there exist species-specific and sex-specific neurological mechanisms sensitive to nicotine that drive metabolic paradigms.

9.13.5 Reproductive Health

As mentioned above, it is well known that cigarette use can elicit detrimental effects on pregnancy outcome, yet the consequences on exposed offspring are underexplored. Studies using neonatal e-cigarette exposure did not exhibit significant effects on future reproductive fitness in females (Wetendorf et al. 2019). However, gestational nicotine exposure was identified to cause long-term effects on ovaries. Ovarian primordial follicles were reduced and elevated apoptosis was observed in granulosa cells and pre-antral follicles in mice (Musanejad et al. 2021). In addition, nicotine exposure caused smaller ovarian vessels with decreased angiogenic signaling, upregulated ovarian apoptosis, and impaired proliferation (Petrik et al. 2009). Furthermore, nicotine was identified to elicit activation of ovarian proinflammatory cytokines and oxidative stress levels with decreased levels of ovarian mast cells (Freitas et al. 2025). Outside gestation, juvenile exposure of nicotine can impair ovarian structures (Rajikin et al. 2009). These animals exhibited abnormal endoplasmic reticulum with numerous vessels present and mitochondria with the absence of cristae, suggesting the occurrence of severe ovarian perturbations (Rajikin et al. 2009). Thus, the ovarian environment is sensitive to the presence of nicotine neonatally and in adulthood.

In neonatally exposed male rodent offspring, cigarettes have exhibited significant consequences on reproductive function. Exposure to cigarettes in utero impaired sperm counts and

Table 9.11 Effect of nicotine exposure on offspring metabolic outcomes in animal studies

Study	Year	Primary measures	Species	Conditions	Results
Wetendorf et al. (2019)	2019	Weight, implantation, serum levels, RNA microarray, immunohistochemistry	Mouse ($n = 5$)	E-cigarette via inhalation	Reduced weight gain in offspring
Saad et al. (2018)	2018	Organ weight, blood glucose, plasma triglyceride, cytokine analysis	Mouse ($n = 10$)	4 cigarettes/day via inhalation	Increased liver weight and blood glucose levels; glucose intolerance; increased plasma triglycerides; liver fibrosis
Somm et al. (2008)	2008	Weight, histology, fat deposition, physical activity	Rat ($n = 10$)	3 mg/kg/day nicotine via osmotic pump	Increased epididymal adipose; adipocyte hypertrophy; glucose intolerance; insulin resistance
Chen et al. (2018)	2018	Weight, RT-PCR	Mouse ($n = 6$–8)	E-cigarette 18 mg/mL via inhalation	Upregulated weights and brain metabolic regulators without nicotine
Bruin et al. (2007)	2007	Apoptosis, histology, immunohistochemistry	Rat ($n = 5$–12)	1 mg/kg/day nicotine bitartrate via subcutaneous injection	Exposure throughout lactation impaired glucose tolerance and caused permanent beta cell loss
Bruin et al. (2008a)	2008	Mitochondria structure/function, glucose tolerance, electron microscopy, oxidative stress	Rat ($n = 5$–12)	1 mg/kg/day nicotine bitartrate via subcutaneous injection	Impaired pancreatic mitochondria and beta cells; glucose intolerance; islet cell oxidative stress increase; increased insulin granules
Bruin et al. (2008c)	2008	Immunohistochemistry, oxidative stress	Rat ($n = 5$–12)	1 mg/kg/day nicotine bitartrate via subcutaneous injection	Elevated islet cell oxidative stress
Bruin et al. (2012)	2012	Apoptosis, histology, immunohistochemistry	Rat ($n = 5$–12)	1 mg/kg/day nicotine bitartrate via subcutaneous injection	Beta cell loss; increased apoptosis
Raez-Villanueva et al. (2022)	2021	Apoptosis, oxidative stress, mitochondrial function, methylation	Rat ($n = 5$–6)	1 mg/kg/day nicotine bitartrate via subcutaneous injection	Impaired pancreatic epigenetic modifiers
Holloway et al. (2005)	2005	Serum insulin, apoptosis	Rat ($n = 5$–6)	1 mg/kg/day nicotine bitartrate via subcutaneous injection	Increased growth; dysglycemia; decreased serum insulin; increased beta cell apoptosis
Grove et al. (2001)	2001	RT-PCR, immunohistochemistry, plasma levels, body/organ weight, amniotic fluid	Rhesus ($n = 4$–7)	1.5 mg/kg/day nicotine tartrate via osmotic minipump	Reduced birth weight; reduced postnatal leptin; increase in pro-opiomelanocortin (POMC) expression in brain; elevated metabolism in nicotine exposed

sperm motility in male offspring with defects in seminiferous tubule development that persisted to the second generation (Lee et al. 2018). Nicotine exposure also caused spermatid retention and overall hypospermia in a rat model that was transient, as these defects resolved by 26 weeks of age

Table 9.12 Effect of nicotine exposure on offspring reproductive health in animal studies

Study	Year	Primary measures	Species	Conditions	Results
Pabarja et al. (2021)	2021	Histology, semen analysis, RT-PCR	Mouse ($n = 7$–9)	1 mg/kg/day nicotine tartrate via intraperitoneal injection	Impaired testes and sperm; elevated reactive oxygen species
Musanejad et al. (2021)	2021	Body/organ weight, histology, follicle count	Mouse ($n = 8$–35)	1 mg/kg/day nicotine via subcutaneous injection	Smaller placentas; decreased weight; decrease in primordial ovarian follicles; upregulated apoptosis in pre-antral follicles and granulosa cells
Anto et al. (2016)	2016	Body/organ weight, litter size, RT-PCR, semen morphology, testosterone level	Mouse ($n = 10$)	20 mg/kg/day nicotine	Decreased growth and litter number; decreased testosterone and testicular weight; impaired sperm number and morphology
Lichtensteiger and Schlumpf (1985)	1985	Testosterone level, saccharin preference	Rat ($n = 3$–22)	25 μg/100 g × hour nicotine via osmotic minipump	Decreased plasma testosterone
Lagunov et al. (2011)	2011	Histology, semen analysis	Rat ($n = 5$–35)	1 mg/kg nicotine bitartrate via subcutaneous injection	Spermatid retention; hypospermia
Petrik et al. (2009)	2009	Histology, apoptosis, vascularization	Rat ($n = 5$–7)	1 mg/kg nicotine bitartrate via subcutaneous injection	Smaller ovarian vessel area and density; decreased angiogenic signaling pathway; impaired proliferation and increased apoptosis in ovary
Freitas et al. (2025)	2025	Oxidative stress, cytokine levels, Western blot, immunohistochemistry	Rat ($n = 10$)	2 mg/kg/day nicotine via osmotic minipump	Increased ovarian malondialdehyde levels; decreased ovarian mast cells; increased ovarian pro-inflammatory markers
Paccola et al. (2014)	2014	Cholesterol levels, testosterone levels, histology, immunohistochemistry	Rat ($n = 5$–105)	2 mg/kg/day nicotine via	Increased testosterone; increased leydig cell size; reduced lipid droplets

(Table 9.12) (Lagunov et al. 2011). In addition, nicotine caused increases in testosterone and cholesterol in male rat offspring at 12 weeks of age (Paccola et al. 2014). Furthermore, these animals exhibited larger Leydig cells with lessened appearances of lipid droplets, which could indicate disrupted steroidogenesis. In mice, these studies were confirmed as seminiferous tubules were decreased in diameter after in utero and lactation exposure (Pabarja et al. 2021). Further, sperm viability, count, and motility parameters were all significantly decreased with nicotine exposure. Sperm DNA fragmentation was also elevated and showed upregulated levels of malondialdehyde, a common indicator of oxidative stress. Regulators of methylation and acetylation marks were also abnormally expressed in sperm cells of in utero-*exposed* offspring. Additionally, exposure to higher levels of nicotine (20 mg/kg/day) during gestation impaired testosterone levels, testes weight, and sperm morphology and number (Anto et al. 2016). In regards to neonatal e-cigarette exposure, e-cigarette vapors with 24 mg/mL nicotine elicited only mild, insignificant impairments on litter number and weight in the F2 generation (Wetendorf et al. 2019). Thus, nicotine, especially increased levels of nicotine, can exhibit rampant deleterious effects on testes morphology and sperm function. One caveat of animal studies is that the dose is often supraphysiologic.

9.14 Harm Reduction of Gestational Nicotine Exposure

As neonatal nicotine and tobacco exposure can drive deleterious effects on offspring, multiple studies have tested the incorporation of pharmaceuticals and dietary supplements to rescue these harmful phenotypes. Rosiglitazone, a thiazolidinedione and peroxisome proliferator-activated receptor g (PPARg) agonist, restored ovarian vessel dysfunction and apoptosis in a neonatal nicotine exposure model in rats (Petrik et al. 2009). It was also used to prevent dysglycemia and decrease insulin resistance with metformin postnatally on neonatal nicotine-exposed rats (Holloway et al. 2011). Additionally, in rhesus macaques, vitamin C supplementation during pregnancy restored lung function and placental blood flow volume and abnormal placental features in nicotine-exposed pregnancies, subsequently in successful clinical trials (Proskocil et al. 2005; Graham and Papandonatos 2008; McEvoy et al. 2023; Shorey-Kendrick et al. 2021). The use of antioxidant compounds has also been tested to reverse the impact of neonatal nicotine and tobacco exposure. A mixture of antioxidants was fed to dams to reverse impairments on beta cell loss and apoptosis (Bruin et al. 2012). In addition, the antioxidant L-carnitine demonstrated partial rescue of metabolic regulators in male brains exposed to cigarettes in utero (Chen et al. 2018). Furthermore, L-carnitine was identified to rescue global DNA methylation increases in kidney tissue (Stangenberg et al. 2019) and protect from metabolic deficits, including increased liver weight and fibrosis, elevated blood glucose and triglyceride levels at adulthood (Saad et al. 2018). Supplementation of alpha Lipoic acid during gestation ameliorated the negative male reproductive effects observed in offspring of gestational nicotine exposure, including reduced testosterone levels, testes size, sperm morphology, and sperm number (Anto et al. 2016). Thus, supplementation of the diet can be used to reverse some effects of gestational nicotine exposure.

9.15 Postnatal to Adulthood Health Outcomes

9.15.1 Growth Outcomes

Embryonic exposure of zebrafish to nicotine resulted in significant dose-dependent changes in the size of the craniofacial skeleton via reduction in cartilage size, with cranial neural crest cells showing the highest sensitivity, assessed 4 days post-fertilization (Borrego-Soto and Eberhart 2022). Nicotine exposure during embryonic development causes delays in secondary spinal motoneuron development, accompanied by persistent changes in swimming behavior (Svoboda et al. 2002) and enhanced motor output (Thomas et al. 2009).

Gestational exposure to nicotine in mice leads to changes in mandibular structure and length of the molars (Durham et al. 2019), with defects in palate structure characterized by persistent midline epithelial seams (Ozturk et al. 2016), reminiscent of tobacco smoke-induced non-syndromic cleft lip or cleft palate in humans (Honein et al. 2007; Li et al. 2010; Sabbagh et al. 2015). In rats, nicotine exposure from gestational day 11 to 20 resulted in delayed chondrogenesis accompanied by inhibition of matrix synthase in fetal growth plates and repression of IGF-1 signaling (Deng et al. 2013).

Studies of physical development in rats have shown no consistent effects on pinna detachment or incisor eruption. Fur growth is delayed, and there are some reports of delays in eye opening. Sexual maturation is most often normal, but sex-dependent acceleration has been reported (Sobrian and Holson 2011; Paulson et al. 1994). There are inconsistent findings regarding the effects of prenatal nicotine exposure on birthweight in rodent models (Zhang et al. 2022). Decreased birth weight may be associated with decreased postnatal weight gain, but the differences are recovered before or during adolescence (Sobrian and Holson 2011). Other studies have reported persistent weight gain with prenatal nicotine exposure, which may be altered by exposure paradigms (Table 9.13) (Sobrian and Holson 2011; Behl et al. 2013).

Prenatal nicotine exposure alters pancreatic weight, morphology, and beta cell survival in rats (Holloway et al. 2005; Bruin et al. 2007, 2008b, c; Somm et al. 2008, 2009). Reduced hypothalamic leptin signaling has been demonstrated in rats (Oliveira et al. 2009, 2010) and reduced leptin levels and lower adrenal and pancreas weights in rhesus macaques (Grove et al. 2001). Prenatal nicotine exposure impairs glucose tolerance in rats, though fasting insulin levels vary (Holloway et al. 2005; Bruin et al. 2007, 2008a; Somm et al. 2008; Behl et al. 2013). Male offspring exposed to nicotine during gestation (Somm et al. 2008), during lactation (Oliveira et al. 2010), or both (Holloway et al. 2005; Bruin et al. 2007, 2008a) have shown impairment in glucose homeostasis and insulin resistance (Holloway et al. 2005; Bruin et al. 2007, 2008a; Somm et al. 2008) or insulin resistance index (Oliveira et al. 2010), findings that were consistent regardless of dose, administration route, and timing of exposure (Behl et al. 2013). One study found evidence for intergenerational transmission of increased insulin resistance, which persisted in the F2 generation male offspring (Holloway et al. 2007). Nicotine exposure is most detrimental during gestation and lactation, with no effects post-weaning (Swislocki et al. 1997; Swislocki 2003; Jose et al. 2009; Swislocki and Fakiri 2008).

Adult male rats exposed to nicotine through gestation and weaning exhibit alterations in early adipogenesis along with increased expression of adipogenic and lipogenic genes, including within the liver, with enhanced susceptibility to later obesity (Fan et al. 2016). Another study in rats also showed elevated circulating and hepatic triglycerides with increased expression of fatty acid synthase, a key enzyme responsible for the synthesis of triglycerides in the liver (Ma et al. 2014). In mice, maternal nicotine exposure resulted in metabolic dysfunction consistent with the promotion of fatty liver disease, mediated by PI3k/Akt activation and Srebp1c and Ppara suppression. The observed insulin resistance and altered lipid metabolism occurred regardless of whether the mice were fed a normal or high-fat diet post-weaning (Huang et al. 2021).

9.15.2 Neurodevelopmental Impairments and Behavioral Abnormalities in Post-pubertal Offspring

Animal models show that prenatal and early postnatal exposure to nicotine can persistently alter brain development, including cholinergic, dopaminergic, and serotonergic neurotransmission (Sobrian and Holson 2011; Cohen and George 2013). Nicotine disrupts synaptic plasticity, neuronal maturation, and brain volume (Jamshed et al. 2020). In 5- to 6-month-old zebrafish, embryonic exposure to nicotine results in increased motor activity (Borrego-Soto and Eberhart 2022; Mora-Zamorano et al. 2016) and reduced shoaling behavior (Borrego-Soto and Eberhart 2022). Male mice show attention and working memory deficits with gestational nicotine exposure (Zhang et al. 2018). Increased hyperactivity, impulsivity, and anxiety-like behavior have commonly been observed as an outcome of prenatal nicotine exposure, and these are often associated with changes in dopamine and serotonin signaling (Elliott and Grunberg 2006).

Depressive-like behaviors in rats are often tested using sucrose/sugar/saccharin preference to measure anhedonia, and female offspring of untreated mothers normally consume more of the sweet solution than do their male littermates; contestably, prenatal nicotine exposure mitigates this normal sexually dimorphic behavior (Lichtensteiger and Schlumpf 1985; King and Stocco 2011; Sobrian et al. 2003). Tests for anxiety-like behaviors in rats and in mice have shown that males prenatally exposed to nicotine seem to be more vulnerable (Sikic et al. 2022).

Studies compare prenatal tobacco smoke extract (TSE) to nicotine, including secondhand exposure doses. Rats exposed to TSE or nicotine

Table 9.13 Effect of nicotine exposure on offspring growth in animal studies

Study	Year	Primary measures	Species	Conditions	Results
Durham et al. (2019)	2019	Morphologic assessment, histology, cell death	Mouse ($n = 15$)	50–200 µM nicotine via drinking water	Altered physiology, increased molar proliferation, decreased molar apoptosis
Ozturk et al. (2016)	2016	Morphologic assessment, genetic microarray	Mouse ($n = 202$)	1.5, 3.0, and 4.5 mg/kg/d nicotine via osmotic micropump	Developmental retardation, still birth, low birth weight, gene downregulation, and altered palatal size
Huang et al. (2021)	2021	Serum levels, ELISA, histology, immunohistochemistry, western blot,	Mouse ($n = 22$)	2 mg/kg nicotine via subcutaneous injection	Lipid metabolism disorder, insulin resistance,
Freitas et al. (2025)	2025	Oxidative stress, cytokine levels, Western blot, immunohistochemistry	Rat ($n = 10$)	2 mg/kg/day nicotine via osmotic minipump	Increased ovarian MDA levels; decreased ovarian mast cells; increased ovarian pro-inflammatory markers
Somm et al. (2008)	2008	Weight, histology, fat deposition, physical activity	Rat ($n = 10$)	3 mg/kg/day nicotine via osmotic pump	Increased epididymal adipose; adipocyte hypertrophy; glucose intolerance; insulin resistance
Paulson et al. (1994)	1994	Weight and behavioral tests	Rat ($n = 10$)	Smokeless tobacco extract (6 mg/kg nicotine) via oral gavage	Maternal and offspring weight gain, negative geotaxis
Swislocki (2003)	2003	Weight, blood pressure, glucose and insulin levels	Rat ($n = 28$)	25 mg/kg nicotine orally via chow	No significant effect on hypertension
Swislocki and Fakiri (2008)	2008	Weight, plasma levels, blood pressure	Rat ($n = 20$)	50 mg/kg nicotine orally via chow	No significant effect on glucose, insulin, free fatty acid, and leptin response
Bruin et al. (2007)	2007	Apoptosis, histology, immunohistochemistry	Rat ($n = 5$–12)	1 mg/kg/day nicotine bitartrate via subcutaneous injection	Exposure throughout lactation impaired glucose tolerance and caused permanent beta cell loss
Oliveira et al. (2009)	2009	Body composition, lipid profile, hormone determination	Rat ($n = 6$)	6 mg/kg nicotine via osmotic minipump	Higher adiposity, hyperleptinemia, and secondary hypothyroidism
Oliveira et al. (2010)	2010	Western blot, insulin sensitivity, tissue glycogen content, and morphometric analysis	Rat ($n = 6$)	6 mg/kg nicotine via osmotic minipump	Increased body fat, increased insulinemia and insulin resistance
Bruin et al. (2008a)	2008	Mitochondria structure/ function, glucose tolerance, electron microscopy, oxidative stress	Rat ($n = 5$–12)	1 mg/kg/day nicotine bitartrate via subcutaneous injection	Impaired pancreatic mitochondria and beta cells; glucose intolerance; islet cell oxidative stress increase; increased insulin granules
Bruin et al. (2008b)	2008	Enzyme quantification, Ros production, Western blot	Rat ($n = 3$–10)	1 mg/kg/day nicotine via subcutaneous injection	Increased carbonyl formation
Holloway et al. (2005)	2005	Serum insulin, apoptosis	Rat ($n = 5$–6)	1 mg/kg/day nicotine bitartrate via subcutaneous injection	Increased growth; dysglycemia; decreased serum insulin; increased beta cell apoptosis

(continued)

Table 9.13 (continued)

Study	Year	Primary measures	Species	Conditions	Results
Holloway et al. (2007)	2007	Glucose homeostasis	Rat ($n = 6–8$)	1 mg/kg/day nicotine via subcutaneous injection	Elevated fasting serum insulin and enhanced total insulin response
Ma et al. (2014)	2014	Triglyceride levels, RT-PCR, western blot, chromatin immunoprecipitation	Rat ($n = 4–7$)	1 mg/kg nicotine bitartrate via subcutaneous injection	Elevated triglycerides, increased fatty acid synthase, increased liver protein expression, histone acetylation
Fan et al. (2016)	2016	Weight, adipogenesis, lipogenesis, histology, RT-PCR, computed tomography scan,	Rat ($n = 8$)	2.0 mg/kg nicotine via subcutaneous injection	Adipogenic/lipogenic gene overexpression, increased weight, higher serum lipids
Jose et al. (2009)	2009	Blood glucose and glycogen levels, porphobilinogen-synthase activity, body/organ weight	Rat ($n = 36$)	5 mg/kg/day nicotine via subcutaneous injection	Reduced body and liver weight, decreased glycogen
Swislocki et al. (1997)	1997	Weight, blood pressure, glucose and insulin levels	Rat ($n = 11$)	50 mg/kg nicotine via intraperitoneal injection	Hypertension
Grove et al. (2001)	2001	RT-PCR, immunohistochemistry, plasma levels, body/organ weight, amniotic fluid	Rhesus ($n = 4–7$)	1.5 mg/kg/day nicotine tartrate via osmotic minipump	Reduced birth weight; reduced postnatal leptin; increase in pro-opiomelanocortin expression in brain; elevated metabolism in nicotine exposed
Thomas et al. (2009)	2009	Bends/minute, photomicrographs,	Zebrafish	1–30 μM nicotine via media	Musculature bends, altered physiology
Svoboda et al. (2002)	2002	Field test, morphology, photomicorographs, immunohistochemistry	Zebrafish	33 μM nicotine via media	Altered nervous system
Borrego-Soto and Eberhart (2022)	2022	Morphology, shoaling response, exposure level, organ weight	Zebrafish	12.5–50 μM nicotine via media	Altered maternal heart and thymus weight

during gestation showed hyperactivity and cognitive deficits, with stronger effects from TSE. Nicotine and TSE outcome measures were highly correlated, but effects were much higher with the TSE (Hall et al. 2016). In vitro studies show TSE promotes larger but fewer neurons, while nicotine affects differentiation with milder effects (Slotkin et al. 2014). Impairment of presynaptic acetylcholine activity was observed most prominently with TSE but also with nicotine exposure in multiple brain regions of the exposed rats, evaluated longitudinally, with decreased cholinergic receptors. Nicotinic acetylcholine receptors increased in the nicotine-only groups along with an increase in choline acetyltransferase (a constitutive marker of acetylcholine nerve terminals), but decreased in the tobacco smoke exposure group, with a lesser increase in choline acetyltransferase in males and a reduction in females (Slotkin et al. 2014).

Prenatal exposure to tobacco smoking is known to increase the risk of nicotine addiction for the exposed offspring (Elliott and Grunberg 2006). Rodent models have been used to study this increased risk and potential mechanisms. Mice prenatally exposed to nicotine later showed increased nicotine preference, especially males. The nicotine-exposed offspring preferentially consumed the nicotine-containing solution as opposed to the saccharin-exposed offspring. The

Table 9.14 Effect of nicotine exposure on post-pubertal neurodevelopment and behavioral outcomes in animal studies

Study	Year	Primary measures	Species	Conditions	Results
Zhang et al. (2018)	2018	Locomotor activity, spontaneous alternation, recognition, and latency to fall	Mouse ($n = 10$)	100 μg/mL nicotine via drinking water	Deficit in attention and memory
Klein et al. (2003)	2003	Water preference, behavior	Mouse ($n = 4$–5)	50 μg/mL nicotine via drinking water	Increased nicotine preference
Hall et al. (2016)	2016	Maze, locomotor activity, object recognition,	Rat ($n = 8$–10)	2 mg/kg nicotine, tobacco smoke extract 0.18 mg/kg via osmotic minipump	Disrupted cognitive/ behavioral function, hyperactivity, memory deficit
Slotkin et al. (2015)	2015	Synaptic markers, growth effects, acetylcholine receptor binding, serotonin receptor binding	Rat ($n = 8$–10)	Tobacco smoke extract 2 mg/kg via osmotic minipump	Impaired cholinergic activity,
Slotkin et al. (2006)	2006	Acetylcholine receptor binding, serotonin receptor binding	Rat ($n = 10$)	6 mg/kg nicotine via osmotic minipump	Damage to serotonin receptors
Sobrian et al. (2003)	2003	Maze, sucrose preference/ intake, locomotor activity	Rat ($n = 66$)	Nicotine 2.5–5 mg/kg via subcutaneous injection	Altered sucrose preference/uptake, altered behavior
Abreu-Villaca et al. (2004)	2004	Weight, acetylcholine receptor binding, cholinergic activity	Rat ($n = 10$)	6 mg/kg nicotine via subcutaneous injection	Acetylcholine receptor upregulation, cholinergic hypoactivity, altered nicotine response
Borrego-Soto and Eberhart (2022)	2022	Morphology, shoaling response, exposure level, organ weight	Zebrafish	12.5–50 μM nicotine via media	Altered maternal heart and thymus weight

nicotine-seeking behavior was most prominent in males (Table 9.14) (Klein et al. 2003).

Pregnant female rats were exposed to nicotine through gestation, and the offspring were then exposed to nicotine again during adolescence (postnatal day 30 to 47.5) to levels approximating that in smokers (Abreu-Villaca et al. 2004). In animals exposed prenatally, there were persistent cholinergic deficits to adulthood. Adolescent nicotine exposure resulted in marked upregulation of nicotinic acetylcholine receptors while suppressing cholinergic activity. Prenatal exposure lessened this adolescent's upregulation of nicotinic acetylcholine receptors in response to nicotine and exacerbated the cholinergic hypoactivity. These same patterns of changes were also evident with serotonin (Slotkin et al. 2015), along with altering serotonin synaptic communication with changes in serotonin receptor levels and induction of adenylyl cyclase through adolescence (Slotkin et al. 2006). Prenatal nicotine alters adolescent neurochemistry, increasing susceptibility to later nicotine use (Abreu-Villaca et al. 2004).

9.15.3 Offspring Sex Differences

When sex differences in offspring birthweight have been reported, it is usually males that have lower birthweights (Sobrian and Holson 2011). In mouse studies, male offspring are more likely to exhibit anxiety and compulsive behaviors, and there are sex-specific differences in expression of glutamate pathway genes, while attention-deficit/hyperactivity-disorder-like behaviors are sex-independent (Polli et al. 2020).

There are conflicting reports of sex differences in cognitive impairment in rodent models of prenatal nicotine exposure, thought to be attributable to differences in the route or gestational window of the exposure (Sikic et al. 2022). Testing multiple defined nicotine exposure windows from gestational day (GD) 0 to postnatal day 7 in mice showed that all windows of exposure resulted in some cognitive deficits, but only females exhibited working memory deficits when they were exposed from GD0 to postnatal day 0 or from GD14 to postnatal day 0. Only males exposed from GD0 to postnatal day 7, GD14 to postnatal day 7, or GD0 to postnatal day 0 showed deficits in attention using the object-based attention task (Alkam et al. 2013). Female rats exposed from GD3 to exhaustion of the 28-day osmotic minipump used showed more prominent reductions in acquisition and retention of avoidance learning (Vaglenova et al. 2004; Vaglenova et al. 2008).

In rat studies, developmental nicotine exposure resulted in female-specific cardiac anatomical defects evident in adolescent animals, including decreased left ventricle mass, smaller left ventricular outflow diameter, and decreased posterior wall thickness. In these same studies, both exposed males and females showed an increase in contractility and enhanced myocyte tension-generating capacity (Flanigan et al. 2024).

9.16 Conclusion

Both THC and nicotine exposure during pregnancy can lead to significant disruptions in fetal development, with long-term consequences for offspring's health. Prenatal THC exposure is associated with impacts to neurodevelopment, metabolism, cardiovascular function, and reproductive health, with sex-specific vulnerabilities that persist into adulthood. Similarly, nicotine-containing cigarettes and e-cigarette vapors have been linked to deficits in pulmonary, neurological, behavioral, cardiac, renal, and epigenetic systems, largely driven by oxidative stress responses across multiple organ tissues. Although animal models have been instrumental in uncovering these effects, much remains unknown about the precise mechanisms underlying these disruptions.

Notably, there is a lack of animal studies examining the combined effects of prenatal THC and nicotine exposure, despite high rates of co-use among pregnant individuals. Co-exposure could potentially have synergistic or additive effects on fetal development, yet few models have been developed to systematically study these interactions. Moreover, modern patterns of polysubstance use remain understudied in preclinical systems. Expanding animal models to address these real-world use patterns is essential to understanding the full scope of developmental risk. The animal models discussed provide a foundation to study both the individual and synergistic effects of THC and nicotine on fetal development.

The evolving landscape of cannabis and nicotine use, particularly with new product formulations and changing social perceptions, underscores the need for continued research. Despite significant advances, further studies are required to refine our understanding of how these substances interact with fetal development, particularly in the context of poly-substance exposure and modern delivery methods. Animal models will continue to serve as critical tools in elucidating these mechanisms and informing public health policies aimed at reducing the risks associated with prenatal THC and nicotine exposure.

References

Abrams R, Cook C, Davis K, Niederreither K, Jaeger M, Szeto H (1985) Plasma delta-9-tetrahydrocannabinol in pregnant sheep and fetus after inhalation of smoke from a marijuana cigarette. Alcohol Drug Res. 6(5): 361–369

Abreu-Villaca Y, Seidler FJ, Tate CA, Cousins MM, Slotkin TA (2004) Prenatal nicotine exposure alters the response to nicotine administration in adolescence: effects on cholinergic systems during exposure and withdrawal. Neuropsychopharmacology. 29(5): 879–890. https://doi.org/10.1038/sj.npp.1300401

Abu-Qare AW, Elmasry E, Abou-Donia MB (2003) A role for P-glycoprotein in environmental toxicology. J Toxicol Environ Health B Crit Rev. 6(3):279–288. https://doi.org/10.1080/10937400306466

Abuse S (2019) Mental health services administration. 2018 national survey on drug use and health: methodological summary and definitions. Center for

Behavioral Health Statistics and Quality. Substance Abuse and Mental Health Services Administration, Rockville

Ahmed KT, Amin MR, Shah P, Ali DW (2018) Motor neuron development in zebrafish is altered by brief (5-hr) exposures to THC (Δ9-tetrahydrocannabinol) or CBD (cannabidiol) during gastrulation. Sci Rep. 8(1):10518. https://doi.org/10.1038/s41598-018-28689-z

Ainiti D-F, Lykeridou A, Nanou C, Deltsidou A (2023) Cannabis use during pregnancy and its effect on the fetus, newborn and later childhood: a systematic review. Eur J Midwifery. 7(August):1–9. https://doi.org/10.18332/ejm/168727

Akingbade G, Ijomone O, Adelakun S, Enaibe B (2021) Histological and biochemical alterations in the superior colliculus and lateral geniculate nucleus of juvenile rats following prenatal exposure to marijuana smoke. Basic Clin Neurosci. 12(6):745–758. https://doi.org/10.32598/bcn.2021.1701.1

Alkam T, Kim HC, Mamiya T, Yamada K, Hiramatsu M, Nabeshima T (2013) Evaluation of cognitive behaviors in young offspring of C57BL/6 J mice after gestational nicotine exposure during different time-windows. Psychopharmacology (Berl). 230(3):451–463. https://doi.org/10.1007/s00213-013-3175-9

Allen S, Natale BV, Ejeckam AO, Lee K, Hardy DB, Natale DRC (2024) Cannabidiol exposure during rat pregnancy leads to labyrinth-specific vascular defects in the placenta and reduced fetal growth. Cannabis Cannabinoid Res. 9(3):766–780. https://doi.org/10.1089/can.2023.0166

Anto SK, Koyada N, Khan S, Jena G (2016) alpha-Lipoic acid attenuates transplacental nicotine-induced germ cell and oxidative DNA damage in adult mice. J Basic Clin Physiol Pharmacol. 27(6):585–593. https://doi.org/10.1515/jbcpp-2015-0151

Antonucci R, Contu P, Porcella A, Atzeni C, Chiappe S (2004) Intrauterine smoke exposure: a new risk factor for bronchopulmonary dysplasia? J Perinat Med. 32(3):272–277. https://doi.org/10.1515/JPM.2004.051

Archie SR, Sifat AE, Mara D, Ahn Y, Akter KA, Zhang Y et al (2023) Impact of in-utero electronic cigarette exposure on neonatal neuroinflammation, oxidative stress and mitochondrial function. Front Pharmacol. 14:1227145. https://doi.org/10.3389/fphar.2023.1227145

Arredondo J, Hall LL, Ndoye A, Nguyen VT, Chernyavsky AI, Bercovich D et al (2003) Central role of fibroblast α3 nicotinic acetylcholine receptor in mediating cutaneous effects of nicotine. Lab Invest 83(2):207–225. https://doi.org/10.1097/01.LAB.0000053917.46614.12

Asch RH, Smith CG (1986) Effects of delta 9-THC, the principal psychoactive component of marijuana, during pregnancy in the rhesus monkey. J Reprod Med. 31(12):1071–1081

Authement AK, Isoherranen N (2024) The impact of pregnancy and associated hormones on the pharmacokinetics of Δ(9)-tetrahydrocannabinol. Expert Opin Drug Metab Toxicol. 20(1–2):73–93. https://doi.org/10.1080/17425255.2024.2309213

Baglot SL, VanRyzin JW, Marquardt AE, Aukema RJ, Petrie GN, Hume C et al (2022) Maternal-fetal transmission of delta-9-tetrahydrocannabinol (THC) and its metabolites following inhalation and injection exposure during pregnancy in rats. J Neurosci Res. 100(3): 713–730. https://doi.org/10.1002/jnr.24992

Bailey J, Cunny H, Paule M, Slikker W Jr (1987) Fetal disposition of Δ9-tetrahydrocannabinol (THC) during late pregnancy in the rhesus monkey. Toxicol Appl Pharmacol 90(2):315–321

Barker DJ (2007) The origins of the developmental origins theory. J Intern Med. 261(5):412–417. https://doi.org/10.1111/j.1365-2796.2007.01809.x

Barra NG, Lisyansky M, Vanduzer TA, Raha S, Holloway AC, Hardy DB (2017) Maternal nicotine exposure leads to decreased cardiac protein disulfide isomerase and impaired mitochondrial function in male rat offspring. J Appl Toxicol. 37(12):1517–1526. https://doi.org/10.1002/jat.3503

Beggiato S, Borelli AC, Tomasini MC, Morgano L, Antonelli T, Tanganelli S et al (2017) Long-lasting alterations of hippocampal GABAergic neurotransmission in adult rats following perinatal Δ9-THC exposure. Neurobiol Learn Mem. 139:135–143. https://doi.org/10.1016/j.nlm.2016.12.023

Beggiato S, Ieraci A, Tomasini MC, Schwarcz R, Ferraro L (2020) Prenatal THC exposure raises kynurenic acid levels in the prefrontal cortex of adult rats. Prog Neuro-Psychopharmacol Biol Psychiatry. 100:109883. https://doi.org/10.1016/j.pnpbp.2020.109883

Behl M, Rao D, Aagaard K, Davidson TL, Levin ED, Slotkin TA et al (2013) Evaluation of the association between maternal smoking, childhood obesity, and metabolic disorders: a national toxicology program workshop review. Environ Health Perspect. 121(2): 170–180. https://doi.org/10.1289/ehp.1205404

Benevenuto SG, Domenico MD, Martins MAG, Costa NS, de Souza ARL, Costa JL et al (2017) Recreational use of marijuana during pregnancy and negative gestational and fetal outcomes: an experimental study in mice. Toxicology. 376:94–101. https://doi.org/10.1016/j.tox.2016.05.020

Benowitz NL, Hukkanen J, Jacob P 3rd. (2009) Nicotine chemistry, metabolism, kinetics and biomarkers. Handb Exp Pharmacol. 192:29–60. https://doi.org/10.1007/978-3-540-69248-5_2

Bergmann KE, Bergmann RL, Von Kries R, Bohm O, Richter R, Dudenhausen JW et al (2003) Early determinants of childhood overweight and adiposity in a birth cohort study: role of breast-feeding. Int J Obes Relat Metab Disord. 27(2):162–172. https://doi.org/10.1038/sj.ijo.802200

Black T, Baccetto SL, Barnard IL, Finch E, McElroy DL, Austin-Scott FVL et al (2023) Characterization of cannabinoid plasma concentration, maternal health, and cytokine levels in a rat model of prenatal Cannabis smoke exposure. Sci Rep 13(1):21070. https://doi.org/10.1038/s41598-023-47861-8

Borrego-Soto G, Eberhart JK (2022) Embryonic nicotine exposure disrupts adult social behavior and craniofacial development in zebrafish. Toxics. 10(10). https://doi.org/10.3390/toxics10100612

Breit KR, Rodriguez CG, Lei A, Thomas JD (2020) Combined vapor exposure to THC and alcohol in pregnant rats: Maternal outcomes and pharmacokinetic effects. Neurotoxicol Teratol. 82:106930. https://doi.org/10.1016/j.ntt.2020.106930

Brinchmann BC, Vist GE, Becher R, Grimsrud TK, Elvsaas I, Underland V et al (2023) Use of Swedish smokeless tobacco during pregnancy: a systematic review of pregnancy and early life health risk. Addiction. 118(5):789–803. https://doi.org/10.1111/add.16114

Bruin JE, Kellenberger LD, Gerstein HC, Morrison KM, Holloway AC (2007) Fetal and neonatal nicotine exposure and postnatal glucose homeostasis: identifying critical windows of exposure. J Endocrinol. 194(1):171–178. https://doi.org/10.1677/JOE-07-0050

Bruin JE, Petre MA, Raha S, Morrison KM, Gerstein HC, Holloway AC (2008a) Fetal and neonatal nicotine exposure in Wistar rats causes progressive pancreatic mitochondrial damage and beta cell dysfunction. PLoS One. 3(10):e3371. https://doi.org/10.1371/journal.pone.0003371

Bruin JE, Petre MA, Lehman MA, Raha S, Gerstein HC, Morrison KM et al (2008b) Maternal nicotine exposure increases oxidative stress in the offspring. Free Radic Biol Med. 44(11):1919–1925. https://doi.org/10.1016/j.freeradbiomed.2008.02.010

Bruin JE, Gerstein HC, Morrison KM, Holloway AC (2008c) Increased pancreatic beta-cell apoptosis following fetal and neonatal exposure to nicotine is mediated via the mitochondria. Toxicol Sci. 103(2):362–370. https://doi.org/10.1093/toxsci/kfn012

Bruin JE, Woynillowicz AK, Hettinga BP, Tarnopolsky MA, Morrison KM, Gerstein HC et al (2012) Maternal antioxidants prevent beta-cell apoptosis and promote formation of dual hormone-expressing endocrine cells in male offspring following fetal and neonatal nicotine exposure. J Diabetes. 4(3):297–306. https://doi.org/10.1111/j.1753-0407.2012.00195.x

Bush D, Goniewicz ML (2015) A pilot study on nicotine residues in houses of electronic cigarette users, tobacco smokers, and non-users of nicotine-containing products. Int J Drug Policy. 26(6):609–611. https://doi.org/10.1016/j.drugpo.2015.03.003

Calkins K, Devaskar SU (2011) Fetal origins of adult disease. Curr Probl Pediatr Adolesc Health Care. 41(6):158–176. https://doi.org/10.1016/j.cppeds.2011.01.001

Carty DR, Thornton C, Gledhill JH, Willett KL (2017) Developmental effects of cannabidiol and Δ9-Tetrahydrocannabinol in zebrafish. Toxicol Sci 162(1):137–145. https://doi.org/10.1093/toxsci/kfx232

Castro EM, Lotfipour S, Leslie FM (2023) Nicotine on the developing brain. Pharmacol Res. 190:106716. https://doi.org/10.1016/j.phrs.2023.106716

Cella M, Leguizamón GF, Sordelli MS, Cervini M, Guadagnoli T, Ribeiro ML et al (2008) Dual effect of anandamide on rat placenta nitric oxide synthesis. Placenta. 29(8):699–707. https://doi.org/10.1016/j.placenta.2008.05.003

Chan YL, Saad S, Pollock C, Oliver B, Al-Odat I, Zaky AA et al (2016) Impact of maternal cigarette smoke exposure on brain inflammation and oxidative stress in male mice offspring. Sci Rep. 6:25881. https://doi.org/10.1038/srep25881

Chan YL, Oliver BG, Chen H (2020) What lessons have we learnt about the impact of maternal cigarette smoking from animal models? Clin Exp Pharmacol Physiol. 47(2):337–344. https://doi.org/10.1111/1440-1681.13182

Chellian R, Behnood-Rod A, Bruijnzeel DM, Wilson R, Pandy V, Bruijnzeel AW (2021) Rodent models for nicotine withdrawal. J Psychopharmacol. 35(10):1169–1187. https://doi.org/10.1177/02698811211005629

Chen H, Li G, Chan YL, Nguyen T, van Reyk D, Saad S et al (2018) Modulation of neural regulators of energy homeostasis, and of inflammation, in the pups of mice exposed to e-cigarettes. Neurosci Lett. 684:61–66. https://doi.org/10.1016/j.neulet.2018.07.001

Cherian SV, Kumar A, Estrada YMRM (2020) E-cigarette or vaping product-associated lung injury: a review. Am J Med. 133(6):657–663. https://doi.org/10.1016/j.amjmed.2020.02.004

Cohen A, George O (2013) Animal models of nicotine exposure: relevance to second-hand smoking, electronic cigarette use, and compulsive smoking. Front Psychiatry. 4:41. https://doi.org/10.3389/fpsyt.2013.00041

Conner SN, Bedell V, Lipsey K, Macones GA, Cahill AG, Tuuli MG (2016) Maternal marijuana use and adverse neonatal outcomes: a systematic review and meta-analysis. Obstet Gynecol. 128(4):713–723. https://doi.org/10.1097/aog.0000000000001649

Crosland BA, Garg B, Bandoli GE, Mandelbaum AD, Hayer S, Ryan KS et al (2024) Risk of adverse neonatal outcomes after combined prenatal cannabis and nicotine exposure. JAMA Netw Open. 7(5):e2410151-e. https://doi.org/10.1001/jamanetworkopen.2024.10151

Cui Y, Shooshtari S, Forget EL, Clara I, Cheung KF (2014) Smoking during pregnancy: findings from the 2009–2010 Canadian Community Health Survey. PLoS One. 9(1):e84640. https://doi.org/10.1371/journal.pone.0084640

Cupo L, Dominguez-Cancino KA, Nazif-Munoz JI, Chakravarty MM (2024) Prenatal cannabis exposure in the clinic and laboratory: what do we know and where do we need to go? Drug Alcohol Depend Rep. 13:100282. https://doi.org/10.1016/j.dadr.2024.100282

de Salas-Quiroga A, García-Rincón D, Gómez-Domínguez D, Valero M, Simón-Sánchez S, Paraíso-Luna J et al (2020) Long-term hippocampal interneuronopathy drives sex-dimorphic spatial memory impairment induced by prenatal THC exposure. Neuropsychopharmacology. 45(5):877–886. https://doi.org/10.1038/s41386-020-0621-3

Deng Y, Cao H, Cu F, Xu D, Lei Y, Tan Y et al (2013) Nicotine-induced retardation of chondrogenesis through down-regulation of IGF-1 signaling pathway to inhibit matrix synthesis of growth plate chondrocytes in fetal rats. Toxicol Appl Pharmacol. 269(1):25–33. https://doi.org/10.1016/j.taap.2013.02.008

Dinis-Oliveira RJ (2016) Metabolomics of Δ9-tetrahydrocannabinol: implications in toxicity. Drug Metab Rev. 48(1):80–87

Duko B, Bedaso A, Dachew BA, Newnham E, Gebremedhin AT, Tessema G et al (2024) The effect of maternal prenatal tobacco smoking on offspring academic achievement: a systematic review and meta-analysis. Addict Behav 153:107985. https://doi.org/10.1016/j.addbeh.2024.107985

Durham EL, Balog C, Howie RN, Boyce MA, Arand JR, Warren G et al (2019) Effects of nicotine exposure on murine mandibular development. PLoS One. 14(6):e0218376. https://doi.org/10.1371/journal.pone.0218376

Elliott BM, Grunberg NE (2006) Prenatal nicotine exposure and animal behavior. In: Miller MW (ed) Brain development: normal processes and the effects of alcohol and nicotine. Oxford University Press, New York, pp 329–340

ElSohly MA, Mehmedic Z, Foster S, Gon C, Chandra S, Church JC (2016) Changes in cannabis potency over the last 2 decades (1995–2014): analysis of current data in the United States. Biol Psychiatry. 79(7):613–619. https://doi.org/10.1016/j.biopsych.2016.01.004

ElSohly MA, Chandra S, Radwan M, Majumdar CG, Church JC (2021) A comprehensive review of cannabis potency in the united states in the last decade. Biol Psychiatry Cogn Neurosci Neuroimaging. 6(6):603–606. https://doi.org/10.1016/j.bpsc.2020.12.016

England LJ, Bunnell RE, Pechacek TF, Tong VT, McAfee TA (2015) Nicotine and the developing human: a neglected element in the electronic cigarette debate. Am J Prev Med. 49(2):286–293. https://doi.org/10.1016/j.amepre.2015.01.015

Fan J, Zhang WX, Rao YS, Xue JL, Wang FF, Zhang L et al (2016) Perinatal nicotine exposure increases obesity susceptibility in adult male rat offspring by altering early adipogenesis. Endocrinology. 157(11):4276–4286. https://doi.org/10.1210/en.2016-1269

Fernández-Trapero M, Pérez-Díaz C, Espejo-Porras F, de Lago E, Fernández-Ruiz J (2020) Pharmacokinetics of Sativex® in dogs: towards a potential cannabinoid-based therapy for canine disorders. Biomolecules. 10(2):279

Ferriero DM (2004) Neonatal brain injury. N Engl J Med. 351(19):1985–1995. https://doi.org/10.1056/NEJMra041996

Flanigan EG, Farman GP, Dennis MR, Wollman L, Van Den Berg M, Granzier H et al (2024) Developmental nicotine exposure alters cardiovascular structure and function in neonatal and juvenile rats. Am J Physiol Heart Circ Physiol. 327(6):H1442–H1H54. https://doi.org/10.1152/ajpheart.00558.2024

Fonseca BM, Correia-da-Silva G, Taylor AH, Lam PM, Marczylo TH, Konje JC et al (2012) Characterisation of the endocannabinoid system in rat haemochorial placenta. Reprod Toxicol. 34(3):347–356. https://doi.org/10.1016/j.reprotox.2012.05.036

Frau R, Miczán V, Traccis F, Aroni S, Pongor CI, Saba P et al (2019) Prenatal THC exposure produces a hyperdopaminergic phenotype rescued by pregnenolone. Nat Neurosci 22(12):1975–1985. https://doi.org/10.1038/s41593-019-0512-2

Freitas IMM, Santos ID, Souza JC, Souza GS, Fischer LW, Da Silva RA et al (2025) Maternal exposure to nicotine causes oxidative stress and inflammatory changes in the ovaries of rats' adult offspring. Reprod Toxicol. 132:108839. https://doi.org/10.1016/j.reprotox.2025.108839

Freudenthal RI, Martin J, Wall ME (1972) Distribution of delta 9-tetrahydrocannabinol in the mouse. Br J Pharmacol. 44(2):244–249. https://doi.org/10.1111/j.1476-5381.1972.tb07260.x

Gabrielsson J, Gumbleton M (1993) Kinetics of nicotine and its metabolites in animals. In: Gorrod JW, Wahren J (eds) Nicotine and related alkaloids: absorption, distribution, metabolism and excretion. Springer, Dordrecht, pp 181–195

Gao YJ, Holloway AC, Su LY, Takemori K, Lu C, Lee RM (2008) Effects of fetal and neonatal exposure to nicotine on blood pressure and perivascular adipose tissue function in adult life. Eur J Pharmacol. 590(1–3):264–268. https://doi.org/10.1016/j.ejphar.2008.05.044

Geber WF, Schramm LC (1969) Effect of marihuana extract on fetal hamsters and rabbits. Toxicol Appl Pharmacol. 14(2):276–282. https://doi.org/10.1016/0041-008x(69)90108-2

Gillies R, Lee K, Vanin S, Laviolette SR, Holloway AC, Arany E et al (2020) Maternal exposure to Δ9-tetrahydrocannabinol impairs female offspring glucose homeostasis and endocrine pancreatic development in the rat. Reprod Toxicol 94:84–91. https://doi.org/10.1016/j.reprotox.2020.04.070

Ginsburg BC, Hruba L, Zaki A, Javors MA, McMahon LR (2014) Blood levels do not predict behavioral or physiological effects of Δ9-tetrahydrocannabinol in rhesus monkeys with different patterns of exposure. Drug Alcohol Depend 139:1–8

Giovenco DP, Spillane TE, Lee HM, Ali N, Little RMP, Rahman SN et al (2025) Retail availability of oral nicotine pouches in 3 US cities: a geographic analysis. Nicotine Tob Res. https://doi.org/10.1093/ntr/ntae312

Goniewicz ML, Knysak J, Gawron M, Kosmider L, Sobczak A, Kurek J et al (2014) Levels of selected carcinogens and toxicants in vapour from electronic cigarettes. Tob Control. 23(2):133–139. https://doi.org/10.1136/tobaccocontrol-2012-050859

Gorrod JW, Jenner P (1975) Chapter 2—The metabolism of tobacco alkaloids. In: Hayes WJ (ed) Essays in toxicology. Elsevier, pp 35–78

Graham AL, Papandonatos GD (2008) Reliability of internet- versus telephone-administered questionnaires in a diverse sample of smokers. J Med Internet Res. 10(1): e8. https://doi.org/10.2196/jmir.987

Greco ER, Engineer A, Saiyin T, Lu X, Zhang M, Jones DL et al (2022) Maternal nicotine exposure induces congenital heart defects in the offspring of mice. J Cell Mol Med. 26(11):3223–3234. https://doi.org/10.1111/jcmm.17328

Grove KL, Sekhon HS, Brogan RS, Keller JA, Smith MS, Spindel ER (2001) Chronic maternal nicotine exposure alters neuronal systems in the arcuate nucleus that regulate feeding behavior in the newborn rhesus macaque. J Clin Endocrinol Metab. 86(11): 5420–5426. https://doi.org/10.1210/jcem.86.11.8033

Gruslin A, Cesta CE, Bell M, Qing Q, Petre MA, Holloway AC (2009) Effect of nicotine exposure during pregnancy and lactation on maternal, fetal, and postnatal rat IGF-II profile. Reprod Sci. 16(9): 875–882. https://doi.org/10.1177/1933719109337038

Gunn J, Rosales C, Center K, Nuñez A, Gibson S, Christ C et al (2016) Prenatal exposure to cannabis and maternal and child health outcomes: a systematic review and meta-analysis. BMJ Open. 6(4):e009986

Habayeb OM, Taylor AH, Bell SC, Taylor DJ, Konje JC (2008) Expression of the endocannabinoid system in human first trimester placenta and its role in trophoblast proliferation. Endocrinology. 149(10): 5052–5060. https://doi.org/10.1210/en.2007-1799

Hall BJ, Cauley M, Burke DA, Kiany A, Slotkin TA, Levin ED (2016) Cognitive and behavioral impairments evoked by low-level exposure to tobacco smoke components: comparison with nicotine alone. Toxicol Sci. 151(2):236–244. https://doi.org/10.1093/toxsci/kfw042

Holloway AC, Lim GE, Petrik JJ, Foster WG, Morrison KM, Gerstein HC (2005) Fetal and neonatal exposure to nicotine in Wistar rats results in increased beta cell apoptosis at birth and postnatal endocrine and metabolic changes associated with type 2 diabetes. Diabetologia. 48(12):2661–2666. https://doi.org/10.1007/s00125-005-0022-5

Holloway AC, Kellenberger LD, Petrik JJ (2006) Fetal and neonatal exposure to nicotine disrupts ovarian function and fertility in adult female rats. Endocrine. 30(2): 213–216. https://doi.org/10.1385/ENDO:30:2:213

Holloway AC, Cuu DQ, Morrison KM, Gerstein HC, Tarnopolsky MA (2007) Transgenerational effects of fetal and neonatal exposure to nicotine. Endocrine. 31(3):254–259. https://doi.org/10.1007/s12020-007-0043-6

Holloway AC, Hettinga BP, Gerstein HC (2011) Effect of combining rosiglitazone with either metformin or insulin on beta-cell mass and function in an animal model of Type 2 diabetes characterized by reduced beta-cell mass at birth. J Diabetes. 3(1):74–81. https://doi.org/10.1111/j.1753-0407.2010.00101.x

Holloway AC, Salomon A, Soares MJ, Garnier V, Raha S, Sergent F et al (2014) Characterization of the adverse effects of nicotine on placental development: in vivo and in vitro studies. Am J Physiol Endocrinol Metab. 306(4):E443–E456. https://doi.org/10.1152/ajpendo.00478.2013

Honein MA, Rasmussen SA, Reefhuis J, Romitti PA, Lammer EJ, Sun L et al (2007) Maternal smoking and environmental tobacco smoke exposure and the risk of orofacial clefts. Epidemiology. 18(2):226–233. https://doi.org/10.1097/01.ede.0000254430.61294.c0

Horvath TL, Diano S, Tschop M (2004) Brain circuits regulating energy homeostasis. Neuroscientist. 10(3): 235–246. https://doi.org/10.1177/1073858403262151

Huang SJ, Chen SQ, Lin Y, Yang HY, Ran J, Yan FF et al (2021) Maternal nicotine exposure aggravates metabolic associated fatty liver disease via PI3K/Akt signaling in adult offspring mice. Liver Int. 41(8): 1867–1878. https://doi.org/10.1111/liv.14902

Hukkanen J, Jacob P 3rd, Benowitz NL (2005) Metabolism and disposition kinetics of nicotine. Pharmacol Rev. 57(1):79–115. https://doi.org/10.1124/pr.57.1.3

Hume C, Baglot SL, Javorcikova L, Lightfoot SHM, Scheufen J, Hill MN (2024) Effects of prenatal THC vapor exposure on body weight, glucose metabolism, and feeding behaviors in chow and high-fat diet fed rats. Int J Obes (Lond). 48(7):981–992. https://doi.org/10.1038/s41366-024-01512-8

Hutchings DE, Martin BR, Gamagaris Z, Miller N, Fico T (1989) Plasma concentrations of delta-9-tetrahydrocannabinol in dams and fetuses following acute or multiple prenatal dosing in rats. Life Sci. 44(11): 697–701

Idänpään-Heikkilä J, Fritchie GE, Englert LF, Ho BT, McIsaac WM (1969) Placental transfer of tritiated-1-Delta-9-tetrahydrocannabinol. N Engl J Med. 281(6): 330. https://doi.org/10.1056/nejm196908072810620

Jamshed L, Perono GA, Jamshed S, Holloway AC (2020) Early life exposure to nicotine: postnatal metabolic, neurobehavioral and respiratory outcomes and the development of childhood cancers. Toxicol Sci. 178(1):3–15. https://doi.org/10.1093/toxsci/kfaa127

Jensen TK, Henriksen TB, Hjollund NH, Scheike T, Kolstad H, Giwercman A et al (1998) Adult and prenatal exposures to tobacco smoke as risk indicators of fertility among 430 Danish couples. Am J Epidemiol 148(10):992–997. https://doi.org/10.1093/oxfordjournals.aje.a009576

Jose AS, Franciscato C, Sonego F, Figueiro M, Thiesen FV, Garcia SC et al (2009) Sensitivity of young rats to nicotine exposure: physiological and biochemical parameters. Ecotoxicol Environ Saf. 72(1):242–247. https://doi.org/10.1016/j.ecoenv.2008.03.010

Joubert BR, Felix JF, Yousefi P, Bakulski KM, Just AC, Breton C et al (2016) DNA methylation in newborns and maternal smoking in pregnancy: genome-wide consortium meta-analysis. Am J Hum Genet. 98(4): 680–696. https://doi.org/10.1016/j.ajhg.2016.02.019

Kenney SP, Kekuda R, Prasad PD, Leibach FH, Devoe LD, Ganapathy V (1999) Cannabinoid receptors and their role in the regulation of the serotonin transporter in human placenta. Am J Obstet Gynecol. 181(2): 491–497. https://doi.org/10.1016/s0002-9378(99)70583-1

Kim YS, Li Y, Yuan J, Borg JP, Sun X, Dey SK (2021) Cannabinoid and planar cell polarity signaling converges to direct placentation. Proc Natl Acad Sci U S A. 118(38). https://doi.org/10.1073/pnas.2108201118

King SR, Stocco DM (2011) Steroidogenic acute regulatory protein expression in the central nervous system. Front Endocrinol (Lausanne). 2:72. https://doi.org/10.3389/fendo.2011.00072

Klein LC, Stine MM, Pfaff DW, Vandenbergh DJ (2003) Laternal nicotine exposure increases nicotine preference in periadolescent male but not female C57B1/6 J mice. Nicotine Tob Res. 5(1):117–124. https://doi.org/10.1080/14622200307257

Kozlenkov A, Jaffe AE, Timashpolsky A, Apontes P, Rudchenko S, Barbu M et al (2017) DNA methylation profiling of human prefrontal cortex neurons in heroin users shows significant difference between genomic contexts of hyper- and hypomethylation and a younger epigenetic age. Genes (Basel). 8(6). https://doi.org/10.3390/genes8060152

Lagunov A, Anzar M, Sadeu JC, Khan MI, Bruin JE, Woynillowicz AK et al (2011) Effect of in utero and lactational nicotine exposure on the male reproductive tract in peripubertal and adult rats. Reprod Toxicol. 31(4):418–423. https://doi.org/10.1016/j.reprotox.2010.12.004

Lankas GR, Wise LD, Cartwright ME, Pippert T, Umbenhauer DR (1998) Placental P-glycoprotein deficiency enhances susceptibility to chemically induced birth defects in mice. Reprod Toxicol. 12(4):457–463. https://doi.org/10.1016/s0890-6238(98)00027-6

Lassen TH, Madsen M, Skovgaard LT, Strandberg-Larsen K, Olsen J, Andersen AM (2010) Maternal use of nicotine replacement therapy during pregnancy and offspring birthweight: a study within the Danish National Birth Cohort. Paediatr Perinat Epidemiol. 24(3):272–281. https://doi.org/10.1111/j.1365-3016.2010.01104.x

Lauterstein DE, Tijerina PB, Corbett K, Akgol Oksuz B, Shen SS, Gordon T et al (2016) Frontal cortex transcriptome analysis of mice exposed to electronic cigarettes during early life stages. Int J Environ Res Public Health. 13(4):417. https://doi.org/10.3390/ijerph13040417

Lawrence J, Xiao D, Xue Q, Rejali M, Yang S, Zhang L (2008) Prenatal nicotine exposure increases heart susceptibility to ischemia/reperfusion injury in adult offspring. J Pharmacol Exp Ther. 324(1):331–341. https://doi.org/10.1124/jpet.107.132175

Le HH, Shorey-Kendrick LE, Hinds MT, McCarty OJT, Lo JO, Anderson DEJ (2024) Effects of in utero exposure to Δ-9-tetrahydrocannabinol on cardiac extracellular matrix expression and vascular transcriptome in rhesus macaques. Am J Physiol-Heart Circ Physiol. 327(3):H701–HH14. https://doi.org/10.1152/ajpheart.00181.2024

Lee HJ, Choi NY, Park YS, Lee SW, Bang JS, Lee Y et al (2018) Multigenerational effects of maternal cigarette smoke exposure during pregnancy on sperm counts of F1 and F2 male offspring. Reprod Toxicol. 78:169–177. https://doi.org/10.1016/j.reprotox.2018.04.011

Lee K, Laviolette SR, Hardy DB (2021) Exposure to Δ9-tetrahydrocannabinol during rat pregnancy leads to impaired cardiac dysfunction in postnatal life. Pediatr Res. 90(3):532–539. https://doi.org/10.1038/s41390-021-01511-9

Lei F, Wang W, Fu Y, Wang J, Zheng Y (2018) Oxidative stress and mitochondrial dysfunction in parafacial respiratory group induced by maternal cigarette smoke exposure in rat offspring. Free Radic Biol Med. 129:169–176. https://doi.org/10.1016/j.freeradbiomed.2018.09.003

Lei F, Wang W, Fu Y, Wang J, Zheng Y (2021) Oxidative stress in retrotrapezoid nucleus/parafacial respiratory group and impairment of central chemoreception in rat offspring exposed to maternal cigarette smoke. Reprod Toxicol. 100:35–41. https://doi.org/10.1016/j.reprotox.2020.12.017

Lei A, Breit KR, Thomas JD (2023) Prenatal alcohol and tetrahydrocannabinol exposure: effects on spatial and working memory. Front Neurosci 17. https://doi.org/10.3389/fnins.2023.1192786

Li YF, Langholz B, Salam MT, Gilliland FD (2005) Maternal and grandmaternal smoking patterns are associated with early childhood asthma. Chest. 127(4):1232–1241. https://doi.org/10.1378/chest.127.4.1232

Li Z, Liu J, Ye R, Zhang L, Zheng X, Ren A (2010) Maternal passive smoking and risk of cleft lip with or without cleft palate. Epidemiology. 21(2):240–242. https://doi.org/10.1097/EDE.0b013e3181c9f941

Li Y, Xiao D, Dasgupta C, Xiong F, Tong W, Yang S et al (2012) Perinatal nicotine exposure increases vulnerability of hypoxic-ischemic brain injury in neonatal rats: role of angiotensin II receptors. Stroke. 43(9): 2483–2490. https://doi.org/10.1161/STROKEAHA.112.664698

Li Y, Xiao D, Yang S, Zhang L (2013) Promoter methylation represses AT2R gene and increases brain hypoxic-ischemic injury in neonatal rats. Neurobiol Dis. 60:32–38. https://doi.org/10.1016/j.nbd.2013.08.011

Li G, Saad S, Oliver BG, Chen H (2018) Heat or burn? Impacts of intrauterine tobacco smoke and e-cigarette vapor exposure on the offspring's health outcome. Toxics. 6(3). https://doi.org/10.3390/toxics6030043

Li G, Chan YL, Nguyen LT, Mak C, Zaky A, Anwer AG et al (2019) Impact of maternal e-cigarette vapor exposure on renal health in the offspring. Ann N Y Acad Sci. 1452(1):65–77. https://doi.org/10.1111/nyas.14174

Li Y, Dewar A, Kim YS, Dey SK, Sun X (2020) Pregnancy success in mice requires appropriate cannabinoid receptor signaling for primary decidua formation. Elife. 9. https://doi.org/10.7554/eLife.61762

Lichtensteiger W, Schlumpf M (1985) Prenatal nicotine affects fetal testosterone and sexual dimorphism of saccharin preference. Pharmacol Biochem Behav. 23(3):439–444. https://doi.org/10.1016/0091-3057(85)90018-8

Lin C, Yon JM, Hong JT, Lee JK, Jeong J, Baek IJ et al (2014) 4-O-methylhonokiol inhibits serious embryo anomalies caused by nicotine via modulations of oxidative stress, apoptosis, and inflammation. Birth Defects Res B Dev Reprod Toxicol. 101(2):125–134. https://doi.org/10.1002/bdrb.21092

Liu J, Naeem E, Tian J, Lombardi V, Kwong K, Akbari O et al (2013) Sex-specific perinatal nicotine-induced asthma in rat offspring. Am J Respir Cell Mol Biol. 48(1):53–62. https://doi.org/10.1165/rcmb.2011-0344OC

Lo JO, Schabel MC, Roberts VH, Morgan TK, Rasanen JP, Kroenke CD et al (2015) Vitamin C supplementation ameliorates the adverse effects of nicotine on placental hemodynamics and histology in nonhuman primates. Am J Obstet Gynecol. 212(3):370e1–370e8. https://doi.org/10.1016/j.ajog.2014.12.042

Lo JO, Shaw B, Robalino S, Ayers CK, Durbin S, Rushkin MC et al (2024) Cannabis use in pregnancy and neonatal outcomes: a systematic review and meta-analysis. Cannabis Cannabinoid Res. 9(2):470–485. https://doi.org/10.1089/can.2022.0262

Luck W, Nau H, Hansen R, Steldinger R (1985) Extent of nicotine and cotinine transfer to the human fetus, placenta and amniotic fluid of smoking mothers. Dev Pharmacol Ther. 8(6):384–395. https://doi.org/10.1159/000457063

Luján MÁ, Young-Morrison R, Aroni S, Katona I, Melis M, Cheer JF (2024) Dynamic overrepresentation of accumbal cues in food- and opioid-seeking rats after prenatal THC exposure. Sci Adv 10(45):eadq5652. https://doi.org/10.1126/sciadv.adq5652

Ma N, Nicholson CJ, Wong M, Holloway AC, Hardy DB (2014) Fetal and neonatal exposure to nicotine leads to augmented hepatic and circulating triglycerides in adult male offspring due to increased expression of fatty acid synthase. Toxicol Appl Pharmacol. 275(1): 1–11. https://doi.org/10.1016/j.taap.2013.12.010

Mallock N, Schulz T, Malke S, Dreiack N, Laux P, Luch A (2024) Levels of nicotine and tobacco-specific nitrosamines in oral nicotine pouches. Tob Control. 33(2):193–199. https://doi.org/10.1136/tc-2022-057280

Mannekote Thippaiah S, Iyengar SS, Vinod KY (2021) Exo-and endo-cannabinoids in depressive and suicidal behaviors. Front Psychiatry 12:636228

Mao C, Wu J, Xiao D, Lv J, Ding Y, Xu Z et al (2009) The effect of fetal and neonatal nicotine exposure on renal development of AT(1) and AT(2) receptors. Reprod Toxicol. 27(2):149–154. https://doi.org/10.1016/j.reprotox.2009.01.012

Marchand G, Masoud AT, Govindan M, Ware K, King A, Ruther S et al (2022) Birth outcomes of neonates exposed to marijuana in utero: a systematic review and meta-analysis. JAMA Netw Open. 5(1): e2145653. https://doi.org/10.1001/jamanetworkopen.2021.45653

Margham J, McAdam K, Forster M, Liu C, Wright C, Mariner D et al (2016) Chemical composition of aerosol from an e-cigarette: a quantitative comparison with cigarette smoke. Chem Res Toxicol. 29(10): 1662–1678. https://doi.org/10.1021/acs.chemrestox.6b00188

Maritz GS, Harding R (2011) Life-long programming implications of exposure to tobacco smoking and nicotine before and soon after birth: evidence for altered lung development. Int J Environ Res Public Health. 8(3):875–898. https://doi.org/10.3390/ijerph8030875

Martin JA, Osterman MJK, Driscoll AK (2023) Declines in cigarette smoking during pregnancy in the United States, 2016–2021. NCHS

Martinez S, Garcia-Meric P, Millet V, Aymeric-Ponsonnet M, Alagha K, Dubus JC (2015) Tobacco smoke in infants with bronchopulmonary dysplasia. Eur J Pediatr. 174(7):943–948. https://doi.org/10.1007/s00431-015-2491-y

Martínez-Peña AA, Lee K, Petrik JJ, Hardy DB, Holloway AC (2021) Gestational exposure to Δ(9)-THC impacts ovarian follicular dynamics and angiogenesis in adulthood in Wistar rats. J Dev Orig Health Dis. 12(6): 865–869. https://doi.org/10.1017/s2040174420001282

Martínez-Peña AA, Lee K, Pereira M, Ayyash A, Petrik JJ, Hardy DB et al (2022) Prenatal exposure to Delta-9-tetrahydrocannabinol (THC) alters the expression of miR-122-5p and its target Igf1r in the adult rat ovary. Int J Mol Sci 23(14):8000

Marzouk H, Awaad A, Abo-Eleneen R, El-Bakry A (2022) Effects of experimentally induced nicotine on the liver of neonatal albino rat. Adv Anim Vet Sci. 10(1): 151–159

Matta SG, Balfour DJ, Benowitz NL, Boyd RT, Buccafusco JJ, Caggiula AR et al (2007) Guidelines on nicotine dose selection for in vivo research. Psychopharmacology (Berl). 190(3):269–319. https://doi.org/10.1007/s00213-006-0441-0

McEvoy CT, Spindel ER (2017) Pulmonary effects of maternal smoking on the fetus and child: effects on lung development, respiratory morbidities, and life long lung health. Paediatr Respir Rev. 21:27–33. https://doi.org/10.1016/j.prrv.2016.08.005

McEvoy CT, Shorey-Kendrick LE, Milner K, Harris J, Vuylsteke B, Cunningham M et al (2023) Effect of vitamin C supplementation for pregnant smokers on offspring airway function and wheeze at age 5 years: follow-up of a randomized clinical trial. JAMA Pediatr. 177(1):16–24. https://doi.org/10.1001/jamapediatrics.2022.4401

Methaneethorn J, Naosang K, Kaewworasut P, Poomsaidorn C, Lohitnavy M (2020) Development of a physiologically-based pharmacokinetic model of Δ9-Tetrahydrocannabinol in mice, rats, and pigs. Eur J Drug Metab Pharmacokinet. 45(4):487–494. https://doi.org/10.1007/s13318-020-00616-6

Metz TD, Stickrath EH (2015) Marijuana use in pregnancy and lactation: a review of the evidence. Am J Obstet Gynecol 213(6):761–778

Mills A, Dakhlallah D, Ranpara A, Goldsmith WT, Chantler PD, Huang YW et al (2025) Pregnancy and postpartum effects of electronic cigarettes on maternal health and vascular function in the fourth trimester. Cardiovasc Toxicol. https://doi.org/10.1007/s12012-025-09961-x

Moellmer SA, Hagen OL, Farhang PA, Duke VR, Fallon ME, Hinds MT et al (2024) Effects of in utero delta-9-tetrahydrocannabinol (THC) exposure on fetal and infant musculoskeletal development in a preclinical nonhuman primate model. PLoS One. 19(7):e0306868. https://doi.org/10.1371/journal.pone.0306868

Mohsenzadeh Y, Rahmani A, Cheraghi J, Pyrani M, Asadollahi K (2014) Prenatal exposure to nicotine in pregnant rat increased inflammatory marker in newborn rat. Mediators Inflamm. 2014:274048. https://doi.org/10.1155/2014/274048

Monfort A, Ferreira E, Leclair G, Lodygensky GA (2022) Pharmacokinetics of cannabis and its derivatives in animals and humans during pregnancy and breastfeeding. Front Pharmacol 13. https://doi.org/10.3389/fphar.2022.919630

Moore CF, Stiltner JW, Davis CM, Weerts EM (2022) Translational models of cannabinoid vapor exposure in laboratory animals. Behav Pharmacol. 33(2&3):63–89. https://doi.org/10.1097/fbp.0000000000000592

Mora-Zamorano FX, Svoboda KR, Carvan MJ 3rd (2016) The nicotine-evoked locomotor response: a behavioral paradigm for toxicity screening in zebrafish (Danio rerio) embryos and eleutheroembryos exposed to methylmercury. PLoS One. 11(4):e0154570. https://doi.org/10.1371/journal.pone.0154570

Morrow LA, Wagner BD, Ingram DA, Poindexter BB, Schibler K, Cotten CM et al (2017) Antenatal determinants of bronchopulmonary dysplasia and late respiratory disease in preterm infants. Am J Respir Crit Care Med. 196(3):364–374. https://doi.org/10.1164/rccm.201612-2414OC

Mosier HD Jr, Jansons RA (1972) Distribution and fate of nicotine in the rat fetus. Teratology. 6(3):303–311. https://doi.org/10.1002/tera.1420060308

Murru E, Carta G, Manca C, Verce M, Everard A, Serra V et al (2024) Impact of prenatal THC exposure on lipid metabolism and microbiota composition in rat offspring. Heliyon. 10(15). https://doi.org/10.1016/j.heliyon.2024.e35637

Musanejad E, Haghpanah T, Mirzaie V, Ezzatabadipour M (2021) Effects of ethanol and nicotine co-administration on follicular atresia and placental histo-morphology in the first-generation mice pups during intrauterine development and lactation periods. Toxicol Rep. 8:793–803. https://doi.org/10.1016/j.toxrep.2021.03.033

Natale BV, Gustin KN, Lee K, Holloway AC, Laviolette SR, Natale DRC et al (2020) Δ9-tetrahydrocannabinol exposure during rat pregnancy leads to symmetrical fetal growth restriction and labyrinth-specific vascular defects in the placenta. Sci Rep 10(1):544. https://doi.org/10.1038/s41598-019-57318-6

National Academies of Sciences, Engineering, and Medicine, Health and Medicine Division, Board on Population Health and Public Health Practice et al (2017) The health effects of cannabis and cannabinoids: the current state of evidence and recommendations for research. National Academies Press

Navarro D, Gasparyan A, Navarrete F, Manzanares J (2024) Fetal cannabinoid syndrome: behavioral and brain alterations of the offspring exposed to dronabinol during gestation and lactation. Int J Mol Sci 25(13):7453

Nemeth O, Sipos L, Matrai P, Szathmari-Meszaros N, Ivanyi D, Simon F et al (2024) Snus use in adolescents: a threat to oral health. J Clin Med. 13(14). https://doi.org/10.3390/jcm13144235

Neuman A, Hohmann C, Orsini N, Pershagen G, Eller E, Kjaer HF et al (2012) Maternal smoking in pregnancy and asthma in preschool children: a pooled analysis of eight birth cohorts. Am J Respir Crit Care Med. 186(10):1037–1043. https://doi.org/10.1164/rccm.201203-0501OC

NIDA (2024) Cannabis (Marijuana)

Noel A, Yilmaz S, Farrow T, Schexnayder M, Eickelberg O, Jelesijevic T (2023) Sex-specific alterations of the lung transcriptome at birth in mouse offspring prenatally exposed to vanilla-flavored e-cigarette aerosols and enhanced susceptibility to asthma. Int J Environ Res Public Health. 20(4). https://doi.org/10.3390/ijerph20043710

O'Connor RJ (2012) Non-cigarette tobacco products: what have we learnt and where are we headed? Tob Control. 21(2):181–190. https://doi.org/10.1136/tobaccocontrol-2011-050281

Oke SL, Lee K, Papp R, Laviolette SR, Hardy DB (2021) In utero exposure to Δ9-Tetrahydrocannabinol leads to postnatal catch-up growth and dysmetabolism in the adult rat liver. Int J Mol Sci 22(14):7502

Oliveira E, Moura EG, Santos-Silva AP, Fagundes AT, Rios AS, Abreu-Villaca Y et al (2009) Short- and long-term effects of maternal nicotine exposure during lactation on body adiposity, lipid profile, and thyroid function of rat offspring. J Endocrinol. 202(3): 397–405. https://doi.org/10.1677/JOE-09-0020

Oliveira E, Moura EG, Santos-Silva AP, Pinheiro CR, Lima NS, Nogueira-Neto JF et al (2010) Neonatal nicotine exposure causes insulin and leptin resistance and inhibits hypothalamic leptin signaling in adult rat offspring. J Endocrinol. 206(1):55–63. https://doi.org/10.1677/JOE-10-0104

Olyaei AF, Campbell LR, Roberts VHJ, Lo JO (2022) Animal models evaluating the impact of prenatal exposure to tobacco and marijuana. Clin Obstet Gynecol. 65(2):334–346. https://doi.org/10.1097/grf.0000000000000693

Orellana JA, Busso D, Ramirez G, Campos M, Rigotti A, Eugenin J et al (2014) Prenatal nicotine exposure enhances Cx43 and Panx1 unopposed channel activity in brain cells of adult offspring mice fed a high-fat/cholesterol diet. Front Cell Neurosci. 8:403. https://doi.org/10.3389/fncel.2014.00403

Orzabal MR, Lunde-Young ER, Ramirez JI, Howe SYF, Naik VD, Lee J et al (2019) Chronic exposure to e-cig aerosols during early development causes vascular dysfunction and offspring growth deficits. Transl Res. 207:70–82. https://doi.org/10.1016/j.trsl.2019.01.001

Ozturk F, Sheldon E, Sharma J, Canturk KM, Otu HH, Nawshad A (2016) Nicotine exposure during pregnancy results in persistent midline epithelial seam with improper palatal fusion. Nicotine Tob Res. 18(5):604–612. https://doi.org/10.1093/ntr/ntv227

Pabarja A, Ganjalikhan Hakemi S, Musanejad E, Ezzatabadipour M, Nematollahi-Mahani SN, Afgar A et al (2021) Genetic and epigenetic modifications of F1 offspring's sperm cells following in utero and lactational combined exposure to nicotine and ethanol. Sci Rep. 11(1):12311. https://doi.org/10.1038/s41598-021-91739-6

Paccola CC, Neves FM, Cipriano I, Stumpp T, Miraglia SM (2014) Effects of prenatal and lactation nicotine exposure on rat testicular interstitial tissue. Andrology. 2(2):175–185. https://doi.org/10.1111/j.2047-2927.2013.00168.x

Palpant NJ, Hofsteen P, Pabon L, Reinecke H, Murry CE (2015) Cardiac development in zebrafish and human embryonic stem cells is inhibited by exposure to tobacco cigarettes and e-cigarettes. PLoS One. 10(5): e0126259. https://doi.org/10.1371/journal.pone.0126259

Park B, Gibbons HM, Mitchell MD, Glassa M (2003) Identification of the CB1 cannabinoid receptor and fatty acid amide hydrolase (FAAH) in the human placenta. Placenta. 24(5):473–478. https://doi.org/10.1053/plac.2002.0926

Paulson RB, Shanfeld J, Vorhees CV, Cole J, Sweazy A, Paulson JO (1994) Behavioral effects of smokeless tobacco on the neonate and young Sprague Dawley rat. Teratology. 49(4):293–305. https://doi.org/10.1002/tera.1420490409

Peng H, Li H, Wei Y, Zhang R, Chang X, Meng L et al (2023) Effects of prenatal exposure to THC on hippocampal neural development in offspring. Toxicol Lett 374:48–56. https://doi.org/10.1016/j.toxlet.2022.12.007

Perlin E, Smith CG, Nichols AI, Almirez R, Flora KP, Cradock J et al (1985) Disposition and bioavailability of various formulations of tetrahydrocannabinol in the rhesus monkey. J Pharm Sci 74(2):171–174

Persaud TV, Ellington AC (1967) Cannabis in early pregnancy. Lancet. 2(7529):1306. https://doi.org/10.1016/s0140-6736(67)90416-3

Persaud TV, Ellington AC (1968) Teratogenic activity of cannabis resin. Lancet. 2(7564):406–407. https://doi.org/10.1016/s0140-6736(68)90626-0

Peterson CS, Baglot SL, Sallam NA, Mina S, Hill MN, Borgland SL (2024) Oral pre- and early postnatal cannabis exposure disinhibits ventral tegmental area dopamine neuron activity but does not influence cocaine preference in offspring in mice. J Neurosci Res. 102(7):e25369. https://doi.org/10.1002/jnr.25369

Petrik JJ, Gerstein HC, Cesta CE, Kellenberger LD, Alfaidy N, Holloway AC (2009) Effects of rosiglitazone on ovarian function and fertility in animals with reduced fertility following fetal and neonatal exposure to nicotine. Endocrine. 36(2):281–290. https://doi.org/10.1007/s12020-009-9229-4

Polli FS, Scharff MB, Ipsen TH, Aznar S, Kohlmeier KA, Andreasen JT (2020) Prenatal nicotine exposure in mice induces sex-dependent anxiety-like behavior, cognitive deficits, hyperactivity, and changes in the expression of glutamate receptor associated-genes in the prefrontal cortex. Pharmacol Biochem Behav. 195: 172951. https://doi.org/10.1016/j.pbb.2020.172951

Proskocil BJ, Sekhon HS, Clark JA, Lupo SL, Jia Y, Hull WM et al (2005) Vitamin C prevents the effects of prenatal nicotine on pulmonary function in newborn monkeys. Am J Respir Crit Care Med. 171(9): 1032–1039. https://doi.org/10.1164/rccm.200408-1029OC

Raez-Villanueva S, Debnath A, Hardy DB, Holloway AC (2022) Prenatal nicotine exposure leads to decreased histone H3 lysine 9 (H3K9) methylation and increased p66shc expression in the neonatal pancreas. J Dev Orig Health Dis. 13(2):156–160. https://doi.org/10.1017/S2040174421000283

Rajikin MH, Latif ES, Mar MR, Mat Top AG, Mokhtar NM (2009) Deleterious effects of nicotine on the ultrastructure of oocytes: role of gamma-tocotrienol. Med Sci Monit. 15(12):BR378–83

Rehan VK, Liu J, Naeem E, Tian J, Sakurai R, Kwong K et al (2012) Perinatal nicotine exposure induces asthma in second generation offspring. BMC Med. 10:129. https://doi.org/10.1186/1741-7015-10-129

Rehan VK, Liu J, Sakurai R, Torday JS (2013) Perinatal nicotine-induced transgenerational asthma. Am J

Physiol Lung Cell Mol Physiol. 305(7):L501–L507. https://doi.org/10.1152/ajplung.00078.2013

Roberts RM, Green JA, Schulz LC (2016) The evolution of the placenta. Reproduction. 152(5):R179–R189. https://doi.org/10.1530/rep-16-0325

Roberts VHJ, Schabel MC, Boniface ER, D'Mello RJ, Morgan TK, Terrobias JJD et al (2022) Chronic prenatal delta-9-tetrahydrocannabinol exposure adversely impacts placental function and development in a rhesus macaque model. Sci Rep 12(1):20260. https://doi.org/10.1038/s41598-022-24401-4

Robinson GI, Ye F, Lu X, Laviolette SR, Feng Q (2024) Maternal Delta-9-Tetrahydrocannabinol exposure induces abnormalities of the developing heart in mice. Cannabis Cannabinoid Res. 9(1):121–133. https://doi.org/10.1089/can.2022.0180

Roeder NM, Penman SL, Richardson BJ, Wang J, Freeman-Striegel L, Khan A et al (2024) Vaporized Δ9-THC in utero results in reduced birthweight, increased locomotion, and altered wake-cycle activity dependent on dose, sex, and diet in the offspring. Life Sci 340:122447. https://doi.org/10.1016/j.lfs.2024.122447

Rouzer SK, Sreeram A, Miranda RC (2024) Reduced fetal cerebral blood flow predicts perinatal mortality in a mouse model of prenatal alcohol and cannabinoid exposure. BMC Pregnancy Childbirth. 24(1):263. https://doi.org/10.1186/s12884-024-06436-9

Roy TS, Seidler FJ, Slotkin TA (2002) Prenatal nicotine exposure evokes alterations of cell structure in hippocampus and somatosensory cortex. J Pharmacol Exp Ther. 300(1):124–133. https://doi.org/10.1124/jpet.300.1.124

Ryan KS, Mahalingaiah S, Campbell LR, Roberts VHJ, Terrobias JJD, Naito CS et al (2021) The effects of delta-9-tetrahydrocannabinol exposure on female menstrual cyclicity and reproductive health in rhesus macaques. F&S Sci 2(3):287–294. https://doi.org/10.1016/j.xfss.2021.05.001

Ryan KS, Karpf JA, Chan CN, Hagen OL, McFarland TJ, Urian JW et al (2024) Prenatal delta-9-tetrahydrocannabinol exposure alters fetal neurodevelopment in rhesus macaques. Sci Rep. 14(1):5808. https://doi.org/10.1038/s41598-024-56386-7

Saad S, Al-Odat I, Chan YL, McGrath KC, Pollock CA, Oliver BG et al (2018) Maternal L-carnitine supplementation improves glucose and lipid profiles in female offspring of dams exposed to cigarette smoke. Clin Exp Pharmacol Physiol. 45(7):694–703. https://doi.org/10.1111/1440-1681.12921

Sabbagh HJ, Hassan MH, Innes NP, Elkodary HM, Little J, Mossey PA (2015) Passive smoking in the etiology of non-syndromic orofacial clefts: a systematic review and meta-analysis. PLoS One. 10(3): e0116963. https://doi.org/10.1371/journal.pone.0116963

SAMHSA (2023) National survey on drug use and health

Sandini TM, Onofrychuk TJ, Roebuck AJ, Hammond SA, Udenze D, Hayat S et al (2023) Repeated exposure to High-THC cannabis smoke during gestation alters sex ratio, behavior, and amygdala gene expression of sprague dawley rat offspring. eNeuro. 10(11). https://doi.org/10.1523/eneuro.0100-23.2023

Sarikahya MH, Cousineau S, De Felice M, Lee K, KKW W, MV DV et al (2022) Prenatal THC exposure induces sex-dependent neuropsychiatric endophenotypes in offspring and long-term disruptions in fatty-acid signaling pathways directly in the mesolimbic circuitry. eneuro. 9(5): ENEURO.0253–22.2022. https://doi.org/10.1523/ENEURO.0253-22.2022

Sarikahya MH, Cousineau SL, De Felice M, Szkudlarek HJ, Wong KKW, DeVuono MV et al (2023) Prenatal THC exposure induces long-term, sex-dependent cognitive dysfunction associated with lipidomic and neuronal pathology in the prefrontal cortex-hippocampal network. Mol Psychiatry 28(10):4234–4250. https://doi.org/10.1038/s41380-023-02190-0

Scheline R (1978) Mammalian metabolism of plant xenobiotics. Academix, London/New York

Seaton MJ, Vesell ES (1993) Variables affecting nicotine metabolism. Pharmacol Ther. 60(3):461–500. https://doi.org/10.1016/0163-7258(93)90032-9

Sekhon HS, Jia Y, Raab R, Kuryatov A, Pankow JF, Whitsett JA et al (1999) Prenatal nicotine increases pulmonary α7 nicotinic receptor expression and alters fetal lung development in monkeys. J Clin Invest 103(5):637–647

Sekhon HS, Keller JA, Benowitz NL, Spindel ER (2001) Prenatal nicotine exposure alters pulmonary function in newborn rhesus monkeys. Am J Respir Crit Care Med. 164(6):989–994. https://doi.org/10.1164/ajrccm.164.6.2011097

Shea AK, Steiner M (2008) Cigarette smoking during pregnancy. Nicotine Tob Res. 10(2):267–278. https://doi.org/10.1080/14622200701825908

Shorey-Kendrick LE, McEvoy CT, O'Sullivan SM, Milner K, Vuylsteke B, Tepper RS et al (2021) Impact of vitamin C supplementation on placental DNA methylation changes related to maternal smoking: association with gene expression and respiratory outcomes. Clin Epigenetics. 13(1):177. https://doi.org/10.1186/s13148-021-01161-y

Shorey-Kendrick LE, Roberts VHJ, D'Mello RJ, Sullivan EL, Murphy SK, McCarty OJT et al (2023a) Prenatal delta-9-tetrahydrocannabinol exposure is associated with changes in rhesus macaque DNA methylation enriched for autism genes. Clin Epigenetics 15(1): 104. https://doi.org/10.1186/s13148-023-01519-4

Shorey-Kendrick L, Roberts VH, Sullivan E, Terrobias JJ, Spindel E, Lo J (2023b) Prenatal THC exposure alters placental and offspring DNA methylation in rhesus macaques. Am J Obstet Gynecol 228(1):S59. https://doi.org/10.1016/j.ajog.2022.11.079

Shorey-Kendrick LE, Crosland BA, Schabel MC, Messaoudi I, Guo M, Drake MG et al (2025) Effects of maternal edible THC consumption on offspring lung growth and function in a rhesus macaque model. Am J

Physiol Lung Cell Mol Physiol. 328(3):L463–Ll77. https://doi.org/10.1152/ajplung.00360.2024

Siddiqui AR, Gold EB, Yang X, Lee K, Brown KH, Bhutta ZA (2008) Prenatal exposure to wood fuel smoke and low birth weight. Environ Health Perspect. 116(4):543–549. https://doi.org/10.1289/ehp.10782

Sikic A, Frie JA, Khokhar JY, Murray JE (2022) Sex differences in the behavioural outcomes of prenatal nicotine and tobacco exposure. Front Neurosci. 16: 921429. https://doi.org/10.3389/fnins.2022.921429

Singh SP, Mishra NC, Rir-Sima-Ah J, Campen M, Kurup V, Razani-Boroujerdi S et al (2009) Maternal exposure to secondhand cigarette smoke primes the lung for induction of phosphodiesterase-4D5 isozyme and exacerbated Th2 responses: rolipram attenuates the airway hyperreactivity and muscarinic receptor expression but not lung inflammation and atopy. J Immunol. 183(3):2115–2121. https://doi.org/10.4049/jimmunol.0900826

Singh SP, Gundavarapu S, Smith KR, Chand HS, Saeed AI, Mishra NC et al (2013) Gestational exposure of mice to secondhand cigarette smoke causes bronchopulmonary dysplasia blocked by the nicotinic receptor antagonist mecamylamine. Environ Health Perspect. 121(8):957–964. https://doi.org/10.1289/ehp.1306611

Singh SP, Chand HS, Gundavarapu S, Saeed AI, Langley RJ, Tesfaigzi Y et al (2015) HIF-1alpha plays a critical role in the gestational sidestream smoke-induced bronchopulmonary dysplasia in mice. PLoS One. 10(9):e0137757. https://doi.org/10.1371/journal.pone.0137757

Singh SP, Chand HS, Langley RJ, Mishra N, Barrett T, Rudolph K et al (2017) Gestational exposure to sidestream (secondhand) cigarette smoke promotes transgenerational epigenetic transmission of exacerbated allergic asthma and bronchopulmonary dysplasia. J Immunol. 198(10):3815–3822. https://doi.org/10.4049/jimmunol.1700014

Slotkin TA, Seidler FJ, Qiao D, Aldridge JE, Tate CA, Cousins MM et al (2005) Effects of prenatal nicotine exposure on primate brain development and attempted amelioration with supplemental choline or vitamin C: neurotransmitter receptors, cell signaling and cell development biomarkers in fetal brain regions of rhesus monkeys. Neuropsychopharmacology. 30(1): 129–144. https://doi.org/10.1038/sj.npp.1300544

Slotkin TA, Tate CA, Cousins MM, Seidler FJ (2006) Prenatal nicotine exposure alters the responses to subsequent nicotine administration and withdrawal in adolescence: serotonin receptors and cell signaling. Neuropsychopharmacology. 31(11):2462–2475. https://doi.org/10.1038/sj.npp.1300988

Slotkin TA, Card J, Stadler A, Levin ED, Seidler FJ (2014) Effects of tobacco smoke on PC12 cell neurodifferentiation are distinct from those of nicotine or benzo[a]pyrene. Neurotoxicol Teratol. 43:19–24. https://doi.org/10.1016/j.ntt.2014.03.002

Slotkin TA, Skavicus S, Card J, Stadler A, Levin ED, Seidler FJ (2015) Developmental neurotoxicity of tobacco smoke directed toward cholinergic and serotonergic systems: more than just nicotine. Toxicol Sci. 147(1):178–189. https://doi.org/10.1093/toxsci/kfv123

Smith D, Aherrera A, Lopez A, Neptune E, Winickoff JP, Klein JD et al (2015) Adult behavior in male mice exposed to e-cigarette nicotine vapors during late prenatal and early postnatal life. PLoS One. 10(9): e0137953. https://doi.org/10.1371/journal.pone.0137953

Sobrian SK, Holson RR (2011) Effects of pre- and neonatal nicotine exposure in rodents: inconsistent evidence. ILAR J. 52(3):251–294. https://doi.org/10.1093/ilar.52.3.251

Sobrian SK, Marr L, Ressman K (2003) Prenatal cocaine and/or nicotine exposure produces depression and anxiety in aging rats. Prog Neuropsychopharmacol Biol Psychiatry. 27(3):501–518. https://doi.org/10.1016/S0278-5846(03)00042-3

Sofuoglu M, LeSage MG (2012) The reinforcement threshold for nicotine as a target for tobacco control. Drug Alcohol Depend. 125(1–2):1–7. https://doi.org/10.1016/j.drugalcdep.2012.04.023

Somm E, Schwitzgebel VM, Vauthay DM, Camm EJ, Chen CY, Giacobino JP et al (2008) Prenatal nicotine exposure alters early pancreatic islet and adipose tissue development with consequences on the control of body weight and glucose metabolism later in life. Endocrinology. 149(12):6289–6299. https://doi.org/10.1210/en.2008-0361

Somm E, Schwitzgebel VM, Vauthay DM, Aubert ML, Huppi PS (2009) Prenatal nicotine exposure and the programming of metabolic and cardiovascular disorders. Mol Cell Endocrinol. 304(1–2):69–77. https://doi.org/10.1016/j.mce.2009.02.026

Stangenberg S, Nguyen LT, Chan YL, Zaky A, Pollock CA, Chen H et al (2019) Maternal L-carnitine supplementation ameliorates renal underdevelopment and epigenetic changes in male mice offspring due to maternal smoking. Clin Exp Pharmacol Physiol. 46(2):183–193. https://doi.org/10.1111/1440-1681.13038

Sun M, Kingdom J, Baczyk D, Lye SJ, Matthews SG, Gibb W (2006) Expression of the multidrug resistance P-glycoprotein, (ABCB1 glycoprotein) in the human placenta decreases with advancing gestation. Placenta. 27(6–7):602–609. https://doi.org/10.1016/j.placenta.2005.05.007

Sun X, Xie H, Yang J, Wang H, Bradshaw HB, Dey SK (2010) Endocannabinoid signaling directs differentiation of trophoblast cell lineages and placentation. Proc Natl Acad Sci U S A. 107(39):16887–16892. https://doi.org/10.1073/pnas.1010892107

Suter M, Ma J, Harris A, Patterson L, Brown KA, Shope C et al (2011) Maternal tobacco use modestly alters correlated epigenome-wide placental DNA methylation and gene expression. Epigenetics. 6(11): 1284–1294. https://doi.org/10.4161/epi.6.11.17819

Svoboda KR, Vijayaraghavan S, Tanguay RL (2002) Nicotinic receptors mediate changes in spinal motoneuron development and axonal pathfinding in embryonic zebrafish exposed to nicotine. J Neurosci. 22(24): 10731–10741. https://doi.org/10.1523/JNEUROSCI.22-24-10731.2002

Swislocki AL (2003) Smokeless nicotine administration does not result in hypertension or a deterioration in glucose tolerance or insulin sensitivity in juvenile rats. Metabolism. 52(1):67–72. https://doi.org/10.1053/meta.2003.50006

Swislocki AL, Fakiri Z (2008) Smokeless nicotine exposure has no lasting effect on fasting or postglucose circulation leptin in young rats. Metab Syndr Relat Disord. 6(4):257–262. https://doi.org/10.1089/met.2008.0017

Swislocki AL, Tsuzuki A, Tait M, Khuu D, Fann K (1997) Smokeless nicotine administration is associated with hypertension but not with a deterioration in glucose tolerance in rats. Metabolism. 46(9):1008–1012. https://doi.org/10.1016/s0026-0495(97)90270-5

Talhout R, Schulz T, Florek E, van Benthem J, Wester P, Opperhuizen A (2011) Hazardous compounds in tobacco smoke. Int J Environ Res Public Health. 8(2): 613–628. https://doi.org/10.3390/ijerph8020613

Tarasi B, Cornuz J, Clair C, Baud D (2022) Cigarette smoking during pregnancy and adverse perinatal outcomes: a cross-sectional study over 10 years. BMC Public Health. 22(1):2403. https://doi.org/10.1186/s12889-022-14881-4

Thomas LT, Welsh L, Galvez F, Svoboda KR (2009) Acute nicotine exposure and modulation of a spinal motor circuit in embryonic zebrafish. Toxicol Appl Pharmacol. 239(1):1–12. https://doi.org/10.1016/j.taap.2008.08.023

Tong VT, Dietz PM, Morrow B, D'Angelo DV, Farr SL, Rockhill KM et al (2013) Trends in smoking before, during, and after pregnancy—pregnancy risk assessment monitoring system, United States, 40 sites, 2000–2010. MMWR Surveill Summ. 62(6):1–19

Torrens A, Vozella V, Huff H, McNeil B, Ahmed F, Ghidini A et al (2020) Comparative pharmacokinetics of Δ9-tetrahydrocannabinol in adolescent and adult male mice. J Pharmacol Exp Ther 374(1):151–160

Traccis F, Serra V, Sagheddu C, Congiu M, Saba P, Giua G et al (2021) Prenatal THC does not affect female mesolimbic dopaminergic system in preadolescent rats. Int J Mol Sci 22(4):1666

Tsai CY, Chou HC, Chen CM (2021) Perinatal nicotine exposure alters lung development and induces HMGB1-RAGE expression in neonatal mice. Birth Defects Res. 113(7):570–578. https://doi.org/10.1002/bdr2.1840

Tutka P, Mosiewicz J, Wielosz M (2005) Pharmacokinetics and metabolism of nicotine. Pharmacol Rep. 57(2): 143–153

Tutka P, Dempsey DA, Jacob P 3rd, Benowitz NL, Kroetz DL (2008) Nicotine metabolism in pregnant and non-pregnant rabbits. Nicotine Tob Res. 10(8):1385–1390. https://doi.org/10.1080/14622200802238878

Vaglenova J, Birru S, Pandiella NM, Breese CR (2004) An assessment of the long-term developmental and behavioral teratogenicity of prenatal nicotine exposure. Behav Brain Res. 150(1–2):159–170. https://doi.org/10.1016/j.bbr.2003.07.005

Vaglenova J, Parameshwaran K, Suppiramaniam V, Breese CR, Pandiella N, Birru S (2008) Long-lasting teratogenic effects of nicotine on cognition: gender specificity and role of AMPA receptor function. Neurobiol Learn Mem. 90(3):527–536. https://doi.org/10.1016/j.nlm.2008.06.009

van der Veen F, Fox H (1982) The effects of cigarette smoking on the human placenta: a light and electron microscopic study. Placenta. 3(3):243–256. https://doi.org/10.1016/s0143-4004(82)80002-7

Volkow ND, Han B, Compton WM, Blanco C (2017) Marijuana use during stages of pregnancy in the United States. Ann Intern Med. 166(10):763–764

Walayat A, Li Y, Zhang Y, Fu Y, Liu B, Shao XM et al (2021) Fetal e-cigarette exposure programs a neonatal brain hypoxic-ischemic sensitive phenotype via altering DNA methylation patterns and autophagy signaling pathway. Am J Physiol Regul Integr Comp Physiol. 321(5):R791–R801. https://doi.org/10.1152/ajpregu.00207.2021

Wang T, Chen M, Yan YE, Xiao FQ, Pan XL, Wang H (2009) Growth retardation of fetal rats exposed to nicotine in utero: possible involvement of CYP1A1, CYP2E1, and P-glycoprotein. Environ Toxicol. 24(1): 33–42. https://doi.org/10.1002/tox.20391

Ward RM, Varner MW (2019) Principles of pharmacokinetics in the pregnant woman and fetus. Clins Perinatol. 46(2):383–398

Weimar HV, Wright HR, Warrick CR, Brown AM, Lugo JM, Freels TG et al (2020) Long-term effects of maternal cannabis vapor exposure on emotional reactivity, social behavior, and behavioral flexibility in offspring. Neuropharmacology. 179:108288. https://doi.org/10.1016/j.neuropharm.2020.108288

Weinberg CR, Wilcox AJ, Baird DD (1989) Reduced fecundability in women with prenatal exposure to cigarette smoking. Am J Epidemiol. 129(5):1072–1078. https://doi.org/10.1093/oxfordjournals.aje.a115211

Wetendorf M, Randall LT, Lemma MT, Hurr SH, Pawlak JB, Tarran R et al (2019) E-cigarette exposure delays implantation and causes reduced weight gain in female offspring exposed in utero. J Endocr Soc. 3(10): 1907–1916. https://doi.org/10.1210/js.2019-00216

Whittington JR, Simmons PM, Phillips AM, Gammill SK, Cen R, Magann EF et al (2018) The use of electronic cigarettes in pregnancy: a review of the literature. Obstet Gynecol Surv. 73(9):544–549. https://doi.org/10.1097/OGX.0000000000000595

Wideroe M, Vik T, Jacobsen G, Bakketeig LS (2003) Does maternal smoking during pregnancy cause childhood overweight? Paediatr Perinat Epidemiol. 17(2): 171–179. https://doi.org/10.1046/j.1365-3016.2003.00481.x

Wieslander G, Norback D, Lindgren T (2001) Experimental exposure to propylene glycol mist in aviation emergency training: acute ocular and respiratory effects. Occup Environ Med. 58(10):649–655. https://doi.org/10.1136/oem.58.10.649

Wong MK, Barra NG, Alfaidy N, Hardy DB, Holloway AC (2015a) Adverse effects of perinatal nicotine exposure on reproductive outcomes. Reproduction. 150(6): R185–R193. https://doi.org/10.1530/REP-15-0295

Wong MK, Nicholson CJ, Holloway AC, Hardy DB (2015b) Maternal nicotine exposure leads to impaired disulfide bond formation and augmented endoplasmic reticulum stress in the rat placenta. PLoS One. 10(3): e0122295. https://doi.org/10.1371/journal.pone.0122295

Xepapadaki P, Manios Y, Liarigkovinos T, Grammatikaki E, Douladiris N, Kortsalioudaki C et al (2009) Association of passive exposure of pregnant women to environmental tobacco smoke with asthma symptoms in children. Pediatr Allergy Immunol. 20(5): 423–429. https://doi.org/10.1111/j.1399-3038.2008.00820.x

Xiao D, Huang X, Yang S, Zhang L (2011) Antenatal nicotine induces heightened oxidative stress and vascular dysfunction in rat offspring. Br J Pharmacol. 164(5):1400–1409. https://doi.org/10.1111/j.1476-5381.2011.01437.x

Young-Wolff KC, Ray GT, Alexeeff SE, Adams SR, Does MB, Ansley D et al (2021) Rates of prenatal Cannabis use among pregnant women before and during the COVID-19 pandemic. JAMA. 326(17):1745–1747. https://doi.org/10.1001/jama.2021.16328

Young-Wolff KC, Adams SR, Alexeeff SE, Zhu Y, Chojolan E, Slama NE et al (2024) Prenatal Cannabis use and maternal pregnancy outcomes. JAMA Intern Med 184(9):1083–1093. https://doi.org/10.1001/jamainternmed.2024.3270

Zhang L, Spencer TJ, Biederman J, Bhide PG (2018) Attention and working memory deficits in a perinatal nicotine exposure mouse model. PLoS One. 13(5): e0198064. https://doi.org/10.1371/journal.pone.0198064

Zhang Y, Angley M, Qi X, Lu L, D'Alton ME, Kahe K (2022) Maternal electronic cigarette exposure in relation to offspring development: a comprehensive review. Am J Obstet Gynecol MFM. 4(5):100659. https://doi.org/10.1016/j.ajogmf.2022.100659

Maternal Caffeine Consumption and Pregnancy Outcomes

10

Jack E. James

Abstract

Caffeine, a habit-forming substance of no nutritional value, is consumed daily by most pregnant women. This focused narrative review examines evidence of association between maternal caffeine consumption and negative pregnancy outcomes, and assesses whether current advice guidelines are consistent with the available evidence. The majority finding from original empirical studies, systematic reviews, and meta-analyses is that maternal consumption of caffeine is reliably associated with serious negative pregnancy outcomes and negative outcomes in offspring. Evidence of harm is strong for miscarriage, stillbirth, and low birth weight and/or small for gestational age, while being less strong for childhood acute leukemia, childhood overweight and obesity, and childhood behavioural and neurocognitive development. In contrast, preterm birth appears not to be at increased risk. Many studies report significant dose-response associations indicative of causation and the absence of a threshold of consumption below which associations are absent. In general, findings are robust to threats from potential confounding and misclassification. Notwithstanding compelling grounds to the contrary, national and international authorities continue to suggest that "moderate" caffeine consumption during pregnancy is safe. Rather, pregnant women and women contemplating pregnancy should be advised not to consume coffee, tea, sodas, or energy drinks that contain caffeine.

Keywords

Caffeine · Pregnancy outcomes · Miscarriage · Stillbirth · Low birth weight

10.1 Maternal Caffeine Consumption and Pregnancy Outcomes

Caffeine is the most widely consumed psychoactive substance in history, with more than 80% of people worldwide being regular consumers (Heckman et al. 2010; James 1997). Indeed, caffeine is unusual among psychoactive compounds in being a staple of the daily diet of most people, including pregnant women (Frary et al. 2005; Fulgoni III et al. 2015). Although average consumption varies between countries, studies have repeatedly confirmed that pregnant women mirror the consumption patterns of the wider population.

J. E. James (✉)
Reykjavík University, Reykjavík, Iceland
e-mail: jack@ru.is

A. N. Bukiya, D. W. Ali (eds.), *Molecular Mechanisms and Lifelong Consequences of Prenatal Exposure to Psychoactive Substances*, Advances in Experimental Medicine and Biology 1500,
https://doi.org/10.1007/978-3-032-12741-9_10

For example, 82% of pregnant women in the United States (Hoyt et al. 2014) and 91% in France (Galéra et al. 2016) reported being regular consumers of the drug. In addition to an extensive body of original empirical research, the relevant literature consists of a substantial number of systematic reviews and meta-analyses. By dealing with the topic primarily from the perspective of a narrative review, this chapter aims to conceptually integrate original research findings with the findings of previous reviews. Before examining the wide range of caffeine-related pregnancy outcomes that have attracted the attention of researchers, context is provided by first considering patterns of usage and key aspects of caffeine pharmacology.

10.1.1 Main Sources of Caffeine and Patterns of Consumption

Caffeine occurs naturally in several plant species, where it serves as a toxin to defend against predation by insects (Ashihara and Crozier 2001). Current human usage transcends almost every social barrier, including age, gender, geography, and culture (Gilbert 1984). No other psychoactive substance, including nicotine, alcohol, and all the illicit drugs past and present, exceeds caffeine for the extent of daily consumption. A common but erroneous belief, sometimes implied in advertisements for caffeine products, is that caffeine has always been widely present in the human diet. In fact, it was not until after European colonization in the seventeenth and eighteenth centuries that caffeine products, previously unavailable to most people, became widely accessible (James 1991). Thus, from an evolutionary perspective, the ubiquitous presence of caffeine in the human diet is a recent phenomenon.

The main dietary sources of caffeine are beverages, principally coffee, tea, sodas, and energy drinks (see Mayo Clinic 2025, for estimates of the average caffeine content of each). The tea plant is indigenous to regions of China, South Asia, and India (Harler 1964). Written accounts in China of tea leaves being used to brew a beverage date from about 350 CE, and by about 600 CE, tea had been introduced to Japan from China (Shalleck 1981). It is unclear, however, to what extent tea was consumed by the general population of either country during these early periods. In the seventeenth century, the Dutch introduced tea to Europe and America, and today, tea is cultivated commercially in many countries. Coffee is indigenous to Ethiopia, from where it was transported for cultivation to Arabia in the fifteenth century (Roden 1977; Smith 1985a, b). By the early sixteenth century, the practice had been established in the Islamic world of extracting caffeine by infusing ground roasted beans. The Dutch brought coffee plants to Europe in the early seventeenth century and established plantations in the Dutch East Indies (now Indonesia). Further colonization by other European powers led to new and extensive plantations being established in the West Indies, Latin America, Africa, and India.

By the late eighteenth century, coffee replaced tea in popularity in the United States, and today coffee is the main source of caffeine globally. Tea continues to be consumed more widely but qualifies as the second main source because its caffeine content is generally lower than that of coffee (James 1997). Soda drinks (i.e., carbonated soft drinks) are an important source of the drug, and the main source for some consumers. The more recently developed so-called "energy" drinks are also increasing in importance as a source of caffeine. Whereas the caffeine in sodas and energy drinks sometimes partly derives from plant products included in their manufacture (e.g., cacao, cola nut, guarana), most of the caffeine content of such drinks is added in refined form. As such, those products are explicitly designed to be psychoactive and hence (as discussed below) habit-forming.

Other common sources of caffeine include cocoa and chocolate (in both solid and beverage form), but the caffeine content of these is generally low and represents a negligible fraction of the total amount of caffeine consumed. In addition, although the daily intake of caffeine from sources specific to certain regions (e.g., maté in parts of South America) may be substantial for individual consumers and local communities, the overall intake from such sources is small relative to total global consumption of the drug. Similarly, some medications, both prescribed and over the counter, contain as much as 200 mg per tablet or capsule (the approximate equivalent of 1–2 cups of coffee or 3–4 cups of tea), and could be an important (even the main) source of caffeine for some individuals. However, for the general population caffeine-containing medications are typically taken intermittently, or not at all, thereby contributing little to total population caffeine intake.

Although consumption patterns of the various main sources of caffeine may change during the lifespan (e.g., an individual may switch from drinking sodas during childhood to coffee in adulthood), exposure to caffeine is essentially lifelong for most people. Indeed, the first exposure for most people precedes birth. Because most pregnant women consume caffeine and caffeine readily crosses the placenta (Darakjian and Kaddoumi 2019; Goldstein and Warren 1962; Horning et al. 1975; James and Paull 1985; Kimmel et al. 1984; Van't Hoff 1982), most newborns will have encountered the drug in utero (Brazier and Salle 1981; Dumas et al. 1982; Van't Hoff 1982). Exposure is also frequently experienced during infancy, due to caffeine being present in the breast milk of lactating mothers (James 1991). Self-administration of the drug commonly begins in childhood, particularly by way of sodas, with consumption tending to consolidate during adolescence and early adulthood when intake from other caffeine beverages typically begins. Thereafter, usage, especially by way of coffee and tea, is inclined to stabilize, generally undergoing little change for the remainder of life (James 1997). This unparalleled level of exposure introduces multipliers in relation to caffeine's possible impact on health and well-being. On one hand, the effects of lifelong use have the potential to accumulate over the lifespan of individuals. On the other hand, considering the near-universal consumption of caffeine, the cumulative impact, even if effects are small at the level of individuals, may be unexpectedly large when assessed across entire populations (Rose 1992; James 2016).

10.1.2 Pharmacology of Caffeine

Caffeine belongs to a family of purine derivatives termed methylated xanthines (also referred to as methylxanthines or xanthines). At room temperature, caffeine is a white odorless powder with a bitter taste (Vitzthum 1976). The drug was first isolated from green coffee beans in 1820 by Ferdinand Runge in Germany, and later was found to be present in a variety of other plant species (e.g., tea, maté, cacao). Figure 10.1 shows the structure of caffeine (1, 3, 7-trimethylxanthine) and its three primary dimethylxanthine metabolites in humans, namely, paraxanthine, theobromine, and theophylline (James 1997). Following oral ingestion, caffeine is rapidly absorbed into the bloodstream from the gastrointestinal tract (Arnaud 1987). Approximately 90% of the caffeine contained in a cup of coffee is cleared from the stomach within 20 min (Chvasta and Cooke 1971), and peak plasma concentration is typically reached within about 40–60 min (Rall 1990). The drug is readily distributed throughout the body, and the concentrations in blood are highly correlated with those found in the brain, saliva, breast milk, semen, amniotic fluid, and fetal tissue. Caffeine has an elimination half-life of about 5 h in adults (Pfeifer and Notari 1988), and typical consumption patterns result in plasma concentrations that remain pharmacologically active for most of the waking hours. In healthy adults, caffeine is virtually completely transformed by the liver, with less than 5% of the ingested compound being recoverable in urine (Somani and Gupta 1988). Although the beverages and foods that contain caffeine may have constituents (e.g., sugar, milk) that possess nutritional value, caffeine itself has no nutritional value.

When caffeine is consumed during pregnancy, the fetus is exposed to concentrations of the drug approximating systemic levels in the mother (Darakjian and Kaddoumi 2019; Horning et al. 1975). The extent of diffusion of caffeine from maternal to fetal circulation is indicated by the presence of caffeine in fetal hair, with concentrations in the hair of newborns being found to correlate well with maternal caffeine

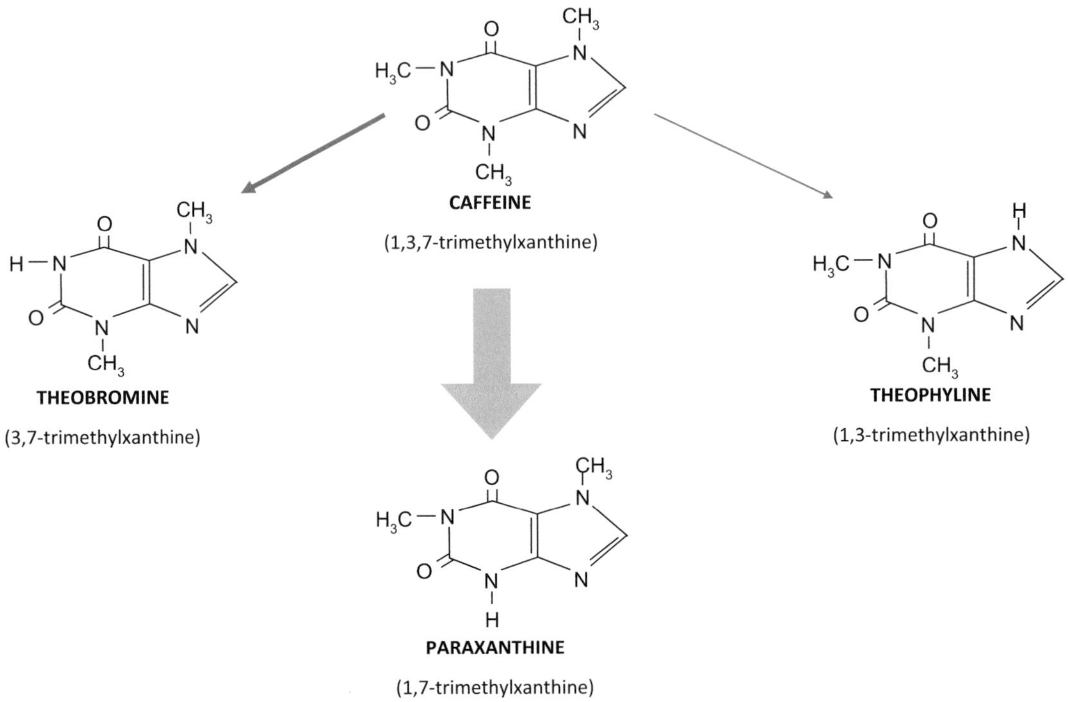

Fig. 10.1 Caffeine and its dimethylated metabolites in humans (*arrow widths* indicate approximate relative proportions of the metabolites in plasma)

consumption (Lehtonen et al. 2021). In adults, caffeine is metabolized principally by cytochrome P450 enzymes (monooxygenase and xanthine oxidase enzymes) in the liver. However, because the P450 enzyme system remains undeveloped during infancy (Parsons and Neims 1981; Pearlman et al. 1989), the kidneys are the main route of excretion in newborns with more than 80% of the drug passing unchanged in urine compared to less than 5% in the urine of adults (Shrestha and Jawa 2017; Somani and Gupta 1988). Notwithstanding differences between individuals, the average elimination half-life of caffeine at birth appears to be about 100 h (Aldridge et al. 1979). Elimination half-life decreases progressively so that by about eight months postnatally, it begins to approximate the average adult rate of 5 h (Aldridge et al. 1979), although complete maturation of the different pathways of caffeine metabolism does not occur before about one year of age (Carrier et al. 1988).

In utero, fetal caffeine clearance depends on maternal metabolism, the rate of which changes during pregnancy. Whereas clearance of caffeine in the first trimester is comparable to that of the non-pregnant state, the rate slows to one-half and then to about one-third during the second and third trimesters, respectively (Aldridge et al. 1981; Yu et al. 2016). The principal mechanism responsible for the reduced rate of caffeine clearance during pregnancy appears to be downregulation of caffeine metabolizing CYP1A2 enzyme (Darakjian and Kaddoumi 2019; Grosso and Bracken 2005). In general, the half-life of caffeine in pregnant women increases from the usual adult rate in the first trimester to about 18 hours by the 38th week of pregnancy (Knutti et al. 1982; Sasaki et al. 2017). Symptoms of nausea and vomiting that frequently accompany pregnancy-related changes in hormonal milieu and the associated reduced rate of caffeine clearance help to explain the observation that women often spontaneously reduce their intake of caffeine when pregnant (Aldridge et al. 1981). Reduced intake means that plasma caffeine concentrations are more likely to be maintained at levels comparable to the pre-pregnant state compared to the appreciably higher levels that would occur if intake remained unchanged.

Main Mechanism of Action Caffeine exerts a variety of pharmacological actions at diverse sites, both centrally and peripherally, which are generally believed to be due mostly to competitive blockade of adenosine receptors (Dunwiddie and Masino 2001). Adenosine is a neuromodulator that acts on specific cell-surface receptors distributed throughout the body (Bush et al. 1989; Cunha et al. 2008; Marangos and Boulenger 1985; Momoi et al. 2008). Because of similarities in the molecular structure of caffeine and adenosine, caffeine occupies adenosine receptor sites, with A_1 and A_{2A} receptors appearing to be the primary targets. Adenosine has important modulatory functions throughout intrauterine development and especially during the first trimester (Glaser et al. 2024; Rivkees and Wendler 2011, 2017). Table 10.1 summarizes some of adenosine's main actions, which generally entail inhibition of physiological activity. Caffeine blocks adenosine receptors, producing effects broadly opposite to those summarized in Table 10.1 (Biaggioni et al. 1991; Franchetti et al. 1994; LeBlanc and Soucy 1994; North et al. 2018). Animal and human studies combined show that caffeine's effects include maintenance of transmitter release in the CNS (anti-somnolent effect), constriction of cerebral and coronary blood vessels, renal diuresis, respiratory bronchodilation, and gastrointestinal acid secretion (Biaggioni et al. 1991; Franchetti et al. 1994; LeBlanc and Soucy 1994; North et al. 2018). In addition, A_1 and A_{2A} receptors interact in functionally important ways with dopamine receptors (Ferré 2016; Garrett and Holtzman 1994), and caffeine stimulates secretion of the catecholamine stress hormones of epinephrine and norepinephrine (Lane et al. 2002). In turn, elevated catecholamine levels have the potential to increase placental vasoconstriction and increase fetal heart rate (Kirkinen et al. 1983), leading to disrupted fetal heart oxygenation (Resch and Papp 1983).

Physical Dependence Repeated exposure to caffeine, such as occurs in the context of dietary use, generally leads to the development of physical dependence, evidenced by the appearance of behavioural, physiological, and subjective withdrawal effects following abrupt cessation of intake (Griffiths et al. 2003; James and Rogers 2005; Juliano and Griffiths 2004; Lane and Phillips-Bute 1998; Walters and Lesk 2016). The mechanism responsible for caffeine physical dependence is generally believed to involve adenosine. Repeated exposure to caffeine, including dietary use, is thought to result in an increased number of adenosine receptors and/or enhanced affinity, resulting in hypersensitivity during abstinence (Biaggioni et al. 1991; Paul et al. 1993; von Borstel and Wurtman 1982). Sleepiness, lethargy, and headache are common symptoms of caffeine withdrawal (Evans and Griffiths 1991; Galletly et al. 1989; Griffiths et al. 1990; Hughes et al. 1991; James 1998; Lane 1997; Lane et al. 2007; Phillips-Bute and Lane 1998), and cessation of as little as 100 mg (one cup of coffee) per day, and possibly less, can produce symptoms (e.g., Lieberman et al. 1987; Smit and Rogers 2000). Effects may be felt within about 12–16 h, generally peaking at around 24–48 h and abating within 3–5 days, though potentially persisting for up to a

Table 10.1 Some acute biological effects of adenosine[a]

Biological system	Effects
Central nervous system	Decreased transmitter release, sedation
Cardiovascular	Dilated cerebral and coronary blood vessels
Renal	Antidiuresis
Respiratory	Bronchoconstriction
Gastrointestinal	Inhibition of acid secretion
Metabolic	Inhibition of lipolysis

[a]By blocking adenosine receptors, caffeine has effects broadly opposite to those summarized above

week (Griffiths et al. 1986; Hughes et al. 1992, 1993). Notably, decreases in psychomotor performance, not necessarily discernible to the individual, are detectable in laboratory tests after as little as 6–8 hours since caffeine was last ingested (Heatherley et al. 2005).

Major systems of medical (World Health Organization 2024) and psychiatric (American Psychiatric Association 2022) diagnosis give formal recognition to caffeine's physical dependence and associated withdrawal effects. At the same time, while repeated consumption leads to rapid development of physical dependence, it is important to acknowledge that the "addictive" potential of caffeine is less than that of classic drugs of abuse (e.g., alcohol, amphetamines, cocaine, opioids). Indeed, relevant empirical research shows that relatively simple strategies (in particular, "caffeine fading") are effective in enabling those who wish to reduce or eliminate a habit of caffeine consumption to succeed in so doing without undue discomfort (Foxx and Rubinoff 1979; James et al. 1985, 1988). In that context, it should be acknowledged that the concentration of caffeine is typically low in decaffeinated coffee and tea, hot chocolate, chocolate bars, chocolate confectionery, and chocolate cake. Accordingly, advice guidelines intended to limit consumption need only target the specific caffeine beverages of coffee, tea, energy drinks, caffeine-containing sodas, and regionally prevalent beverages such as maté, which collectively account for almost all the caffeine that is regularly consumed.

Understanding caffeine withdrawal helps to explain the popularity of caffeine, which is widely attributed to perceived consumer benefits such as increased alertness and performance. For example, a survey of 1248 college students revealed a host of purported effects, including increased wakefulness, concentration, and physical energy, as well as elevated mood (Lieberman et al. 2015). However, it is a mistake to assume that such reports solely reflect the primary effects of the drug. Rather, the "enhancements" perceived by many are largely attributable to reversal of negative withdrawal effects caused by physical dependence (James 2005; James and Keane 2007; Rogers et al. 2013). Even brief periods of caffeine abstinence can produce feelings of sleepiness, degraded concentration, diminished physical energy, and negative mood. In that regard, the "benefits" consumers report are to a substantial degree illusory. That is, subjective wellbeing, having been degraded by caffeine withdrawal, is restored to levels the individual would experience were they not a caffeine consumer in the first place, with little net benefit attributable to the drug.

10.2 Pregnancy Outcomes: Empirical Evidence

Maternal caffeine consumption has been researched in reference to diverse negative pregnancy outcomes and negative outcomes in offspring, including pregnancy that ends in fetal loss due to miscarriage/spontaneous abortion and stillbirth, fetal growth, including low birth weight/small for gestational age, premature/preterm birth, postnatal childhood acute leukemia, childhood overweight and obesity, and childhood behavioural and neurocognitive development.

10.2.1 Miscarriage

Specific terminology referring to fetal loss may vary. While the terms *miscarriage* and *spontaneous abortion* are generally used to refer to the spontaneous loss of a fetus that occurs earlier rather than later in pregnancy, the convention concerning the length of the period may vary between the first 20 to 28 weeks of gestation. Of the two terms, *miscarriage* has come to be more widely adopted in preference to *spontaneous abortion*, in part because of possible confusion over the use of *abortion* to refer to the intentional termination of a pregnancy. Fetal loss that occurs after 20 to 28 weeks of gestation, depending on whichever cutoff period is used to define miscarriage, is referred to as *stillbirth* (discussed below).

There is a high degree of consistency regarding the association between maternal caffeine consumption and miscarriage reported in observational studies (i.e., epidemiological investigations that employ a non-experimental design). Table 10.2 summarizes 10 such studies published since 2000, nine of which reported significant associations between caffeine and increased risk of miscarriage. The nine reports of positive findings comprised five that employed a prospective cohort design (Gaskins et al. 2018; Khoury et al. 2004; Purdue-Smithe et al. 2019; Wen et al. 2001; Weng et al. 2008) and four studies that employed a case-control design (Cnattingius et al. 2000; Giannelli et al. 2003; Rasch 2003; Stefanidou et al. 2011). The one inconsistent result was from a cross-sectional study (Savitz et al. 2008) in which a "suggestive" association was reckoned to be due to recall bias. Notably, however, no such suspicion regarding recall bias arises in relation to the prospective design of the five cohort studies, all of which reported significant caffeine-related increased risk for miscarriage.

It has been suggested that the observed association between maternal caffeine consumption and miscarriage could be due to confounding from pregnancy-induced nausea, which is less frequent in pregnancies that miscarry than those that go full-term (Stein and Susser 1991). The speculation is indeed plausible given that women who experience nausea tend to reduce their caffeine intake during pregnancy more than those who do not experience the same level of nausea (Aldridge et al. 1981). Thus, it could be that nausea-related "loss of taste" for caffeine rather than reduced caffeine per se is the basis for the observed positive correlation between higher caffeine use and miscarriage. However, notwithstanding the plausibility of the nausea hypothesis, support is lacking among empirical studies that took into account nausea experienced during pregnancy (e.g., Giannelli et al. 2003; Wen et al. 2001).

Table 10.3 shows that a high level of consistency is also present in the findings of meta-analyses of caffeine and miscarriage, wherein all seven of the studies listed reported a significant caffeine-related increased risk (Ayoub and Yaseen 2022; Chen et al. 2016; Fernandes et al. 1998; Greenwood et al. 2014; Jafari et al. 2022; Li et al. 2015a; Lyngsø et al. 2017). Estimates of overall risk vary between studies in part because of differences in the cutoff points chosen regarding the amount of daily caffeine intake. Lyngsø et al. (2017), for example, found that women who consumed 100 mg caffeine per day compared to those who consumed no caffeine during pregnancy experienced an increased risk for miscarriage of 8%. In the same study, women who reported consuming 300 mg and 600 mg caffeine per day evidenced an increased risk for miscarriage of 37% and 132%, respectively. Studies that specifically examined dose–response associations consistently reported significantly increased risk. For each increment of 100 mg caffeine consumed per day, Chen et al. (2016) reported increased risk of 7% (95% CI: 1.03–1.12) for prospective studies, Greenwood et al. (2014) reported 14% (95% CI: 1.10–1.19) for cohort and case-control studies combined, and Jafari et al. (2022) reported 14% (1.03–1.26) and 26% (1.12–1.41) for cohort and case-control studies, respectively.

10.2.2 Stillbirth

Findings for stillbirth were largely consistent. Table 10.2 shows that five of six observational studies reported caffeine-related increased risk for stillbirth (Bech et al. 2006; Greenwood et al. 2010; Heazell et al. 2021; Matijasevich et al. 2006; Wisborg et al. 2003). The level of increased risk for high caffeine-consuming women was variously reported to be approximately two-fold (95% CI: 1.23–4.41) (Matijasevich et al. 2006), three-fold (95% CI: 1.5–5.9) (Wisborg et al. 2003), and five-fold (95% CI: 1.6–16.4) (Greenwood et al. 2010) after adjustment for potential confounders. Notably, the sole inconsistent study reporting a non-significant result for stillbirth (loss after 20 weeks of pregnancy) reported significantly increased risk for miscarriage (loss before 20 weeks) (Gaskins et al. 2018). The two meta-analyses summarized in Table 10.3

Table 10.2 Summary of original observational studies of maternal caffeine consumption and pregnancy outcomes published since year 2000

Authors	Year	Study design	Country	*N*	Key findings
Miscarriage					
Cnattingius et al.	2000	Case-control	Sweden	562 cases 953 controls	Maternal caffeine consumption associated with increased risk, not confounded by pregnancy-related symptoms, and present in nonsmokers (plasma cotinine confirmed)
Wen et al.	2001	Prospective cohort	USA	650	Maternal caffeine consumption associated with increased risk, not confounded by pregnancy-related symptoms. Results for women experiencing and those not experiencing nausea were examined separately, showing caffeine-related ($\geq$300 vs. <20 mg per day) increased risk in the former
Giannelli et al.	2003	Case-control	United Kingdom	160 cases 314 controls	Maternal caffeine consumption ($\leq$150 mg vs. >300 mg per day) doubled miscarriage risk, not confounded by pregnancy-related symptoms, with most participants being nonsmokers
Rasch	2003	Case-control	Denmark	330 cases 1168 controls	Maternal caffeine consumption ($\geq$375 mg per day) associated with increased risk independent of alcohol consumption and smoking status
Khoury et al.	2004	Prospective cohort	USA	191	Maternal caffeine consumption among women with Type 1 diabetes associated with a 4.5-fold increased risk, not confounded by smoking status. Caffeine-related risk estimated to be greater than that attributable to smoking
Savitz et al.	2008	Cross-sectional	USA	2407	"Suggestive" caffeine-related increased risk, discounted due to suspected recall bias
Weng et al.	2008	Prospective cohort	USA	1063	Maternal caffeine consumption associated with increased risk, more pronounced in nonsmokers and not confounded by pregnancy-related symptoms
Stefanidou et al.	2011	Case-control	Italy	52 cases 260 controls	Maternal caffeine consumption associated with a dose-response increased risk of *sine causa* recurrent miscarriage of nearly 3-fold for each 100 mg increase in daily caffeine intake, not confounded by pregnancy-related symptoms or smoking status
Gaskins et al.	2018	Prospective cohort	USA	11,072	Maternal caffeine consumption of average less than 200 mg per day associated with increased risk, including never smokers, and not confounded by pregnancy-related symptoms
Purdue-Smithe et al.	2019	Prospective cohort	USA	1228	Maternal caffeine consumption (biomarker confirmed) associated with increased risk, with no minimum safe threshold of consumption, and not confounded by pregnancy-related symptoms
Stillbirth					
Wisborg et al.	2003	Prospective cohort	Denmark	18,478	Maternal caffeine consumption associated with increased risk, with similar magnitude for smokers and nonsmokers

(continued)

Table 10.2 (continued)

Authors	Year	Study design	Country	*N*	Key findings
Bech et al.	2006	Case-control	Denmark	142 cases 157 controls	Maternal caffeine consumption associated with increased risk, irrespective of genotype for caffeine metabolism
Matijasevich et al.	2006	Case-control	Uruguay	382 cases 792 controls	Maternal caffeine consumption associated with increased risk, with similar magnitude for smokers and nonsmokers, independent of pregnancy-related symptoms
Greenwood et al.	2010	Prospective cohort	United Kingdom	2643	Compared to maternal consumption of less than 100 mg caffeine per day, 300+ mg per day was associated with a five fold (95% CI: 1.6–16.4) increased risk, not confounded by smoking or pregnancy-related symptoms
Gaskins et al.	2018	Prospective cohort	USA	11,072	Caffeine consumption not associated with increased risk
Heazell et al.	2021	Case-control	United Kingdom	290 cases 729 controls	Maternal caffeine consumption associated with a significantly increased risk for each increment of 100 mg caffeine consumed per day up to ≥300 mg per day
Low birth weight (LBW) and/or small for gestational age (SGA)					
Klebanoff et al.	2002	Prospective cohort	USA	2515	Maternal caffeine consumption (biomarker confirmed) associated with increased risk of SGA in women who smoked
Clausson et al.	2002	Prospective cohort	Sweden	953	Maternal caffeine consumption not associated with LBW or SGA
Bracken et al.	2003	Prospective cohort	USA	2291	Decreased birth weight of 28 g associated with each increment of 100 mg per day in maternal caffeine
CARE Study Group	2008	Prospective cohort	UK	2635	Maternal caffeine consumption associated with decreased birth weight, not confounded by smoking status (salivary cotinine confirmed), with no identifiable threshold of consumption below which the association was absent
Bakker et al.	2010	Prospective cohort	Netherlands	7346	Maternal caffeine consumption not associated with LBW. High intake (≥6 cups of coffee per day) associated with increased risk of SGA
Sengpiel et al.	2013	Prospective cohort	Norway	59,123	Maternal caffeine consumption associated with LBW and SGA
Hoyt et al.	2014	Case-control	USA	648 cases 7295 controls	Maternal caffeine consumption associated with SGA
Bech et al.	2015	Prospective cohort	Denmark	71,000	Maternal caffeine consumption associated with increased risk of LBW and SGA for both smokers and nonsmokers
Del Castillo et al.	2015	Cross-sectional	Spain	1175	Maternal caffeine consumption of >115 mg per day compared to no consumption associated with LBW after adjustment for potential confounders including tobacco and alcohol
Okubo et al.	2015	Prospective cohort	Japan	858	Maternal caffeine consumption not associated with LBW or SGA
Voerman et al.	2016	Prospective cohort	Netherlands	7857	Maternal caffeine consumption (<2 vs. ≥6 cups of coffee per day) associated with LBW

(continued)

Table 10.2 (continued)

Authors	Year	Study design	Country	*N*	Key findings
Chen et al.	2018	Prospective cohort	Ireland	941	Maternal caffeine consumption associated with LBW for both coffee and tea
Kobayashi et al.	2019	Prospective cohort	Japan	94,876	Increased risk of SGA of 18% (95% CI: 1.10–1.27) for the highest vs. lowest quartile of maternal caffeine consumption
Modzelewska et al.	2019	Prospective cohort	Norway	67,569	Maternal caffeine consumption associated with increased SGA risk
Kukkonen et al.	2024	Prospective cohort	Finland	2007	First trimester maternal caffeine consumption >50 mg per day associated with increased SGA risk
Preterm birth					
Bracken et al.	2003	Prospective cohort	USA	2291	Maternal caffeine consumption not associated with increased risk
Chiaffarino et al.	2006	Case-control	Italy	502 cases 1966 controls	Maternal caffeine consumption not associated with increased risk
Del Castillo et al.	2015	Cross-sectional	Spain	1175	Maternal caffeine consumption not associated with increased risk
Okubo et al.	2015	Prospective cohort	Japan	858	Increased risk of 28% (95% CI: 1.03–1.58) for each increment of 100 mg caffeine consumed per day
Chen et al.	2018	Prospective cohort	Ireland	941	Increased risk of 174% (95% CI: 1.05–7.16) and 156% (95% CI: 1.14–5.75) comparing the highest and lowest caffeine intake categories for coffee and tea, respectively
Kobayashi et al.	2019	Prospective cohort	Japan	94,876	Increased risk of 94% (95% CI: 1.12–3.37) for the highest vs. Lowest quartile of maternal caffeine consumption
Sindiani et al.	2020	Case-control	Jordan	314 cases 796 controls	Maternal caffeine consumption not associated with increased risk
Childhood acute leukemia					
Menegaux et al.	2007	Case-control	France	472 cases 567 controls	No overall association, but evidence of maternal caffeine consumption of >3 cups per day associated with increased risk among nonsmokers
Milne et al.	2011	Case-control	Australia	337 cases 697 controls	No overall association, but evidence of "higher" levels of maternal caffeine consumption associated with increased risk among nonsmokers
Bonaventure et al.	2013	Case-control	France	764 cases 1681 controls	Maternal caffeine consumption associated with increased risk
Orsi et al.	2015	Case-control	France	747 cases 1421 controls	Role of maternal coffee consumption reported to be "unclear"
Milne et al.	2018	Case-control	Australia, France, Greece, USA	2552 cases 4876 controls	Maternal caffeine consumption (>2 cups per day vs. no coffee) associated with increased risk
Karalexi et al.	2019	Case-control	France, Greece, Germany, USA	554 cases 1419 controls	Maternal caffeine consumption of >1 cup per day associated with increased risk

(continued)

Table 10.2 (continued)

Authors	Year	Study design	Country	*N*	Key findings
Madsen et al.	2020	Prospective cohort	Denmark	141,216	Maternal caffeine consumption not associated with increased risk
Childhood overweight and obesity					
Li et al.	2015	Prospective cohort	USA	615	Maternal caffeine consumption associated with a dose-response increased risk of childhood obesity at 15 years follow-up
Klebanoff and Keim	2015	Case-control	USA	1986 cases 1986 controls	Maternal caffeine consumption not associated with risk of childhood obesity at 4 and 7 years
Voerman et al.	2016	Prospective cohort	Netherlands	7857	Maternal caffeine consumption associated with increased risk of childhood overweight at 6 years
Papadopoulou et al.	2018	Prospective cohort	Norway	50,943	Maternal caffeine consumption associated with increased risk of childhood overweight up to 8 years
Chen et al.	2019	Prospective cohort	Ireland	558	Maternal caffeine consumption associated with increased risk of childhood adiposity and obesity at 5 and 9 years

both reported significant associations, with overall caffeine-related increased risk of stillbirth for each additional 100 mg daily intake of the drug estimated to be 9% (95% CI: 1.02–1.12) in one review (Chen et al. 2016) and 19% (95% CI: 1.05–1.35) in the other (Greenwood et al. 2014).

Questions regarding possible caffeine-related genetic predisposition were examined in a study that tested the hypothesis that "slow metabolizers" are at increased risk (Bech et al. 2006). Among various polymorphisms of the genes that encode enzymes responsible for caffeine metabolism, no single genotype was associated with risk. However, a combination of three separate genes that contribute to a slower rate of caffeine metabolism was found to be associated with an almost two-fold increased risk compared with other genotype combinations.

10.2.3 Fetal Growth: Low Birth Weight (LBW) and/or Small for Gestational Age (SGA)

It has long been known that caffeine in the diet of pregnant rodents contributes to lower fetal weight (Dunlop and Court 1981; Fujii and Nishimura 1972; Gilbert and Pistey 1973; Momoi et al. 2008; Thayer and Kensler 1973). Although animal experiments have tended to involve levels of caffeine exposure greater than that typical of the consumption patterns of humans, overall findings have been largely complementary. Table 10.2 summarizes 15 observational studies comprised of 13 cohort studies, one case-control study, and one cross-sectional study. These, in turn, divide between five that reported results for LBW alone (Bracken et al. 2003; CARE Study Group 2008; Chen et al. 2018; Del Castillo et al. 2015; Voerman et al. 2016), five for SGA alone (Hoyt et al. 2014; Klebanoff et al. 2002; Kobayashi et al. 2019; Kukkonen et al. 2024; Modzelewska et al. 2019), and five for both outcomes (Bakker et al. 2010; Bech et al. 2015; Clausson et al. 2002; Okubo et al. 2015; Sengpiel et al. 2013).

Of the ten studies reporting results for LBW, seven reported caffeine-related increased risk (Bracken et al. 2003; Bech et al. 2015; CARE Study Group 2008; Chen et al. 2018; Del Castillo et al. 2015; Sengpiel et al. 2013; Voerman et al. 2016) and three reported no association (Bakker et al. 2010; Clausson et al. 2002; Okubo et al. 2015). Of ten studies reporting results for SGA, eight reported caffeine-related increased risk (Bakker et al. 2010; Bech et al. 2015; Hoyt et al. 2014; Klebanoff et al. 2002; Kobayashi et al.

Table 10.3 Summary of caffeine-related percentage increased risk of harm (95% CI) for diverse negative pregnancy outcomes reported in meta-analyses published since 1998

Authors	Year	Increased risk % (95% CI)	Consumption (mg per day)[a]
Miscarriage			
Fernandes et al.	1998	36 (1.29–1.45)	<150 vs. ≥150
Greenwood et al.	2014	14 (1.10–1.19)	Per 100
Li et al.	2015a	32 (1.24–1.40)	<150 vs. ≥150
Chen et al.	2016	7 (1.03–1.12)	Per 100
Lyngsø et al.	2017	8 (1.03–1.13)	0 vs. 100
		37 (1.19–1.57)	0 vs. 300
		132 (1.62–3.31)	0 vs. 600
Ayoub and Yaseen	2022	65 (1.46–1.87)	≤150 vs. >150
Jafari et al.	2022	Cohort studies 14 (1.03–1.26)	Per 100
		Case-control studies 26 (1.12–1.41)	
Stillbirth			
Greenwood et al.	2014	19 (1.05–1.35)	Per 100
Chen et al.	2016	9 (1.02–1.16)	Per 100
Low birth weight/small for gestational age			
Fernandes et al.	1998	51 (1.39–1.63)	<150 vs. ≥150
Santos et al.	1998	29 (1.18–1.41)/24 (1.05–1.43)	None/low vs. high
Chen et al.	2014	13 (1.06–1.21)	Per 100
Greenwood et al.	2014	7 (1.01–1.12)/10 (1.06–1.14)	Per 100
Rhee et al.	2015	38 (1.10–1.73)	Lowest vs. highest
Jin and Qiao	2021	33 (1.12–1.57)	Lowest vs. highest
Soltani et al.	2022	70 (CI: 1.19–2.43)	Lowest vs. highest
Premature/preterm birth			
Santos et al.	1998	"Indeterminate"	None/low vs. high
Maslova et al.	2010	No "important" association	Lowest vs. highest
Greenwood et al.	2014	No association	Per 100
Childhood acute leukemia			
Milne et al.	2011	67 (1.20–2.32)	None vs. 3+ cups coffee
Cheng et al.	2014	72 (1.32–2.16)	None/lowest vs. highest
Thomopoulos et al.	2015	57 (1.16–2.11)	Lowest vs. highest
Childhood overweight and obesity			
Jin and Qiao	2021	39 (1.15–1.69)	Lowest vs highest
		31% (95% CI: 1.11, 1.55)	Per 100

[a]Level of maternal caffeine consumption (mg per day), if given, reported to have been used as the basis for estimating risk of harm

2019; Kukkonen et al. 2024; Modzelewska et al. 2019; Sengpiel et al. 2013) and two reported no association (Clausson et al. 2002; Okubo et al. 2015). That is, of the 15 studies of LBW and/or SGA summarized in Table 10.2, all but two reported caffeine-related increased risk for one or both LBW and SGA. Addressing the question of comparative risk from other substances, the CARE Study Group (2008) reported that the caffeine-related risk for LBW was comparable to the risk associated with maternal consumption of alcohol.

Notwithstanding occasional null results, the substantial consistency in findings from original observational studies of LBW and SGA is reflected in the findings of meta-analyses. Of the seven meta-analyses listed in Table 10.3, all reported results for LBW (Chen et al. 2014; Fernandes et al. 1998; Greenwood et al. 2014; Jin and Qiao 2021; Rhee et al. 2015; Santos et al. 1998; Soltani et al. 2022) and two reported results for SGA (Greenwood et al. 2014; Santos et al. 1998). All seven meta-analyses reported positive associations between maternal caffeine consumption and increased risk for LBW and/or SGA. Dose–response analyses for LBW yielded estimates of increased risk for each additional 100 mg er day of caffeine intake of 7% (95% CI: 1.01–1.12) (Greenwood et al. 2014) and 13% (1.06–1.21) (Chen et al. 2014). For SGA, a dose–response association of 10% (95 % CI 1.06–1.14) per 100 mg increased daily intake was reported (Greenwood et al. 2014).

Taken as a whole, the relevant literature has led to increasingly unequivocal conclusions. For example, an early systematic review concluded that there was tentative support for the conclusion that caffeine contributes to fetal growth restriction and low birth weight (James and Paull 1985). The authors of that review highlighted various methodological limitations in the then extant literature and called for more research employing improved methods for measuring caffeine exposure and better controls against potential confounders, especially concurrent alcohol and tobacco use. An updated review published six years later concluded that the evidence had strengthened (James 1991), and another review published after a further six years concluded that the evidence had become "strong" (James 1997). Subsequent empirical findings confirm that conclusion. Moreover, consistent reports of a dose–response relation and the absence of a threshold effect provide additional compelling evidence of a causal relation between maternal caffeine consumption and impaired fetal development. Thus, despite some inconsistencies in earlier published findings, studies conducted over recent decades provide broadly consistent evidence for concluding that maternal caffeine consumption contributes to impaired fetal growth.

10.2.4 Premature/Preterm Birth

Table 10.2 shows that of seven observational studies, three reported that maternal caffeine consumption was associated with increased risk of preterm birth (Chen et al. 2018; Kobayashi et al. 2019; Okubo et al. 2015), and four reported no association (Bracken et al. 2003; Chiaffarino et al. 2006; Del Castillo et al. 2015; Sindiani et al. 2020). Of the three meta-analyses listed in Table 10.3, one reported that high heterogeneity within the published data prevented computation of reliable pooled estimates (Santos et al. 1998), and two concluded that maternal caffeine consumption appears not to increase the risk of preterm birth (Greenwood et al. 2014; Maslova et al. 2010). Conversely, it might be noted that publication of all three meta-analyses preceded the three observational studies that reported significant associations (Chen et al. 2018; Kobayashi et al. 2019; Okubo et al. 2015).

10.2.5 Childhood Acute Leukemia

Table 10.2 summarizes findings from seven studies of caffeine-related risk of childhood leukemia, including acute lymphocytic (lymphoblastic) leukemia (ALL), which accounts for about 75% of childhood leukemias and is the most common cause of death from cancer in children, and acute myeloid leukemia (AML) which accounts for most of the remaining cases of childhood leukemia (Hunger and Mullighan 2015). Three of six case-control studies reported evidence of significant associations with either ALL or AML (Bonaventure et al. 2013; Karalexi et al. 2019; Milne et al. 2018). Among the remaining three case-control studies, two found no overall association while reporting evidence of association for nonsmoking mothers who reported relatively high caffeine consumption (Menegaux et al. 2007; Milne et al. 2011). An interaction with smoking is plausible in that smoking is known to accelerate caffeine metabolism, thereby offering smokers potential limited protection against the harmful effects of caffeine (Milne et al. 2011). The remaining case-control study reported that the association between maternal caffeine consumption and risk of childhood acute leukemia was "unclear" (Orsi et al. 2015), and the sole prospective cohort study reported no association (Madsen et al. 2020).

Notwithstanding mixed results from the observational studies summarized in Table 10.2, all three meta-analyses summarized in Table 10.3 concluded that maternal caffeine consumption is associated with increased risk of childhood acute leukemia. This includes the findings of a meta-analysis reported in the same article which presented equivocal findings for a case-control study the authors had also undertaken (Milne et al. 2011). One of the two more recent meta-analyses reported that high maternal caffeine consumption was associated with a 72% (95% CI: 1.32–2.16) increased risk for acute leukemia overall (Cheng et al. 2014), and increased risks of 65% (95% CI: 1.28–2.12) and 58% (95% CI: 1.20–2.08) for ALL and AML, respectively. The remaining meta-analysis reported broadly similar increased risks of 57% (95% CI: 1.16–2.11) for acute leukemia overall and 43% (95% CI: 1.22–1.68) for ALL, while reporting a substantially larger increased risk of 152% (95% CI: 1.59–3.57) for AML (Thomopoulos et al. 2015).

10.2.6 Childhood Overweight and Obesity

Animal studies have shown that maternal caffeine exposure is associated with long-term changes in metabolic functions under the control of the hypothalamic-pituitary-adrenal axis (Li et al. 2015b; Xu et al. 2012). Such changes affect regulation by adenosine and/or its receptors involved in development (Buscariollo et al. 2014; Rivkees and Wendler 2011), while also influencing placental expression and transport of leptins essential for regulating appetite (Wu et al. 2015). Consequently, the role of maternal caffeine in childhood overweight and obesity has emerged as an area of focus in recent human research.

Table 10.2 summarizes the findings of four cohort studies (Chen et al. 2019; Li et al. 2015a; Papadopoulou et al. 2018; Voerman et al. 2016) and one case-control study (Klebanoff and Keim 2015). With one exception, the studies reported significant associations between maternal caffeine consumption and increased risk of childhood overweight, adiposity, and/or obesity. The inconsistent finding was reported in the case-control study, which used data collected more than 50 years ago (Klebanoff and Keim 2015). A dose–response association was reported in one study, with children of mothers whose caffeine consumption was highest (≥150 mg of caffeine per day) experiencing a greater than twofold overall increased risk of obesity (OR: 2.37; CI: 1.24–4.52) at age five years compared to children of mothers who consumed no caffeine during pregnancy (Li et al. 2015a).

A systematic review of relevant literature concluded that maternal caffeine consumption is associated with increased risk of childhood obesity (Frayer and Kim 2020). That conclusion was confirmed by a more recent meta-analysis (Jin and Qiao 2021), which found the association to be dose-related (see Table 10.3). Specifically, risk of childhood obesity was found to increase by more than 30% for each additional 100 mg/day caffeine consumed during pregnancy. Based on their respective analyses, the authors of both the systematic review (Frayer and Kim 2020) and the meta-analysis (Jin and Qiao 2021) suggested that "complete avoidance" of caffeine during pregnancy may be appropriate.

10.2.7 Childhood Behavioural and Neurocognitive Development

Rodent Experimental Studies Strong confirmation of the high biological plausibility of harm from maternal caffeine exposure to human behavioral and neurocognitive development can be found in early rodent studies (Grimm and Frieder 1988; Nakamoto et al. 1991). For example, Grimm and Frieder (1988) exposed pregnant rat dams to daily doses of 0.15, 0.30, or 0.45 mg/ml caffeine in drinking water for the last 7 days of gestation. Compared to untreated controls, offspring exposed to the low dose (0.15 mg/ml) evidenced hyperactivity in an open-field task, and offspring exposed to the high dose

(0.45 mg/ml) evidenced disruption to complex visual and auditory discrimination learning. Foreshadowing later observational research with humans (Chen et al. 2019; Li et al. 2015b; Papadopoulou et al. 2018; Voerman et al. 2016), Grimm and Frieder (1988) reported that the medium (0.30 mg/ml) and high (0.45 mg/ml) doses also led to increased weight observable at 35 days, with weight gains becoming progressively greater as the animals aged.

The Grimm and Frieder (1988) findings are all the more salient when the caffeine doses they used are compared to typical human exposures. With the caveat that the translation of caffeine dosing in animal studies to human consumption patterns is complex and approximate, a dose of 0.30 mg/ml in drinking water was estimated by Silva et al. (2013) to produce plasma concentrations of caffeine in rat dams comparable to those found in the blood of humans drinking 3–4 cups of coffee per day. On the other hand, Li et al. (2018) estimated the same dose (0.30 mg/ml) of caffeine in drinking water to be comparable to the human consumption of about two cups of coffee per day. Thus, bearing in mind the approximate nature of such estimates, the Grimm and Frieder (1988) "low" dose of 0.15 mg/ml and possibly the "medium" dose of 0.30 mg/ml, could be considered comparable to the levels of exposure often cited as "safe" and "moderate" for human pregnancies. In that vein, the 0.45 mg/ml dose would be comparable to intake widely considered "high" but not uncommon among pregnant women.

Table 10.4 summarizes key findings from five more rodent studies (Fazeli et al. 2017; Li et al. 2018; Silva et al. 2013; Soellner et al. 2009; Zappettini et al. 2019), all of which found evidence of harm. For example, Soellner et al. (2009) exposed pregnant rat dams to either plain tap water or caffeinated tap water throughout gestation, in contrast to the Grimm and Frieder (1988) study, which limited exposure to the latter stages of pregnancy. The level of caffeine exposure in the Soellner et al. (2009) study was estimated to be the human equivalent of 2 to 3 cups of coffee per day. Adult male and female offspring of dams exposed to caffeine during pregnancy exhibited memory and learning impairments in object recognition and spatial learning tasks. The findings were interpreted as suggesting developmental changes in the expression and/or function of adenosine receptors within the hippocampus and prefrontal cortex, leading to long-term alterations in memory and learning. Long-term effects were also reported by Silva et al. (2013), who exposed mouse dams to 0.30 mg/ml caffeine in drinking water throughout gestation and lactation. Compared to untreated controls, adult offspring of treated animals showed increased excitability in hippocampal circuits and associated sequelae, including increased susceptibility to seizures.

Fazeli et al. (2017) also reported increased seizure susceptibility in a study in which caffeine in drinking water was intended to mimic human consumption of approximately three cups of coffee per day. Compared to control offspring, the formation and activity of cortical networks were found to be impaired in offspring of caffeine-exposed mouse dams. In another study that sought to mimic human consumption patterns with the use of 0.30 mg/ml caffeine in drinking water, Zappettini et al. (2019) were careful to parallel human exposure before and during pregnancy until full-term birth, taking account of both the time span of caffeine exposure and the amount of caffeine consumed. Electrophysiological recordings of hippocampal CA1 pyramidal cells in vitro revealed caffeine-related changes likely to increase the risk for early onset of dementia-associated pathology. In addition, Li et al. (2018) reported that expression of adenosine A_1 and A_{2A} receptors was impaired in fetal and neonatal brain among offspring of rat dams exposed to 20 mg/kg caffeine (compared to saline) administered twice daily via subcutaneous injection. The same study also reported that learning and memory were impaired in adult offspring exposed to caffeine in utero.

In summary, animal studies have repeatedly confirmed the decades-long inference of high biological plausibility of harm for behavioural

Table 10.4 Summary of experimental animal and human prospective cohort studies of maternal caffeine consumption and childhood behavioural and neurocognitive development

Authors	Year	Main aim	Method	Key findings
Experimental studies with rodents				
Soellner et al.	2009	Effects of chronic prenatal exposure to caffeine on cognitive performance in adult male and female offspring	Pregnant rat dams were exposed via drinking water to the human equivalent of 2 to 3 cups of coffee per day throughout pregnancy, and offspring were compared to the offspring of caffeine-free dams	Compared to untreated controls, adult male and female offspring of caffeine-exposed dams exhibited impaired cognition, including 24-h memory retention in novel object recognition and spatial learning in a maze task. Findings were suggestive of developmental changes in the adenosine-receptor functioning in the hippocampus and prefrontal cortex, leading to long-term alterations in memory and learning
Silva et al.	2013	Effects of maternal exposure to caffeine, as an adenosine modulator, on offspring neural development	Offspring of mouse dams exposed to 0.30 mg/ml caffeine in drinking water during pregnancy and lactation were compared to offspring of caffeine-free dams	Compared to untreated controls, caffeine-exposed offspring showed delayed migration and insertion of *g*-aminobutyric acid (GABA) neurons into the hippocampal circuitry during the first postnatal week, and increased neuronal network excitability and susceptibility to seizures. Adult offspring displayed loss of hippocampal GABA neurons and cognitive deficits
Fazeli et al.	2017	The construction and activity of cortical networks in offspring of dams exposed to effects of caffeine during pregnancy and the early postnatal period	Female mice were exposed to caffeine in drinking water in concentrations mimicking human consumption of 3 cups of coffee per day	Compared to controls, caffeine-exposed offspring showed impaired brain development, including altered construction of GABAergic neuronal networks in the primary visual cortex at postnatal days 6–7, increased synaptic activity *in vitro* and elevated network activity *in vivo* in the primary visual cortex, altered *in vivo* hippocampal network activity from the neonatal period until adulthood, and increased seizure susceptibility
Li et al.	2018	Effects of maternal caffeine exposure on neurocognitive functions	Rat dams received subcutaneous injections of 20 mg/kg caffeine or saline twice daily throughout pregnancy. Measurements were taken of fetal and	Compared to saline-treated controls, caffeine-exposed offspring showed fetal growth restriction; long-term impairment in learning and memory; intrauterine

(continued)

Table 10.4 (continued)

Authors	Year	Main aim	Method	Key findings
			offspring body and brain weight, learning- and memory-related receptors, and learning and memory in adult offspring	programming dysfunction of adenosine receptors; and impairment of subunits of down-stream protein-binding systems in fetal, neonatal, and adult brain
Zappettini et al.	2019	The long-term consequences of early-life exposure to caffeine for Alzheimer's disease-like pathology	Using a rodent model of Alzheimer's disease (THY-Tau22 transgenic mice), the exposure schedule involved caffeine in drinking water intended to mimic the amount and time span of the human consumption of caffeine before and throughout gestation	Caffeine-exposed offspring showed deficits in spatial learning and memory earlier than untreated controls, and disordered electrophysiological recordings suggestive of early onset of Alzheimer's disease-like pathology
Human prospective cohort studies				
Linnet et al.	2009	Associations between maternal coffee exposure and risk of hyperkinetic disorder and attention deficit hyperactivity disorder (ADHD)	24,068 Danish children, including 88 children aged 3–12 years with hyperkinetic disorder and/or ADHD	High maternal caffeine consumption (10+ cups of coffee per day) reported at 16 weeks of gestation was associated with a threefold increased risk of hyperkinetic disorder and ADHD. After adjustment for confounders, the risk decreased to RR 2.3 (95% CI 0.9–5.9) and was no longer statistically significant
Bekkhus et al.	2010	Associations between maternal caffeine consumption and inattention/ overactivity suggestive of ADHD	25,343 Norwegian mothers and their 18-month-old children	After adjustment for potential confounders, caffeine in the form of soft drinks but not coffee or tea, reported at 17 and 30 weeks of gestation, was found to be associated with inattention/ overactivity
Loomans et al.	2012	Associations between maternal caffeine consumption and offspring behavioural problems	3439 children in The Netherlands assessed at age 5–6 years via mother- and teacher-reported problem behaviour	After adjustment for potential confounders, maternal caffeine consumption reported at 16 weeks of gestation was not associated with a higher risk for behaviour problems or with suboptimal prosocial behaviour
Galéra et al.	2016	Associations between maternal caffeine consumption and impaired cognitive development in offspring	1083 French mother-child pairs followed from pregnancy to when the children were aged 5.5 years	After adjustment for potential confounders, there was a significant caffeine-related association with reduced childhood IQ of nearly one full IQ point per additional 100 mg/day of maternal caffeine intake assessed before pregnancy and after delivery

(continued)

Table 10.4 (continued)

Authors	Year	Main aim	Method	Key findings
Klebanoff and Keim	2015	Associations between maternal serum paraxanthine (the primary metabolite of caffeine) and offspring IQ and problem behaviour	2197 children in the United States assessed at ages 4 and 7 years	After adjustment for potential confounders, no statistically significant associations were reported between maternal serum paraxanthine, measured at "early pregnancy" (<20 weeks) and "third trimester" (>26 weeks), and either IQ or problem behaviour
Del-Ponte et al.	2016	Associations between maternal consumption of caffeine during pregnancy and childhood ADHD	3485 Brazilian children assessed at age 11 years	After adjustment for potential confounders, maternal caffeine consumption, assessed by interview after delivery, was not associated with ADHD
Mikkelsen et al.	2017	Associations between maternal caffeine consumption and offspring behavioural and psychiatric disorders	47,491 Danish mother-child pairs	After adjustment for potential confounders, maternal caffeine consumption reported at 15 weeks gestation was reported to be associated with increased risk of a range of behavioural and psychiatric disorders
Berglundh et al.	2021	Associations between maternal caffeine consumption and childhood neurodevelopment	64,189 Norwegian children assessed at ages 6 and 18 months, and 3, 5 and 8 years	After adjustment for potential confounders, maternal caffeine consumption reported at 22 weeks of gestation yielded no consistent associations with childhood neurodevelopment at any age
Christensen et al.	2021	Associations between maternal caffeine consumption and childhood neurodevelopment	9157 children in the United States assessed at 9–10 years using magnetic resonance imaging (MRI)	After adjustment for potential confounders, MRI revealed caffeine-related alterations in brain microstructures associated with maternal caffeine consumption reported "throughout gestation"

and neurocognitive development from maternal caffeine exposure. The studies summarized in Table 10.4 report a wide range of caffeine-related disruption to brain function and structure, and associated developmental impairment in behaviour and cognition. Whereas there may have been a tendency to discount earlier similar findings due to pregnant animals being exposed to levels of caffeine higher than the levels resulting from human consumption patterns, most of the studies summarized in Table 10.4 were careful to use regimens of caffeine intake that mimicked typical human exposure. As such, animal findings have been important in raising awareness of potential harm from maternal caffeine consumption for child development.

Human Observational Studies Table 10.4 summarizes key findings from nine prospective cohort studies of potential caffeine-related harm to childhood behavioural and neurocognitive development. It is evident from the table that diversity of investigatory approach and inconsistency in reported findings represent major challenges to interpreting the evidence. In an early study of attention deficit hyperactivity disorder (ADHD), Linnet et al. (2009) reported that high maternal caffeine consumption (defined as 10+ cups of coffee per day) was associated with a threefold increased risk of ADHD-related behavior among 24,068 Danish children aged between 3 and 12 years. However, the estimated risk was reduced to a level that no longer represented a statistically significant difference when adjustment was made for confounders, including cigarette smoking, alcohol consumption, age of mother, gestational age, presence of psychiatric disorder among parents and siblings, education level, and employment status.

Bekkhus et al. (2010) reported a significant association for ADHD-related behavior among 25,343 Norwegian children aged 18 months. In this instance, however, increased risk was observed for maternal consumption of soft drinks but not coffee and tea, leading the authors to suggest that caffeine was unlikely to be responsible for the reported association. At the same time, the authors cautioned that the children may have been "too young" for caffeine-related effects to be reliably observed. In a study of 3439 Dutch children, Loomans et al. (2012) reported that maternal caffeine consumption was unrelated to mother and teacher ratings of ADHD-related behavior among children aged 5 to 6 years. Absence of association was also reported by Klebanoff and Keim (2015) in the United States for 2197 children aged 4 and 7 years, and by Del-Ponte et al. (2016) for 3458 Brazilian children aged 11 years. Conversely, in a larger study of 47,491 Danish children aged 11 years, Mikkelsen et al. (2017) reported that high maternal caffeine consumption, defined as 8+ cups of coffee per day assessed at 15 weeks of pregnancy, was associated with increased risk for a range of behavioural and psychiatric disorders, including ADHD-related behavior.

In the same study that reported no association for ADHD-related behavior, Klebanoff and Keim (2015) found no association between maternal caffeine consumption and intelligence quotient (IQ) in children aged 4 and 7 years. Conversely, Galéra et al. (2016) reported a significant association between maternal caffeine consumption and lower IQ among 1083 French children aged 5.5 years. Reasons for the discrepant findings were debated in an exchange of letters without the respective groups (Bernard et al. 2016; Klebanoff and Keim 2016) reaching an agreement. Bernard et al. (2016) reasoned that a combination of the two sets of results supported the conclusion that a causal link exists between high caffeine exposure and lower childhood IQ. In reply, Klebanoff and Keim (2016) reiterated their belief "that the amount of caffeine consumed by most pregnant women … is not likely to be associated with reduced child cognition" (p. 873).

Berglundh et al. (2021) examined the association between maternal caffeine consumption and impaired neurodevelopment, including motor development, behavior problems, and language difficulties among 64,189 Norwegian children aged 6 and 18 months, and 3, 5, and 8 years, and found no consistent associations. Conversely, Christensen et al. (2021) in the United States examined maternal caffeine consumption and regional brain microstructure among 9157 children aged 9 to 10 years. Maternal exposure was measured dichotomously to create an exposed group of women who reported consuming caffeine more than once a week throughout pregnancy and a group comprised of women who reported consuming caffeine less than once a week. Magnetic resonance imaging (MRI) indicated microstructure alterations of "critical fibre tracts" among children of the exposed group of mothers compared with children of control mothers.

Confirming the general pattern of findings summarized in Table 10.4, a recent systematic review concluded that methodological diversity and inconsistent results prevent firm conclusions regarding potential negative effects of maternal caffeine consumption for childhood neurobehavioral development (Santana et al. 2024). No one set of factors can explain all the inconsistencies. Notably, studies to date have been few and have involved participants in different countries with varying patterns of caffeine consumption. In addition, apart from being prospective in nature, studies have employed widely differing investigatory approaches. There has been little consistency in the measurement of maternal caffeine exposure; the population samples examined have differed greatly in size, children have been assessed at different ages, and different behavioural and neurocognitive developmental outcomes have been examined.

10.3 Discussion

Without ignoring discrepant results, the findings of original observational studies summarized in Table 10.2 reveal a high level of consistency, which is also reflected in the conclusions of the 23 meta-analyses summarized in Table 10.3. Specifically, maternal caffeine consumption was reported to be associated with increased risk by all seven meta-analyses of miscarriage, in both of two meta-analyses for stillbirth, in all seven meta-analyses for LBW and/or SGA, and in all three meta-analyses for childhood acute leukemia. Significant increased risk was also reported in the sole meta-analysis for childhood overweight and obesity. Additionally, consistency was reported for premature/preterm birth, wherein all three meta-analyses found maternal caffeine consumption to be *not* associated with increased risk. Conversely, as summarized in Table 10.4, firm conclusions are precluded in relation to human studies of childhood neurobehavioral development due to heterogeneity in both methodology and findings. In summary, evidence of harm is strong for miscarriage, stillbirth, and low birth weight and/or small for gestational age. Evidence for childhood acute leukemia and childhood overweight and obesity is less strong, and less again for childhood behavioral and neurocognitive developmental impairment.

Consistent evidence of harm has clear implications for the framing of advice about caffeine consumption for mothers and mothers-to-be. Consequently, it is imperative that the veracity of the evidence is closely scrutinized, not least in relation to the question of causation. Likelihood of causation, rather than mere association, is indicated by the many reports of observed dose–response relationships between the amount of caffeine consumed during pregnancy and risk of negative pregnancy outcomes and negative outcomes in offspring. Causation is also implied by multiple reports of no threshold of consumption below which associations are absent. Overall, then, the likelihood of causation is supported by a compelling body of evidence, both theoretical (i.e., biological plausibility) and empirical, including strong consensus among observational studies and meta-analyses of dose–response relationships and reported absence of threshold effects.

10.3.1 Is the Evidence of Harm from Maternal Caffeine Consumption Valid?

Notwithstanding the large body of consistent evidence of caffeine-related negative pregnancy outcomes and negative outcomes in offspring, questions persist as to the validity of the evidence. At this juncture, it is imperative to consider the decades-long involvement of interested parties in industry. In the late 1970s, the United States Food and Drug Administration (FDA) announced the possible removal of caffeine from its list of food additives "generally recognized as safe" (GRAS). That threat elicited an immediate response from soft drink manufacturers, which led to the founding of the International Life Sciences Institute (ILSI) (James 1994, 2002; Pendergrast 1999). Headquartered in Washington, DC, ILSI expanded rapidly to include an extensive global network of corporate members with interests beyond caffeine. Today, "membership is open to all companies active in the food or food-related sector, as well as companies engaged in the manufacture of medicinal products and products for human consumption and producers of ingredients [including agrochemicals] used in the food supply chain" (https://ilsi.eu/community/our-members/). While describing itself as a "nonprofit federation dedicated to generating and advancing emerging science," ILSI has come to be widely recognized for its sustained attempts to influence public policy in favour of industry interests to the detriment of public health (Demortain 2018; Greenhalgh 2019, 2021; Grimm 2016; James 2002; MacDonald 2001; Mialon et al. 2024; Steele et al. 2020, 2022; Strassheim and Loer 2019; Zeltner 2000). Once mobilized to counter the threat that caffeine may be removed from the FDA's GRAS list, ILSI was well-positioned to counter new threats, such as a 1980 FDA warning about caffeine and pregnancy (Goyan 1980). ILSI influence has been brought to bear primarily through its Caffeine Working Group and a multitude of affiliated industry organizations, including the American Beverage Association and the National Coffee Association. A recurring feature of industry-affiliated commentary has been the promotion of a spurious narrative that seeks to portray evidence of caffeine-related harm as untrustworthy. For example, one review concluded that the "evidence does not support *a positive relationship* between caffeine consumption and adverse reproductive or perinatal outcomes" (Peck et al. 2010, p. 2573, emphasis added), while in a similar vein another concluded that daily consumption of caffeine is "*not associated* with adverse reproductive and developmental effects" (Wikoff et al. 2017, p. 637, emphasis added). Yet, the self-same industry-affiliated commentaries cannot escape acknowledging that maternal caffeine consumption *is* associated with (i.e., has a "positive relationship" with) negative pregnancy outcomes. What these ILSI-affiliated authors (e.g., Peck et al. 2010; Wikoff et al. 2017) have sought to do is to *conflate* association with causation. That is, legitimate questions about *causation* have been used to make false claims about absence of *association*, when all commentators (including those who wish to discredit the evidence) agree that multiple caffeine-associated negative pregnancy outcomes are an established fact.

As for legitimate questions about causation, the main threats to causal inference of harm from maternal caffeine consumption are generally recognized to be potential confounding from extraneous variables, and possible misclassification of exposure and outcome variables. However, contrary to claims by ILSI-affiliated authors (Doepker et al. 2016, 2018; Peck et al. 2010; Wikoff et al. 2017) that the relevant studies may be characterized as having employed poor methodology, caffeine and pregnancy as a field of research is noteworthy for the effort that has been invested in the search for and control of potential confounders. Additionally, objective measurement has also often been used to minimize the risk of misclassification. Regarding potential confounding, diverse demographic variables, behavior patterns, and living environments have been repeatedly examined, including age at conception, health status, pregnancy history, use of oral contraceptives, smoking, alcohol, other substance use, exposure to pollutants, maternal body mass, physical activity, religion, education, and occupation. Among the many potential confounders, those accepted as being most likely, and the ones highlighted in ILSI-affiliated publications (Doepker et al. 2016, 2018; Peck et al. 2010; Wikoff et al. 2017), are pregnancy symptoms (also referred to as pregnancy signal symptoms), potential recall bias, maternal cigarette smoking, and approaches to measuring caffeine consumption.

Pregnancy Symptoms Symptoms such as nausea and vomiting in early pregnancy are predictive of a healthy pregnancy, and (as mentioned above) are often accompanied by a spontaneous reduction in caffeine intake (Meyer et al. 1994; Sapra et al. 2017). Accordingly, it has long been hypothesized that the association between negative pregnancy outcomes and maternal caffeine consumption could be due to a tendency among women who experience few symptoms of pregnancy and are at higher risk of experiencing negative pregnancy outcomes to also consume more caffeine (Stein and Susser 1991). However, that hypothesis has been extensively examined and has been repeatedly disconfirmed in diverse studies spanning more than three decades (Boylan et al. 2013; Gaskins et al. 2018; Giannelli et al. 2003; Matijasevich et al. 2006; Purdue-Smithe et al. 2019; Stefanidou et al. 2011; Stein and Susser 1991; Wen et al. 2001; Weng et al. 2008).

Recall Bias Recall bias in relation to amount of caffeine consumed during pregnancy has long been offered as a possible source of confounding, especially by commentators with caffeine-industry affiliations (Doepker et al. 2016, 2018; Peck et al. 2010; Wikoff et al. 2017). However, considering the large body of prospective cohort studies in which caffeine exposure was measured, sometimes involving confirmation by objective biomarkers, before conception and/or during early pregnancy, before knowledge of pregnancy outcomes, recall bias is not a plausible challenge to evidence of harm from maternal caffeine consumption.

Maternal Smoking Prospective measurement, sometimes involving the use of biomarkers, has shown that cigarette smoking is an unlikely source of serious confounding. Indeed, concerns about smoking as a source of confounding may be considered conclusively disconfirmed by the frequent reports of significant caffeine-related negative pregnancy outcomes in nonsmokers and never smokers (Bech et al. 2015; CARE Study Group 2008; Cnattingius et al. 2000; Gaskins et al. 2018; Giannelli et al. 2003; Greenwood et al. 2010; Khoury et al. 2004; Matijasevich et al. 2006; Menegaux et al. 2007; Milne et al. 2011; Stefanidou et al. 2011; Weng et al. 2008; Wisborg et al. 2003).

Measuring Caffeine Consumption Notwithstanding the likely absence of recall bias, lack of consistency in the specific methods used to measure caffeine consumption during pregnancy could account for inconsistencies in findings. In most studies, caffeine intake during pregnancy was assessed by means of a self-report questionnaire, administered in person or by mail. Typically, participants were asked to report the number of servings (e.g., cups, mugs, glasses, or bottles) of caffeine beverages (typically, coffee, tea, caffeinated soft drinks, and energy drinks), with responses often being aggregated to derive estimates of milligrams of caffeine consumed per day. In some studies, participants reported information concerning the method of preparation (e.g., instant, espresso, percolated, or filtered coffee). Studies often provided little or no information concerning the reliability and validity of the measurements used, although there are notable exceptions (e.g., Modzelewska et al. 2019; Sengpiel et al. 2013). Only infrequently have observational studies employed an objective biomarker of caffeine exposure in the form of serum paraxanthine, the primary metabolite of caffeine. That omission, which has been typical even in studies that obtained blood samples for other purposes, is disappointing given that the relevant testing protocols for measuring paraxanthine in blood and saliva are well-established and routine. While the absence is regrettable and may explain some inconsistencies in findings, failure to objectively measure caffeine intake is not a credible ground for dismissing the persistent and extensive body of positive associations reported to exist between maternal caffeine consumption and negative pregnancy outcomes and negative outcomes in offspring.

10.3.2 Are Randomized Controlled Trials the Solution?

Notwithstanding the record of strong controls against potential confounding in the extant body of observational studies of caffeine and pregnancy, it is reasonable to consider whether the research would yield clearer answers were randomized controlled trials employed. That question was the subject of a meta-analysis (Jahanfar and Jaafar 2015), which identified only one relevant study (Bech et al. 2007) in which coffee-consuming women at about the twentieth week of pregnancy were randomly assigned to two groups. The women were supplied with coffee (either regular or decaffeinated) and asked to consume the supplied coffee in place of their usual product. From the results, the authors concluded that a "moderate reduction in caffeine intake in the second half of pregnancy has no effect on birth weight or length of gestation" (Bech et al. 2007, p. 5). However, the trial results are of doubtful value due to several limitations. Notably, the trial is relevant only to questions about potential outcomes attributable to caffeine consumption during the latter stages of pregnancy. In contrast, virtually all the relevant science agrees that caffeine-related disruption of adenosine modulation is a threat to the developing fetus throughout pregnancy and perhaps especially in the first trimester of pregnancy (Darakjian and Kaddoumi 2019; Grosso and Bracken 2005).

In addition, there was evidently a substantial level of participant noncompliance to the requirements of the study. Specifically, participants reported drinking coffee other than that which had been supplied, and only about half in both groups returned diaries in which they had been requested to record their caffeine intake (Bech et al. 2007). Furthermore, in addition to questioning the soundness of the Bech et al. (2007) study, Jahanfar and Jaafar (2015) raised the more general question concerning the ethicality of involving pregnant women in randomized controlled trials of caffeine. They argued that such studies "would be unethical if a harmful outcome could be anticipated" (p. 11) for pregnant women who might otherwise have discontinued coffee consumption but were encouraged by the study protocol to continue consuming coffee.

10.3.3 The Persistent Disjunction Between Empirical Findings and Advice Guidelines

Early Concerns Knowledge of caffeine pharmacology provides strong theoretical justification for questioning whether consumption of the drug during pregnancy poses risks. That the developing fetus of a caffeine-consuming mother-to-be is exposed to concentrations of the drug equal to systemic levels in the mother heightens the salience of the question. Moreover, caffeine has no known nutritional benefit for either mother or baby. Thus, it is unsurprising that recognition of the high theoretical plausibility of harm and absence of benefit encouraged early experimentation with rodents (mice and rats). That research has revealed a range of caffeine-induced fetal abnormalities, including cleft palate, ectrodactyly (absent or deformed digits), and skeletal malformations (Fujii and Nishimura 1972; Nishimura and Nakai 1960; Palm et al. 1978; Terada and Nishimura 1975). As mentioned above, responding to early findings, the FDA issued a warning advising pregnant women to restrict or eliminate coffee consumption (Goyan 1980). The warning elicited wide discussion, including sustained opposition from caffeine-beverage industries (James 2002). Many comments focused on the fact that animal studies often used caffeine doses exceeding the levels typical of human dietary intake (Thayer and Palm 1975), thereby drawing into question the adequacy of the animal models that had been used to test the potential harm of caffeine for humans.

Indeed, early epidemiologic studies typically reported little by way of significant associations between caffeine and/or coffee consumption and birth defects of the kind reported in animal studies (Furuhashi et al. 1985; Kurppa et al. 1983; Linn et al. 1982; McDonald et al. 1992; Rosenberg et al. 1982). The inference, which continues to be widely accepted, is that typical patterns of caffeine consumption are an unlikely cause of physical birth defects in humans. However, the comfort that inference has encouraged ignores the fact that *teratology*, the scientific study of conditions caused by the interruption or alteration of normal development, includes not only the study of congenital morphological defects but also the study of diverse physical outcomes, including fatalities, as well as less obvious behavioural and emotional anomalies. Moreover, the usual safety standard employed by the FDA in relation to the human consumption of food additives is one-hundredth the maximum safe level of exposure in animals (Renwick 1993), a margin of safety that for decades has "proven to be reliably protective of public health" (Rulis and Levitt 2009, p. 5). By that standard, virtually any pattern of regular caffeine consumption by a woman who is pregnant would be viewed as putting her unborn child at risk. Thus, notwithstanding questions regarding the generalizability of animal findings to humans, the implication is clear: Applying the FDA's usual standards, pregnant women should abstain from caffeine. Furthermore, claims regarding possible non-generalizability of animal findings tend to ignore recent animal research in which caffeine exposure levels have been carefully chosen to mimic human consumption patterns (e.g., Fazeli et al. 2017; Zappettini et al. 2019).

The Current Situation As mentioned, much current advice about maternal caffeine consumption is guided by the idea that "moderate" caffeine consumption during pregnancy is safe. However, recommendations advising "moderation" are without a scientific foundation. For example, the US Dietary Guidelines Advisory Committee used a meta-analysis by Greenwood et al. (2014) as its main source for concluding that the "risk of miscarriage, stillbirth, low birth weight, and SGA births is minimal" (DGAC 2015, p. 303). Yet, the very evidence reviewed by the Advisory Committee shows that its claim of "minimal" risk is misleading. Neither Greenwood et al. (2014) nor the DGAC (2015) attempted to estimate the potential burden of disease implied by the risk estimates the former reported and the latter accepted. When such estimates are attempted, the cumulative population effects on the outcomes reported by Greenwood et al. (2014) are shown to be anything but "minimal."

Part of the problem here is that the contribution of moderate caffeine consumption to negative pregnancy outcomes and negative outcomes in offspring does not leave an indelible footprint in its wake. Thus, it is important to stress that for those who have experienced a negative pregnancy outcome, caffeine is but one of a plethora of potential contributing factors. There is simply no basis for making a specific assessment about the possible contribution of caffeine at the level of the individual case. Conversely, it is equally important to understand that whereas caffeine-related increased risk of harm may be relatively small at the individual level, even a small increased individual risk when aggregated across populations may be far from trivial (James 2016). Geoffrey Rose, the eminent British epidemiologist, expressed the relevant principle well when he stated, "A population-wide preventive measure [in this instance, avoidance of caffeine during pregnancy] may offer a disappointingly trivial benefit to individuals, but yet its cumulative benefit for the population as a whole can be unexpectedly large" (Rose 1992, p. 102).

As such, it is instructive to hypothesize what might be the population impact if all pregnant women consumed caffeine at the widely reputed moderate level of 200 mg per day. Note that this level of consumption is less than the 300 mg per day, which the DGAC (2020) claims in its revised *Dietary Guidelines for Americans, 2020–2025*, "*usually* does not adversely affect the infant" (emphasis added, p. 118). Using the Greenwood et al. (2014) estimates of caffeine-related harm, Table 10.5 summarizes computational steps for estimating the possible population impact on the four major negative outcomes of miscarriage, stillbirth, LBW, and SGA. The table predicts that were this hypothesized scenario to occur, the population-wide "safe" level of consumption could be responsible for 347,488 negative pregnancy outcomes per year in the United States alone, adding about one quarter to the current yearly total. While any such computational process is subject to inflationary or deflationary error, the estimated total in this instance might reasonably be considered an underestimate of the total potential harm. This is because the estimated harmful outcomes itemized in Table 10.5 relate to only four specified outcomes, while ignoring childhood acute leukemia and childhood overweight/obesity, for which there is good evidence of caffeine-related harm, and other possible negative outcomes that have yet to be identified.

Although the *2020–2025 Guidelines* (DGAC 2020) claim that maternal caffeine consumption of 300 mg per day "usually" has no adverse effects, there is a hint of circumspection in the

Table 10.5 Summary of estimated negative pregnancy outcomes in the hypothetical event that all pregnant women consumed caffeine at reputedly "moderate and safe" levels

	(i)	(ii)	(iii)	(iv)	(v)
Outcome	Risk (%) per 100 mg[a] (95% CI)	Risk (%) at 200 mg[b] (column (i) × 2)	Incidence of events (%)	Total number of events	Caffeine-related events (product of columns (ii) and (iv))
Miscarriage	14 (10–19)	28	16.67[c]	circa 1,000,000[c]	280,000
Stillbirth	19 (5–35)	38	0.6[d]	24,000[e]	9120
LBW	7 (1–12)	14	8.28[f]	331,200[e]	46,368
SGA	10 (6–14)	20	1.5[g]	60,000[e]	12,000
				1,415,200	347,488

Note. The contents of this table are a compilation of statistics from different sources, and are broadly representative of the more than 60 million women in the United States between the ages of 15 and 44 years (Martin et al. 2017, 2018)
[a]Greenwood et al. (2014) as part of dose-response associations having no threshold of caffeine intake below which negative events were absent
[b]Extrapolating from Greenwood et al. (2014) estimated risk for maternal caffeine consumption at the widely endorsed "safe" level of 200 mg per day
[c]Estimates of incidence of pregnancy "loss" are inevitably approximate. Among roughly 6 million pregnancies per year in the United States, an estimated one-third end in loss comprised of 1 million each of miscarriages and induced abortions (Curtin et al. 2013; Sapra et al. 2017)
[d]Percentage of all births (Hoyert and Gregory 2016)
[e]Product of column (iii) and the approximate total of 4 million births
[f]Percentage of all births (Martin et al. 2017)
[g]Percentage of all births (Ewing et al. 2017)
LBW low birth weight, *SGA* small for gestational age

advice. Namely, the *Guidelines* state that women "who could be or who are pregnant should consult their healthcare providers for advice concerning caffeine consumption" (DGAC 2020, p. 118). We may guess that this revision of earlier, less equivocal advice is an attempt at caution, possibly reflecting growing awareness of evidence of harm associated with maternal caffeine consumption. However, such equivocation is disappointing, especially when viewed in the context of the DGAC's (2020) self-proclaimed aim to provide clear and direct dietary advice. Moreover, despite this issue being of relevance to most women, FDA advice is equally marred by procrastination. Currently, it advises "if you're pregnant, trying to become pregnant, or breastfeeding, we recommend talking to your health care provider about whether you need to limit caffeine consumption" (FDA 2024, p. 1). As such, both the DGAC (2020) and FDA (2024) have opted to transfer responsibility to an ill-defined group of "healthcare providers," the large majority of whom may be assumed to have limited specialist knowledge of the topic. On the contrary, most are likely to have been exposed to the "moderation" narrative, which, if anything, encourages complacency regarding maternal caffeine consumption.

Notwithstanding current prevarication within some quarters, something approaching a consensus has emerged among other major authorities wherein a limit of 200 mg caffeine per day is currently widely advised. For example, the American College of Obstetricians and Gynecologists advises that "moderate caffeine consumption [of] less than 200 milligrams per day" (ACOG 2024). Similarly, the European Food Safety Authority states that maternal caffeine consumption of up to 200 mg per day during pregnancy does "not give rise to safety concerns for the fetus" (EFSA 2024), and the UK National Health Service advises pregnant women to consume "no more than 200 mg per day" (NHS 2024). While a proportion of pregnant women consume little or no caffeine, many throughout the world regularly consume more than the reputedly safe level of 200 mg caffeine per day (Galéra et al. 2016; Hoyt et al. 2014; Lehtonen et al. 2021). For example, 41% of a cohort of pregnant women in Finland were found to be consuming more than the EFSA recommended maximum of 200 mg per day (Lehtonen et al. 2021) and 25% of a cohort of pregnant Dutch women were found to be consuming more than 250 mg caffeine per day (Loomans et al. 2012). Despite evidence of the absence of a threshold of consumption below which caffeine is safe, current guidelines may encourage complacency regarding maternal caffeine consumption by promulgating a mistaken belief in reputed safe levels of intake.

Misinformation and Bias As argued above, it is important to remain alert to industry's role in promoting misinformation about the reputed safety of caffeine consumed during pregnancy. In addition to the sanitized accounts that have appeared in industry-affiliated publications (e.g., Doepker et al. 2016, 2018; Peck et al. 2010; Wikoff et al. 2017), industry groups, such as ISLI, have long sought to influence public policy through direct engagement with national and global health authorities (e.g., Demortain 2018; Greenhalgh 2019, 2021; Grimm 2016; James 2002; MacDonald 2001; Mialon et al. 2024; Steele et al. 2020, 2022; Strassheim and Loer 2019; Zeltner 2000). Such attempts by well-funded sources to skew scientific knowledge in favour of for-profit vested interests must be resisted. The public's stake in women's health is of a magnitude that calls for calm reflection and preparedness for sober engagement with the evidence concerning caffeine-related negative pregnancy outcomes and negative outcomes in offspring (James 2021a, b).

Future Research For the present, it is not possible to be highly prescriptive about preferred directions for future research. Animal experimentation offers the substantial advantage of permitting controlled manipulations of caffeine exposure and should be pursued with a view to informing researchers concerning relatively unexplored areas of potential harm in humans (e.g., harm to fetal brain structures). Alas, comparable levels of experimental control, such as may be achieved in randomized controlled trials with humans, although theoretically possible, are unlikely to be conducted due to questionable ethicality (Jahanfar and Jaafar 2015). Consequently, advances in the field are likely to depend on continued epidemiological investigation. Here, much benefit would accrue with the adoption of reliable and validated standardized measurement protocols for assessing caffeine exposure, such as has been in use for some time in the Norwegian Mother and Child Cohort Study (Modzelewska et al. 2019; Sengpiel et al. 2013). Similarly, continued vigilance concerning the control of potential confounders is important, including, where possible the use of biological indicators of exposure, not only for caffeine, but also for the use of other substances such as nicotine and alcohol.

However, it was *not* the intention of the present review to dwell on specifics concerning directions and possible improvements for future research. Doing so risks encouraging further prevarication and delay regarding a public health matter which, based on existing knowledge, requires urgent action. The published evidence reviewed here shows beyond reasonable doubt that maternal caffeine consumption is a likely cause of a host of negative pregnancy outcomes and negative outcomes in offspring. Whereas new and improved knowledge is always welcome (e.g., further study of possible harm to childhood neurobehavioral development), immediate action in the public health sphere is warranted based on existing knowledge of harm. Chronic exposure during pregnancy to chemical substances of any description is always cause for concern. Caffeine, a substance possessing no nutritional value, is consumed daily by most pregnant women. Accordingly, drawing upon well-founded extant knowledge, public health guidance advising avoidance of caffeine during pregnancy can and should be implemented as a matter of urgency.

10.4 Conclusions

The findings of a large corpus of research comprising original studies, systematic reviews, and meta-analyses may be broadly summarized as follows: Caffeine consumed during pregnancy possesses high biological plausibility of harm; evidence of harm has been revealed in numerous human observational studies; there is strong agreement among systematic reviews and meta-analyses of caffeine-induced negative pregnancy outcomes and negative outcomes in offspring; findings have been shown to be robust to threats from confounding and measurement misclassification; dose-response associations have been frequently reported; and multiple studies have reported that there is no threshold of caffeine consumption below which negative pregnancy outcomes and negative outcomes in offspring are absent. Evidence of harm is strong in relation to miscarriage, stillbirth, and low birth weight and/or small for gestational age; somewhat less strong for childhood acute leukemia; with further indications of possible harm for childhood overweight and obesity. Of the major outcomes reviewed, findings for preterm birth alone indicate little or no increased risk, whereas further studies are needed to establish whether maternal caffeine consumption is harmful for childhood neurobehavioral development. Thus, the principal finding of the present review is that maternal caffeine consumption is a source of serious harm. Evidence of harm provides compelling grounds for rejecting current advice regarding the reputed safety of "moderate" caffeine consumption during pregnancy. Rather, pregnant women and women contemplating pregnancy should be advised to desist from consuming caffeine beverages.

Conflict of Interest The author states that there is no conflict of interest.

References

Aldridge A, Aranda JV, Neims MD (1979) Caffeine metabolism in the newborn. Clin Pharmacol Ther 25: 447–453

Aldridge A, Bailey J, Neims AH (1981) The disposition of caffeine during and after pregnancy. Semin Perinatol 5: 310–314

American College of Obstetricians and Gynecologists (ACOG) (2024) How much coffee can I drink while I'm pregnant? https://www.acog.org/womens-health/experts-and-stories/ask-acog/how-much-coffee-can-i-drink-while-pregnant. Accessed 13 Nov 2024.

American Psychiatric Association (2022) Diagnostic and statistical manual of mental disorders, fifth edition revised (DSM-5-TR). American Psychiatric Association, Washington, DC

Arnaud MJ (1987) The pharmacology of caffeine. Prog Drug Res 31:273–313

Ashihara H, Crozier A (2001) Caffeine: A well known but little mentioned compound in plant science. Trends Plant Sci 6:407–413

Ayoub A, Yaseen M (2022) Relationship between caffeine or coffee consumption and miscarriage: findings from systematic review and meta-analysis. J Health Inform Dev Ctries 16(1)

Bakker R, Steegers EA, Obradov A et al (2010) Maternal caffeine intake from coffee and tea, fetal growth, and the risks of adverse birth outcomes: the Generation R Study. Am J Clin Nutr 91:1691–1698

Bech BH, Autrup H, Nohr EA et al (2006) Stillbirth and slow metabolizers of caffeine: comparison by genotypes. Int J Epidemiol 35:948–953

Bech BH, Obel C, Henriksen TB, Olsen J (2007) Effect of reducing caffeine intake on birth weight and length of gestation: randomised controlled trial. BMJ 334:409

Bech BH, Frydenberg M, Henriksen TB et al (2015) Coffee consumption during pregnancy and birth weight: does smoking modify the association? J Caffeine Res 5:65–72

Bekkhus M, Skjøthaug T, Nordhagen R, Borge AI (2010) Intrauterine exposure to caffeine and inattention/overactivity in children. Acta Paediatrica 99:925–928

Berglundh S, Vollrath M, Brantsæter AL et al (2021) Maternal caffeine intake during pregnancy and child neurodevelopment up to eight years of age: results from the Norwegian Mother, Father and Child Cohort Study. Eur J Nutr 60:791–780

Bernard JY, Heude B, Galéra C (2016) Maternal caffeine intake during pregnancy and child cognition and behavior at 4 and 7 years of age. Am J Epidemiol 183:871–872

Biaggioni I, Paul S, Puckett A, Arzubiaga C (1991) Caffeine and theophylline as adenosine receptor antagonists in humans. J Pharmacol Exp Ther 258: 588–593

Bonaventure A, Rudant J, Goujon-Bellec S et al (2013) Childhood acute leukemia, maternal beverage intake during pregnancy, and metabolic polymorphisms. Cancer Causes Control 24:783–793

Boylan SM, Greenwood DC, Alwan N et al (2013) Does nausea and vomiting of pregnancy play a role in the association found between maternal caffeine intake and fetal growth restriction? Matern Child Health J 17:601–608

Bracken MB, Triche EW, Belanger K, Hellenbrand K, Leaderer BP (2003) Association of maternal caffeine consumption with decrements in fetal growth. Am J Epidemiol 157:456–466

Brazier JL, Salle B (1981) Conversion of theophylline to caffeine by the human fetus. Semin Perinatol 5:315–320

Buscariollo DL, Fang X, Greenwood V et al (2014) Embryonic caffeine exposure acts via A1 adenosine receptors to alter adult cardiac function and DNA methylation in mice. PloS One 9:e87547

Bush A, Busst CM, Clarke B, Barnes PJ (1989) Effect of infused adenosine on cardiac output and systemic resistance in normal subjects. Br J Clin Pharmacol 27:165–171

CARE Study Group (2008) Maternal caffeine intake during pregnancy and risk of fetal growth restriction: a large prospective observational study. BMJ 337:a233

Carrier O, Pons G, Rey E et al (1988) Maturation of caffeine metabolic pathways in infancy. Clin Pharmacol Ther 44:45–151

Chen LW, Wu Y, Neelakantan N et al (2014) Maternal caffeine intake during pregnancy is associated with risk of low birth weight: a systematic review and dose response meta-analysis. BMC Med 12:174

Chen LW, Wu Y, Neelakantan N et al (2016) Maternal caffeine intake during pregnancy and risk of pregnancy loss: a categorical and dose–response meta-analysis of prospective studies. Public Health Nutr 19:1233–1244

Chen LW, Fitzgerald R, Murrin CM et al (2018) Associations of maternal caffeine intake with birth outcomes: results from the Lifeways Cross Generation Cohort Study. Am J Clin Nutr 108:1301–1308

Chen L-W, Murrin CM, Mehegan J et al (2019) Maternal, but not paternal or grandparental, caffeine intake is associated with childhood obesity and adiposity: the Lifeways Cross-Generation Cohort Study. Am J Clin Nutr 109:1648–1655

Cheng J, Su H, Zhu R et al (2014) Maternal coffee consumption during pregnancy and risk of childhood acute leukemia: a metaanalysis. Am J Obstet Gynecol 210: 151–1e1

Chiaffarino F, Parazzini F, Chatenoud L et al (2006) Coffee drinking and risk of preterm birth. Eur Clin Nutr 60:610–613

Christensen ZP, Freedman EG, Foxe JJ (2021) Caffeine exposure in utero is associated with structural brain alterations and deleterious neurocognitive outcomes in 9–10 year old children. Neuropharmacology 186: 108479

Chvasta TE, Cooke AR (1971) Absorption and emptying of caffeine from the human stomach. Gastroenterology 61:838–843

Clausson B, Granath F, Ekbom A et al (2002) Effect of caffeine exposure during pregnancy on birth weight and gestational age. Am J Epidemiol 155:429–436

Cnattingius S, Signorello LB, Anneren G et al (2000) Caffeine intake and the risk of first-trimester spontaneous abortion. N Engl J Med 343:1839–1845

Cunha RA, Ferré S, Vaugeois J-M, Chen J-F (2008) Potential therapeutic interest of adenosine A_{2A} receptors in psychiatric disorders. Curr Pharm Des 14:1512–1524

Curtin SC, Abma JC, Ventura SJ, Henshaw SK (2013) Pregnancy rates for U.S. women continue to drop. National Center for Health Statistics Data Brief, No. 136. Centers for Disease Control and Prevention, Washington, DC

Darakjian LI, Kaddoumi A (2019) Physiologically based pharmacokinetic/pharmacodynamic model for caffeine disposition in pregnancy. Mol Pharmaceutics 16: 1340–1349

Del Castillo N, Jiménez-Moleón JJ, Olmedo-Requena R et al (2015) Perinatal outcomes of prematurity and birth weight according to maternal caffeine consumption. Nutr Hosp 32:2658–2664

Del-Ponte B, Santos IS, Tovo-Rodrigues L et al (2016) Caffeine consumption during pregnancy and ADHD at the age of 11 years: a birth cohort study. BMJ Open 6: e012749

Demortain D (2018) Are scientists agents of corporate power on public policy? Corporations and the use of science for diffuse lobbying strategies. Paper presented at the Pervasive powers, corporate authority and public policy conference. Université Paris-Dauphine, Paris

Dietary Guidelines Advisory Committee (DGAC) (2015) Scientific report of the 2015 Dietary Guidelines Advisory Committee: Advisory report to the Secretary of Health and Human Services and the Secretary of Agriculture. U.S. Department of Agriculture, Agricultural Research Service, Washington, DC. https://health.gov/sites/default/files/2019-09/Scientific-Report-of-the-2015-Dietary-Guidelines-Advisory-Committee.pdf

Dietary Guidelines Advisory Committee (DGAC) Dietary Guidelines for Americans, 2020–2025 (2020) US Department of Agriculture and US Department of Health and Human Services, 9th Edition December 2020. https://www.dietaryguidelines.gov/sites/default/files/2021-03/Dietary_Guidelines_for_Americans-2020-2025.pdf

Doepker C, Lieberman HR, Smith AP et al (2016) Caffeine: friend or foe? Annu Rev Food Sci Technol 7: 117–137

Doepker C, Franke K, Myers E et al (2018) Key findings and implications of a recent systematic review of the potential adverse effects of caffeine consumption in healthy adults, pregnant women, adolescents, and children. Nutrients 10:1536. https://doi.org/10.3390/nu10101536

Dumas M, Gouyon JB, Tenenbaum D et al (1982) Systematic determination of caffeine plasma concentrations at birth in preterm and full-term infants. Dev Pharmacol Therap 4:182–186

Dunlop M, Court JM (1981) Effects of maternal caffeine ingestion on neonatal growth in rats. Neonatology 39: 178–184

Dunwiddie TV, Masino SA (2001) The role and regulation of adenosine in the central nervous system. Annu Rev Neurosci 24:31–55

European Food Safety Authority (EFSA) (2024) Caffeine. https://www.efsa.europa.eu/en/topics/topic/caffeine. Accessed 13 Nov 2024

Evans SM, Griffiths RR (1991) Dose-related caffeine discrimination in normal volunteers: individual differences in subjective effects and self-reported cues. Behav Pharmacol 2:345–356

Ewing AC, Ellington SR, Shapiro-Mendoza CK et al (2017) Full-term small-for-gestational-age newborns in the US: characteristics, trends, and morbidity. Matern Child Health J 21:786–796

Fazeli W, Zappettini S, Marguet SL et al (2017) Early-life exposure to caffeine affects the construction and activity of cortical networks in mice. Exp Neurol 295:88–103

Fernandes O, Sabharwal M, Smiley T et al (1998) Moderate to heavy caffeine consumption during pregnancy and relationship to spontaneous abortion and abnormal fetal growth: a meta-analysis. Reprod Toxicol 12:435–444

Ferré S (2016) Mechanisms of the psychostimulant effects of caffeine: Implications for substance use disorders. Psychopharmacol 233:1963–1979

Foxx RM, Rubinoff A (1979) Behavioral treatment of caffeinism: Reducing excessive coffee drinking. J App Behav Anal 12:344–355

Franchetti P, Messini L, Cappellacci L et al (1994) 8-Azaxanthine derivatives as antagonists of adenosine receptors. J Med Chem 37:2970–1975

Frary CD, Johnson RK, Wang MQ (2005) Food sources and intakes of caffeine in the diets of persons in the United States. J Am Diet Assoc 105:110–113

Frayer NC, Kim Y (2020) Caffeine intake during pregnancy and risk of childhood obesity: a systematic review. Int J MCH AIDS 9(3):364

Fujii T, Nishimura H (1972) Adverse effects of prolonged administration of caffeine on rat fetus. Toxicol Appl Pharmacol 22:449–457

Fulgoni VL III, Keast DR, Lieberman HR (2015) Trends in intake and sources of caffeine in the diets of US adults: 2001–2010. Am J Nutr 101:1081–1087

Furuhashi N, Sato S, Suzuki M et al (1985) Effects of caffeine ingestion during pregnancy. Gynecol Obstet Invest 19:187–191

Galéra C, Bernard JY, van der Waerden J et al (2016) Prenatal caffeine exposure and child IQ at age 5.5 years: the EDEN mother-child cohort. Biol Psychiatry 80:720–726

Galletly DC, Fennelly M, Whitwam JG (1989) Does caffeine withdrawal contribute to postanaesthetic morbidity? Lancet 1:1335

Garrett BE, Holtzman SG (1994) D1 and D2 dopamine receptor antagonists block caffeine-induced stimulation of locomotor activity in rats. Pharmacol Biochem Behav 47:89–94

Gaskins AJ, Rich-Edwards JW, Williams PL et al (2018) Pre-pregnancy caffeine and caffeinated beverage intake and risk of spontaneous abortion. Eur J Nutr 57:107–117

Giannelli M, Doyle P, Roman E et al (2003) The effect of caffeine consumption and nausea on the risk of miscarriage. Paediatr Perinatal Epidemiol 17:316–323

Gilbert RM (1984) Caffeine consumption. In: Spiller GA (ed) The methylxanthine beverages and foods: chemistry, consumption, and health effects. Alan R. Liss, New York, pp 185–214

Gilbert EF, Pistey WR (1973) Effect on the offspring of repeated caffeine administration to pregnant rats. Reproduction 34:495–499

Glaser T, Martins P, Beco R et al (2024) Impairment of adenosine signalling disrupts early embryo development: unveiling the underlying mechanisms. Front Pharmacol 14:1328398

Goldstein A, Warren R (1962) Passage of caffeine into human gonadal and fetal tissue. Biochem Pharmacol 11:166–168

Goyan J (1980) Food and Drug Administration news release, no. P80-36, Washington DC

Greenhalgh S (2019) Making China safe for coke: how Coca-Cola shaped obesity science and policy in China. BMJ 364:k5050

Greenhalgh S (2021) Inside ILSI. J Health Politics Policy Law 46(2):235–276

Greenwood DC, Alwan N, Boylan S et al (2010) Caffeine intake during pregnancy, late miscarriage and stillbirth. Eur J Epidemiol 25:275–280

Greenwood DC, Thatcher NJ, Ye J et al (2014) Caffeine intake during pregnancy and adverse birth outcomes: a systematic review and dose–response meta-analysis. Eur J Epidemiol 29:725–734

Griffiths RR, Bigelow GE, Liebson IA (1986) Human coffee drinking: reinforcing and physical dependence producing effects of caffeine. J Pharmacol Exp Ther 239:416–425

Griffiths RR, Evans SM, Heishman SJ et al (1990) Low-dose caffeine physical dependence in humans. J Pharmacol Exp Ther 255:1123–1132

Griffiths RR, Juliano LM, Chausmer AL (2003) Caffeine: pharmacology and clinical effects. In: Graham AW, Schultz TK, Mayo-Smith MF, Ries RK, Wilford BB (eds) Principles of addiction medicine, 3rd edn. American Society of Addiction Medicine, Chevy Chase, pp 134–193

Grimm H-U (2016) Information-domination in the European food industry: focus on Germany. In: Steier G, Patel K (eds) International food law and policy. Springer, Cham, pp 3–30

Grimm VE, Frieder B (1988) Prenatal caffeine causes long lasting behavioral and neurochemical changes. Int J Neurosci 41(1-2):15–28

Grosso LM, Bracken MB (2005) Caffeine metabolism, genetics, and perinatal outcomes: a review of exposure assessment considerations during pregnancy. Ann Epidemiol 15:460–466

Harler CR (1964) The culture and marketing of tea, 3rd edn. Oxford University Press, London

Heatherley SV, Hayward RC, Seers HE, Rogers PJ (2005) Cognitive and psychomotor performance, mood, and pressor effects of caffeine after 4, 6 and 8 h caffeine abstinence. Psychopharmacol 178:461–470

Heazell AE, Timms K, Scott RE et al (2021) Associations between consumption of coffee and caffeinated soft drinks and late stillbirth: findings from the Midland and North of England stillbirth case-control study. Eur J Obstet Gynecol Reprod Biol 256:471–477

Heckman MA, Weil J, Gonzalez de Mejia E (2010) Caffeine (1, 3, 7-trimethylxanthine) in foods: a comprehensive review on consumption, functionality, safety, and regulatory matters. J Food Sci 75:77–87

Horning MG, Butler CM, Nowlin J, Hill RB (1975) Drug metabolism in the human neonate. Life Sci 16:651–671

Hoyert DL, Gregory ECW (2016) Cause of fetal death: data from the fetal death report, 2014. National vital statistics reports, vol 65, no 7. Centers for Disease Control and Prevention, Washington, DC. https://www.cdc.gov/nchs/data/nvsr/nvsr65/nvsr65_07.pdf

Hoyt AT, Browne M, Richardson S et al (2014) Maternal caffeine consumption and small for gestational age births: results from a population-based case–control study. Matern Child Health J 18:1540–1551

Hughes JR, Higgins ST, Bickel WK et al (1991) Caffeine self-administration, withdrawal, and adverse effects among coffee drinkers. Archiv Gen Psychiatry 48: 611–617

Hughes JR, Oliveto AH, Helzer JE et al (1992) Should caffeine abuse, dependence or withdrawal be added to DSM-IV and ICD-10? Am J Psychiatry 149:33–40

Hughes JR, Oliveto AH, Bickel WK et al (1993) Caffeine self-administration and withdrawal: incidence, individual differences and interrelationships. Drug Alcohol Depend 32:239–246

Hunger SP, Mullighan CG (2015) Acute lymphoblastic leukemia in children. N Engl J Med 373:1541–1552

Jafari A, Naghshi S, Shahinfar H et al (2022) Relationship between maternal caffeine and coffee intake and pregnancy loss: a grading of recommendations assessment, development, and evaluation-assessed, dose-response meta-analysis of observational studies. Front Nutr 9:886224

Jahanfar S, Jaafar SH (2015) Effects of restricted caffeine intake by mother on fetal, neonatal and pregnancy outcomes. Cochrane Database Syst Rev Issue 6: CD006965. https://doi.org/10.1002/14651858.CD006965.pub4

James JE (1991) Caffeine and health. Academic, London

James JE (1994) Caffeine, health and commercial interests. Addiction 89:1595–1599

James JE (1997) Understanding caffeine: a biobehavioral analysis. Sage, Thousand Oaks

James JE (1998) Acute and chronic effects of caffeine on performance, mood, headache, and sleep. Neuropsychobiol 38:32–41

James JE (2002) 'Third-party' threats to research integrity in public–private partnerships. Addiction 97:1251–1255

James JE (2004) A critical review of dietary caffeine and blood pressure: a relationship that should be taken more seriously. Psychosom Med 66:63–71

James JE (2005) Caffeine-induced enhancement of cognitive performance: confounding due to reversal of withdrawal effects. Aust J Psychol 57:197–200

James JE (2016) The health of populations. Elsevier-Academic Press, London

James JE (2021a) Maternal caffeine consumption and pregnancy outcomes: A narrative review with implications for advice to mothers and mothers-to-be. BMJ Evid Based Med 26(3):114–115

James JE (2021b) Caffeine and pregnancy: the need for calm reflection. Reply to Murphy et al. [Letter]. BMJ Evid Based Med 25. Available: https://ebm.bmj.com/content/26/3/114.responses#caffeine-and-pregnancy-the-need-for-calm-reflection-reply-to-murphy-et-al

James JE, Keane MA (2007) Caffeine, sleep and wakefulness: implications of new understanding about withdrawal reversal. Hum Psychopharmacol Clin Exp 22: 549–558

James JE, Paull I (1985) Caffeine and human reproduction. Rev Environ Health 7:151–167

James JE, Rogers PJ (2005) Effects of caffeine on performance and mood: withdrawal reversal is the most plausible explanation. Psychopharmacol 182:1–8

James JE, Stirling KP, Hampton BAM (1985) Caffeine fading: behavioral treatment of caffeine abuse. Behav Ther 16:15–27

James JE, Paull I, Cameron-Traub E et al (1988) Biochemical validation of self-reported caffeine consumption during caffeine fading. J Behav Med 11:15–30

Jin F, Qiao C (2021) Association of maternal caffeine intake during pregnancy with low birth weight, childhood overweight, and obesity: a meta-analysis of cohort studies. Int J Obes 45(2):279–287

Juliano LM, Griffiths RR (2004) A critical review of caffeine withdrawal: Empirical validation of symptoms and signs, incidence, severity, and associated features. Psychopharmacol 176:1–29

Karalexi MA, Dessypris N, Clavel J et al (2019) Coffee and tea consumption during pregnancy and risk of childhood acute myeloid leukemia: a Childhood Leukemia International Consortium (CLIC) study. Cancer Epidemiol 62:101581

Khoury JC, Miodovnik M, Buncher CR et al (2004) Consequences of smoking and caffeine consumption during pregnancy in women with type 1 diabetes. J Matern Fetal Neonatal Med 15:44–50

Kimmel CA, Kimmel GL, White CG et al (1984) Blood flow changes and conceptual development in pregnant rats in response to caffeine. Fundam Appl Toxicol 4: 240–247

Kirkinen P, Jouppila P, Koivula A et al (1983) The effect of caffeine on placental and fetal blood flow in human pregnancy. Am J Obstet Gynecol 147:939–942

Klebanoff MA, Keim SA (2015) Maternal serum paraxanthine during pregnancy and offspring body mass index at ages 4 and 7 years. Epidemiol 26:185–191

Klebanoff MA, Keim SA (2016) Maternal caffeine intake during pregnancy and child cognition and behavior at 4 and 7 years of age. Am J Epidemiol 183:872–873

Klebanoff MA, Levine RJ, Clemens JD, Wilkins DG (2002) Maternal serum caffeine metabolites and small-for-gestational age birth. Am J Epidemiol 155: 32–37

Knutti R, Rothweiler H, Schlatter C (1982) Effect of pregnancy on the pharmacokinetics of caffeine. Eur J Clin Pharmacol 21:121–126

Kobayashi S, Sata F, Murata K et al (2019) Dose-dependent associations between prenatal caffeine consumption and small for gestational age, preterm birth, and reduced birthweight in the Japan Environment and Children's Study. Paediatr Perinat Epidemiol 33:185–194

Kukkonen A, Hantunen S, Voutilainen A et al (2024) Maternal caffeine intake during pregnancy and the risk of delivering a small for gestational age baby: Kuopio Birth Cohort. Arch Gynecol Obstet 310:359–368

Kurppa K, Holmberg PC, Kuosma E, Saxen L (1983) Coffee consumption during pregnancy and selected congenital malformations: a nation wide case-control study. Am J Public Health 73:1397–1399

Lane JD (1997) Effects of brief caffeine deprivation on mood, symptoms, and psychomotor performance. Pharmacol Biochem Behav 58:203–208

Lane JD, Phillips-Bute BG (1998) Caffeine deprivation affects vigilance performance and mood. Physiol Behav 65:171–175

Lane JD, Pieper CF, Phillips-Bute BG et al (2002) Caffeine affects cardiovascular and neuroendocrine activation at work and home. Psychosom Med 64:595–603

Lane JD, Hwang AL, Feinglos MN, Surwit RS (2007) Exaggeration of postprandial hyperglycemia in patients with type 2 diabetes by administration of caffeine in coffee. Endocrine Pract 13:239–243

LeBlanc J, Soucy J (1994) Hormonal dose–response to an adenosine receptor agonist. Can J Physiol Pharmacol 72:113–116

Lehtonen A, Uusitalo L, Auriola S et al (2021) Caffeine content in newborn hair correlates with maternal dietary intake. Eur J Nutr 60:193–201

Li J, Zhao H, Song JM et al (2015a) A meta-analysis of risk of pregnancy loss and caffeine and coffee consumption during pregnancy. Int J Gynaecol Obstet 130:116–122

Li J, Luo H, Wu Y et al (2015b) Gender-specific increase in susceptibility to metabolic syndrome of offspring rats after prenatal caffeine exposure with post-weaning high-fat diet. Toxicol Applied Pharmacol 284:345–353

Li Y, Zhang W, Shi R et al (2018) Prenatal caffeine damaged learning and memory in rat offspring mediated by ARs/PKA/CREB/BDNF pathway. Physiol Res 67:975–983

Lieberman HR, Wurtman RJ, Emde GG et al (1987) The effects of low doses of caffeine on human performance and mood. Psychopharmacol 92:308–312

Lieberman H, Marriott B, Judelson D et al (2015) Intake of caffeine from all sources including energy drinks and reasons for use in US college students. FASEB J 29: 392–391

Linn S, Schoenbaum SC, Monson RR et al (1982) No association between coffee consumption and adverse outcomes of pregnancy. NEJM 306:141–145

Linnet KM, Wisborg K, Secher NJ et al (2009) Coffee consumption during pregnancy and the risk of hyperkinetic disorder and ADHD: a prospective cohort study. Acta Paediatrica 98:173–179

Loomans EM, Hofland L, Van der Stelt O et al (2012) Caffeine intake during pregnancy and risk of problem behavior in 5-to 6-year-old children. Pediatrics 130: e305–e313

Lyngsø J, Ramlau-Hansen CH, Bay B et al (2017) Association between coffee or caffeine consumption and fecundity and fertility: A systematic review and dose-response meta-analysis. Clin Epidemiol 9:699–719

MacDonald R (2001) WHO says tobacco industry "used" institute to undermine its policies. BMJ 322:576

Madsen CN, Henriksen TB, Ramlau-Hansen CH et al (2020) Coffee intake during pregnancy and childhood acute leukemia – a cohort study. Cancer Epidemiol 67: 101747

Marangos PJ, Boulenger JP (1985) Basic and clinical aspects of adenosinergic neuromodulation. Neurosci Biobehav Rev 9:421–430

Martin JA, Hamilton BE, Osterma MJK et al (2017) Births: final data for 2015. National Vital Statistics Reports, vol 66, no 1. Centers for Disease Control and Prevention, Washington, DC. https://www.cdc.gov/nchs/data/nvsr/nvsr66/nvsr66_01.pdf

Martin JA, Hamilton BE, Osterma MJK et al (2018) Births: final data for 2017. National Vital Statistics Reports, vol 67, no 8. Centers for Disease Control

and Prevention, Washington, DC. https://www.cdc.gov/nchs/data/nvsr/nvsr67/nvsr67_08-508.pdf
Maslova E, Bhattacharya S, Lin SW, Michels KB (2010) Caffeine consumption during pregnancy and risk of preterm birth: a meta-analysis. Am J Clin Nutr 92: 1120–1132
Matijasevich A, Barros FC, Santos IS, Yemini A (2006) Maternal caffeine consumption and fetal death: a case–control study in Uruguay. Paediatr Perinat Epidemiol 20:100–109
Mayo Clinic (2025) Caffeine content for coffee, tea, soda and more. https://www.mayoclinic.org/healthy-lifestyle/nutrition-and-healthy-eating/in-depth/caffeine/art-20049372. Accessed 10 Apr 2025
McDonald AD, Armstrong BG, Sloan M (1992) Cigarette, alcohol, and coffee consumption and congenital defects. Am J Public Health 82:91–93
Menegaux F, Ripert M, Hémon D, Clavel J (2007) Maternal alcohol and coffee drinking, parental smoking and childhood leukaemia: a French population-based case–control study. Paediatr Perinat Epidemiol 21:293–299
Meyer LC, Peacock JL, Bland JM, Anderson HR (1994) Symptoms and health problems in pregnancy: their association with social factors, smoking, alcohol, caffeine and attitude to pregnancy. Paediatr Perinat Epidemiol 8:145–155
Mialon M, Serodio PM, Crosbie E et al (2024) Conflicts of interest for members of the US 2020 Dietary Guidelines Advisory Committee. Public Health Nutr 27(1):e69:1–13
Mikkelsen SH, Obel C, Olsen J et al (2017) Maternal caffeine consumption during pregnancy and behavioral disorders in 11-year-old offspring: a Danish National Birth Cohort study. J Pediatrics 189:120–127
Milne E, Royle JA, Bennett LC et al (2011) Maternal consumption of coffee and tea during pregnancy and risk of childhood ALL: results from an Australian case–control study. Cancer Causes Control 22:207–218
Milne E, Greenop KR, Petridou E et al (2018) Maternal consumption of coffee and tea during pregnancy and risk of childhood all: a pooled analysis from the Childhood Leukemia International Consortium. Cancer Causes Control 29:539–550
Modzelewska D, Bellocco R, Elfvin A et al (2019) Caffeine exposure during pregnancy, small for gestational age birth and neonatal outcome: results from the Norwegian Mother and Child Cohort Study. BMC Pregnancy Childbirth 19:1–11
Momoi N, Tinney JP, Liu LJ et al (2008) Modest maternal caffeine exposure affects developing embryonic cardiovascular function and growth. Am J Physiol Heart Circulatory Physiol 294:H2248–H2256
Nakamoto T, Roy G, Gottschalk SB et al (1991) Lasting effects of early chronic caffeine feeding on rats' behavior and brain in later life. Physiol Behav 49(4):721–727
Nishimura H, Nakai K (1960) Congenital malformations in offspring of mice treated with caffeine. Exp Biol Med 104:140–142
North KC, Chang J, Bukiya AN, Dopico AM (2018) Extra-endothelial TRPV1 channels participate in alcohol and caffeine actions on cerebral artery diameter. Alcohol 73:45–55
Okubo H, Miyake Y, Tanaka K et al (2015) Maternal total caffeine intake, mainly from Japanese and Chinese tea, during pregnancy was associated with risk of preterm birth: the Osaka Maternal and Child Health Study. Nutr Res 35:309–316
Orsi L, Rudant J, Ajrouche R et al (2015) Parental smoking, maternal alcohol, coffee and tea consumption during pregnancy, and childhood acute leukemia: the ESTELLE study. Cancer Causes Control 26:1003–1017
Palm PE, Arnold EP, Rachwall PC et al (1978) Evaluation of the teratogenic potential of fresh-brewed coffee and caffeine in the rat. Toxicol Appl Pharmacol 44:1–16
Papadopoulou E, Botton J, Brantsater A-L et al (2018) Maternal caffeine intake during pregnancy and childhood growth and overweight: results from a large Norwegian prospective observational cohort study. BMJ Open 8:e018895
Parsons WD, Neims AH (1981) Prolonged half-life of caffeine in healthy term newborn infants. J Pediatr 98:640–641
Paul S, Kurunwune B, Biaggioni I (1993) Caffeine withdrawal: apparent heterologous sensitization to adenosine and prostacyclin actions in human platelets. J Pharmacol Exp Ther 267:838–843
Pearlman SA, Duran C, Wood MA (1989) Caffeine pharmacokinetics in preterm infants older than 2 weeks. Dev Pharmacol Ther 12:65–69
Peck JD, Leviton A, Cowan LD (2010) A review of the epidemiologic evidence concerning the reproductive health effects of caffeine consumption: a 2000–2009 update. Food Chem Toxicol 48:2549–2576
Pendergrast M (1999) Uncommon grounds: the history of coffee and how it transformed our world. Basic Books, New York
Pfeifer RW, Notari RE (1988) Predicting caffeine plasma concentrations resulting from consumption of food or beverages: a simple method and its origin. Drug Intelligence Clin Pharm 22:953–959
Phillips-Bute BG, Lane JD (1998) Caffeine withdrawal symptoms following brief caffeine deprivation. Physiol Behav 63:35–39
Purdue-Smithe AC, Kim K, Schisterman EF et al (2019) Caffeinated beverage intake and serum caffeine metabolites and risk of pregnancy loss. Fertil Steril 112:e27
Rall TW (1990) Drugs used in the treatment of asthma. The methylxanthines, cromolyn sodium, and other agents. In: Gilman AG, Rall TW, Nies AS, Taylor P (eds) Goodman and Gilman's the pharmacological basis of therapeutics. Pergamon, New York, pp 618–637
Rasch V (2003) Cigarette, alcohol, and caffeine consumption: risk factors for spontaneous abortion. Acta Obstet Gynecol Scand 82:182–188

Renwick AG (1993) Data-derived safety factors for the evaluation of food additives and environmental contaminants. Food Addit Contam 10(3):275–305
Resch BA, Papp JG (1983) Effects of caffeine on the fetal heart. Am J Obstet Gynecol 146:231–232
Rhee J, Kim R, Kim Y (2015) Maternal caffeine consumption during pregnancy and risk of low birth weight: a dose-response meta-analysis of observational studies. PloS One 10:e0132334
Rivkees SA, Wendler CC (2011) Adverse and protective influences of adenosine on the newborn and embryo: implications for preterm white matter injury and embryo protection. Pediatr Res 69:271–278
Rivkees SA, Wendler CC (2017) Long-term consequences of disrupting adenosine signalling during embryonic development. Mol Asp Med 55:110–117
Robertson D, Wade D, Workman R et al (1981) Tolerance to the humoral and hemodynamic effects of caffeine in man. J Clin Invest. 67:1111–1117
Roden C (1977) Coffee. Faber & Faber, London
Rogers PJ, Heatherley SV, Mullings EL, Smith JE (2013) Faster but not smarter: effects of caffeine and caffeine withdrawal on alertness and performance. Psychopharmacol 226:229–240
Rose G (1992) The strategy of preventive medicine. Oxford University Press, Oxford
Rosenberg L, Mitchell AA, Shapiro S, Slone D (1982) Selected birth defects in relation to caffeine-containing beverages. JAMA 247:1429–1432
Rulis AM, Levitt JA (2009) FDA'S food ingredient approval process: Safety assurance based on scientific assessment. Regul Toxicol Pharmacol 53(1):20–31
Santana AB, Spelta LEW, Martinez-Sobalvarro JV et al (2024) Prenatal caffeine consumption and neurobehavioral disorders: a systematic review. Reprod Toxicol 108563
Santos IS, Victora CG, Huttly S, Morris S (1998) Caffeine intake and pregnancy outcomes: a meta-analytic review. Cad Saude Publica 14(3):523–530
Sapra KJ, Joseph KS, Galea S et al (2017) Signs and symptoms of early pregnancy loss: a systematic review. Reprod Sci 24:502–513
Sasaki S, Limpar M, Sata F et al (2017) Interaction between maternal caffeine intake during pregnancy and CYP1A2 C164A polymorphism affects infant birth size in the Hokkaido study. Pediatr Res 82:19–28
Savitz DA, Chan RL, Herring AH et al (2008) Caffeine and miscarriage risk. Epidemiol 19:55–62
Sengpiel V, Elind E, Bacelis J et al (2013) Maternal caffeine intake during pregnancy is associated with birth weight but not with gestational length: results from a large prospective observational cohort study. BMC Med. 11:1–18
Shalleck J (1981) Tea. Viking, New York
Shrestha B, Jawa G (2017) Caffeine citrate: is it a silver bullet in neonatology? Pediatr Neonatol 58(5): 391–397
Silva CG, Métin C, Fazeli W et al (2013) Adenosine receptor antagonists including caffeine alter fetal brain development in mice. Sci Transl Med 5:197–204
Sindiani AM, Khader Y, Amarin Z (2020) The association between coffee and tea consumption during pregnancy and preterm delivery: case-control study. J Multidiscip Health 13:2011–2019
Smit HJ, Rogers PJ (2000) Effects of caffeine on cognitive performance, mood and thirst in lower and higher caffeine consumers. Psychopharmacol 152:167–173
Smith AW (1985a) Introduction. In: Clarke RJ, Macrae R (eds) Coffee. Volume 1: Chemistry. Elsevier Applied Science, London, pp 1–41
Smith RF (1985b) A history of coffee. In: Clifford MN, Willson KC (eds) Coffee: botany, biochemistry and production of beans and beverage. Croom-Helm, London, pp 1–12
Soellner DE, Grandys T, Nuñez JL (2009) Chronic prenatal caffeine exposure impairs novel object recognition and radial arm maze behaviors in adult rats. Behavioural brain research 14;205(1):191–9
Soltani S, Salari-Moghaddam A, Saneei P et al (2022) Maternal caffeine consumption during pregnancy and risk of low birth weight: a dose–response meta-analysis of cohort studies. Crit Rev Food Sci Nutr 63(2): 224–233
Somani SM, Gupta P (1988) Caffeine: A new look at an age-old drug. Int J Clin Pharmacol Ther Toxicol 26: 521–533
Steele S, Ruskin G, Stuckler D (2020) Pushing partnerships: corporate influence on research and policy via the International Life Sciences Institute. Public Health Nutr 23(11):2032–2040
Steele S, Sarcevic L, Ruskin G, Stuckler D (2022) Confronting potential food industry "front groups": case study of the International Food Information Council's nutrition communications using the UCSF food industry documents archive. Glob Health 18(1): 16–25
Stefanidou EM, Caramellino L, Patriarca A, Menato G (2011) Maternal caffeine consumption and sine causa recurrent miscarriage. Eur J Obstet Gynecol Reprod Biol 158:220–224
Stein Z, Susser M (1991) Miscarriage, caffeine, and the epiphenomena of pregnancy: the causal model. Epidemiol 2:163–167
Strassheim H, Loer K (2019) Who are the policymakers and what are their interests? In: Ewert B, Loer K (eds) Behavioural policies for health promotion and disease prevention. Palgrave Pivot, Cham, pp 73–92
Terada M, Nishimura H (1975) Mitigation of caffeine induced teratogenicity in mice by prior chronic caffeine ingestion. Teratol 12:79–82
Thayer PS, Kensler CJ (1973) Exposure of four generations of mice to caffeine in drinking water. Toxicol Appl Pharmacol 25:169–179
Thayer P, Palm P (1975) A current assessment of mutagenic and teratogenic effects of caffeine. Crit Rev Toxicol 5:345–380

Thomopoulos TP, Ntouvelis E, Diamantaras AA et al (2015) Maternal and childhood consumption of coffee, tea and cola beverages in association with childhood leukemia: a meta-analysis. Cancer Epidemiol 39: 1047–1059

United Kingdom National Health Service (NHS) (2024) Foods to avoid in pregnancy. https://www.nhs.uk/pregnancy/keeping-well/foods-to-avoid/. Accessed 13 Nov 2024.

United States Food and Drug administration (FDA) (2024) Spilling the beans: how much caffeine is too much? https://www.fda.gov/consumers/consumer-updates/spilling-beans-how-much-caffeine-too-much. Accessed 13 Nov 2024.

Van't Hoff W (1982) Caffeine in pregnancy. Lancet 319: 1020

Vitzthum OG (1976) Chemie und bearbeitung des kaffees. In: Eichler O (ed) Kaffee und coffein, 2nd edn. Springer, Berlin, pp 3–64

Voerman E, Jaddoe VW, Gishti O et al (2016) Maternal caffeine intake during pregnancy, early growth, and body fat distribution at school age. Obes 24:1170–1177

von Borstel RW, Wurtman RJ (1982) Caffeine withdrawal enhances sensitivity to physiologic level of adenosine in vivo. Federation Proc. 41:1669

Walters ER, Lesk VE (2016) The effect of prior caffeine consumption on neuropsychological test performance: a placebo-controlled study. Dement Geriatr Cogn Disord 41:146–151

Wen W, Shu XO, Jacobs DR Jr, Brown JE (2001) The associations of maternal caffeine consumption and nausea with spontaneous abortion. Epidemiol 12:38–42

Weng X, Odouli R, Li DK (2008) Maternal caffeine consumption during pregnancy and the risk of miscarriage: a prospective cohort study. Am J Obstet Gynecol 198: 279–2e1

Wikoff D, Welsh BT, Henderson R et al (2017) Systematic review of the potential adverse effects of caffeine consumption in healthy adults, pregnant women, adolescents, and children. Food Chem Toxicol 109: 585–648

Wisborg K, Kesmodel U, Bech BH et al (2003) Maternal consumption of coffee during pregnancy and stillbirth and infant death in first year of life: prospective study. BMJ 326:420

World Health Organization (2024) International classification of diseases, eleventh revision (ICD-11). World Health Organization, Geneva. https://icd.who.int/browse/2024-01/mms/en

Wu YM, Luo HW, Kou H et al (2015) Prenatal caffeine exposure induced a lower level of fetal blood leptin mainly via placental mechanism. Toxicol Appl Pharmacol 289:109–1016

Xu D, Zhang B, Liang G et al (2012) Caffeine-induced activated glucocorticoid metabolism in the hippocampus causes hypothalamic-pituitary-adrenal axis inhibition in fetal rats. PLoS One 7:e44497

Yu T, Campbell SC, Stockmann C et al (2016) Pregnancy-induced changes in the pharmacokinetics of caffeine and its metabolites. J Clin Pharmacol 56:590–596

Zappettini S, Faivre E, Ghestem A et al (2019) Caffeine consumption during pregnancy accelerates the development of cognitive deficits in offspring in a model of tauopathy. Front Cell Neurosci 13. https://doi.org/10.3389/fncel.2019.00438

Zeltner T (2000) Tobacco company strategies to undermine tobacco control activities at the World Health Organization. Report of the committee of experts on tobacco industry documents, pp 229–243

11 Animal Models of Prenatal Opioid Exposure: Insights into Impaired Neurodevelopment

Chelsea B. Valery, Nethra K. Madurai, and Lauren L. Jantzie

Abstract

With opioids being increasingly prescribed and illicit opioids being misused, substance use disorder has become a growing public health concern. The impacts of the opioid epidemic have been devastating, especially for pregnant people, infants, and children. Pre- and perinatal opioid exposure is complex. Opioids affect multiple body systems and have detrimental effects on the placenta, brain, and immune system. Pharmacological properties make each class of opioid unique, thereby compounding effects on development based on the type, receptors engaged, or combination of drugs used. Accordingly, animal models are necessary to elucidate the mechanisms, pathways, and developmental processes affected by opioid exposure during and after pregnancy. However, the complexity of opioid use in humans means that preclinical modeling is also complicated with variation by species type, duration, and timing of exposure, and combinations of opioids studied. In this chapter, we present a summary of numerous, intricate preclinical models of perinatal opioid exposure. Specifically, we discuss (1) the inherent variability and difficulty in modeling complex patterns of opioid use by pregnant and peripartum people, (2) provide background on opioids and their receptors, and (3) present evidence for long-term changes in brain structure and function secondary to prenatal opioid exposure. Together, we emphasize the significant immunological, structural, and cognitive changes documented in animals and humans after opioid exposure to highlight the potential for translatability and illustrate a path forward for improved mechanistic and therapeutic discovery.

C. B. Valery · N. K. Madurai
Neonatal-Perinatal Medicine, Department of Pediatrics, Johns Hopkins University School of Medicine, Baltimore, MD, USA

Department of Neurosurgery, Johns Hopkins University School of Medicine, Baltimore, MD, USA
e-mail: nethra@jhmi.edu

L. L. Jantzie (✉)
Neonatal-Perinatal Medicine, Department of Pediatrics, Johns Hopkins University School of Medicine, Baltimore, MD, USA

Department of Neurosurgery, Johns Hopkins University School of Medicine, Baltimore, MD, USA

Department of Neurology, Johns Hopkins University School of Medicine, Baltimore, MD, USA

Kennedy Krieger Institute, Baltimore, MD, USA

Neurosciences Intensive Care Nursery (NICN), Johns Hopkins Children's Center, Baltimore, MD, USA
e-mail: ljantzie@jhmi.edu

A. N. Bukiya, D. W. Ali (eds.), *Molecular Mechanisms and Lifelong Consequences of Prenatal Exposure to Psychoactive Substances*, Advances in Experimental Medicine and Biology 1500,
https://doi.org/10.1007/978-3-032-12741-9_11

Keywords

Methadone · Inflammation · Cognition · Brain injury · MRI

11.1 Introduction

The Center for Disease Control estimates the total economic burden of opioid misuse to be 78.5 billion USD annually, highlighting the impact of the opioid epidemic on health, social, and financial well-being (Florence et al. 2016, 2021). As the epidemic has advanced, opioids have become increasingly used and misused. The rates of substance and opioid use disorder (SUD and OUD, respectively) during pregnancy have surged, resulting in significantly increased incidence of pre- and perinatal opioid exposure (POE) (Hirai et al. 2021). Both pediatric and adult health outcomes are negatively impacted by POE, which includes the misuse of illicit opioids such as heroin, prescription opioids such as oxycodone, morphine, codeine, and medications intended to manage OUD, such as methadone and buprenorphine (Ogunyankin 2020; Patrick et al. 2015a, 2017; McQueen and Murphy-Oikonen 2016). The consequences of untreated OUD and substance misuse in pregnancy are well defined. Pregnant people affected by SUD are at risk for adverse pregnancy outcomes, including fetal growth restriction, placental abruption, preterm birth, respiratory depression, white matter injury, neurodevelopmental abnormalities, neonatal opioid withdrawal syndrome (NOWS), and neonatal death (Merhar et al. 2019; Ragsdale et al. 2024).

The rates of NOWS, a well-recognized consequence of POE, have increased fivefold in the last decade. NOWS occurs in ~5.8 infants in every 1000-hospital births (Patrick et al. 2015b). This results in individual, familial, and societal burdens alongside an estimated economic encumbrance of 1.5 billion dollars in hospital charges that is mainly shouldered by Medicaid (Patrick et al. 2015b; Committee opinion no 711 2017; Haight et al. 2018; Schiff and Patrick 2017). Opioids rapidly cross the placenta with direct impact on the central nervous system (CNS) (Sirnes et al. 2017; Nekhayeva et al. 2005). While withdrawal is easily diagnosed in infants and the symptoms of NOWS are clearly defined, it has recently become apparent that the adverse effects of POE on neurodevelopment and health extend far beyond a withdrawal syndrome. Significantly, not all infants with POE and at risk for brain damage and later life neurodevelopmental disability exhibit NOWS (Sirnes et al. 2017; Nekhayeva et al. 2005).

Current clinical guidelines suggest that medication-assisted treatment for OUD is safer for both women and neonates than abstinence or withdrawal during pregnancy (Committee opinion no 711 2017; Rausgaard et al. 2020). However, these medications were integrated into clinical practice without randomized control trials and long-term follow-up in the children (Jones et al. 2010; Boardman et al. 2022). Indeed, the safety of opioids during pregnancy, including the use of methadone and buprenorphine to manage OUD, has primarily been evaluated in observational studies, with no mechanistic evaluations of postnatal sequelae (Committee opinion no 711 2017; Nezvalová-Henriksen et al. 2011; Broussard et al. 2011; Andersen et al. 2020). Long-term, longitudinal, population-based studies on the effects of POE are still lacking, however meta analyzes demonstrate worse cognitive, psychomotor, behavioral, attentional and executive functioning in children born to women on opioid maintenance therapy during pregnancy compared to children without prenatal exposure (Andersen et al. 2020; Corsi et al. 2020). Indeed, mounting clinical (Boardman et al. 2022; Oei et al. 2017; Schlagal et al. 2021; Sundelin Wahlsten and Sarman 2013; Azuine et al. 2019; Oei 2018; Yeoh et al. 2019) and preclinical evidence (Schlagal et al. 2021; Jantzie et al. 2020; Newville et al. 2020; Kongstorp et al. 2020; Grecco et al. 2021; Oberoi et al. 2019; Tan et al. 2018; Velasco et al. 2021) suggest that mechanistic evaluation of the effects of methadone and buprenorphine on the developing brain, coupled with long-term outcome studies are desperately needed. This is essential because, despite improved pregnancy outcomes, infants exposed to methadone or buprenorphine are microcephalic, have reduced whole brain, basal ganglia, and cerebellar volumes (Sirnes et al. 2017), reduced cortical thickness (Merhar et al. 2019, 2021a; Broussard et al. 2011; Schlagal et al. 2021; Binder and Vavrinková 2008; Hunt et al. 2008), and impaired white matter development (Boardman et al. 2022; Monnelly et al. 2018; Walhovd et al. 2010, 2012; Mactier et al. 2014; Mactier and Hamilton 2020; Peterson et al. 2020). Microstructural brain injury is detected on magnetic resonance imaging (MRI), and impaired neurodevelopment is a lasting consequence in these children (Boardman et al. 2022; Sundelin Wahlsten and Sarman 2013; Monnelly et al. 2018, 2019; Walhovd et al. 2010, 2012; Mactier et al. 2014; Mactier and Hamilton 2020; Peterson et al. 2020; Nygaard et al. 2018). Indeed, these changes are often visualized in our own patients along with elevated placental inflammatory biomarkers.

In adults, opioids impair brain function and cognitive skills acutely (Oei et al. 2017; Younger et al. 2011; Wallin et al. 2021). By contrast, effects on the developing brain are long-lasting (Oei et al. 2017; Caritis and Panigrahy 2019). Children with POE are at higher risk for impaired executive function, attention deficit hyperactivity disorder (ADHD), difficulties with information processing, and impaired psychomotor and behavioral outcomes (Sundelin Wahlsten and Sarman 2013; Azuine et al. 2019; Nygaard et al. 2018; Schwartz et al. 2021; Conradt et al. 2019; Guo et al. 1994; Konijnenberg and Melinder 2015; Baldacchino et al. 2015; Konijnenberg et al. 2016). They also have a greater likelihood of being impaired in two or more functional domains at school-age compared to non-opioid-exposed children, and carry their risk for educational delay throughout the duration of their school years (Boardman et al. 2022; Oei et al. 2017; Sundelin Wahlsten and Sarman 2013; Oei 2018; Lee et al. 2019, 2020a, b). Especially in older children, decreased composite cognition, psychomotor performance, language proficiency, fine motor skills, hand-eye coordination, executive function, and attention are significant concerns (Boardman et al. 2022; Oei et al. 2017; Younger et al. 2011; Wallin et al. 2021; Caritis and Panigrahy 2019; Lee et al. 2020a; Welton et al. 2019; Arter et al. 2021). In preclinical literature, there is a dearth of knowledge on the direct effects of opioids on developing neural circuitry and the cellular and molecular mechanisms of POE (Caritis and Panigrahy 2019). This almost complete lack of preclinical knowledge is particularly serious,and egregious given the potential individual and societal consequences of having an expanding population of children with lifelong cognitive and behavioral issues. Most distressing, there is no scientifically sound equipoise or mechanistic evaluations supporting either the use of methadone or buprenorphine for pregnant women with OUD (Rausgaard et al. 2020; Jones et al. 2010; Binder and Vavrinková 2008; Caritis and Panigrahy 2019; Jones et al. 2005; Tobon et al. 2019). Most prior preclinical research is 3–4 decades old·(Zagon and McLaughlin 1978; Zagon and McLaughlin 1977; McLaughlin et al. 1978), and neglects the role of the developing immune system, glia, and neural network structure/function. Older studies suggested detrimental effects of opioids on neuro-ontogeny and neural biochemistry (Patrick et al. 2017; Haight et al. 2018; Schiff and Patrick 2017; Sirnes et al. 2017; Schlagal et al. 2021). Opioids increase dopamine neurons in the ventral tegmental area, providing key mechanistic insight into the development of attentional and impulsivity disorders in adolescence (Schlagal et al. 2021; Kongstorp et al. 2020). Opioids also alter neurogenesis, cortical progenitors, corticogenesis, and neuronal electrophysiology (Schlagal et al. 2021; Grecco et al. 2021; Tan et al. 2018; Jurga et al. 2016). The relationship between opioid exposure, neural circuitry changes, and psychosocial factors is complex (Jansson et al. 2011, 2012, 2017; Velez et al. 2018; Kaltenbach et al. 2018; Bakhireva et al. 2019). and cumulatively emphasize the importance of evaluating brain architecture, neural topology, and cognition in preclinical studies of POE that aim to gain mechanistic insight.

Given the complexity of POE, animal models and translationally relevant preclinical platforms are necessary to elucidate how cellular and molecular changes are related to long-term behavioral, cognitive, and neurological deficits. These animal models can vary in the species used, opioid type, drug administration methods, and length of exposure. Indeed, each model approach has its own strengths and weaknesses. While human studies of opioid exposure are important and essential, animal models and pre-clinical approaches allow for a controlled environment where researchers can isolate the effects of specific opioids, dosing regimens, and exposure durations—factors that are difficult to manipulate in human studies. Additionally, confounding variables like polysubstance use, socioeconomic factors, and genetic and epigenetic changes can be controlled. Understanding the mechanistic impact of opioid-induced injury, including neuroinflammation, immune modulations, changes in neural transmission, and neurochemistry, neuronal cell death, and synaptic plasticity in neonates, may inform the care of all those affected by the opioid epidemic. Thus, to understand the current landscape of preclinical models, we will review the pharmacology of opioids and their receptors, the relationship between receptor activation, inflammation, and neural development, contemporary animal models of POE, and the neurodevelopmental outcomes in each.

11.2 Opioid Pharmacology and Mechanisms of Action

Opioid Receptors: Opioid receptors are a part of the body's internal regulation of pain, reward, stress, and motivation. The activation of these receptors by endogenous or exogenous opioids results in a chemical cascade that reduces neuronal excitability and provides analgesia. The effectiveness of opioid receptor agonism to modulate pain led to the development of synthetic opioid receptor modulators. However, the reliance on opioids and the lack of alternatives for pain management has led to them being overprescribed and increasingly misused and abused. To understand the widespread impact and therapeutic potential of opioid receptors targeted pharmacology, it is important to explore pain processing and homeostatic opioid-driven signal transduction.

Pain processing typically begins with activation of nociceptors in peripheral tissues. These nociceptors are activated by strong, harmful stimuli that then propagate along the primary afferents to the dorsal root and trigeminal ganglia, and then to the brainstem, thalamus, and other cortical structures. As noxious stimuli ascend through this pathway, there are regions like the periaqueductal gray, hypothalamus, and amygdala in the descending pain modulatory circuit that can alter pain perception. Notably, there is a significant central component to pain, including phantom pain phenomena and nociplastic pain, that occurs in the absence of peripheral nociceptor activation. Opioid receptors regulate pain circuitry and activity. These G-protein-coupled receptors are the targets of both endogenous opioid peptides and synthetic opioid derivatives in both the central and peripheral nervous systems. Their activation not only modulates pain responses, but also functions in stress regulation, reward pathways, respiration, and other essential physiological responses (Valentino and Volkow 2018; Kieffer et al. 1992; Minami et al. 1993; Chen et al. 1993). In mice, opioid receptors on neural cells appear as early as embryonic day 11.5 (E11.5), and the activation of these receptors directs neural development (Zhu et al. 1998). One important neurodevelopmental non-neuronal modulatory target is oligodendrocytes (OLs). Oligodendrocyte precursor cells (OPCs) appear at E12.5 in mice and E14 in rats in the periventricular zones (Bergles and Richardson 2015). As both OPCs and mature oligodendrocytes express opioid receptors, their activation can modulate early brain development, including OL proliferation, migration, differentiation, and myelin wrapping in both gray and white matter structures (Velasco et al. 2021; Vestal-Laborde et al. 2014).

There are at least three opioid receptor types, including mu (MOR), delta (DOR), and kappa (KOR) receptors (Velasco et al. 2021; Valentino and Volkow 2018; Kieffer et al. 1992; Minami et al. 1993; Chen et al. 1993; Zhu et al. 1998;

Bergles and Richardson 2015; Vestal-Laborde et al. 2014). MORs are the most abundant receptors in the CNS and are densely populated in brain regions responsible for pain, stress, and reward, such as the somatosensory cortex, spinal dorsal horns, and the limbic system. MORs function in the reward pathway through inhibition of GABAergic input from the rostromedial tegmental nucleus and, less so, the nucleus accumbens, leading to an increase in the firing rate of the dopaminergic cells in the ventral tegmental area (VTA). This signal transduction underlies motivation-based behavior (Matsui et al. 2014). MORs modulate pain through inhibition of GABA release in the periaqueductal gray matter and raphe nuclei (Li et al. 2016), which in turn reduces the nociceptive signals from the periphery to the thalamus (Birdsong et al. 2019). Both endogenous opioids like beta-endorphins, endomorphins, and enkephalins and exogenous opioids like morphine, fentanyl, and oxycodone (McDonald and Lambert 2005; Eshleman et al. 2020) produce these effects through an affinity for MORs in the midbrain and direct inhibition in the periphery. MORs also play a role in respiratory, cardiovascular, and gastrointestinal function. Indeed, respiratory depression is a risk of opioid use, among other unwanted side effects. Buprenorphine is a partial agonist of MORs, which limits the negative, peripheral side effects associated with MOR activation, such as respiratory depression through a "ceiling effect" where increasing the dosage beyond a certain point does not increase pharmacological effect (Gudin and Fudin 2020; Infantino et al. 2021).

Delta opioid receptors (DORs), like MORs, are widely expressed throughout the CNS in the cortical regions, olfactory bulb, amygdala, and striatum, along with the dorsal root ganglion in the periphery (Peng et al. 2012; Chu Sin Chung et al. 2015) DORs also have important roles in chronic pain, anxiety, and depression (Pradhan et al. 2010; Gaveriaux-Ruff et al. 2011; Jin et al. 2022). In the normal state, DORs are sequestered in neurons. However, during chronic pain, sustained opioid exposure, or with inflammation, DORs are inserted into the neuronal membrane (Patwardhan et al. 2005; Cahill et al. 2022) and can be activated by DOR agonists. DORs exert acute anxiogenic effects through the DOR1 subtype, while DOR2 membrane insertion and subsequent activation reduce anxiety-like behaviors in persistent pain states (Zhou et al. 2021). DOR1 activation in the central nucleus of the amygdala specifically inhibits anxiogenic and anxiolytic signals from the parabrachial nucleus and basolateral amygdala, respectively. DOR2, on the other hand, only inhibits the anxiogenic inputs from the parabrachial nucleus (Zhou et al. 2021). Enkephalins are endogenous agonists of DORs, but exogenous agonists like fentanyl and morphine also have an affinity for this receptor type, although less than the affinity for MORs (McDonald and Lambert 2005).

KORs are expressed in both primary afferents of the periphery and CNS regions, including the nucleus accumbens, ventral tegmental area, dorsal raphe nucleus, and amygdala (Snyder et al. 2018; Crowley and Kash 2015). KORs function in analgesia and can treat pruritus (Kim et al. 2022; Wang et al. 2021) through the inhibition of calcium influx (Snyder et al. 2018). While the activation of KORs is not associated with respiratory depression, negative side effects include dysphoria, stress, and depression. Dynorphins, stress-induced neuropeptides, are endogenous KOR agonists (Gomes et al. 2020). KOR activation in the dorsal raphe nucleus increases depression in part by inhibiting excitatory inputs onto serotonergic neurons and reducing extracellular serotonin (Lemos et al. 2012). Interestingly, KOR signaling includes both a G-protein and a β-arrestin pathway important when considering alternatives to MORs. The G-protein pathway mediates analgesia, while the β-arrestin pathway is responsible for the negative effects of KORs. Indeed, blocking this second pathway in the development of pain medications may decrease associated side effects (Valentino and Volkow 2018; Bruchas and Chavkin 2010; Morgenweck et al. 2015). This type of KOR agonists are candidates for restricted peripheral administration to decrease pain and neurogenic inflammation. They may be beneficial and have fewer negative side effects as agonists can activate KORs located in the peripheral dorsal root ganglion (Snyder et al. 2018).

Placental Development Placental development begins shortly after blastocyst implantation into the endometrium of the uterine wall and functions as the bridge between the fetus and maternal circulatory systems. Contact between the outer layer of the blastocyst, called the trophoblast, and the endometrium, forms layers in the chorion called syncytiotrophoblast and cytotrophoblast that trigger the release of hCG enzymes that break down the endometrial wall. From here, the cytotrophoblast layer pushes into the syncytiotrophoblast layer in a finger-like pattern to form primary chorionic villi. As the villi continue to branch and organize, capillary beds grow, and the placenta is formed, allowing the influx of oxygen and nutrients and the removal of waste.

The placenta is fully formed and functional by 10–12 weeks in humans, but continues to grow throughout pregnancy. In rodents, placental development continues until a few days before birth and is considered functional at mid-gestation, roughly embryonic day 11. Opioid exposure can disrupt this process in the early stages of development. Maternal methadone use has been associated with delayed villous maturation, a prelude to stillbirth, where the placental villi do not develop properly and placental efficiency is reduced (Serra et al. 2017). While the placenta regulates the substances that traverse the maternal-fetal axis, it is an incomplete barrier that allows opioids to enter fetal circulation. Once opioids cross the fetal blood–brain barrier, they bind to opioid receptors in the CNS, including immature neurons, oligodendrocytes, and microglia. This premature or excessive activation by exogenous opioids can disturb the delicate balance of fetal brain development that governs myelination, synaptogenesis, and neurogenesis. These changes can interfere with typical neurodevelopmental processes and potentially lead to altered brain microstructure, impaired anatomical and functional connectivity, and long-term deficits in cognitive and executive function.

Placental Involvement Opioid receptors are expressed in placental tissue, and when activated by exogenous opioids, can cause placental dysfunction. Specifically, activation of opioid receptors can cause deficits in angiogenesis, poor vascularization and hypoxia. Through their action on MORs, opioids cause vasoconstriction (Kopecky et al. 2000). This constriction reduces blood flow to the placenta and the developing fetus, leading to hypoxia and ischemia. This reduced placental blood flow can result in less oxygen and fewer nutrients reaching the fetus, which can catalyze intrauterine growth restriction (IUGR) and precipitate low birth weight. Notably, there is an established relationship between MOR activation and nitric oxide (NO) release (Mantione et al. 2010). NO levels are an important factor in the placental vascular development that is necessary to support blood flow to the growing fetus. Disruption of this balance may impact fetal neural development through changes in vessel caliber, oxygen saturation and direct impact on neural cells themselves (Patrick et al. 2015b; Humphries et al. 2023).

Placental Transcriptomics and Epigenomics Post-opioid Exposure Transcriptomics analyzes RNA expression (both mRNA and miRNA) while epigenomics focuses on modifications along the DNA, such as methylation and acetylation, that ultimately affects gene and protein expression. Environmental factors can influence placental transcriptomics and epigenomics (Diez-Ahijado et al. 2024; Lapehn and Paquette 2022; Apicella et al. 2019; Sainty et al. 2023). Elegant studies have revealed that gene expression in the placenta can be altered by opioid exposure and cause negative downstream effects in placental function and fetal development (Radhakrishna et al. 2021a; Sadovsky et al. 2023). In these studies, differentially expressed and methylated genes in opioid-exposed placental tissue compared to controls were involved in immune function, neuronal development, and cellular replication (Sousa et al. 2025). Notably, NOWS-associated methylation differences have been found in many solute carrier (SLC) transporters, ATP-binding cassette (ABC) transporters, and phosphorylated kinase C (PKC) genes that function in oxidative-stress response and impulsivity. Accordingly, these methylation changes have been proposed as biomarkers of NOWS with clinical utility (Radhakrishna et al. 2021b, 2024).

Studies of placental genetics in opioid-exposed mice showed sex specific expression patterns, with female opioid-exposed placentae having an upregulation of genes in the carcinoembryonic antigen (CEA), prolactin (prl), and trophoblast-specific protein (tpbp) families (Green et al. 2020). The enrichment of these genes in the female placenta may offer a mechanism for additional protection against maternal stressors (Bu et al. 2016). In comparison, male placental genes associated with opioid exposure include downregulation in specific ribosomal proteins, which may explain sex-linked differences in prenatal opioid exposure (Green et al. 2020; Madurai et al. 2024; Nygaard et al. 2015).

In the examination of the effects of oxycodone on the mouse placenta, a decrease is seen in the ratio of cells in the parietal trophoblast giant cell (pTGC) region compared to both the labyrinth (LA) and spongiotrophoblast (spongioTB) regions (Green et al. 2020). pTGC plays an important role in implantation and modulates uterine natural killer cells, which are important for maternal artery remodeling (Lawless et al. 2023; Robson et al. 2012). These changes in the opioid exposed placental transcriptome suggest impaired placental function that could negatively impact cellular placental structure, fetal brain development, and susceptibility to later withdrawal. Opioid induced epigenomic changes in placentae have also been shown in genes responsible for immune regulation (Sousa et al. 2025) and within the ABCB1 promoter (Townsel et al. 2025) Interestingly, the ABCB1 gene (also known as the multidrug resistance 1 gene) is responsible for an ATP-dependent transporter that moves molecules, including drugs, toxins and lipids out of cells and into the extracellular environment. A decrease in methylation within this promoter is associated with severe NOWS, as the transporter that is encoded by this gene returns opioid molecules to the maternal bloodstream, thereby increasing blood concentrations (Townsel et al. 2025; Nanovskaya et al. 2005; Walker et al. 2017). Analyses of cord blood and serum also reveal increases in the methylation of mu-opioid receptor promoters (OPRM1) that are associated with more severe NOWS (Wachman et al. 2014). Taken together, it is clear that the neonatal epigenetic and transcriptomic profile is changed after opioid exposure, and that these stressors impact fetal development and can impart a higher risk for severe NOWS and lasting structural and functional changes.

The crossing of opioids through the placenta can affect the molecular mechanisms of synaptogenesis through downregulation of AMPAR and NMDAR mRNA expression in the nucleus accumbens. In animal models, morphine temporally alters GluR1-4, NR1, and NR2A-D subunit expression. Specifically, morphine decreases the mRNA expression of these AMPAR and NMDAR subunits, together with post-synaptic density protein 95 (PSD-95), robustly in the nucleus accumbens and throughout other regions of the mesolimbic system (Wu et al. 2018) at both postnatal day 14 (P14) P14 and P30. Molecularly, synaptic complexes between PSD-95 and these glutamatergic receptor subunits control calcium flux, synaptogenesis, synaptic pruning, and neuronal survival. Cumulatively, this can impact cognition and impact reward-seeking behavior, learning, and memory (Wu et al. 2018). PSD-95 anchors AMPARs and NMDARs to the post-synaptic density, an important component in long-term potentiation and synaptic plasticity that underlies learning and memory (Haight et al. 2018; Ravi et al. 2022; Migaud et al. 1998). Overall, disruption in glutamate receptor signaling and GABAergic signal transduction as described above, has implications for cognition and neuronal excitability, including epileptiform activity. These are dominant clinical symptoms in NOWS and in disorders of neurodevelopment affecting cognition, pain processing, and executive function.

Immune Activation Opioid receptors are expressed on peripheral immune cells such as

T-cells, macrophages, and natural killer cells (Brejchova et al. 2020) that can migrate into the CNS during profound inflammation. Opioid receptors are also expressed on resident CNS immune cells, including microglia, astrocytes, and oligodendrocytes, where their activation plays a role in immunomodulation through proinflammatory chemokine mediation. Neuroinflammation occurs when astrocytes and microglia, the glial immune modulators in the CNS, are activated and release cytokines, chemokines, and reactive oxygen species to initiate an immune response in the CNS. This process is intended to be neuroprotective or to facilitate neurorepair after injury, but chronic, persistent, or exaggerated immune responses can damage the CNS. In fetal development, exogenous opioid exposure disrupts this delicate balance, leading to immune priming that causes sustained immune hyperreactivity (Jantzie et al. 2020; Newville et al. 2020). Coupled with neuroinflammation, this is also linked to the dysfunction of the blood-brain barrier, reduction in myelin basic protein, and changes in the ratio between phosphorylated neurofilament and total neurofilament, markers of myelination and axon dysfunction (Jantzie et al. 2020). Inflammatory cytokines, such as tumor necrosis factor-alpha (TNF-α) and interleukins (ILs), can compromise the integrity of the blood-brain barrier, making the brain more susceptible to toxins and pathogens.

Activation of Toll-Like Receptors by Opioids and Propagation of Inflammation An important relationship between opioids and sustained inflammation mediated by Toll-Like 4 receptors (TLR4) has been proposed in the mature CNS (Jurga et al. 2016; Hutchinson et al. 2012; Lewis et al. 2012), but it is completely untested in the immature CNS. TLR4 signaling in the mature CNS occurs in response to endogenous, semisynthetic, and fully synthetic opioids, including methadone, morphine, buprenorphine, and oxycodone (Jacobsen et al. 2014). Opioids bind to TLR4 coupled with myeloid differentiation protein 2 (MD-2), resulting in the assembly of a TLR4 oligomer, NFkB activation, and a downstream central immune response (Wang et al. 2012). This activity specifically increases major pro-inflammatory cytokines like interleukin 1-beta (IL-1b), tumor necrosis factor alpha (TNFa), interleukin 6 (IL-6), and the chemokines monocyte chemoattractant protein-1 (MCP-1/CCL2) and (C-X-C) motif ligand 1 (CXCL1) (Coller and Hutchinson 2012). Notably, opioids also activate NFkB via opioid receptors, and activation of NFkB signaling upregulates transcription of opioid receptors and peptides, propagating a detrimental intracellular signaling cascade (Seney et al. 2021; Sawaya et al. 2009; Wang et al. 2004; Rehni et al. 2008; Chen et al. 2007). The opioid induced activation of TLR4 (Dye et al. 2025; Gabr et al. 2021), also stimulates the secretion of neuroexcitatory, proinflammatory cytokines that cause hyperexcitability in pain transmission pathways and subsequent hyperalgesia (Hutchinson et al. 2010; Watkins et al. 2009). Indeed, TLR4 activation, alongside canonical reward pathway stimulation, is also thought to play a significant role in pattern recognition and habit reinforcement through long-term potentiation and synaptic plasticity (Rizzo et al. 2018).

In adults, microglia have been identified as key contributors to opioid-induced neuroplasticity (Seney et al. 2021; Ryu et al. 2021; Zhang et al. 2020), and are suggested as the cellular bridge between opioids and the neural-immune system. Indeed, seminal studies show opioid-induced glial activation opposes opioid analgesia in the mature CNS and enhances opioid tolerance, dependence, and reward (Watkins et al. 2009; Hutchinson et al. 2008). The relationship between methadone, buprenorphine, and TLR4 has not been examined fully in POE, however. Using a rat model of POE with an intact maternal-placental-fetal axis, it has been demonstrated that POE negatively affects multiple aspects of CNS development and shares features of a profound neuroinflammatory disease defined by microglial activation, immune cell recruitment, myelin loss, and changes in functional and anatomical connectivity (Jantzie et al. 2020; Newville et al. 2020; Vasan et al. 2021). Similarly, both methadone and buprenorphine induce a TLR4-dependent immune response that results in profound upregulation of pro-inflammatory mediators in the placental-fetal-brain axis and induce immune cell priming and hyperactivity that results well into the postnatal period, with impacts to critical periods in development.

It is important to note that both methadone and buprenorphine cross the fetal-placental axis, exposing the developing fetus to exogenous opioids during critical periods of brain and immune system development (Monnelly et al. 2018). Using preclinical approaches, differential pharmacology can be used to exploit the stereoselective properties of opioid receptors and TLR4. Unlike classical opioid receptors, TLR4 can be selectively activated or blocked by (+)-isomers (Hutchinson et al. 2007, 2008, 2012; Wang et al. 2012; Watkins et al. 2009; Grace et al. 2015). Opioid receptors do not bind (+)-methadone, (+)-morphine, (+)-naltrexone, and (+)-naloxone. Only (+)-opioids bind and potentiate TLR4 inflammatory signal transduction. On the other hand, (+)-naloxone and (+)-naltrexone block TLR4 and downstream production of inflammatory mediators. Specifically, (+)-isomers such as (+)-naloxone bind MD-2 to diminish NFkB activation and lower IL-1b, TNFa, and IL-6 synthesis. This pharmacology can be exploited in animal models and in vitro to understand opioid-receptor dependent and independent effects to develop targeted therapeutic approaches for POE and NOWS, and improving outcome after opioid exposure.

11.3 Animal Models of Prenatal Opioid Exposure

While the majority of opioid exposure models are conducted in rodents, there are also established models in invertebrates, zebrafish, tadpoles, chicks, sheep, pigs, dogs, and non-human primates (Byrnes and Vassoler 2018; Ding and Ko 2021). Understanding placental structure and function in different animal models is important to effectively model POE. It is also essential to overcome the translational barrier of emerging therapeutics and diagnostic or prognostic biomarkers. Rodent models are widely utilized for factors including, but not limited to, similarities in reward-seeking pathways, ability to self-administer opioids and other pharmacotherapies, and species-conserved presence of each opioid receptor subtype. Non-human primates have particular translational value as their more complex behavioral responses and closer biological relationship to humans have the potential to develop drugs targeting substance use disorders (Banks et al. 2017). Morphine was the first opioid utilized in these animal models, although buprenorphine, methadone, oxycodone, and illicit opioids like fentanyl and heroin are used in modern experimental approaches (Robinson and Wallace 2001; Castellano and Ammassari-Teule 1984; Davis et al. 2010; Chiang et al. 2010; Alipio et al. 2021; Wang and Han 2009; Hornburg et al. 2023). Buprenorphine is specifically salient in models of OUD as it is a transition medication used for pregnant individuals with opioid disorders, as immediate cessation of drug use can cause preterm labor. The half-life, molecular size, and even lipid solubility can affect both the duration of effect and overall bioavailability of the opioid and the subsequent neural effects. Each opioid ligand also has varying affinity for the different opioid receptor types, making this an important consideration in animal model design. An excellent review by Julia Ferrante and Julie Blendy has thoroughly covered opioid pharmacology and is an exemplary resource in understanding this aspect of prenatal opioid models (Ferrante and Blendy 2024).

Placental Organization Differences Placental classification can be based on two categories: villi distribution and the number of placental layers between maternal and fetal blood. The villi are finger-like projections between the chorion and endometrium that facilitate the transfer of oxygen and nutrients to the fetus. Villi distribution can be classified as diffuse, cotyledonary, zonary, or discoid (Imakawa and Nakagawa

2017). Diffuse villi are evenly distributed along the choroid surface and are seen in horses and pigs. Cotyledonary villi are distributed in individual circular clusters known as cotyledons in animals like sheep, also known as ruminants. Zonary villi are distributed in a band around the center of the choroid in animals like dogs and cats. Discoid villi are concentrated into one disc-like shape and are seen in rodents and primates, including humans (Imakawa and Nakagawa 2017; Khorami-Sarvestani et al. 2024). The number of layers between the uterus and fetal sac can be epitheliochorial (six layers of separation) in pigs and horses, endotheliochorial (five layers of separation) in dogs and cats, or hemochorial (three layers of separation) in rodents and primates. A lesser degree of separation between fetal and maternal bloodstreams, like what is found in hemochorial animals, results in a faster transfer of nutrients to the fetus, but this also includes the increased transfer of harmful substances like opioids. These differences are crucial in the context of opioid exposure research, where the efficiency of placental transfer and the degree of trophoblast invasion affect both drug exposure levels and fetal vulnerability. Sheep models of perinatal opioid exposure may suffer from major differences in placental organization, with a lack of significant trophoblast invasion of the uterus seen in human development, limiting the translational potential to human pregnancies (Barry and Anthony 2008). On the other hand, rodent and non-human primate models have the most similarity with the human placenta, but non-human primate models benefit from the fact that the brain is not underdeveloped at the time of birth. Rodents, while not identical to human fetal development, offer a practical alternative to non-human primate models with the option for large-scale studies, as rodents share key placental features with humans. Specifically, rodents have a hemichorial discoid placenta like humans. For these reasons and the popularity of rodent models in opioid exposure studies, rodent studies will be discussed in greater detail below.

Routes of Exposure During embryonic exposure, pregnant dams are administered opioids through treated water, intravenously, via self-administration, implantation of a minipump, or direct injection. Considering the translatability of rat and mouse models, rodents born at postnatal day 0 are equivalent to the third trimester of human development (Semple et al. 2013). To account for this physiological difference, opioids must be administered postnatally in these rodent models through intraperitoneal injection to pups or continued administration to the dam and introduction through the dam's milk. However, models that rely on opioid transfer through milk only may be inaccurate as transfer through lactation is variable throughout the intended exposure period. This variability can lead to inconsistent blood levels of opioids in pups, potentially masking, delaying, or exaggerating the symptoms of NOWS. Cumulatively, this may impact observation of later life changes in neurodevelopment. To avoid the ambiguity associated with opioids transferred through lactation from an opioid exposed dam, some animal models employ cross-fostering, where pups are fostered by an opioid naive dam. This ensures that continued opioid exposure through milk is completely eliminated, and withdrawal symptoms can be accurately observed, and the connections between exposure alone and exposure plus withdrawal can be studied in detail.

Length of Exposure Timing of initial opioid administration varies, as some models begin prior to or early in gestation when the opioid receptors are first developing in the CNS. Others target a specific developmental period, such as the timepoint that is equivalent to the human second and third trimester, when the bulk of human neurodevelopment is occurring. In the development of an animal model, it is important to recognize that many individuals are taking opioids before getting pregnant. With roughly 40% of US pregnancies being unplanned, women who use opioids, prescribed or otherwise, could be exposing their fetus to opioids very early during a critical period of development (Rossen et al.

2023). Pregnant people with opioid use disorders may transition to maintenance drugs like methadone or buprenorphine up to the time of delivery, a necessary consideration in designing animal models. It is also common for pregnant women with substance use disorder to use a combination of drugs; to model this polysubstance use, some animal models utilize multiple drugs (i.e. cannabinoids, ethanol, selective serotonin reuptake inhibitors, anti-psychotics, amphetamine, xylazine) to understand the neurological changes associated with multidrug perinatal opioid exposure.

Maternal Behavior in Animal Models Opioid exposure can reduce maternal caregiving behaviors such as pup retrieval, nesting, licking, and nursing (Dye et al. 2025). These behavioral changes in dams can be a contributing factor to the decrease in body size seen in opioid exposed pups. There is also some support for increased anxiety-like behaviors in opioid exposed pups, and in fact, a study that separated buprenorphine exposed pups from their dam for 2 hours per day found decreased anxiety-like behaviors (Nyberg et al. 2024).

Limitations of Animal Models Single-opiate models are primarily used in research so that outcomes can be appropriately ascribed to a singular drug type. However, this does not accurately recapitulate maternal opioid use, as there is a greater likelihood of polysubstance use with opioid use disorder. Major considerations are presented in Fig. 11.1.

11.4 Insights Gained from Neuroimaging: Lasting Consequences of Opioid Exposure

Imaging studies reveal that prenatal opioid exposure affects aspects of fetal brain development, including brain volume (Merhar et al. 2021a; Taylor et al. 2023; Wu et al. 2025), myelination (Walhovd et al. 2012; Vestal-Laborde et al. 2014; Sanchez et al. 2008), functional connectivity (Radhakrishnan et al. 2021; Merhar et al. 2021b; Chin et al. 2023), and neurogenesis (Wu et al. 2014). In adult humans, even short-term opioid exposure negatively impacts brain volumes. The infant brain is at a greater risk of volumetric changes as a result of opioid exposure during gestation, with decreased volumes seen specifically in the deep gray matter, thalamus, subthalamic nucleus, insular white matter, and brainstem (Merhar et al. 2021a). These changes begin during fetal development as opposed to infants exposed to opioids postnatally after normal fetal development, underscoring the importance of timing in opioid exposure on structural changes, cognition, and neurodevelopment.

White Matter Volume Decreased white matter volumes could be associated with the myelination changes associated with perinatal opioid exposure and with decreased fractional anisotropy (Chin et al. 2023). Oligodendrocytes, the myelinating cells of the CNS, contain both MORs and KORs, with KORs expressed only on mature oligodendrocytes (Knapp et al. 1998). Activation of these oligodendritic opioid receptors by antagonists such as buprenorphine (a KOR antagonist) could alter oligodendrocyte generation and subsequent myelination. MOR activation by various agonists like methadone can accelerate oligodendrocyte maturation, which could alter the time-sensitive myelination processes and disrupt the connectivity in the developing brain (Sanchez et al. 2008). In fact, in an animal model of both therapeutic and supratherapeutic levels of buprenorphine, there was a reduced thickness of the myelin sheath and changes in axonal maturation and caliber (Sanchez et al. 2008).

Gray Matter Volume The decrease in gray matter volumes could be attributed to decreases in neurogenesis, increased apoptosis, and reductions in dendritic spine density seen in opioid exposure (Wu et al. 2014; Robinson et al. 2002; Liao et al. 2005). In a study examining heroin exposure, an increase in activation of capsase-3 and Bcl2-associated X protein (Bax) and profound cell death were noted (Wang and Han 2009). Significantly, the activation of these apoptotic pathways could have negative consequences for learning

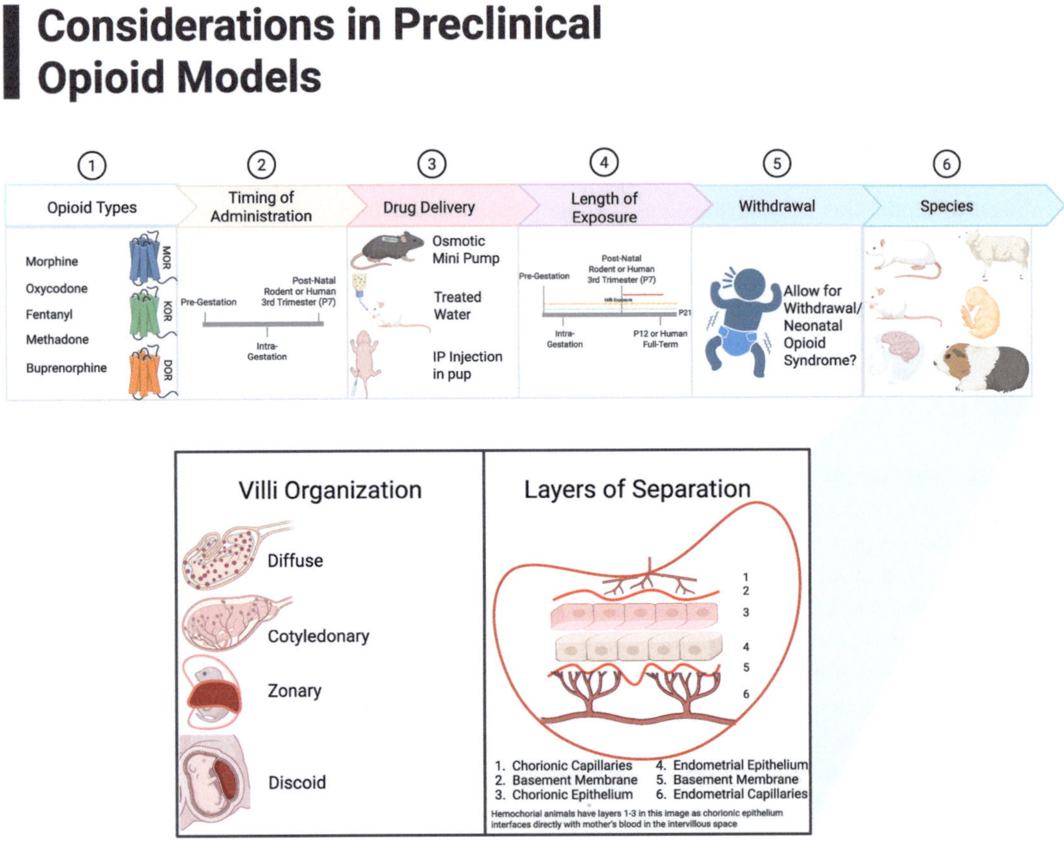

Fig. 11.1 Key considerations in designing a preclinical opioid model include (1) opioid type(s), (2) timing of administration, (3) drug delivery mechanism, (4) the length of exposure, (5) whether withdrawal is allowed through the separation of pups to non-opioid exposed dams, and/or (6) species used. Placental structure and function are unique for each species and is categorized by macrostructure, villi organization, and layer of separation between fetal and maternal circulation

and memory, as the connection between synapse number, volume, complexity of neural arbor, and architecture is well established.

Functional Connectivity Alterations in functional connectivity on fMRI have also been reported in several neuroimaging studies, with a diffuse decrease in functional connectivity across gray matter regions (Chin et al. 2023). In a pilot study of resting-state MRI in opioid-exposed infants, an increase in connectivity between the right amygdala and medial prefrontal cortex was observed (Radhakrishnan et al. 2021; Salzwedel et al. 2015). As the amygdala is involved in the regulation of emotion, motivation, and behavior, changes in functional connections in the developing infant could be associated with negative outcomes. Both diffuse and localized functional connectivity alteration in the developing brain may be related to neurocognitive function as these neural networks support many cognitive domains including behavior.

11.5 Developmental Pathology

POE has been consistently linked to adverse cognitive and neurodevelopmental outcomes in infants. Children exposed to opioids in utero are at increased risk for cognitive delays that persist into early childhood and beyond. Studies have reported impairments in executive function, attention, working memory, language development, and overall IQ scores when compared to non-exposed peers (Jantzie et al. 2020; Monnelly et al. 2019; Schwartz et al. 2021; Alipio et al. 2021; Muthukumar et al. 2022). These deficits could be affected by postnatal environmental factors, such as maternal mental health, low socioeconomic status, changes in primary caregiver, level of maternal interaction, and, as such, studies should try to parse out the possible effect of various confounding environmental variables. Controlled longitudinal studies, such as those conducted by Messinger et al. on maternal lifestyle, have shown that these confounding variables could intensify the significance of opioid exposure on some cognitive and behavioral outcomes, and as such, adequate analysis controlling for covariates is necessary in opioid exposure studies (Messinger et al. 2004; Cotton et al. 2017). These findings underscore the importance of considering external factors when evaluating developmental outcomes in children with POE and acknowledge that environment and other sociodemographic factors play a substantive role in shaping long-term developmental outcomes.

It has been established that prenatal opioid exposure has sustained effects on brain structure and function, including smaller whole brain volumes in young adults ages 17–22 (Nygaard et al. 2018), and neural abnormalities like these could account for the cognitive differences observed in these offspring. In mice initially given oxycodone before conception and then switched to buprenorphine after confirmed pregnancy, behavioral changes post-exposure involved hyperactivity (Schlagal et al. 2021). Hyperactivity in rodents was tested in this study through an open field, where more risk-taking behavior, like traveling in the center of an open field, is associated with lower anxiety levels, and higher movement speed is associated with hyperactivity. Mice exposed in utero to fentanyl also experienced a sustained increase in anxiety-like behavior as tested in an elevated plus maze at P35 (Alipio et al. 2021). In the cohort of mice exposed to both a classical opioid and a medicine for OUD, alterations in the number of dopaminergic neurons in the ventral tegmental area were also reported, and these changes may be related to the hyperactive phenotype (Schlagal et al. 2021). ADHD symptoms like hyperactivity are also increased in human adolescents with prenatal opioid exposure, emphasizing the utility of animal models in recapitulating the human condition (Monnelly et al. 2018; Schwartz et al. 2021).

In addition to microstructural brain injury, opioid exposure also has a marked and lasting effect on learning, memory, and executive control (Fig. 11.2). Using a touchscreen cognitive assessment platform, adult methadone exposed animals were tested on their ability to associate an image with a reward and their ability to change these associations during a reversal learning stage. Opioid exposed animals not only had difficulty learning the association, but they also perseverated on previously learned associations more than controls, demonstrating impairments in associative learning and executive functioning (Jantzie et al. 2020; Muthukumar et al. 2022). In a prenatal opioid exposure model utilizing morphine, juvenile rats showed impaired spatial memory in a Y-maze test, which may be associated with observed changes in the dentate gyrus (Niu et al. 2009). Each opioid type can have varying effects on behavior and development, a well-described point in an opioid review by Ferrante and Blendy (2024), which further illustrates the difficulties in understanding the effects of polydrug exposure. While there are varying conclusions drawn based on the opioid type used, there is consistent reporting of cognitive and behavioral deficits, supporting a similar theme: prenatal opioid exposure disrupts molecular pathways of fetal development, brain structure, and neurocognitive outcomes, with lasting consequences, regardless of the presence of NOWS symptoms. These findings underscore the critical importance of well-designed animal models that not only capture the pharmacological diversity of opioids but also reflect developmental trajectories seen in humans.

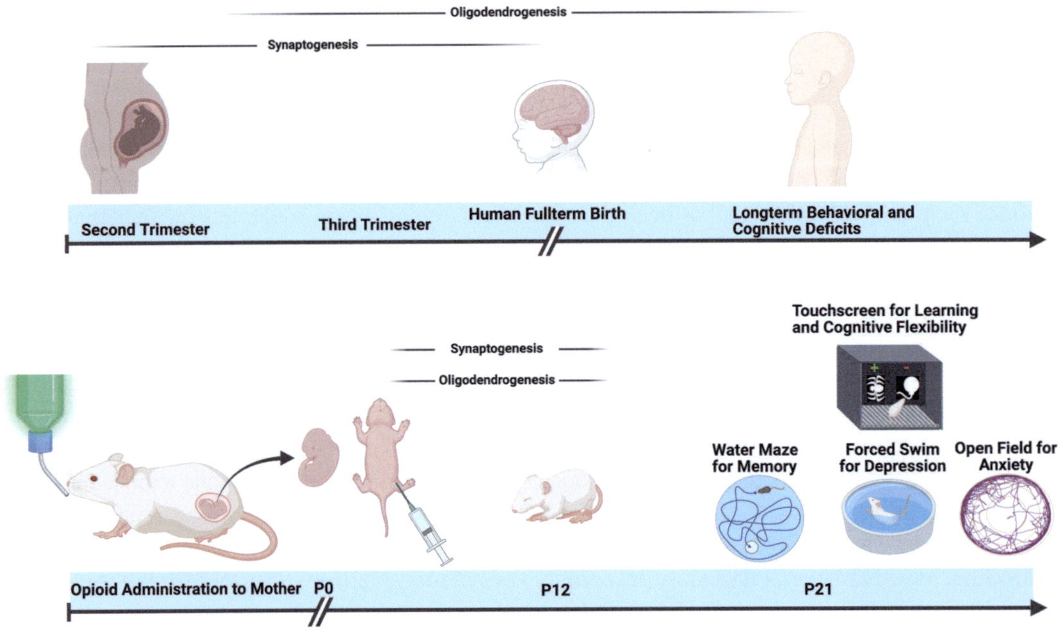

Fig. 11.2 Developmental timeline differences between rats and humans, including cell type maturation, and neurocognitive and behavioral testing in rodents

11.6 Conclusion

These detrimental outcomes underscore the urgent need to better understand the full scope of the impact of POE on neonates. While much is known about the negative effects of opioid exposure, the cellular and molecular mechanisms underlying changes in brain structure and function, and prominent throughout gestation, are still not well described. Taken together, these data highlight the need for translational animal modeling that incorporates long-term outcome measures that assess brain structure and function through adulthood and the entire lifespan. To maximize model translatability, variations in clinical presentation, including co-exposures, maternal condition, and potential sex differences, should be accounted for. Critically, animal models that not only reproduce the acute NOWS symptoms but also account for the variable consequences in the long-term neurocognitive and behavioral outcomes are key in the effort to improve clinical care. The integration of animal model findings with clinical evidence will improve the ability to identify therapeutic targets and/or potential biomarkers. The use of preclinical models also uniquely affords the opportunity to explore possible biomarkers, along with structural and neuroimmunological alterations associated with POE, that would likely remain inaccessible in purely human studies. Ultimately, advancements in animal models of POE will allow for a better understanding of the observed pathophysiology while also informing efforts for prevention, intervention, and reducing the overall burden of OUD and POE.

References

Alipio JB, Brockett AT, Fox ME, Tennyson SS, deBettencourt CA, El-Metwally D, Francis NA, Kanold PO, Lobo MK, Roesch MR et al (2021) Enduring consequences of perinatal fentanyl exposure in mice. Addict Biol 26(2):e12895

Andersen JM, Høiseth G, Nygaard E (2020) Prenatal exposure to methadone or buprenorphine and long-term outcomes: a meta-analysis. Early Hum Dev 143: 104997

Apicella C, Ruano CSM, Méhats C, Miralles F, Vaiman D (2019) The role of epigenetics in placental development and the etiology of preeclampsia. Int J Mol Sci 20(11):2837. https://doi.org/10.3390/ijms20112837

Arter S, Lambert J, Brokman A, Fall N (2021) Diagnoses during the first three years of life for children with prenatal opioid exposure and neonatal abstinence syndrome using a large maternal infant data hub. J Pediatr Nurs 61:34–39

Azuine RE, Ji Y, Chang H, Kim Y, Ji H, DiBari J, Hong X, Wang G, Singh GK, Pearson C et al (2019) Prenatal risk factors and perinatal and postnatal outcomes associated with maternal opioid exposure in an urban, low-income, multiethnic US population. JAMA Netw Open 2(6):e196405

Bakhireva LN, Holbrook BD, Shrestha S, Leyva Y, Ashley M, Cano S, Lowe J, Stephen JM, Leeman L (2019) Association between prenatal opioid exposure, neonatal opioid withdrawal syndrome, and neurodevelopmental and behavioral outcomes at 5–8 months of age. Early Hum Dev 128:69–76

Baldacchino A, Arbuckle K, Petrie DJ, McCowan C (2015) Erratum: Neurobehavioral consequences of chronic intrauterine opioid exposure in infants and preschool children: a systematic review and meta-analysis. BMC Psychiatry 15:134–135

Banks ML, Czoty PW, Negus SS (2017) Utility of nonhuman primates in substance use disorders research. Ilar J 58(2):202–215

Barry JS, Anthony RV (2008) The pregnant sheep as a model for human pregnancy. Theriogenology 69(1): 55–67

Bergles DE, Richardson WD (2015) Oligodendrocyte development and plasticity. Cold Spring Harb Perspect Biol 8(2):a020453

Binder T, Vavrinková B (2008) Prospective randomised comparative study of the effect of buprenorphine, methadone and heroin on the course of pregnancy, birthweight of newborns, early postpartum adaptation and course of the neonatal abstinence syndrome (NAS) in women followed up in the outpatient department. Neuro Endocrinol Lett 29(1):80–86

Birdsong WT, Jongbloets BC, Engeln KA, Wang D, Scherrer G, Mao T (2019) Synapse-specific opioid modulation of thalamo-cortico-striatal circuits. Elife 8. https://doi.org/10.7554/eLife.45146

Boardman JP, Mactier H, Devlin LA (2022) Opioids and the developing brain: time to rethink perinatal care for infants of opioid-dependent mothers. Arch Dis Child Fetal Neonatal Ed 107(1):98–104

Brejchova J, Holan V, Svoboda P (2020) Expression of opioid receptors in cells of the immune system. Int J Mol Sci 22(1):315. https://doi.org/10.3390/ijms22010315

Broussard CS, Rasmussen SA, Reefhuis J, Friedman JM, Jann MW, Riehle-Colarusso T, Honein MA (2011) National Birth Defects Prevention Study. Maternal treatment with opioid analgesics and risk for birth defects. Am J Obstet Gynecol 204(4):314.e1,314.11

Bruchas MR, Chavkin C (2010) Kinase cascades and ligand-directed signaling at the kappa opioid receptor. Psychopharmacology (Berl) 210(2):137–147

Bu P, Alam SMK, Dhakal P, Vivian JL, Soares MJ (2016) A prolactin family paralog regulates placental adaptations to a physiological stressor. Biol Reprod 94(5):107

Byrnes EM, Vassoler FM (2018) Modeling prenatal opioid exposure in animals: current findings and future directions. Front Neuroendocrinol 51:1–13

Cahill CM, Holdridge SV, Liu SS, Xue L, Magnussen C, Ong E, Grenier P, Sutherland A, Olmstead MC (2022) Delta opioid receptor activation modulates affective pain and modality-specific pain hypersensitivity associated with chronic neuropathic pain. J Neurosci Res 100(1):129–148

Caritis SN, Panigrahy A (2019) Opioids affect the fetal brain: reframing the detoxification debate. Am J Obstet Gynecol 221(6):602–608

Castellano C, Ammassari-Teule M (1984) Prenatal exposure to morphine in mice: enhanced responsiveness to morphine and stress. Pharmacol Biochem Behav 21(1): 103–108

Chen Y, Mestek A, Liu J, Hurley JA, Yu L (1993) Molecular cloning and functional expression of a mu-opioid receptor from rat brain. Mol Pharmacol 44(1):8–12

Chen YL, Law P, Loh HH (2007) Action of NF-kappaB on the delta opioid receptor gene promoter. Biochem Biophys Res Commun 352(3):818–822

Chiang Y, Hung T, Lee CW, Yan J, Ho I (2010) Enhancement of tolerance development to morphine in rats prenatally exposed to morphine, methadone, and buprenorphine. J Biomed Sci 17(1):46

Chin EM, Kitase Y, Madurai NK, Robinson S, Jantzie LL (2023) In utero methadone exposure permanently alters anatomical and functional connectivity: a preclinical evaluation. Front Pediatr 11:1139378

Chu Sin Chung P, Keyworth HL, Martin-Garcia E, Charbogne P, Darcq E, Bailey A, Filliol D, Matifas A, Scherrer G, Ouagazzal A et al (2015) A novel anxiogenic role for the delta opioid receptor expressed in GABAergic forebrain neurons. Biol Psychiatry 77(4):404–415

Coller JK, Hutchinson MR (2012) Implications of central immune signaling caused by drugs of abuse: mechanisms, mediators and new therapeutic approaches for prediction and treatment of drug dependence. Pharmacol Ther 134(2):219–245

Committee opinion no. 711: Opioid use and opioid use disorder in pregnancy. Obstet Gynecol 2017;130(2): e81–94

Conradt E, Flannery T, Aschner JL, Annett RD, Croen LA, Duarte CS, Friedman AM, Guille C, Hedderson MM, Hofheimer JA et al (2019) Prenatal opioid exposure: neurodevelopmental consequences and future research priorities. Pediatrics 144(3)

Corsi DJ, Hsu H, Fell DB, Wen SW, Walker M (2020) Association of maternal opioid use in pregnancy with adverse perinatal outcomes in ontario, canada, from 2012 to 2018. JAMA Netw Open 3(7):e208256

Cotton BP, Lohman MC, Brooks JM, LaGasse LL (2017) Perinatal substance use, residential instability, and negative behavioral outcomes among adolescents: lessons from the maternal lifestyle study. J Child Adolesc Psychiatr Nurs 30(3):149–155

Crowley NA, Kash TL (2015) Kappa opioid receptor signaling in the brain: circuitry and implications for treatment. Prog Neuropsychopharmacol Biol Psychiatry 62:51–60

Davis CP, Franklin LM, Johnson GS, Schrott LM (2010) Prenatal oxycodone exposure impairs spatial learning and/or memory in rats. Behav Brain Res 212(1):27–34

Diez-Ahijado L, Cilleros-Portet A, Fernández-Jimenez N, Fernández MF, Guxens M, Julvez J, Llop S, Lopez-Espinosa M, Subiza-Pérez M, Lozano M et al (2024) Evaluating the association between placenta DNA methylation and cognitive functions in the offspring. Transl Psychiatry 14(1):383

Ding H, Ko M (2021) Translational value of non-human primates in opioid research. Exp Neurol 338:113602

Dye CN, Webb AI, Fankhauser MP, Singleton JJ, Kalathil A, Ringland A, Leuner B, Lenz KM (2025) Peripartum buprenorphine and oxycodone exposure impair maternal behavior and increase neuroinflammation in new mother rats. Brain Behav Immun 124:264–279

Eshleman AJ, Nagarajan S, Wolfrum KM, Reed JF, Nilsen A, Torralva R, Janowsky A (2020) Affinity, potency, efficacy, selectivity, and molecular modeling of substituted fentanyls at opioid receptors. Biochem Pharmacol 182:114293

Ferrante JR, Blendy JA (2024) Advances in animal models of prenatal opioid exposure. Trends Neurosci 47(5): 367–382

Florence CS, Zhou C, Luo F, Xu L (2016) The economic burden of prescription opioid overdose, abuse, and dependence in the united states, 2013. Med Care 54(10):901–906

Florence C, Luo F, Rice K (2021) The economic burden of opioid use disorder and fatal opioid overdose in the united states, 2017. Drug Alcohol Depend 218:108350

Gabr MM, Saeed I, Miles JA, Ross BP, Shaw PN, Hollmann MW, Parat M (2021) Interaction of opioids with TLR4—mechanisms and ramifications. Cancers 13(21)

Gaveriaux-Ruff C, Nozaki C, Nadal X, Hever XC, Weibel R, Matifas A, Reiss D, Filliol D, Nassar MA, Wood JN et al (2011) Genetic ablation of delta opioid receptors in nociceptive sensory neurons increases chronic pain and abolishes opioid analgesia. Pain 152(6):1238–1248

Gomes I, Sierra S, Lueptow L, Gupta A, Gouty S, Margolis EB, Cox BM, Devi LA (2020) Biased signaling by endogenous opioid peptides. Proc Natl Acad Sci U S A 117(21):11820–11828

Grace PM, Maier SF, Watkins LR (2015) Opioid-induced central immune signaling: implications for opioid analgesia. Headache 55(4):475–489

Grecco GG, Mork BE, Huang J, Metzger CE, Haggerty DL, Reeves KC, Gao Y, Hoffman H, Katner SN, Masters AR et al (2021) Prenatal methadone exposure disrupts behavioral development and alters motor neuron intrinsic properties and local circuitry. eLife 10: e66230

Green MT, Martin RE, Kinkade JA, Schmidt RR, Bivens NJ, Tuteja G, Mao J, Rosenfeld CS (2020) Maternal oxycodone treatment causes pathophysiological changes in the mouse placenta. Placenta 100:96–110

Gudin J, Fudin J (2020) A narrative pharmacological review of buprenorphine: a unique opioid for the treatment of chronic pain. Pain Ther 9(1):41–54

Guo X, Spencer JW, Suess PE, Hickey JE, Better WE, Herning RI (1994) Cognitive brain potential alterations in boys exposed to opiates: in utero and lifestyle comparisons. Addict Behav 19(4):429–441

Haight SC, Ko JY, Tong VT, Bohm MK, Callaghan WM (2018) Opioid use disorder documented at delivery hospitalization – United States, 1999–2014. MMWR Morb Mortal Wkly Rep 67(31):845–849

Hirai AH, Ko JY, Owens PL, Stocks C, Patrick SW (2021) Neonatal abstinence syndrome and maternal opioid-related diagnoses in the US, 2010–2017. JAMA 325(2):146–155

Hornburg KJ, Slosky LM, Cofer G, Cook J, Qi Y, Porkka F, Clark NB, Pires A, Petrella JR, White LE et al (2023) Prenatal heroin exposure alters brain morphology and connectivity in adolescent mice. NMR in Biomedicine 36(2):e4842

Humphries A, Simcox K, Howell B (2023) A review of the literature: how does prenatal opioid exposure impact placental health and fetal brain development? Develop Psychobiol 65(3):e22378

Hunt RW, Tzioumi D, Collins E, Jeffery HE (2008) Adverse neurodevelopmental outcome of infants exposed to opiate in-utero. Early Hum Dev 84(1): 29–35

Hutchinson MR, Bland ST, Johnson KW, Rice KC, Maier SF, Watkins LR (2007) Opioid-induced glial activation: mechanisms of activation and implications for opioid analgesia, dependence, and reward. ScientificWorldJournal 7:98–111

Hutchinson MR, Coats BD, Lewis SS, Zhang Y, Sprunger DB, Rezvani N, Baker EM, Jekich BM, Wieseler JL, Somogyi AA et al (2008) Proinflammatory cytokines oppose opioid-induced acute and chronic analgesia. Brain Behav Immun 22(8):1178–1189

Hutchinson MR, Zhang Y, Shridhar M, Evans JH, Buchanan MM, Zhao TX, Slivka PF, Coats BD, Rezvani N, Wieseler J et al (2010) Evidence that opioids may have toll-like receptor 4 and MD-2 effects. Brain Behav Immun 24(1):83–95

Hutchinson MR, Northcutt AL, Hiranita T, Wang X, Lewis SS, Thomas J, van Steeg K, Kopajtic TA, Loram LC, Sfregola C et al (2012) Opioid activation of toll-like receptor 4 contributes to drug reinforcement. J Neurosci 32(33):11187–11200

Imakawa K, Nakagawa S (2017) Chapter four – the phylogeny of placental evolution through dynamic integrations of retrotransposons. Prog Mol Biol Transl Sci 145:89–109

Infantino R, Mattia C, Locarini P, Pastore AL, Maione S, Luongo L (2021) Buprenorphine: far beyond the

"ceiling". Biomolecules 11(6):816. https://doi.org/10.3390/biom11060816
Jacobsen JHW, Watkins LR, Hutchinson MR (2014) Chapter six – discovery of a novel site of opioid action at the innate immune pattern-recognition receptor TLR4 and its role in addiction. Int Rev Neurobiol 118:129–163
Jansson LM, Dipietro JA, Velez M, Elko A, Williams E, Milio L, O'Grady K, Jones HE (2011) Fetal neurobehavioral effects of exposure to methadone or buprenorphine. Neurotoxicol Teratol 33(2):240–243
Jansson LM, Di Pietro JA, Elko A, Williams EL, Milio L, Velez M (2012) Pregnancies exposed to methadone, methadone and other illicit substances, and poly-drugs without methadone: a comparison of fetal neurobehaviors and infant outcomes. Drug Alcohol Depend 122(3):213–219
Jansson LM, Velez M, McConnell K, Spencer N, Tuten M, Jones HE, King VL, Gandotra N, Milio LA, Voegtline K et al (2017) Maternal buprenorphine treatment and fetal neurobehavioral development. Am J Obstet Gynecol 216(5):529.e1–529.e8
Jantzie LL, Maxwell JR, Newville JC, Yellowhair TR, Kitase Y, Madurai N, Ramachandra S, Bakhireva LN, Northington FJ, Gerner G et al (2020) Prenatal opioid exposure: the next neonatal neuroinflammatory disease. Brain Behav Immun 84:45–58
Jin D, Chen H, Huang Y, Chen S, Pan H (2022) Δ-opioid receptors in primary sensory neurons tonically restrain nociceptive input in chronic pain but do not enhance morphine analgesic tolerance. Neuropharmacology 217:109202
Jones HE, Johnson RE, Jasinski DR, O'Grady KE, Chisholm CA, Choo RE, Crocetti M, Dudas R, Harrow C, Huestis MA et al (2005) Buprenorphine versus methadone in the treatment of pregnant opioid-dependent patients: effects on the neonatal abstinence syndrome. Drug Alcohol Depend 79(1): 1–10
Jones HE, Kaltenbach K, Heil SH, Stine SM, Coyle MG, Arria AM, O'Grady KE, Selby P, Martin PR, Fischer G (2010) Neonatal abstinence syndrome after methadone or buprenorphine exposure. N Engl J Med 363(24): 2320–2331
Jurga AM, Rojewska E, Piotrowska A, Makuch W, Pilat D, Przewlocka B, Mika J (2016) Blockade of toll-like receptors (TLR2, TLR4) attenuates pain and potentiates buprenorphine analgesia in a rat neuropathic pain model. Neural Plast 2016:5238730
Kaltenbach K, O'Grady KE, Heil SH, Salisbury AL, Coyle MG, Fischer G, Martin PR, Stine S, Jones HE (2018) Prenatal exposure to methadone or buprenorphine: early childhood developmental outcomes. Drug Alcohol Depend 185:40–49
Khorami-Sarvestani S, Vanaki N, Shojaeian S, Zarnani K, Stensballe A, Jeddi-Tehrani M, Zarnani A (2024) Placenta: an old organ with new functions. Front Immunol 15:1385762
Kieffer BL, Befort K, Gaveriaux-Ruff C, Hirth CG (1992) The delta-opioid receptor: isolation of a cDNA by expression cloning and pharmacological characterization. Proc Natl Acad Sci U S A 89(24):12048–12052
Kim BS, Inan S, Ständer S, Sciascia T, Szepietowski JC, Yosipovitch G (2022) Role of kappa-opioid and mu-opioid receptors in pruritus: peripheral and central itch circuits. Exp Dermatol 31(12):1900–1907
Knapp PE, Maderspach K, Hauser KF (1998) Endogenous opioid system in developing normal and jimpy oligodendrocytes: Mu and kappa opioid receptors mediate differential mitogenic and growth responses. Glia 22(2):189–201
Kongstorp M, Bogen IL, Stiris T, Andersen JM (2020) Prenatal exposure to methadone or buprenorphine impairs cognitive performance in young adult rats. Drug Alcohol Depend 212:108008
Konijnenberg C, Melinder A (2015) Visual selective attention is impaired in children prenatally exposed to opioid agonist medication. Eur Addict Res 21(2):63–70
Konijnenberg C, Sarfi M, Melinder A (2016) Mother-child interaction and cognitive development in children prenatally exposed to methadone or buprenorphine. Early Hum Dev 101:91–97
Kopecky EA, Ryan ML, Barrett JF, Seaward PG, Ryan G, Koren G, Amankwah K (2000) Fetal response to maternally administered morphine. Am J Obstet Gynecol 183(2):424–430
Lapehn S, Paquette AG (2022) The placental epigenome as a molecular link between prenatal exposures and fetal health outcomes through the DOHaD hypothesis. Curr Environ Health Rep 9(3):490–501
Lawless L, Qin Y, Xie L, Zhang K (2023) Trophoblast differentiation: mechanisms and implications for pregnancy complications. Nutrients 15(16):3564. https://doi.org/10.3390/nu15163564
Lee SJ, Woodward LJ, Henderson JMT (2019) Educational achievement at age 9.5 years of children born to mothers maintained on methadone during pregnancy. Plos One 14(10):e0223685
Lee SJ, Bora S, Austin NC, Westerman A, Henderson JMT (2020a) Neurodevelopmental outcomes of children born to opioid-dependent mothers: a systematic review and meta-analysis. Acad Pediatr 20(3):308–318
Lee SJ, Pritchard VE, Austin NC, Henderson JMT, Woodward LJ (2020b) Health and neurodevelopment of children born to opioid-dependent mothers at school entry. J Dev Behav Pediatr 41(1):48–57
Lemos JC, Roth CA, Messinger DI, Gill HK, Phillips PEM, Chavkin C (2012) Repeated stress dysregulates κ-opioid receptor signaling in the dorsal raphe through a p38α MAPK-dependent mechanism. J Neurosci 32(36):12325–12336
Lewis SS, Loram LC, Hutchinson MR, Li C, Zhang Y, Maier SF, Huang Y, Rice KC, Watkins LR (2012) (+)-Naloxone, an opioid-inactive toll-like receptor 4 signaling inhibitor, reverses multiple models of chronic neuropathic pain in rats. J Pain 13(5):498–506

Li C, Sugam JA, Lowery-Gionta E, McElligott ZA, McCall NM, Lopez AJ, McKlveen JM, Pleil KE, Kash TL (2016) Mu opioid receptor modulation of dopamine neurons in the periaqueductal gray/dorsal raphe: a role in regulation of pain. Neuropsychopharmacology 41(8):2122–2132

Liao D, Lin H, Law PY, Loh HH (2005) Mu-opioid receptors modulate the stability of dendritic spines. Proc Natl Acad Sci U S A 102(5):1725–1730

Mactier H, Hamilton R (2020) Prenatal opioid exposure – increasing evidence of harm. Early Hum Dev 150: 105188

Mactier H, Shipton D, Dryden C, Tappin DM (2014) Reduced fetal growth in methadone-maintained pregnancies is not fully explained by smoking or socio-economic deprivation. Addiction 109(3): 482–488

Madurai NK, Jantzie LL, Yen E (2024) Sex differences in neonatal outcomes following prenatal opioid exposure. Front Pediatr 12:1357970

Mantione KJ, Angert RM, Cadet P, Kream RM, Stefano GB (2010) Identification of a μ opiate receptor signaling mechanism in human placenta. Med Sci Monit 16(11):BR347–BR352

Matsui A, Jarvie BC, Robinson BG, Hentges ST, Williams JT (2014) Separate GABA afferents to dopamine neurons mediate acute action of opioids, development of tolerance, and expression of withdrawal. Neuron 82(6):1346–1356

McDonald J, Lambert DG (2005) Opioid receptors. Contin Educ Anaesth Crit Care Pain 5(1):22–25

McLaughlin PJ, Zagon IS, White WJ (1978) Perinatal methadone exposure in rats. effects on body and organ development. Biol Neonate 34(1–2):48–54

McQueen K, Murphy-Oikonen J (2016) Neonatal abstinence syndrome. N Engl J Med 375(25):2468–2479

Merhar SL, Parikh NA, Braimah A, Poindexter BB, Tkach J, Kline-Fath B (2019) White matter injury and structural anomalies in infants with prenatal opioid exposure. AJNR Am J Neuroradiol 40(12):2161–2165

Merhar SL, Kline JE, Braimah A, Kline-Fath B, Tkach JA, Altaye M, He L, Parikh NA (2021a) Prenatal opioid exposure is associated with smaller brain volumes in multiple regions. Pediatr Res 90(2):397–402

Merhar SL, Jiang W, Parikh NA, Yin W, Zhou Z, Tkach JA, Wang L, Kline-Fath BM, He L, Braimah A et al (2021b) Effects of prenatal opioid exposure on functional networks in infancy. Dev Cogn Neurosci 51: 100996

Messinger DS, Bauer CR, Das A, Seifer R, Lester BM, Lagasse LL, Wright LL, Shankaran S, Bada HS, Smeriglio VL et al (2004) The maternal lifestyle study: cognitive, motor, and behavioral outcomes of cocaine-exposed and opiate-exposed infants through three years of age. Pediatrics (Evanston) 113(6): 1677–1685

Migaud M, Charlesworth P, Dempster M, Webster LC, Watabe AM, Makhinson M, He Y, Ramsay MF, Morris RGM, Morrison JH et al (1998) Enhanced long-term potentiation and impaired learning in mice with mutant postsynaptic density-95 protein. Nature 396(6710):433–439

Minami M, Toya T, Katao Y, Maekawa K, Nakamura S, Onogi T, Kaneko S, Satoh M (1993) Cloning and expression of a cDNA for the rat kappa-opioid receptor. FEBS Lett 329(3):291–295

Monnelly VJ, Anblagan D, Quigley A, Cabez MB, Cooper ES, Mactier H, Semple SI, Bastin ME, Boardman JP (2018) Prenatal methadone exposure is associated with altered neonatal brain development. NeuroImage Clin 18:9–14

Monnelly VJ, Hamilton R, Chappell FM, Mactier H, Boardman JP (2019) Childhood neurodevelopment after prescription of maintenance methadone for opioid dependency in pregnancy: a systematic review and meta-analysis. Dev Med Child Neurol 61(7):750–760

Morgenweck J, Frankowski KJ, Prisinzano TE, Aubé J, Bohn LM (2015) Investigation of the role of βarrestin2 in kappa opioid receptor modulation in a mouse model of pruritus. Neuropharmacology 99:600–609

Muthukumar S, Mehrotra K, Fouda M, Hamimi S, Jantzie LL, Robinson S (2022) Prenatal and postnatal insults differentially contribute to executive function and cognition: utilizing touchscreen technology for perinatal brain injury research. Exp Neurol 354:114104

Nanovskaya T, Nekhayeva I, Karunaratne N, Audus K, Hankins GDV, Ahmed MS (2005) Role of P-glycoprotein in transplacental transfer of methadone. Biochem Pharmacol 69(12):1869–1878

Nekhayeva IA, Nanovskaya TN, Deshmukh SV, Zharikova OL, Hankins GDV, Ahmed MS (2005) Bidirectional transfer of methadone across human placenta. Biochem Pharmacol 69(1):187–197

Newville J, Maxwell JR, Kitase Y, Robinson S, Jantzie LL (2020) Perinatal opioid exposure primes the peripheral immune system toward hyperreactivity. Front Pediatr 8:272

Nezvalová-Henriksen K, Spigset O, Nordeng H (2011) Effects of codeine on pregnancy outcome: results from a large population-based cohort study. Eur J Clin Pharmacol 67(12):1253–1261

Niu L, Cao B, Zhu H, Mei B, Wang M, Yang Y, Zhou Y (2009) Impaired in vivo synaptic plasticity in dentate gyrus and spatial memory in juvenile rats induced by prenatal morphine exposure. Hippocampus 19(7): 649–657

Nyberg H, Bogen IL, Nygaard E, Andersen JM (2024) Effects of prenatal exposure to methadone or buprenorphine and maternal separation on anxiety-like behavior in rats. Drug Alcohol Depend 262: 111367

Nygaard E, Moe V, Slinning K, Walhovd KB (2015) Longitudinal cognitive development of children born to mothers with opioid and polysubstance use. Pediatr Res 78(3):330–335

Nygaard E, Slinning K, Moe V, Due-Tønnessen P, Fjell A, Walhovd KB (2018) Neuroanatomical characteristics of youths with prenatal opioid and poly-drug exposure. Neurotoxicol Teratol 68:13–26

Oberoi R, Chu T, Mellen N, Jagadapillai R, Ouyang H, Devlin LA, Cai J (2019) Diverse changes in myelin protein expression in rat brain after perinatal methadone exposure. Acta Neurobiol Exp (Wars) 79(4): 367–373

Oei JL (2018) Adult consequences of prenatal drug exposure. Intern Med J 48(1):25–31

Oei JL, Melhuish E, Uebel H, Azzam N, Breen C, Burns L, Hilder L, Bajuk B, Abdel-Latif ME, Ward M et al (2017) Neonatal abstinence syndrome and high school performance. Pediatrics 139(2):e20162651. https://doi.org/10.1542/peds.2016-2651. Epub 2017 Jan 16

Ogunyankin F (2020) Opioid exposure in newborns: lessons learned from fetal alcohol spectrum disorder. J Public Health Policy 41(4):529–534

Patrick SW, Dudley J, Martin PR, Harrell FE, Warren MD, Hartmann KE, Ely EW, Grijalva CG, Cooper WO (2015a) Prescription opioid epidemic and infant outcomes. Pediatrics 135(5):842–850

Patrick SW, Davis MM, Lehmann CU, Cooper WO (2015b) Increasing incidence and geographic distribution of neonatal abstinence syndrome: United states 2009 to 2012. J Perinatol 35(8):650–655

Patrick SW, Schiff DM, Committee on Substance Use and Prevention (2017) A public health response to opioid use in pregnancy. Pediatrics 139(3):e20164070. https://doi.org/10.1542/peds.2016-4070. Epub 2017 Feb 20

Patwardhan AM, Berg KA, Akopain AN, Jeske NA, Gamper N, Clarke WP, Hargreaves KM (2005) Bradykinin-induced functional competence and trafficking of the delta-opioid receptor in trigeminal nociceptors. J Neurosci 25(39):8825–8832

Peng J, Sarkar S, Chang SL (2012) Opioid receptor expression in human brain and peripheral tissues using absolute quantitative real-time RT-PCR. Drug Alcohol Depend 124(3):223–228

Peterson BS, Rosen T, Dingman S, Toth ZR, Sawardekar S, Hao X, Liu F, Xu D, Dong Z, Peterson JB et al (2020) Associations of maternal prenatal drug abuse with measures of newborn brain structure, tissue organization, and metabolite concentrations. JAMA Pediatr 174(9):831–842

Pradhan AAA, Walwyn W, Nozaki C, Filliol D, Erbs E, Matifas A, Evans C, Kieffer BL (2010) Ligand-directed trafficking of the δ-opioid receptor in vivo: two paths toward analgesic tolerance. J Neurosci 30(49):16459–16468

Radhakrishna U, Nath SK, Vishweswaraiah S, Uppala LV, Forray A, Muvvala SB, Mishra NK, Southekal S, Guda C, Govindamangalam H et al (2021a) Maternal opioid use disorder: placental transcriptome analysis for neonatal opioid withdrawal syndrome. Genomics 113(6):3610–3617

Radhakrishna U, Vishweswaraiah S, Uppala LV, Szymanska M, Macknis J, Kumar S, Saleem-Rasheed-F, Aydas B, Forray A, Muvvala SB et al (2021b) Placental DNA methylation profiles in opioid-exposed pregnancies and associations with the neonatal opioid withdrawal syndrome. Genomics 113(3):1127–1135

Radhakrishna U, Radhakrishnan R, Uppala LV, Muvvala SB, Prajapati J, Rawal RM, Bahado-Singh RO, Sadhasivam S (2024) Prenatal opioid exposure significantly impacts placental protein kinase C (PKC) and drug transporters, leading to drug resistance and neonatal opioid withdrawal syndrome. Front Neurosci. 18: 1442915

Radhakrishnan R, Elsaid NMH, Sadhasivam S, Reher TA, Hines AC, Yoder KK, Saykin AJ, Wu Y (2021) Resting state functional MRI in infants with prenatal opioid exposure—a pilot study. Neuroradiology 63(4): 585–591

Ragsdale AS, Al-Hammadi N, Loux TM, Bass S, Keller JM, Chavan NR (2024) Perinatal substance use disorder: examining the impact on adverse pregnancy outcomes. Eur J Obstet Gynecol Reprod Biol X 22: 100308

Rausgaard NLK, Ibsen IO, Jørgensen JS, Lamont RF, Ravn P (2020) Management and monitoring of opioid use in pregnancy. Acta Obstet Gynecol Scand 99(1): 7–15

Ravi AS, Zeng M, Chen X, Sandoval G, Diaz-Alonso J, Zhang M, Nicoll RA (2022) Long-term potentiation reconstituted with an artificial TARP/PSD-95 complex. Cell Reports 41(2):111483

Rehni AK, Bhateja P, Singh TG, Singh N (2008) Nuclear factor-kappa-B inhibitor modulates the development of opioid dependence in a mouse model of naloxone-induced opioid withdrawal syndrome. Behav Pharmacol 19(3):265–269

Rizzo FR, Musella A, De Vito F, Fresegna D, Bullitta S, Vanni V, Guadalupi L, Stampanoni Bassi M, Buttari F, Mandolesi G et al (2018) Tumor necrosis factor and interleukin-1β modulate synaptic plasticity during neuroinflammation. Neural Plast 2018:8430123

Robinson SE, Wallace MJ (2001) Effect of perinatal buprenorphine exposure on development in the rat. J Pharmacol Exp Ther 298(2):797–804

Robinson TE, Gorny G, Savage VR, Kolb B (2002) Widespread but regionally specific effects of experimenter-versus self-administered morphine on dendritic spines in the nucleus accumbens, hippocampus, and neocortex of adult rats. Synapse 46(4):271–279

Robson A, Harris LK, Innes BA, Lash GE, Aljunaidy MM, Aplin JD, Baker PN, Robson SC, Bulmer JN (2012) Uterine natural killer cells initiate spiral artery remodeling in human pregnancy. Faseb J 26(12): 4876–4885

Rossen LM, Hamilton BE, Abma JC, Gregory ECW, Beresovsky V, Resendez A, Chandra A, Martin JA (2023) Updated methodology to estimate overall and

unintended pregnancy rates in the united states. Vital Health Stat Ser 2(201)
Ryu J, Stone P, Lee S, Payne B, Gorse K, Lafrenaye A (2021) Buprenorphine alters microglia and astrocytes acutely following diffuse traumatic brain injury. Sci Rep 11(1):8620–z
Sadovsky E, Chu T, Barak O, Sadovsky Y, Ouyang Y (2023) The impact of opioids on the transcriptional landscape of human villous trophoblasts. Placenta 143:54–61
Sainty R, Silver MJ, Prentice AM, Monk D (2023) The influence of early environment and micronutrient availability on developmental epigenetic programming: lessons from the placenta. Front Cell Dev Biol 11:1212199
Salzwedel AP, Grewen KM, Vachet C, Gerig G, Lin W, Gao W (2015) Prenatal drug exposure affects neonatal brain functional connectivity. J Neurosci 35(14): 5860–5869
Sanchez ES, Bigbee JW, Fobbs W, Robinson SE, Sato-Bigbee C (2008) Opioid addiction and pregnancy: perinatal exposure to buprenorphine affects myelination in the developing brain. Glia 56(9): 1017–1027
Sawaya BE, Deshmane SL, Mukerjee R, Fan S, Khalili K (2009) TNF alpha production in morphine-treated human neural cells is NF-kappaB-dependent. J Neuroimmune Pharmacol 4(1):140–149
Schiff DM, Patrick SW (2017) Treatment of opioid use disorder during pregnancy and cases of neonatal abstinence syndrome. JAMA Pediatr 171(7):707
Schlagal CR, Dunn TJ, Xu P, Felsing DE, Merritt CR, Manja S, Fox RG, Buffington SA, Saade G, Dineley KT et al (2021) Maternal opioid exposure culminates in perturbed murine neurodevelopment and hyperactive phenotype in adolescence. Neuroscience 463:272–287
Schwartz AN, Reyes LM, Meschke LL, Kintziger KW (2021) Prenatal opioid exposure and ADHD childhood symptoms: a meta-analysis. Children (Basel) 8(2):106. https://doi.org/10.3390/children8020106
Semple BD, Blomgren K, Gimlin K, Ferriero DM, Noble-Haeusslein LJ (2013) Brain development in rodents and humans: Identifying benchmarks of maturation and vulnerability to injury across species. Prog Neurobiol 106–107:1–16
Seney ML, Kim S, Glausier JR, Hildebrand MA, Xue X, Zong W, Wang J, Shelton MA, Phan BN, Srinivasan C et al (2021) Transcriptional alterations in dorsolateral prefrontal cortex and nucleus accumbens implicate neuroinflammation and synaptic remodeling in opioid use disorder. Biol Psychiatry 90(8):550–562
Serra AE, Lemon LS, Mokhtari NB, Parks WT, Catov JM, Venkataramanan R, Caritis SN (2017) Delayed villous maturation in term placentas exposed to opioid maintenance therapy: a retrospective cohort study. Am J Obstetr Gynecol 216(4):418.e1–418.e5
Sirnes E, Oltedal L, Bartsch H, Eide GE, Elgen IB, Aukland SM (2017) Brain morphology in school-aged children with prenatal opioid exposure: a structural MRI study. Early Hum Dev 106–107:33–39
Snyder LM, Chiang MC, Loeza-Alcocer E, Omori Y, Hachisuka J, Sheahan TD, Gale JR, Adelman PC, Sypek EI, Fulton SA et al (2018) Kappa opioid receptor distribution and function in primary afferents. Neuron 99(6):1274,1288.e6
Sousa A, Besong OTO, Wachman EM, Taglauer ES, Beane JE, Kefella Y, Koo JS, Saia K, Jones HE, Zhang H (2025) Placental transcriptome analysis in opioid-exposed versus non-opioid exposed pregnancies. Placenta 162:27–34
Sundelin Wahlsten V, Sarman I (2013) Neurobehavioural development of preschool-age children born to addicted mothers given opiate maintenance treatment with buprenorphine during pregnancy. Acta Paediatr 102(5):544–549
Tan KZ, Cunningham AM, Joshi A, Oei JL, Ward MC (2018) Expression of kappa opioid receptors in developing rat brain – implications for perinatal buprenorphine exposure. Reprod Toxicol 78:81–89
Taylor M, Cheng AB, Hodkinson DJ, Afacan O, Zurakowski D, Bajic D (2023) Body size and brain volumetry in the rat following prolonged morphine administration in infancy and adulthood. Front Pain Res (Lausanne) 4:962783
Tobon AL, Habecker E, Forray A (2019) Opioid use in pregnancy. Curr Psychiatry Rep 21(12):118–114
Townsel C, Truax B, Quaid M, Covault J, Dolinoy DC, Goodrich JM (2025) Increased risk of severe neonatal opioid withdrawal syndrome in pregnancies with low placental ABCB1 DNA methylation. J Perinatol 45(4): 458–464
Valentino RJ, Volkow ND (2018) Untangling the complexity of opioid receptor function. Neuropsychopharmacology 43(13):2514–2520
Vasan V, Kitase Y, Newville JC, Robinson S, Gerner G, Burton VJ, Jantzie LL (2021) Neonatal opioid exposure: public health crisis and novel neuroinflammatory disease. Neural Regen Res 16(3):430–432
Velasco B, Mohamed E, Sato-Bigbee C (2021) Endogenous and exogenous opioid effects on oligodendrocyte biology and developmental brain myelination. Neurotoxicol Teratol 86:107002
Velez ML, McConnell K, Spencer N, Montoya L, Tuten M, Jansson LM (2018) Prenatal buprenorphine exposure and neonatal neurobehavioral functioning. Early Hum Dev 117:7–14
Vestal-Laborde A, Eschenroeder AC, Bigbee JW, Robinson SE, Sato-Bigbee C (2014) The opioid system and brain development: effects of methadone on the oligodendrocyte lineage and the early stages of myelination. Develop Neurosci 36(5):409–421
Wachman EM, Hayes MJ, Lester BM, Terrin N, Brown MS, Nielsen DA, Davis JM (2014) Epigenetic

variation in the mu-opioid receptor gene in infants with neonatal abstinence syndrome. J Pediatr 165(3): 472–478

Walhovd KB, Westlye LT, Moe V, Slinning K, Due-Tønnessen P, Bjørnerud A, van der Kouwe A, Dale AM, Fjell AM (2010) White matter characteristics and cognition in prenatally opiate- and polysubstance-exposed children: a diffusion tensor imaging study. Am J Neuroradiol 31(5):894–900

Walhovd KB, Watts R, Amlien I, Woodward LJ (2012) Neural tract development of infants born to methadone-maintained mothers. Pediatr Neurol 47(1): 1–6

Walker N, Filis P, Soffientini U, Bellingham M, O'Shaughnessy PJ, Fowler PA (2017) Placental transporter localization and expression in the human: The importance of species, sex, and gestational age differences†. Biol Reprod 96(4):733–742

Wallin CM, Bowen SE, Brummelte S (2021) Opioid use during pregnancy can impair maternal behavior and the maternal brain network: a literature review. Neurotoxicol Teratol 86:106976

Wang Y, Han T-Z (2009) Prenatal exposure to heroin in mice elicits memory deficits that can be attributed to neuronal apoptosis. Neuroscience 160(2):330–338

Wang X, Douglas SD, Commons KG, Pleasure DE, Lai J, Ho C, Bannerman P, Williams M, Ho W (2004) A non-peptide substance P antagonist (CP-96,345) inhibits morphine-induced NF-kappa B promoter activation in human NT2-N neurons. J Neurosci Res 75(4):544–553

Wang X, Loram LC, Ramos K, de Jesus AJ, Thomas J, Cheng K, Reddy A, Somogyi AA, Hutchinson MR, Watkins LR et al (2012) Morphine activates neuroinflammation in a manner parallel to endotoxin. Proc Natl Acad Sci U S A 109(16):6325–6330

Wang X, Gou X, Yu X, Bai D, Tan B, Cao P, Qian M, Zheng X, Wang H, Tang P et al (2021) Antinociceptive and antipruritic effects of HSK21542, a peripherally-restricted kappa opioid receptor agonist, in animal models of pain and itch. Front Pharmacol 12:773204

Watkins LR, Hutchinson MR, Rice KC, Maier SF (2009) The "toll" of opioid-induced glial activation: Improving the clinical efficacy of opioids by targeting glia. Trends Pharmacol Sci 30(11):581–591

Welton S, Blakelock B, Madden S, Kelly L (2019) Effects of opioid use in pregnancy on pediatric development and behaviour in children older than age 2: systematic review. Can Fam Physician 65(12):e544–e551

Wu C, Hung C, Shen C, Chen W, Chang C, Pan H, Liao S, Chen C (2014) Prenatal buprenorphine exposure decreases neurogenesis in rats. Toxicol Lett 225(1): 92–101

Wu P, Yang Y, Suen J, Yang YSH, Yang C, Yang S (2018) Long-lasting alterations in gene expression of postsynaptic density 95 and inotropic glutamatergic receptor subunit in the mesocorticolimbic system of rat offspring born to morphine-addicted mothers. Biomed Res Int 2018:5437092

Wu Y, Merhar SL, Bann CM, Newman JE, Kapse K, De Asis-Cruz J, Mack N, De Mauro SB, Ambalavanan N, Davis JM et al (2025) Antenatal opioid exposure and global and regional brain volumes in newborns. JAMA Pediatr 179(6):639–646

Yeoh SL, Eastwood J, Wright IM, Morton R, Melhuish E, Ward M, Oei JL (2019) Cognitive and motor outcomes of children with prenatal opioid exposure: a systematic review and meta-analysis. JAMA Netw Open 2(7): e197025

Younger JW, Chu LF, D'Arcy NT, Trott KE, Jastrzab LE, Mackey SC (2011) Prescription opioid analgesics rapidly change the human brain. Pain 152(8):1803–1810

Zagon IS, McLaughlin PJ (1977) The effects of different schedules of methadone treatment on rat brain development. Exp Neurol 56(3):538–552

Zagon IS, McLaughlin PJ (1978) Perinatal methadone exposure and brain development: a biochemical study. J Neurochem 31(1):49–54

Zhang P, Yang M, Chen C, Liu L, Wei X, Zeng S (2020) Toll-like receptor 4 (TLR4)/opioid receptor pathway crosstalk and impact on opioid analgesia, immune function, and gastrointestinal motility. Front Immunol 11:1455

Zhou W, Li Y, Meng X, Liu A, Mao Y, Zhu X, Meng Q, Jin Y, Zhang Z, Tao W (2021) Switching of delta opioid receptor subtypes in central amygdala microcircuits is associated with anxiety states in pain. J Biol Chem 296:100277

Zhu Y, Hsu MS, Pintar JE (1998) Developmental expression of the mu, kappa, and delta opioid receptor mRNAs in mouse. J Neurosci 18(7):2538–2549

12 Prenatal Opioid Exposure and Neonatal Opioid Withdrawal Syndrome

Alana Painter, Kathryn Westphal, Adriana Herrera,
Emilee Lewis, Alison Sweeney, and Ashley G. Sutton

Abstract

Maternal substance use during pregnancy exposes the fetus to pharmacologic effects and creates the potential for dependence and withdrawal in the neonatal period. Opioids cross the placenta and the fetal blood–brain barrier, resulting in prenatal opioid exposure (POE). The binding of opioids to developing opioid receptors disrupts neurologic, gastrointestinal, and autonomic regulation, leading to the development of neonatal opioid withdrawal syndrome (NOWS), previously referred to as neonatal abstinence syndrome (NAS). The impact of exposure varies by opioid type, dose, duration, and maternal metabolism, resulting in a wide spectrum of neonatal symptoms and severity.

In response to the rising incidence of NOWS during the heroin epidemic, scoring systems, including the Finnegan scale, were developed to guide diagnosis and treatment. Infants with POE whose Finnegan scores reached a particular threshold were treated with pharmacologic therapy (typically morphine), which required a prolonged taper. A more recently defined approach, the Eat, Sleep, Console method, focuses on functional well-being rather than a numeric score. Current best practice for management emphasizes non-pharmacologic interventions such as caregiver presence, skin-to-skin care, and a low-stimulation environment, and reserves pharmacologic therapy for severe symptoms.

While short-term effects of POE are well documented, including prolonged hospitalization and feeding challenges, long-term neurodevelopmental and behavioral outcomes remain under investigation. Further research is essential to refine screening, optimize management strategies, standardize care, and address

A. Painter (✉) · K. Westphal
Department of Pediatrics, College of Medicine, The Ohio State University, Columbus, OH, USA

Division of Pediatric Hospital Medicine, Nationwide Children's Hospital, Columbus, OH, USA
e-mail: Alana.Painter@nationwidechildrens.org

A. Herrera
Division of Pediatric Hospital Medicine, Nationwide Children's Hospital, Columbus, OH, USA

Department of Pediatrics, University of North Carolina at Chapel Hill, School of Medicine, Chapel Hill, NC, USA

Division of Pediatric Hospital Medicine, University of North Carolina Children's Hospital, Chapel Hill, NC, USA

E. Lewis · A. Sweeney · A. G. Sutton
Department of Pediatrics, University of North Carolina at Chapel Hill, School of Medicine, Chapel Hill, NC, USA

Division of Pediatric Hospital Medicine, University of North Carolina Children's Hospital, Chapel Hill, NC, USA
e-mail: agsutton@email.unc.edu

A. N. Bukiya, D. W. Ali (eds.), *Molecular Mechanisms and Lifelong Consequences of Prenatal Exposure to Psychoactive Substances*, Advances in Experimental Medicine and Biology 1500,
https://doi.org/10.1007/978-3-032-12741-9_12

social and health disparities affecting families impacted by POE.

Keywords

Prenatal opioid exposure · Neonatal abstinence syndrome · Neonatal opioid withdrawal syndrome · Finnegan scoring · Eat, Sleep, Console method · Neurodevelopmental outcomes

12.1 Overview

Maternal use of substances during pregnancy exposes the developing fetus to their associated effects, creates a potential for dependence and withdrawal in the neonatal period, and may have long-term sequelae on the child (Bakhireva et al. 2019; Bakhireva et al. 2022; Fujiwara et al. 2023; Gray et al. 2010; Levine & Woodward 2018; Levine et al. 2021; Wouldes & Lester 2023). There can be significant variation in the interval and dosage of maternal medications and substance use, and maternal and fetal exposure can include either prescribed/or illicit substances (Allegaert and Oei 2022). Maternal use and misuse of medications and substances varies widely from intermittent or random use intervals to daily intake or exposure. For certain substances, alcohol, for example, there is clear evidence that in utero exposure is harmful to the fetus and results in a well-described syndrome with a spectrum of effects on developmental and health outcomes (Wang & Cosci 2021). For other substances, including many prescribed medications, the potential impact on the fetus is often unclear or unknown (Benninger et al. 2022; Benninger et al. 2023). At the time of birth, there is an immediate cessation of exposure when the umbilical cord is cut, creating the potential for withdrawal from the compound. Neonatal abstinence syndrome (NAS) is the broad term used to describe newborn neurobehavioral dysregulation from in utero substance exposure, which may or may not include opioids (Roncero et al. 2020; Cestonaro et al. 2022). This may consist of withdrawal from a substance or the direct effects of the substance.

Historically, NAS has frequently become synonymous with infants with prenatal opioid exposure (POE) and the immediate outcomes and clinical findings resulting from infant dependency at birth. Neonatal Opioid Withdrawal Syndrome (NOWS) has more recently been used in the literature to specifically describe infants with signs and symptoms of POE. For clarity, NOWS will be utilized to describe this infant condition, despite the term not being utilized in historical literature. Like many substances, maternal opioid use resulting in POE encompasses a highly variable spectrum of exposure, including prescribed opioids for treatment of acute or chronic conditions during pregnancy, intermittent illicit use of non-prescribed opioids including diverted prescribed or synthetic opioid medications and heroin, and chronic maternal opioid use disorder (OUD) with or without medication assisted treatment (MAT) with prescribed long-acting opioids.

Opioids readily cross both the placenta and the blood–brain barrier, and the exact degree of exposure is dependent on the type of drug (long vs. short acting), timing and duration of exposure, and metabolism in the maternal liver and the placenta (differs for each patient) (Van Hoogdalem et al. 2022). Fetal-to-maternal plasma concentration ratios of 0.5–1.0 have been reported for various opiates. Mu, delta, and kappa opioid receptors are expressed in the human fetus as early as 10–12 weeks of gestation, and expression of these receptors increases with gestational age (Spodnick et al. 2025). Despite variable medications, substances, and metabolism, opioids remain highly available for uptake in fetal opioid receptors that are present in higher proportions in both the gastrointestinal tract and the nervous system than in other tissues (Herlenius and Lagercrantz 2001). Impact on these tissues leads to the most common symptoms associated with NOWS, namely, irritability and dysregulation of these systems, and may also alter development, leading to other medical consequences, such as necrotizing enterocolitis (NEC) and weight faltering (Barnett et al. 2024; Caritis and Panigrahy 2019). In the setting of maternal OUD, there are high rates of polysubstance co-use, which likely have both separate and additive impacts on fetal development and symptoms following birth (Bader et al 2021; Blount et al. 2019). As such, fetal POE results in a wide range of duration and dose of exposure, resulting in a spectrum of symptoms and degree of disrupted state regulation in infants (Hasan et al. 2024).

12.2 Historical Context

Four naturally occurring compounds can be isolated from *P. somniferum,* including morphine, codeine, thebaine, and papaverine. Many semi-synthetic (heroin, dihydromorphone, buprenorphine, oxycodone) and synthetic compounds (fentanyl, methadone) can be derived from these naturally occurring alkaloids. Opioids can be classified by their derivatives or based on their effect at opioid receptors. While the nomenclature has changed several times over history, there are three opioid receptors: mu or MOP, delta or DOP, and kappa or KOP. These receptors are located throughout the central nervous system and peripheral tissues. Opioids act on these receptors as agonists, partial agonists, antagonists, or agonist-antagonists. Opioid agonists interact with a receptor to produce a complete response, antagonists bind to the receptor and produce no response but block an agonist from binding, partial agonists bind receptors and produce a partial response, and agonist-antagonists have both agonist and antagonist activity, which varies based on receptor type (James and Williams 2020).

Ancient writings describe the cultivation of the opium poppy, *Papaver somniferum*, for the use of its active ingredients. The early use of opium as a euphoriant is described as early as 3000 BC, and records of medicinal use date as early as 1500 BC (Brownstein 1993). In 1806, the active ingredient in opium was isolated and named morphine. While descriptions of abuse appeared in Europe in the sixteenth century, the determination of the chemical formula for morphine and the invention of the hypodermic needle in the nineteenth century led to more widespread use.

Congenital morphinism, the term coined to describe infants born to mothers using opiates, first appeared in the literature in 1875, with the definition of "full term infants who appeared normal at birth, then began crying inconsolably on the third day of life; some of these infants were reported to develop generalized seizures" (Perlstein 1947). Initially, these infants were noted to have a high mortality rate, likely due to a lack of modern general neonatal care and outcomes, as well as infants with dependence having associated poor feeding and subsequent hypoglycemia, which resulted in seizures and death.

Heroin, synthesized in 1898, was believed not to cause addiction, and was sold over-the-counter as treatment for colds and influenza (Gomez-Pomar and Finnegan 2018; Offit 2016). With the false impression of safety, heroin was even marketed to pregnant women and infants (Offit 2016). In the early twentieth century, a case series described successful treatment of opium-exposed infants and children with opium in small quantities, directly and/or indirectly through breastmilk (Petty 1912). This early observation influenced the treatment of infants with POE with narcotics.

Maternal opioid use became a critical concern during the heroin epidemic of the 1970s and led to the first modern description of the spectrum of clinical findings of NOWS (Finnegan et al. 1975). Scoring systems, including Finnegan Neonatal Abstinence Scoring System (FNASS), the Lipsitz tool, the Neonatal Narcotic Withdrawal Index, and the Ostrea tool, were developed as a way to identify infants with NOWS and quantify the severity of symptoms. The Finnegan scoring, developed in 1975, was developed as a means to evaluate infants at risk for opiate withdrawal in a uniform manner and variations of this scale became the most commonly used scale for several decades. Diagnostic criteria for NOWS became synonymous with FNASS scoring, resulting in challenges with determining the sensitivity and specificity of this model for assessing and treating infants with opioid dependence. Despite widespread clinical adoption of the FNASS to diagnose and treat NOWS, no consensus has been reached regarding which scoring system should be used, score thresholds for treatment, or frequency of assessments. Despite publication and widespread knowledge of the potential impact on infants related to maternal use, the incidence of NOWS has steadily increased since the 1970s (Patrick et al. 2012).

The epidemiology of POE has evolved significantly in recent decades, reflecting broader trends in opioid use and misuse. Opioid prescriptions for the treatment of chronic pain emerged in the early 2000s. False marketing claims of the non-addictive nature of these medications led to misguided comfort in both the prescribing and use of opioid pain medications. The number of opioid prescriptions for pain in pregnant women increased dramatically. A retrospective cohort study of pregnant women enrolled in Tennessee Medicaid demonstrated that the prevalence of prescribed opioid analgesics doubled from 1995 to 2009 (Epstein 2013). Initial sustained, consistent exposure to long-acting opioids resulting from prescription use changed the pattern of presentation for infants affected by POE, with potential for increased dependency due to regular, and often escalating, opioid dosages compared with obtainment and use of heroin illicitly. Increased prescriptions and poor controls on the amount of pills prescribed per patient resulted in an eruption in the volume of diverted, prescribed narcotics being used, and additionally contributed to increased adult OUD during this era. Due to both the increase in maternal exposure and the nature of the consistent opioid exposure, the rate of NOWS increased in the United States from 1.5 per 1,000 hospital births in 2004 to 6.2 per 1000 live births in 2020 (Hirai et al. 2021). Overall, the number of infants affected by POE is likely underestimated, given that diagnosis is clinical and there is no gold standard objective method to determine infants that are mildly affected by NOWS, but do not require intervention beyond standard care. It is also important to note that the diagnosis of NOWS focuses on the immediate outcome for the infant in the weeks following delivery. There is no current diagnostic category and limited data defining longer-term impacts of POE or the definition of a syndrome of long-term impacts akin to fetal alcohol spectrum disorders for in utero alcohol exposure.

Widespread knowledge of the addictive impacts of prescribed opioids has led to significant tightening and oversight of prescription opioids in the general population, including pregnant women. Fortunately, some data suggest stabilization or decline in OUD due to improved opioid prescribing practices and harm-reduction efforts (Hirai et al. 2021). Concurrently, there has been an evolution in the approach to treatment for stabilizing pregnant women with OUD during pregnancy. Given the high level of potential maternal and fetal morbidity and the vulnerability of the period of pregnancy for mothers with OUD, current recommendations include stabilization with long-acting opioids such as methadone or buprenorphine (Lisonkova et al. 2019). While this has been shown to improve maternal/infant dyad outcomes overall, it additionally contributes to the population of infants with NOWS who have exposure to long-acting opioids with prolonged half-lives and develop symptoms much later than previously described infants with POE from heroin or shorter-acting prescription opioids (Suarez et al. 2022). More recently, exposure to manufactured and synthetic opioids, including fentanyl, that lack any pharmacologic oversight or testing for purity, has impacted both the clinical presentation and management of exposed infants. Heroin and other opioids have been noted to have an increase in fentanyl contamination. Additionally, a large proportion of illicit fentanyl contains other substances that can both increase potency and risk of overdose for adults, but have further potential impacts that are undefined on infants with in-utero exposure (Edinoff et al. 2024).

The highest rates of NOWS are seen in rural areas in the United States (particularly Appalachia and New England) and those economically disadvantaged, where OUD is more prevalent (Mascarenhas et al. 2024). NOWS also disproportionately affects infants born to younger mothers, those with lower socioeconomic status, and those receiving public health insurance (Strahan 2020). While the United States has some of the highest reported rates of NOWS, opioid exposure in utero is a growing issue globally. Differences in opioid prescribing practices, access to addiction treatment, and newborn care protocols contribute to differences in NOWS incidence worldwide (Blandthorn 2018).

12.3 Screening and Diagnosis

The American College of Obstetricians and Gynecologists (ACOG) recommends universal screening for substance use during the first prenatal visit using a validated screening tool (Obstet Gynecol. 2017). This is the preferred method to identify infants with in-utero opioid exposure who would then be at risk for the development of NOWS (Patrick et al. 2020). These screening tools can be completed via a written questionnaire or verbally with the patient, and are preferred over toxicology testing. Commonly used screening tools include the 4P's Plus, NIDA Quick Screen ASSIST (Modified Alcohol, Smoking and Substance Involvement Screening Test), and SURP-P (Substance Use Risk Profile-Pregnancy) scale, which have an 80–90% sensitivity rate for substance use (Bader et al. 2021; Coleman-Cowger et al. 2019; Witt et al. 2017). The CRAFFT is also a validated screening tool appropriate for patients less than 26 years of age (Mascola et al. 2017). The intention behind prenatal screens is primarily to ensure the health and safety of both the mother and the infant by identifying potential substance use that could impact pregnancy outcomes, and provide the opportunity for brief intervention and referral for treatment if appropriate. Despite the recommendation for universal screening for substance use during pregnancy, there is variability in screening rates, but in settings with a standard screening process, 80–90% of patients are screened prenatally (Hostage et al. 2020; Patel et al. 2021 Ulrich et al. 2021; White et al. 2024).

ACOG and the American Academy of Pediatrics (AAP) recommend against routine testing of pregnant women for illicit substances. Concerns with substance use testing include the potential for false positive results, which can have a significant legal impact depending on mandatory reporting laws (Dos Santos et al. 2018). Also, a positive test reflects a specific period in time and provides limited information on the amount of substance used and with what frequency or duration. Additionally, it is possible for the test to not capture certain substances that are not included in the test or are not detected at the time of testing, depending on the date of last use (Lebin and Novick 2022; Mascola et al. 2017). With regard to both perinatal toxicology testing and the legal ramifications of substance use testing, significant racial and ethnic disparities exist (Grigoriadis et al. 2020; Murosko 2022; Pahl et al. 2020). Therefore, these professional societies encourage obtaining consent prior to any toxicology testing being performed perinatally or after the birth of the infant. Toxicology testing can be performed on urine, meconium, or umbilical cord blood. Testing should be reserved for cases in which the results would impact the clinical management of the infant.

Early detection of opioid use during pregnancy is essential for implementing timely interventions that can significantly improve neonatal outcomes and overall maternal-infant health. Early detection facilitates the initiation of medication-assisted treatment (MAT) with buprenorphine or methadone, which has been shown to improve maternal outcomes and reduce the risk of relapse. It also allows for comprehensive antenatal counseling, including education on NOWS, breastfeeding benefits, and postpartum care. This anticipatory guidance prepares parents for the delivery, hospitalization, and potential challenges that may arise. Lastly, early detection can lead to other methods of support, including counseling and social services.

A panel of experts identified two required criteria for the diagnosis of NOWS. The first criterion is known exposure to opioids during pregnancy. This could be reported by the mother or identified on toxicology testing of the mother or infant. The second criteria is the presence of at least two of the most common clinical signs of withdrawal, specifically excessive crying, fragmented sleep, tremors, hypertonia, and gastrointestinal dysfunction (Jilani et al. 2022). The signs and symptoms of NOWS can be similar to other significant pathologies in the newborn.

Sepsis, seizures, respiratory distress, hyperthyroidism, and hypoglycemia are examples of diagnoses that can mimic or accompany NOWS. It is important for the clinician to consider these diagnoses if the newborn is not responding to interventions as expected.

12.4 Presentation

The clinical presentation of NOWS primarily involves dysfunction of the central nervous system, gastrointestinal tract, and/or autonomic system, where fetal opioid receptors are known to be present. Withdrawal from opioids is highly complex in all patients, but understanding the pathophysiology in neonates is further compounded by their neurological immaturity and difficulty separating the effects of prenatal exposure on the developing fetus from the direct effect of dependence and withdrawal after delivery (Kocherlakota 2014; . Infants experience a range of metabolic disturbances, including increased energy expenditure manifesting as hyperphagia (excessive feeding attempts) and weight loss (Biffi et al. 2020). Estimated caloric needs for infants experiencing NOWS are 30–60% higher than unaffected newborns, with increased caloric need to maintain growth estimated to be 150–200 calories per kilogram per day (Hudak et al. 2012). This is partly due to the activation of the hypothalamic-pituitary-adrenal (HPA) axis and the autonomic nervous system, leading to symptoms such as irritability, tremors, and gastrointestinal disturbances like vomiting and diarrhea. Other common clinical manifestations of NOWS include difficulty feeding, excessive sucking, poor weight gain, jitteriness, hyperreflexia, sweating, sneezing, elevated temperatures, tachypnea, frequent yawning, and disruption of normal sleep patterns (Mascarenhas et al. 2024). Many of these manifestations contribute to and are exacerbated by others, including the combination of increased caloric expenditure and hyperphagia and frequent oral motor feeding dysfunction due to poor state regulation and neurologic status. Without intervention, these manifestations can combine to result in significant weight loss and agitation that can worsen withdrawal symptoms overall due to hunger and calorie deficit.

As previously mentioned, not every infant with POE develops clinically significant NOWS. The onset and severity of those affected depend on many factors, including opioid type, amount and timing of exposure, maternal and infant metabolism, and other substance exposure (Cestonaro et al. 2022; Patrick et al. 2020; Straub 2022). In general, the timing of withdrawal reflects the half-life of the opioid. Signs of withdrawal may begin within the first 24 h of life for short-acting opioids, whereas withdrawal from longer-acting opioids like methadone and buprenorphine typically appears in the first 72 h of life but may not emerge for 2–5 days. The acute period of withdrawal typically lasts several days to weeks; however, subacute signs can persist for several months. Disease severity and likelihood of developing clinically significant NOWS have also been shown to increase with higher cumulative doses of prescribed opioids during pregnancy (Straub 2022). Infants exposed to medication to treat OUD generally have less severe NOWS than those exposed to illicit and prescribed opiates prenatally. Among infants with prenatal exposure to medication to treat OUD (most commonly buprenorphine or methadone), those who were methadone-exposed tended to have more severe disease than those who were buprenorphine-exposed (Bakhireva et al. 2022; Suarez et al. 2022; Jones et al. 2010). This difference is attributed to buprenorphine having low intrinsic opioid receptor efficacy as a partial mu-opioid agonist and a kappa-opioid antagonist, compared with methadone, which is a full mu-opioid agonist. In adults with OUD, buprenorphine has a low overdose risk, and patients abruptly discontinuing use do not experience intense withdrawal, as is common with full mu-opioid agonists. These properties presumably translate to decreased overall opioid exposure by POE and, similar to adults, milder symptoms of withdrawal after birth (Jones et al. 2010). However, clinical scenarios exist in which methadone may be utilized to treat OUD for expectant mothers, depending on access to clinics and the degree of opioid dependence, given that buprenorphine has less of an opioid effect overall. Interestingly, overall engagement in prenatal care seems to be protective against severe disease, and, given that mothers being prescribed MAT for OUD are by default connected to care, these combined findings may exponentially improve outcomes for infants. Current research additionally suggests that genetic and epigenetic factors may contribute to an infant's risk of severe disease (Bibi 2023, Roncero et al. 2020). Additionally, NOWS is less likely to occur in infants delivered prematurely, believed to be due to a variety of factors, including increased permeability of the placenta to opioids with increasing gestational age, less cumulative exposure, and differences in opioid accumulation/storage and sensitivity with earlier gestational ages (Kocherlakota 2014).

Polysubstance exposure is common and likely a risk factor for infants being diagnosed with NOWS. Exposure to multiple substances impacts the clinical course of NOWS in both unique and compounding ways. For example, heroin and cocaine can directly impact POE exposure as they cause increased placental permeability, and thus fetal exposure, of some opiates (Kocherlakota 2014). Infants who are withdrawing from another substance in addition to opioid exposure may struggle to cope with the added stress of concurrent withdrawal from multiple substances. Given that most other substances do not have prescribed approaches to assist with weaning from dependence in infants, clinical symptoms can also overlap and result in increased apparent symptoms from POE that overlap with withdrawal from other substances. While many co-exposures have unclear data, prior studies have demonstrated that concurrent exposure to opioids and cocaine and/or cannabis is associated with more severe NOWS (Gray et al. 2010; Gunn et al. 2016; Morris 2022; Munn et al. 2024; Roncero et al. 2020). Additionally, co-exposure to psychiatric medications, including selective serotonin reuptake inhibitors, benzodiazepines, and gabapentin, is associated with more severe NOWS (Kautzky et al 2022; Sanlorenzo et al. 2019; Wang and Cosci 2021).

12.5 Evaluation

Given the risks associated with POE and its effects on the infant after delivery, infants with POE are monitored for signs and symptoms of withdrawal and other consequences of in utero exposure. During the birth hospitalization, infants with POE are monitored for signs of withdrawal shortly after birth, then every three to four hours until discharge. Infants with POE are typically monitored in the mother-infant unit, unless other indications for transfer to a neonatal intensive care unit exist, and assessments are completed in the room alongside the caregiver. Rooming-in of the infant with the caregiver is associated with increased parental presence during hospitalization, higher rates of breastfeeding initiation, reduced need for pharmacologic treatment of withdrawal, fewer total days of opioid treatment if needed, and a shorter length of hospitalization compared with care in separate units (MacMillan 2018; Hahn et al. 2024). The potential need for cardiorespiratory monitoring may limit the ability to room-in in some settings. Limited data suggest it is safe to monitor infants with POE not requiring pharmacotherapy without the use of cardiorespiratory monitors, while cardiorespiratory monitoring may be used for those infants who do require pharmacotherapy (Joshi 2023).

Prenatal opioid exposure (POE) can result in a physiologic dependence for infants, with subsequent withdrawal symptoms following delivery, and may require medical management in neonatal care settings. There are two predominant scoring tools used to guide the diagnosis and treatment of neonatal withdrawal (Grossman 2018; Czynski et al. 2020; Marchand et al. 2022). Despite variability in tools used, each can be successful if used in a standardized way, and the medical team is adequately trained on the tool to improve inter-rater reliability. Historically, the previously mentioned FNASS was the most common scoring tool used in the United States. This tool uses 21 items to evaluate a range of withdrawal symptoms. Each symptom is assigned a score based on the severity at the time of the assessment. A total score of eight or higher on two assessments or a single score of 12 or higher suggests the infant may need pharmacologic treatment. A newer scoring tool is the function-based Eat, Sleep, Console (ESC) method (Grossman et al. 2018). If an infant is unable to eat at least one ounce or breastfeed well, sleep undisturbed for at least one hour, and/or be consoled within 10 min, the medical team then huddles to brainstorm ways to optimize non-pharmacologic care. If an infant continues to have difficulty with these three functions despite optimization of non-pharmacologic care, the infant may need pharmacologic treatment. The evolution of evaluation, as well as variability in scoring and management approach, is reflective of the historical evolution of NOWS identification and diagnosis, and lack of a defined standard outside of immediate symptoms to diagnose onset of the disorder. Both scores and all known evaluation methods for NOWS involve subjectivity and thus have the potential for variability in diagnosis and treatment (Grigoriadis et al. 2020; Pahl et al. 2020). While the FNASS is more focused on the specific disturbances that may point towards opioid withdrawal requiring intervention, the ESC approach is more focused on clinical outcomes to promote progression to successful antenatal transition and discharge. International comparisons of NOWS assessment practices reflect wide differences in both scoring tools and treatment thresholds (Benninger et al. 2023; Grigoriadis et al. 2022; Cestonaro et al. 2022).

12.6 Management

Infants with POE have difficulty with state-regulation and managing stimulation of the extra-uterine environment for many of the reasons discussed previously. As such, much of the care of the infant post-delivery is focused on managing the environment while the infant adjusts to the withdrawal of maternal opioids to limit energy expenditure and help maintain a supportive environment for the infant to transition and obtain self-regulation. Standard components of environmental control of stimuli, typically referred to as non-pharmacologic care, are provided for all opioid exposed infants, regardless of definite NOWS symptoms, in addition to individualized approaches (Allegaert & Oei 2022; Biffi et al. 2020; Roncero et al. 2020). The rationale for this approach is that promoting regulation and limiting environmental stimuli may improve the infant's ability to cope with mild NOWS symptoms and still achieve clinical goals for progression towards discharge. Additionally, infants with NOWS have exaggerated neurologic responses (tremors, exaggerated Moro reflex, hypertonia, irritability) at baseline, and thus limiting provocation of these symptoms can assist in the infant being more easily soothed and promote feeding, which is crucial to successful management of NOWS (Hudak 2012; Gaalema et al. 2012).

Standard practices include maintaining the mother-infant dyad, clustering care, skin-to-skin contact with a caregiver, safe swaddling, promoting the use of pacifiers or thumbs for excessive sucking, maintaining a low stimulation environment, and promoting breastfeeding. Assuming the absence of contraindications, breastfeeding is generally safe for mothers taking prescribed methadone or buprenorphine, especially if the mother has not had a relapse in the last three months and has not been actively using other substances (Wouldes and Lester 2023). Low concentrations of methadone and buprenorphine are excreted in the breast milk and may allow for more gradual opioid withdrawal and minimize NOWS symptoms. Concentration of buprenorphine in breast milk is equivalent to less than 1% of the maternal weight-adjusted dose, and the concentration of methadone in breast milk is equivalent to 2–3% of the maternal weight-adjusted dose (Jansson and Patrick 2019; Jansson et al. 2008, 2016, 2024). Other interventions can be used to directly target the particular symptoms of an infant experiencing withdrawal. For example, an infant with tremors or a hyperactive Moro reflex may benefit from swaddling. Prevention of increased painful stimuli, including barrier cream to prevent skin breakdown from loose stools and swaddling to minimize excoriations of the skin from excessive movement and scratching, can also be beneficial.

Given increased energy expenditure during withdrawal, infants are at risk for excessive weight loss. Ensuring early adequate nutrition to minimize weight loss is part of their initial care. Infants are fed on demand, at a minimum every three hours. If an infant is experiencing excessive weight loss, interventions may include supplementing breastfeeding with formula feeding and fortifying expressed breastmilk or formula to a higher calorie content. If the infant is unable to consume enough calories to meet their energy needs with these interventions or because of other symptoms of withdrawal (i.e., poor coordination, irritability), then nutrition can be supported with nasogastric tube feeds (Levine & Woodward 2018; Wang & Cosci 2021; Biffi et al. 2020). Interventions to minimize withdrawal symptoms also mitigate caloric expenditure and can additionally help promote weight gain.

Historically, infants identified as having clinically significant signs of withdrawal were treated with scheduled doses of morphine, which were slowly weaned as the mainstay of management (Patrick 2020; Davis et al. 2018). Protocols attempted to estimate dose-exposure and need for post-natal opioid and opted for a slow taper to allow for mitigation of withdrawal symptoms. However, a growing body of literature from the current era of the opioid epidemic suggests that due to the complex nature and many contributing factors that impact the severity of NOWS and its response to opioid therapy, this approach was likely not warranted for many infants with POE. Research supports that primarily relying on opioid management of infants with POE results in prolonged postnatal opioid exposure, lengthy hospitalizations resulting in separation of the mother-infant dyad, and increased expenditures (Blount et al. 2019). While this practice continues to exist for certain clinical scenarios, more recent models emphasize non-pharmacologic interventions and the use of as-needed treatment with morphine for NOWS (Benninger et al. 2022; Hahn et al. 2023; Hahn et al. 2024; Marchand et al. 2022; Munn et al. 2024; Kautzky et al. 2022). Scheduled doses of morphine are only initiated after an infant has received several as-needed doses. Occasionally, adjunctive therapy with clonidine and/or phenobarbital is utilized in refractory cases when morphine monotherapy is insufficient to control symptoms. These adjunctive therapies may also target the impacts of polysubstance exposure and components of neurologic immaturity that compound the poor state regulation and withdrawal symptoms from POE. The shift in practice from Finnegan scoring to ESC, and from scheduled to as-needed doses of morphine has been shown to shorten hospital length of stay and decrease pharmacologic use without an increase in adverse events (Young et al. 2023).

The timing of discharge is dependent on successful transition to postnatal life for the infant, including the ability to feed and maintain enough intake for the expected weight trajectory to be normal, achieving state-regulation, and not requiring opioid management of symptoms. Infants were often hospitalized for 30 or more days under prior protocols that resulted in high doses of postnatal opioid administration and prolonged weaning. Under current approaches, many infants do not receive opioid therapy postnatally, and thus observation time can vary depending on clinical and social factors, including the half-life of the opioid resulting in POE, parental support, and assurance of outpatient monitoring of the infant for complications. Given the wide variability of presentation and degree of POE, some infants transition to home care closer to a timeline of a non-opiate-exposed newborn, and others require longer hospitalization for feeding or medication management.

Post-hospital care of an infant with NOWS is important as they are at increased risk of rehospitalization and higher healthcare utilization within the first year of life (Shrestha et al. 2021). Reasons for readmission include a variety of medical and social issues, including higher odds of readmission for lower respiratory infections, seizures, poor growth, traumatic brain injury, and skull fractures (Gaither et al. 2024; Salt et al. 2023; Milliren 2021). These hospitalizations have been described as longer, more expensive, and more likely to require the intensive care unit (Milliren 2021). Findings suggest infants with POE and NOWS need comprehensive post-discharge follow-up and support to address both medical needs and social determinants of health, which could minimize preventable readmissions and optimize outcomes. Interventions may include home visits, social work involvement, lactation support, and efforts to target appointment attendance.

12.7 Outcomes

Short-term outcomes for infants with POE are very clearly defined in the literature and are of interest to clinicians working in the hospital setting, as they assist with transition to home care. Assessed outcomes include those discussed above such as caloric intake and weight trajectory, and also include length of stay (LOS) in the hospital attributable to NOWS, need for admission to a neonatal intensive care unit, total opioid treatment days for infants who receive pharmacotherapy, need for readmission to the hospital after discharge from birth hospitalization, and outcomes of the maternal-infant dyad including risk of maltreatment of the infant or inadequate weight gain following discharge from the hospital.

Length of stay attributable to NOWS varies based on the substance of exposure, screening tool used to monitor the infant for withdrawal, use of nonpharmacologic treatment, and use of pharmacotherapy for the infant. Infants born to mothers on medication-assisted therapy (MAT, including methadone or buprenorphine) had a shorter LOS when compared with infants born to mothers who did not use MAT (Zankl et al. 2021). Use of pharmacotherapy to treat NOWS is associated with increased risk of intensive care admission (and therefore separation of the mother-infant dyad), and increased LOS. A large cluster randomized control trial demonstrated a decrease in time to readiness to discharge with the use of the Eat, Sleep, Consult method versus usual therapy, with no difference in adverse outcome rate (Young et al. 2023).

Prenatal opioid exposure has been associated with differences in head growth and brain structure at birth. Several studies have reported that infants treated for NOWS have a significantly smaller mean head circumference compared to non-opioid-exposed controls. Furthermore, they are more likely to meet criteria for microcephaly (<10th percentile) compared to controls (Towers et al. 2019; Visconti et al. 2015). Head growth is a surrogate for brain growth in utero, so this difference in head circumference may have implications for neurodevelopmental outcomes. POE has also been associated with microstructural alteration in white matter tracts in the brain, independent of head growth (Monnelly 2017). Monnelly and colleagues performed diffused MRI on 20 methadone-exposed and 20 non-exposed newborns and compared fractional anisotropy data between them. Fractional anisotropy is a quantitative measure that assesses the diffusion of water molecules in brain tissue. In the developing brain, water diffusion becomes increasingly directional (anisotropic) as white matter tracts mature. This is due to the growth of axons, myelination, and improved organization of fiber bundles (Mukherjee et al. 2001). Reduced fractional anisotropy reflects disrupted or delayed white matter development, which is important for communication between brain regions. Data from the study by Monnelly et al. (2017) revealed that methadone-exposed newborns had decreased fractional anisotropy, possibly due to opioid-related neurotoxicity or altered neurodevelopmental signaling affecting white matter integrity during critical periods of brain development. Lower fractional anisotropy is associated with poorer neurodevelopmental outcomes (Brown-Lum et al. 2020), which may help explain some observed long-term neurodevelopmental vulnerabilities in infants with POE.

Long-term outcomes from POE and NOWS, including risk of developmental delay, vision impairment, out-of-home placement, neurobehavioral disorders, and mortality, have proven more challenging to investigate. Additionally, POE and other prenatal substance exposures result in increased risk of being born small for gestational age, which, combined with increased immediate caloric needs, can result in longer-term challenges in maintaining adequate growth and nutritional status. Long-term need for nutritional support remains unclear and is an area for future study. Infants born with POE have also been shown, after the immediate newborn stage, to have increased healthcare utilization outside of routine health maintenance (MacMillan 2019). While prior studies suggest an increased risk of the aforementioned long-term outcomes with antenatal opioid exposure, limitations exist. Confounding factors, including maternal polysubstance use, nicotine use, concurrent maternal mental health disorders, and genetic and environmental differences, have interpreted prior studies difficult. Several large-scale studies aim to address the limitations of prior studies in order to better understand the relationship between POE, the treatment of NOWS, and long-term outcomes for the child.

Infants born to mothers with opioid use disorder or those given a NOWS diagnosis are notably at an increased risk of post-neonatal death (between one month and one year of life) compared with infants without these exposures. In the large cohort studies, most deaths were due to ill-defined or unknown causes (Grossarth et al. 2023) that are likely multifactorial. Future research is needed to study the increased risk of post-neonatal mortality further to understand other confounding and causative factors that can be targeted by preventative interventions.

References

Allegaert K, Oei JL (2022) Neonatal abstinence syndrome: prevention, management and outcomes: from birth to adulthood. Children (Basel). 9(8):1151. PMID 36010042

Bader MY, Zaghloul N, Repholz A et al (2021) A retrospective review following the addition of clonidine to a neonatal abstinence syndrome treatment algorithm. Front Pediatr. 9:632836. PMID 34164354

Bakhireva LN, Holbrook BD, Shrestha S et al (2019) Association between prenatal opioid exposure, neonatal opioid withdrawal syndrome, and neurodevelopmental and behavioral outcomes at 5–8 months of age. Early Hum Dev. 128:69–76. PMID 30554024

Bakhireva LN, Sparks A, Herman M, Hund L, Ashley M, Salisbury A (2022) Severity of neonatal opioid withdrawal syndrome with prenatal exposure to serotonin reuptake inhibitors. Pediatr Res. 91(4):867–873. PMID 34588611

Barnett RC, Lewis AN, Gong Q et al (2024) Modulation of intestinal TLR4 expression in infants with neonatal opioid withdrawal syndrome. J Perinatol 44:1125–1131. https://doi.org/10.1038/s41372-023-01859-2

Benninger KL, Richard C, Conroy S et al (2022) One-year neurodevelopmental outcomes after neonatal opioid withdrawal syndrome: a prospective cohort study. Perspect ASHA Spec Interest Groups. 7(4): 1019–1032. PMID 36211832

Benninger KL, McAllister JM, Merhar SL (2023) Neonatal opioid withdrawal syndrome: an update on developmental outcomes. Clin Perinatol. 50(1):17–29. PMID 36868704

Bibi S, Gaddis N, Johnson EO, Lester BM, Kraft W, Singh R, Terrin N, Adeniyi-Jones S, Davis JM (2023) Polygenic risk scores and the need for pharmacotherapy in neonatal abstinence syndrome. Pediatr Res 93 (5):1368–1374. https://doi.org/10.1038/s41390-022-02243-0. Epub 2022 Aug 16. PMID: 35974158; PMCID: PMC9931940

Biffi A, Cantarutti A, Rea F, Locatelli A, Zanini R, Corrao G (2020) Use of antidepressants during pregnancy and neonatal outcomes: an umbrella review of meta-analyses of observational studies. J Psychiatr Res. 124:99–108. PMID 32135392

Blandthorn J, Leung L, Loke Y, Lloyd-Jones DM, Thurman R, Bowman E, Bonomo Y (2018) Prescription opioid use in pregnancy. Aust N Z J Obstet Gynaecol 58(5):494–498. https://doi.org/10.1111/ajo.12823

Blount T, Painter A, Freeman E, Grossman M, Sutton AG (2019) Reduction in length of stay and morphine use for NAS with the "eat, sleep, console" method. Hosp Pediatr. 9(8):615–623. PMID 31285356

Brown-Lum M, Izadi-Najafabadi S, Oberlander TF, Rauscher A, Zwicker JG (2020) Differences in white matter microstructure among children with developmental coordination disorder. JAMA Netw Open. 3(3):e201184. https://doi.org/10.1001/jamanetworkopen.2020.1184

Brownstein MJ (1993) A brief history of opiates, opioid peptides, and opioid receptors. Proc Natl Acad Sci U S A. 90(12):5391–5393. https://doi.org/10.1073/pnas.90.12.5391. PMID:8390660; PMCID: PMC46725

Caritis SN, Panigrahy A (2019) Opioids affect the fetal brain: reframing the detoxification debate. Am J Obstet Gynecol 221(6):602–608. https://doi.org/10.1016/j.ajog.2019.07.022. Epub 2019 Jul 16. PMID: 31323217; PMCID: PMC8150872

Cestonaro C, Menozzi L, Terranova C (2022) Infants of mothers with cocaine use: review of clinical and medico-legal aspects. Children (Basel). 9(1):67. PMID 35053692

Coleman-Cowger V, Oga E, Peters E, Trocin K, Koszowski B, Mark K (2019) Accuracy of three screening tools for prenatal substance use. Obstetr Gynecol 133(5):952–961. https://doi.org/10.1097/AOG.0000000000003230

Czynski AJ, Davis JM, Dansereau LM et al (2020) Neurodevelopmental outcomes of neonates randomized to morphine or methadone for treatment of neonatal abstinence syndrome. J Pediatr. 219:146–151.e1. PMID 31987653

Davis JM, Shenberger J, Terrin N et al (2018) Comparison of safety and efficacy of methadone vs morphine for treatment of neonatal abstinence syndrome: a randomized clinical trial. JAMA Pediatr. 172(8): 741–748. PMID 29913015

Dos Santos JF, de Melo Bastos Cavalcante C, Barbosa FT et al (2018) Maternal, fetal and neonatal consequences associated with the use of crack cocaine during the gestational period: a systematic review and meta-analysis. Arch Gynecol Obstet. 298(3):487–503. PMID 29951712

Edinoff AN, Sall S, Upshaw WC, Spillers NJ, Vincik LY, De Witt AS, Murnane KS, Kaye AM, Kaye AD (2024) Xylazine: a drug adulterant of clinical concern. Curr Pain Headache Rep 28(5):417–426. https://doi.org/10.1007/s11916-024-01211-z. Epub 2024 Mar 20. PMID: 38507135 PMCID: PMC11126434

Epstein RA, Bobo WV, Martin PR, Morrow JA, Wang W, Chandrasekhar R, Cooper WO (2013) Increasing pregnancyrelated use of prescribed opioid analgesics. Ann Epidemiol 23(8):498–503. https://doi.org/10.1016/j.annepidem.2013.05.017. PMID: 23889859; PMCID: PMC3888316

Finnegan LP, Kron RE, Connaughton JF, Emich JP (1975) Assessment and treatment of abstinence in the infant of the drug-dependent mother. Int J Clin Pharmacol Biopharm. 12(1–2):19–32. PMID 1100537

Fujiwara R, Journey M, Al-Doori F et al (2023) Potential neonatal toxicity of new psychoactive substances. Pharmacol Ther 248:108468. PMID 37290575

Gaalema DE, Scott TL, Heil SH et al (2012) Differences in the profile of neonatal abstinence syndrome signs in methadone- versus buprenorphine-exposed neonates. Addiction. 107(Suppl 1):53–62. PMID 23106927

Gaither JR, Drago MJ, Grossman MR, Li Y, Shabanova V, Xu X, Leventhal JM (2024) Hospital readmissions among infants with neonatal opioid withdrawal syndrome. JAMA Netw Open. 7(9):e2435074. https://doi.org/10.1001/jamanetworkopen.2024.35074. PMID: 39316398; PMCID: PMC11423163

Gomez-Pomar E, Finnegan LP (2018) The epidemic of neonatal abstinence syndrome, historical references of its' origins, assessment, and management. Front Pediatr. 6:33. https://doi.org/10.3389/fped.2018.00033. PMID: 29520355; PMCID: PMC5827164

Gray TR, Eiden RD, Leonard KE, Connors GJ, Shisler S, Huestis MA (2010) Identifying prenatal cannabis exposure and effects of concurrent tobacco exposure on neonatal growth. Clin Chem. 56(9):1442–1450. PMID 20628142

Grigoriadis S, Graves L, Peer M et al (2020) Pregnancy and delivery outcomes following benzodiazepine exposure: a systematic review and meta-analysis. Can J Psychiatry. 65(12):821–834. PMID 32148076

Grigoriadis S, Alibrahim A, Mansfield JK, Sullovey A, Robinson GE (2022) Hypnotic benzodiazepine receptor agonist exposure during pregnancy and the risk of congenital malformations and other adverse pregnancy outcomes: a systematic review and meta-analysis. Acta Psychiatr Scand. 146(4):312–324. PMID 35488412

Grossarth S, Osmundson SS, Wiese AD et al (2023) Maternal opioid use disorder and the risk of postneonatal infant mortality. JAMA Pediatr. 177(7):675–683. PMID 37155175

Grossman MR, Lipshaw MJ, Osborn RR, Berkwitt AK (2018) A novel approach to assessing infants with neonatal abstinence syndrome. Hosp Pediatr 8(1):1–6. PMID 29263121

Gunn JKL, Rosales CB, Center KE et al (2016) Prenatal exposure to cannabis and maternal and child health outcomes: a systematic review and meta-analysis. BMJ Open. 6(4):e009986. PMID 27048634

Hahn PD, Melvin P, Graham DA, Ozonoff A, Milliren CE (2023) Association between pharmacologic treatment and hospital utilization at birth among neonatal opioid withdrawal syndrome mother-infant dyads. J Perinatol. 43(3):283–292. PMID 36717607

Hahn PD, Graham DA, Ozonoff A, Milliren CE (2024) Neonatal opioid withdrawal syndrome treatment guidelines and birth hospital utilization. Pediatrics. 154(1):e2023063635. PMID 38899388

Hasan M, Meador KJ, Brothers TN et al (2024) Neurodevelopmental outcomes in children prenatally exposed to opioid maintenance treatment: a population-based study. Pharmacotherapy. 44(10): 770–781. PMID 39415648

Herlenius E, Lagercrantz H (2001) Neurotransmitters and neuromodulators during early human development. Early Hum Dev. 65(1):21–37. https://doi.org/10.1016/s0378-3782(01)00189-x

Hirai AH, Ko JY, Owens PL, Stocks C, Patrick SW (2021) Neonatal abstinence syndrome and maternal opioid-related diagnoses in the us, 2010–2017. JAMA. 325(2):146–155. PMID 33433576

Hostage J, Brock J, Craig W, Sepulveda D (2020) Integrating Screening, Brief Intervention and Referral to Treatment (SBIRT) for substance use into prenatal care. Matern Child Health J 24:412–418. https://doi.org/10.1007/s10995-020-02892-9

Hudak ML, Tan RC, The Committee on Drugs, The Committee on Fetus and Newborn, Frattarelli DAC, Galinkin JL, Green TP, Neville KA, Paul IM, Van Den Anker JN, Papile L-A, Baley JE, Bhutani VK, Carlo WA, Cummings J, Kumar P, Polin RA, Wang KS, Watterberg KL (2012) Neonatal drug withdrawal. Pediatrics 129(2):e540–e560. https://doi.org/10.1542/peds.2011-3212

James A, Williams J (2020) Basic opioid pharmacology – an update. Br J Pain 14(2):115–121. https://doi.org/10.1177/2049463720911986. Epub 2020 Mar 20. PMID: 32537150; PMCID: PMC7265597

Jansson LM, Patrick SW (2019) Neonatal abstinence syndrome. Pediatr Clin North Am. 66(2):353–367. PMID 30819342

Jansson LM, Choo R, Velez ML, Harrow C, Schroeder JR, Shakleya DM, Huestis MA (2008) Methadone maintenance and breastfeeding in the neonatal period. Pediatrics. 121(1):106–114. https://doi.org/10.1542/peds.2007-1182

Jansson LM, Spencer N, McConnell K, Velez M, Tuten M, Harrow CA, Jones HE, Swortwood MJ, Barnes AJ, Scheidweiler KB, Huestis MA (2016) Maternal buprenorphine maintenance and lactation. J Hum Lact. 32(4):675–681. https://doi.org/10.1177/0890334416663198. Epub 2016 Sep 26

Jansson LM, McConnell K, Velez M, Spencer N, Gomonit M, Swortwood MJ (2024) Buprenorphine-naloxone maintenance and lactation. J Hum Lact. 40(1):113–119. https://doi.org/10.1177/08903344231209304. Epub 2023 Nov 29

Jilani SM, Jones HE, Grossman M et al (2022) Standardizing the clinical definition of opioid withdrawal in the neonate. J Pediatr. 243:33–39.e1. PMID 34942181

Jones HE, Kaltenbach K, Heil SH, Stine SM, Coyle MG, Arria AM, O'Grady KE, Selby P, Martin PR, Fischer G (2010) Neonatal abstinence syndrome after methadone or buprenorphine exposure. N Engl J Med. 363(24):2320–2331. https://doi.org/10.1056/NEJMoa1005359. PMID: 21142534; PMCID: PMC3073631

Joshi NS, Flaherman VJ, Halpern-Felsher B, Chung EK, Congdon JL, Lee HC (2023) Admission and care practices in United States well newborn nurseries. Hosp Pediatr 13(3):208–216. https://doi.org/10.1542/hpeds.2022-006882. PMID: 36843483; PMCID: PMC9986853

Kautzky A, Slamanig R, Unger A, Höflich A (2022) Neonatal outcome and adaption after in utero exposure to antidepressants: a systematic review and meta-analysis. Acta Psychiatr Scand. 145(1):6–28. PMID 34486740

Kocherlakota P (2014) Neonatal abstinence syndrome. Pediatrics. 134(2):e547–e561. https://doi.org/10.1542/peds.2013-3524

Lebin LG, Novick AM (2022) Selective serotonin reuptake inhibitors (Ssris) in pregnancy: an updated review on risks to mother, fetus, and child. Curr Psychiatry Rep. 24(11):687–695. PMID 36181572

Levine TA, Woodward LJ (2018) Early inhibitory control and working memory abilities of children prenatally exposed to methadone. Early Hum Dev. 116:68–75. PMID 29195088

Levine TA, Davie-Gray A, Kim HM, Lee SJ, Woodward LJ (2021) Prenatal methadone exposure and child developmental outcomes in 2-year-old children. Dev Med Child Neurol. 63(9):1114–1122. PMID 33462809

Lisonkova S, Richter LL, Ting J, Muraca GM, Wen Q, Mehrabadi A, Mitchell-Foster S, Oviedo-Joekes E, Lyons J (2019) Neonatal abstinence syndrome and associated neonatal and maternal mortality and morbidity. Pediatrics 144(2):e20183664. https://doi.org/10.1542/peds.2018-3664. PMID 31300529

MacMillan KDL, Rendon CP, Verma K, Riblet N, Washer DB, Volpe Holmes A (2018) Association of Rooming-in with Outcomes for neonatal abstinence syndrome: a systematic review and meta-analysis. JAMA Pediatr 172(4):345–351. https://doi.org/10.1001/jamapediatrics.2017.5195. PMID: 29404599; PMCID: PMC5875350

MacMillan KDL (2019) Neonatal abstinence syndrome: review of epidemiology, care models, and current understanding of outcomes. Clin Perinatol. 46(4):817–832. https://doi.org/10.1016/j.clp.2019.08.012. Epub 2019 Aug 14

Marchand G, Masoud AT, Govindan M et al (2022) Birth outcomes of neonates exposed to marijuana in utero: a systematic review and meta-analysis. JAMA Netw Open. 5(1):e2145653. PMID 35084479

Mascarenhas M, Wachman EM, Chandra I, Xue R, Sarathy L, Schiff DM (2024) Advances in the care of infants with prenatal opioid exposure and neonatal opioid withdrawal syndrome. Pediatrics. 153(2):e2023062871. PMID 38178779

Mascola M, Borders A, Terplan M (2017) ACOG Committee Opinion No. 524: opioid use and opioid use disorder in pregnancy. Obstet Gynecol:711

Milliren CE, Melvin P, Ozonoff A (2021) Pediatric hospital readmissions for infants with neonatal opioid withdrawal syndrome, 2016-2019. Hosp Pediatr 11(9):979–988. https://doi.org/10.1542/hpeds.2021-005904

Monnelly VJ, Anblagan D, Quigley A, Cabez MB, Cooper ES, Mactier H, Semple SI, Bastin ME, Boardman JP (2017) Prenatal methadone exposure is associated with altered neonatal brain development. Neuroimage Clin. 18:9–14. https://doi.org/10.1016/j.nicl.2017.12.033. PMID: 29326869; PMCID: PMC5760461

Morris E, Bardsley T, Schulte K, Seidel J, Shakib JH, Buchi KF, Fung CM (2022) Hospital outcomes of infants with neonatal opioid withdrawal syndrome at a tertiary care hospital with high rates of concurrent nonopioid (polysubstance) exposure. Am J Perinatol 39(4):387–393. https://doi.org/10.1055/s-0040-1716490. Epub 2020 Sep 6. PMID: 32892326; PMCID: PMC8632549

Mukherjee P et al (2001) Normal brain maturation during childhood: developmental trends characterized with diffusion-tensor MR imaging. Radiology 221(2):349–358

Munn Z, Pollock D, Stone J et al (2024) The impact of using cannabis during pregnancy on the infant and mother: an overview of systematic reviews, evidence map, targeted updates, and de novo synthesis. Aust N Z J Obstet Gynaecol. PMID 39699257

Murosko D, Paul K, Barfield WD, Montoya-Williams D, Parga-Belinkie J (2022) Equity in policies regarding urine drug testing in infants. NeoReviews 23(11):788–

795. https://doi.org/10.1542/neo.23-10-e788. PMID: 36316251; PMCID: PMC10044569
Obstet Gynecol (2017) Committee opinion no. 711: opioid use and opioid use disorder in pregnancy. Obstet Gynecol. 130(2):e81–e94. PMID 28742676
Offit PA (2016) Pandora's lab: seven stories of science gone wrong. National Geographic, Washington, DC, p 287
Pahl A, Young L, Buus-Frank ME, Marcellus L, Soll R (2020) Non-pharmacological care for opioid withdrawal in newborns. Cochrane Database Syst Rev. 12(12):CD013217. PMID 33348423
Patel E, Bandara S, Saloner B, Stuart E, Goodman D, Terplan M, McCourt A, White S, McGinty W (2021) Heterogeneity in prenatal substance use screening despite universal screening recommendations: findings from the Pregnancy Risk Assessment Monitoring System, 2016–2018. Am J Obstetr Gynecol MFM. 3(5). https://doi.org/10.1016/j.ajogmf.2021.100419
Patrick SW, Schumacher RE, Benneyworth BD, Krans EE, McAllister JM, Davis MM (2012) Neonatal abstinence syndrome and associated health care expenditures: United States, 2000–2009. JAMA. 307(18):1934–1940. PMID 22546608
Patrick SW, Barfield WD, Poindexter BB, Committee on Fetus and Newborn, Committee on Substance Use and Prevention (2020) Neonatal opioid withdrawal syndrome. Pediatrics. 146(5):e2020029074. PMID 33106341
Perlstein MA (1947) Congenital morphinism; a rare cause of convulsions in the newborn. J Am Med Assoc. 135(10):633. https://doi.org/10.1001/jama.1947.62890100006006c
Petty GE (1912) 1 Congenital morphinism, with report of cases. Tex Med J (Austin). 27(9):337–343. PMCID: PMC9642179 PMID: 36956630
Roncero C, Valriberas-Herrero I, Mezzatesta-Gava M, Villegas JL, Aguilar L, Grau-López L (2020) Cannabis use during pregnancy and its relationship with fetal developmental outcomes and psychiatric disorders. A systematic review. Reprod Health. 17(1):25. PMID 32066469
Salt E, Wiggins A, Pick A, Bada H, Howard C, Currie M, Rayens MK (2023) A case-control study comparing rates and diagnoses of hospital readmission in infants affected by neonatal abstinence syndrome. J Matern Fetal Neonatal Med. 36(1):2162820. https://doi.org/10.1080/14767058.2022.2162820
Sanlorenzo LA, Cooper WO, Dudley JA, Stratton S, Maalouf FI, Patrick SW (2019) Increased severity of neonatal abstinence syndrome associated with concomitant antenatal opioid and benzodiazepine exposure. Hosp Pediatr. 9(8):569–575. PMID 31262946
Shrestha S, Roberts MH, Maxwell JR, Leeman LM, Bakhireva LN (2021) Post-discharge healthcare utilization in infants with neonatal opioid withdrawal syndrome. Neurotoxicol Teratol. 86:106975. PMID 33766722
Spodnick MB, McElderry SC, Diaz MR (2025) Opioid receptor signaling throughout ontogeny: shaping neural and behavioral trajectories. Neurosci Biobehav Rev 170:106033. https://doi.org/10.1016/j.neubiorev.2025.106033. Epub 2025 Jan 31. PMID: 39894419; PMCID: PMC11851333
Strahan AE, Guy GP Jr, Bohm M, Frey M, Ko JY (2020) Neonatal abstinence syndrome incidence and health care costs in the United States, 2016. JAMA Pediatr 174(2):200–202. https://doi.org/10.1001/jamapediatrics.2019.4791. PMID: 31841581; PMCID: PMC6990852
Straub L, Huybrechts KF, Hernández-Díaz S, Zhu Y, Vine S, Desai RJ, Gray KJ, Bateman BT (2022) Trajectories of prescription opioid utilization during pregnancy among Prepregnancy chronic users and risk of neonatal opioid withdrawal syndrome. Am J Epidemiol 191 (1):208–219. https://doi.org/10.1093/aje/kwab249. PMID: 34643225; PMCID: PMC8897996
Suarez EA, Huybrechts KF, Straub L, Hernández-Díaz S, Jones HE, Connery HS, Davis JM, Gray KJ, Lester B, Terplan M, Mogun H, Bateman BT (2022) Buprenorphine versus methadone for opioid use disorder in pregnancy. N Engl J Med. 387(22):2033–2044. https://doi.org/10.1056/NEJMoa2203318. PMID 36449419
Towers CV, Hyatt BW, Visconti KC, Chernicky L, Chattin K, Fortner KB (2019) Neonatal head circumference in newborns with neonatal abstinence syndrome. Pediatrics. 143(1):e20180541. https://doi.org/10.1542/peds.2018-0541. Epub 2018 Dec 10
Ulrich M, Memmo E, Cruz A, Heinz A, Iverson R (2021) Implementation of a universal screening process for substance use in pregnancy. Obstetr Gynecol. 137(4): 695–701. https://doi.org/10.1097/AOG.0000000000004305
Van Hoogdalem MW, Wexelblatt SL, Akinbi HT, Vinks AA, Mizuno T (2022) A review of pregnancy-induced changes in opioid pharmacokinetics, placental transfer, and fetal exposure: towards fetomaternal physiologically-based pharmacokinetic modeling to improve the treatment of neonatal opioid withdrawal syndrome. Pharmacol Ther 234:108045, ISSN 0163-7258. https://doi.org/10.1016/j.pharmthera.2021.108045
Visconti KC, Hennessy KC, Towers CV, Howard BC (2015) Chronic opiate use in pregnancy and newborn head circumference. Am J Perinatol. 32(1):27–32. https://doi.org/10.1055/s-0034-1374817. Epub 2014 May 2
Wang J, Cosci F (2021) Neonatal withdrawal syndrome following late in utero exposure to selective serotonin reuptake inhibitors: a systematic review and meta-analysis of observational studies. Psychother Psychosom. 90(5):299–307. PMID 33971648
White A, Afsari M, Balakrishnan H, Chapa E, Kim M, Mehra S, Faucher MA, Miller J, Cordova P, Duryea EL, Nelson DB, Ambia AM, Mcintire DD, Adhikari EH (2024) Implementation of universal screening for

substance use in pregnancy in a public healthcare system. AJOG Glob Rep. 4(3):100384. https://doi.org/10.1016/j.xagr.2024.100384

Witt CE, Rudd KE, Bhatraju P, Rivara FP, Hawes SE, Weiss NS (2017) Neonatal abstinence syndrome and early childhood morbidity and mortality in Washington state: a retrospective cohort study. J Perinatol. 37(10): 1124–1129. https://doi.org/10.1038/jp.2017.106. PMID 28682319

Wouldes TA, Lester BM (2023) Opioid, methamphetamine, and polysubstance use: perinatal outcomes for the mother and infant. Front Pediatr. 11:1305508. PMID 38250592

Young LW, Ounpraseuth ST, Merhar SL et al (2023) Eat, sleep, console approach or usual care for neonatal opioid withdrawal. N Engl J Med. 388(25): 2326–2337. PMID 37125831

Zankl A, Martin J, Davey JG, Osborn DA (2021) Opioid treatment for opioid withdrawal in newborn infants. Cochrane Database Syst Rev. 7(7):CD002059. PMID 34231914

Zhang Y, Gong F, Liu P, He Y, Wang H (2021) Effects of prenatal methamphetamine exposure on birth outcomes, brain structure, and neurodevelopmental outcomes. Dev Neurosci. 43(5):271–280. PMID 34139695

MIX
Papier aus verantwortungsvollen Quellen
Paper from responsible sources
FSC® C105338

If you have any concerns about our products,
you can contact us on
ProductSafety@springernature.com

In case Publisher is established outside the EU,
the EU authorized representative is:
Springer Nature Customer Service Center GmbH
Europaplatz 3, 69115 Heidelberg, Germany

Printed by Libri Plureos GmbH
in Hamburg, Germany